VITAMINS AND HORMONES

VOLUME 33

VITAMINS AND HORMONES

ADVANCES IN RESEARCH AND APPLICATIONS

Edited by

PAUL L. MUNSON
University of North Carolina
Chapel Hill, North Carolina

EGON DICZFALUSY
Karolinska Sjukhuset
Stockholm, Sweden

JOHN GLOVER
University of Liverpool
Liverpool, England

ROBERT E. OLSON
St. Louis University
St. Louis, Missouri

Consulting Editors

ROBERT S. HARRIS
32 Dwhinda Road
Newton, Massachusetts

KENNETH V. THIMANN
University of California, Santa Cruz
Santa Cruz, California

JOHN A. LORAINE
University of Edinburgh
Edinburgh, Scotland

IRA G. WOOL
University of Chicago
Chicago, Illinois

Volume 33

1975

ACADEMIC PRESS   New York   San Francisco   London

A Subsidiary of Harcourt Brace Jovanovich, Publishers

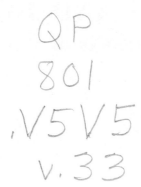

ACADEMIC PRESS, INC.
111 Fifth Avenue, New York, New York 10003

United Kingdom Edition published by
ACADEMIC PRESS, INC. (LONDON) LTD.
24/28 Oval Road, London NW1

LIBRARY OF CONGRESS CATALOG CARD NUMBER: 43–10535

ISBN 0–12–709833–X

PRINTED IN THE UNITED STATES OF AMERICA

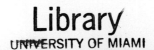

Contents

Endocrine Control of the Prostate
An International Symposium
in Honor of Dr. Charles Huggins

Morphological and Biochemical Parameters of Androgen Effects on Rat Ventral Prostate in Organ Culture

E. E. BAULIEU, C. LE GOASCOGNE, A. GROYER,
T. FEYEL-CABANES, AND P. ROBEL

Polynucleotide Polymerizations and Prostate Proliferation

H. G. WILLIAMS-ASHMAN, B. TADOLINI, J. WILSON,
AND A. CORTI

Hormonal Effects on Cell Proliferation in Rat Prostate

N. BRUCHOVSKY, B. LESSER, E. VAN DOORN, AND S. CRAVEN

Animal Models in the Study of Antiprostatic Drugs

F. Neumann, K.-D. Richter, and Th. Senge

Effects of Hormone–Cytostatic Complexes on the Rat Ventral Prostate *In Vivo* and *In Vitro*

J. G. Forsberg and P. A. Høisæter

Potential Test Systems for Chemotherapeutic Agents against Prostatic Cancer

A. A. Sandberg

Round Table Discussion on the Evaluation of Drugs and Hormones Effective against Prostatic Disease

(*Rapporteur:* H. G. WILLIAMS-ASHMAN)   189

Androgen Metabolism by the Perfused Prostate

K. B. EIK-NES

Production of Testosterone by Prostate and Other Peripheral Tissues in Man

MORTIMER B. LIPSETT

Steroid Hormone Receptors: A Survey

W. I. P. MAINWARING

Androgen Binding and Metabolism in the Human Prostate

A. Attramadal, K. J. Tveter, S. C. Weddington, O. Djöseland, O. Naess, V. Hansson, and O. Torgersen

Testosterone Receptors in the Prostate and Other Tissues

G. Verhoeven, W. Heyns, and P. De Moor

Androgen Binding and Transport in Testis and Epididymis

E. Ritzén, L. Hagenäs, V. Hansson, S. C. Weddington, F. S. French, and S. N. Nayfeh

Androgen Receptors and Androgen-Dependent Initiation of Protein Synthesis in the Prostate

S. Liao, J. L. Tymoczko, E. Castañeda, and T. Liang

Androgen *Receptors* in the Rat Ventral Prostate and Their Hormonal Control

J. P. Blondeau, C. Corpechot, C. Le Goascogne, E. E. Baulieu, and P. Robel

Round Table Discussion on Prostatic *Receptors*

(*Rapporteur:* E. E. Baulieu)

Treatment of Prostatic Carcinoma with Various Types of Estrogen Derivatives

G. Jönsson, A. M. Olsson, W. Luttrop, Z. Cekan, K. Purvis, and E. Diczfalusy

The Nonsurgical Treatment of Prostatic Carcinoma

G. D. CHISHOLM AND E. P. N. O'DONOGHUE

Management of Reactivated Prostatic Cancer

G. P. MURPHY

Androgen Metabolism in Patients with Benign Prostatic Hypertrophy

K.-D. VOIGT, H.-J. HORST, AND M. KRIEG

Nonsurgical Treatment of Human Benign Prostatic Hyperplasia

W. W. SCOTT AND D. S. COFFEY

Thiaminases and Their Effects on Animals

W. Charles Evans

Pellagra and Amino Acid Imbalance

C. Gopalan and Kamala S. Jaya Rao

Myo-inositol Lipids

J. N. Hawthorne and D. A. White

Hormonal Regulation of Cartilage Growth and Metabolism

HAROLD E. LEBOVITZ AND GEORGE S. EISENBARTH

Steroid Hormone *Receptors*

ETIENNE-EMILE BAULIEU, MICHEL ATGER, MARTIN BEST-BELPOMME, PIERRE CORVOL, JEAN-CLAUDE COURVALIN, JAN MESTER, EDWIN MILGROM, PAUL ROBEL, HENRI ROCHEFORT, AND DENISE DE CATALOGNE

Contributors to Symposium

Numbers in parentheses indicate the pages on which the authors' contributions begin.

A. ATTRAMADAL, *Laboratory of Histochemistry, Institute of Pathology, Surgical Department A, and the Laboratory of Endocrinology, Medical Department B, Rikshospitalet, Oslo, Norway* (247)

E. E. BAULIEU, *Unité de Recherches sur le Métabolisme Moléculaire et la Physio-Pathologie des Stéroides de l'Institut National de la Santé et de la Recherche Médicale (Inserm) and ER 125 Cnrs, Département de Chimie Biologique, Faculté de Médecine Paris-Sud, Bicêtre, France* (1, 319, 347)

J. P. BLONDEAU, *Unité de Recherches sur le Métabolisme Moléculaire et la Physio-Pathologie des Stéroides de l'Institut National de la Santé et de la Recherche Médicale (Inserm) and ER 125 Cnrs, Département de Chimie Biologique, Faculté de Médecine Paris-Sud, Bicêtre, France* (319)

N. BRUCHOVSKY, *Department of Medicine, University of Alberta, Edmonton, Alberta, Canada* (61)

E. CASTAÑEDA, *The Ben May Laboratory for Cancer Research and the Department of Biochemistry, University of Chicago, Chicago, Illinois* (297)

Z. CEKAN, *Swedish Medical Research Council, Reproductive Endocrinology Research Unit, Karolinska Sjukhuset, Stockholm, Sweden* (351)

G. D. CHISHOLM, *Institute of Urology and St. Peter's, St. Paul's and St. Philip's Hospitals, Royal Postgraduate Medical School and Hammersmith Hospital, London, England* (377)

D. S. COFFEY, *Departments of Urology, Pharmacology and Experimental Therapeutics, and Oncology, The Johns Hopkins Hospital, Baltimore, Maryland* (439)

C. CORPECHOT, *Unité de Recherches sur le Métabolisme Moléculaire et la Physio-Pathologie des Stéroides de l'Institut National de la Santé et de la Recherche Médicale (Inserm) and ER 125 Cnrs, Département de Chimie Biologique, Faculté de Médecine Paris-Sud, Bicêtre, France* (319)

A. CORTI,* *The Ben May Laboratory for Cancer Research, Departments of Biochemistry and Pharmacological and Physiological Sciences, University of Chicago, Chicago, Illinois* (39)

S. CRAVEN, *Department of Medicine, University of Alberta, Edmonton, Alberta, Canada* (61)

P. DE MOOR, *Laboratorium voor Experimentele Geneeskunde, Rega Instituut, Leuven, Belgium* (265)

E. DICZFALUSY, *Swedish Medical Research Council, Reproductive Endocrinology Research Unit, Karolinska Sjukhuset, Stockholm, Sweden* (351)

O. DJÖSELAND, *Laboratory of Histochemistry, Institute of Pathology, Surgical Department A, and the Laboratory of Endocrinology, Medical Department B, Rikshospitalet, Oslo, Norway* (247)

K. B. EIK-NES, *Department of Biophysics, N.T.H., University of Trondheim, Trondheim, Norway* (193)

T. FEYEL-CABANES, *Unité de Recherches sur le Métabolisme Moléculaire et la Physio-Pathologie des Stéroides de l'Institut National de la Santé et de la Recherche Médicale (Inserm) and ER 125 Cnrs, Département de Chimie Biologique, Faculté de Médecine Paris-Sud, Bicêtre, France* (1)

J. G. FORSBERG, *The Institute of Anatomy and Department of General Surgery, Urology Section, University of Bergen, Bergen, Norway* (137)

F. S. FRENCH, *Departments of Pediatrics and Biochemistry, and Laboratories for Reproductive Biology, University of North Carolina, Chapel Hill, North Carolina* (283)

A. GROYER, *Unité de Recherches sur le Métabolisme Moléculaire et la Physio-Pathologie des Stéroides de l'Institut National de la Santé et de la Recherche Médicale (Inserm) and ER 125 Cnrs, Département de Chimie Biologique, Faculté de Médecine Paris-Sud, Bicêtre, France* (1)

L. HAGENÄS, *Pediatric Endocrinology Unit, Karolinska Sjukhuset, Stockholm, Sweden* (283)

* Present address: Istituto di Chimica Biologica, University of Bologna, Bologna, Italy.

V. HANSSON, *Laboratory of Histochemistry, Institute of Pathology, Surgical Department A, and the Laboratory of Endocrinology, Medical Department B, Rikshospitalet, Oslo, Norway* (247, 283)

W. HEYNS, *Laboratorium voor Experimentele Geneeskunde, Rega Instituut, Leuven, Belgium* (265)

P. A. HØISÆTER, *The Institute of Anatomy and Department of General Surgery, Urology Section, University of Bergen, Bergen, Norway* (137)

H.-J. HORST, *Department of Clinical Chemistry, Medical Clinic, University of Hamburg, Hamburg, Federal Republic of Germany* (417)

G. JÖNSSON, *Department of Urology, University Hospital of Lund, Lund, Sweden* (351)

M. KRIEG, *Department of Clinical Chemistry, Medical Clinic, University of Hamburg, Hamburg, Federal Republic of Germany* (417)

C. LE GOASCOGNE, *Unité de Recherches sur le Métabolisme Moléculaire et la Physio-Pathologie des Stéroides de l'Institut National de la Santé et de la Recherche Médicale (Inserm) and ER 125 Cnrs, Département de Chimie Biologique, Faculté de Médecine Paris-Sud, Bicêtre, France* (1, 319)

B. LESSER, *Department of Medicine, University of Alberta, Edmonton, Alberta, Canada* (61)

T. LIANG, *The Ben May Laboratory for Cancer Research and the Department of Biochemistry, University of Chicago, Chicago, Illinois* (297)

S. LIAO, *The Ben May Laboratory for Cancer Research and the Department of Biochemistry, University of Chicago, Chicago, Illinois* (297)

MORTIMER B. LIPSETT, *The Cancer Center, Inc., Case Western Reserve University School of Medicine, Cleveland, Ohio* (209)

W. LUTTROP, *Department of Urology, University Hospital of Lund, Lund, Sweden* (351)

W. I. P. MAINWARING, *Androgen Physiology Department, Imperial Cancer Research Fund, Lincoln's Inn Fields, London, England* (223)

G. P. MURPHY, *Roswell Park Memorial Institute, New York State Department of Health, State University of New York at Buffalo, Buffalo, New York* (399)

O. Naess, *Laboratory of Histochemistry, Institute of Pathology, Surgical Department A, and the Laboratory of Endocrinology, Medical Department B, Rikshospitalet, Oslo, Norway* (247)

S. N. Nayfeh, *Departments of Pediatrics and Biochemistry, and Laboratories for Reproductive Biology, University of North Carolina, Chapel Hill, North Carolina* (283)

F. Neumann, *Research Laboratories of Schering AG, Department of Endocrinopharmacology, Berlin, Germany* (103)

E. P. N. O'Donoghue, *Institute of Urology and St. Peter's, St. Paul's and St. Philip's Hospitals, Royal Postgraduate Medical School and Hammersmith Hospital, London, England* (377)

A. M. Olsson, *Department of Urology, University Hospital of Lund, Lund, Sweden* (351)

K. Purvis, *Swedish Medical Research Council, Reproductive Endocrinology Research Unit, Karolinska Sjukhuset, Stockholm, Sweden* (351)

K.-D. Richter, *Experimental Animal Department, University of Münster, Münster, Germany* (103)

E. Ritzén, *Pediatric Endocrinology Unit, Karolinska Sjukhuset, Stockholm, Sweden* (283)

Paul Robel, *Unité de Recherches sur le Métabolisme Moléculaire et la Physio-Pathologie des Stéroides de l'Institut National de la Santé et de la Recherche Médicale (Inserm U 33), and ER 125 Cnrs, Département de Chimie Biologique, Faculté de Médecine Paris-Sud, Bicêtre, France* (1, 319)

A. A. Sandberg, *Roswell Park Memorial Institute, Buffalo, New York* (155)

W. W. Scott, *Department of Urology, The Johns Hopkins University School of Medicine, Baltimore, Maryland* (439)

Th. Senge, *Department of Urology, Klinikum, Essen, Germany* (103)

B. Tadolini, *The Ben May Laboratory for Cancer Research, Departments of Biochemistry and Pharmacological and Physiological Sciences, University of Chicago, Chicago, Illinois* (39)

O. Torgersen, *Laboratory of Histochemistry, Institute of Pathology, Surgical Department A, and the Laboratory of Endocrinology, Medical Department B, Rikshospitalet, Oslo, Norway* (247)

K. J. TVETER, *Laboratory of Histochemistry, Institute of Pathology, Surgical Department A, and the Laboratory of Endocrinology, Medical Department B, Rikshospitalet, Oslo, Norway* (247)

J. L. TYMOCZKO, *The Ben May Laboratory for Cancer Research and the Department of Biochemistry, University of Chicago, Chicago, Illinois* (297)

E. VAN DOORN, *Department of Medicine, University of Alberta, Edmonton, Alberta, Canada* (61)

G. VERHOEVEN, *Laboratorium voor Experimentele Geneeskunde, Rega Instituut, Leuven, Belgium* (265)

K.-D. VOIGT, *Department of Clinical Chemistry, Medical Clinic, University of Hamburg, Hamburg, Federal Republic of Germany* (417)

S. C. WEDDINGTON, *Laboratory of Histochemistry, Institute of Pathology, Surgical Department A, and the Laboratory of Endocrinology, Medical Department B, Rikshospitalet, Oslo, Norway* (247, 283)

H. G. WILLIAMS-ASHMAN, *The Ben May Laboratory for Cancer Research, Departments of Biochemistry and Pharmacological and Physiological Sciences, University of Chicago, Chicago, Illinois* (39, 189)

J. WILSON, *The Ben May Laboratory for Cancer Research, Department of Biochemistry and Pharmacological and Physiological Sciences, University of Chicago, Chicago, Illinois* (39)

Contributors of Regular Articles

Numbers in parentheses indicate the pages on which the authors' contributions begin.

MICHEL ATGER, *Unité de Recherches sur le Métabolisme Moléculaire et la Physio-Pathologie des Stéroides de l'Institut National de la Santé et de la Recherche Médicale (Inserm U 33 and U 135), Département de Chimie Biologique, Faculté de Médecine de Bicêtre, Université Paris-Sud, Bicêtre, France* (649)

ETIENNE-EMILE BAULIEU, *Unité de Recherches sur le Métabolisme Moléculaire et la Physio-Pathologie des Stéroides de l'Institut National de la Santé et de la Recherche Médicale (Inserm U 33) and ER 125 Cnrs, Département de Chimie Biologique, Faculté de Médecine de Bicêtre, Université Paris-Sud, Bicêtre, France* (649)

MARTIN BEST-BELPOMME,* *Unité de Recherches sur le Métabolisme Moléculaire et la Physio-Pathologie des Stéroides de l'Institut National de la Santé et de la Recherche Médicale (Inserm U 33), Départemente de Chimie Biologique, Faculté de Médecine de Bicêtre, Université Paris-Sud, Bicêtre, France* (649)

PIERRE CORVOL, *Unité de Recherches sur le Métabolisme Moleculaire et la Physio-Pathologie des Stéroides de l'Institut National de la Santé et de la Recherche Médicale (Inserm U 47), 17 rue du Fer à Moulin, Paris, France*

JEAN-CLAUDE COURVALIN, *Unité de Recherches sur le Métabolisme Moléculaire et la Physio-Pathologie des Stéroides de l'Institut National de la Santé et de la Recherche Médicale (Inserm U 33), Département de Chimie Biologique, Faculté de Médecine de Bicêtre, Université Paris-Sud, Bicêtre, France* (649)

DENISE DE CATALOGNE, *Unité de Recherches sur le Métabolisme Moléculaire et la Physio-Pathologie des Stéroides de l'Institut National de la Santé et de la Recherche Médicale (Inserm U 33), Départmente de Chimie Biologique, Faculté de Médecine de Bicêtre, Université Paris-Sud, Bicêtre, France* (649)

GEORGE S. EISENBARTH, *Departments of Medicine and Physiology, Duke University Medical Center, Durham, North Carolina* (575)

* Present address: Biologie Animale, Paris VI, 12 rue Cuvier, 75005-Paris, France.

W. CHARLES EVANS, *Department of Biochemistry and Soil Science, University College of North Wales, Bangor, Gwynedd, Wales* (467)

C. GOPALAN, *National Institute of Nutrition, Indian Council of Medical Research, Hyderabad, India* (505)

J. N. HAWTHORNE, *Department of Biochemistry, University Hospital and Medical School, Nottingham, England* (529)

KAMALA S. JAYA RAO, *National Institute of Nutrition, Indian Council of Medical Research, Hyderabad, India* (505)

HAROLD E. LEBOVITZ, *Departments of Medicine and Physiology, Duke University Medical Center, Durham, North Carolina* (575)

JAN MESTER, *Unité de Recherches sur le Métabolisme Moléculaire et la Physio-Pathologie des Stéroides de l'Institut National de la Santé et de la Recherche Médicale (Inserm U 33), Départment de Chimie Biologique, Faculté de Médecine de Bicêtre, Université Paris-Sud, Bicêtre, France* (649)

EDWIN MILGROM, *Unité de Recherches sur le Métabolisme Moléculaire et la Physio-Pathologie des Stéroides de l'Institut National de la Santé et de la Recherche Médicale (Inserm U 33 and U 135), Département de Chimie Biologique, Faculté de Médecine de Bicêtre, Université Paris-Sud, Bicêtre, France* (649)

PAUL ROBEL, *Unité de Recherches sur le Métabolisme Moléculaire et la Physio-Pathologie des Stéroides de l'Institut National de la Santé et de la Recherche Médicale (Inserm U 33), and ER 125 Cnrs, Département de Chimie Biologique, Faculté de Médecine de Bicêtre, Université Paris-Sud, Bicêtre, France* (649)

HENRI ROCHEFORT, *Unité Recherches sur le Métabolisme Moléculaire et la Physio-Pathologie des Stéroides de l'Institut National de la Santé et de la Recherche Médicale (Inserm U 58), Montpellier, France* (649)

D. A. WHITE, *Department of Biochemistry, University Hospital and Medical School, Nottingham, England* (529)

Preface

The Editors take pride in presenting the thirty-third volume of *Vitamins and Hormones*.

This volume is composed of two parts. This first section contains the nineteen papers presented at the "International Symposium on Endocrine Control of the Prostate" that was held at Helsingborg, Sweden, June 2 to 4, 1975. Reports of two round table discussions held during the symposium also are included. The symposium honored Professor Charles Huggins, a pioneer in our understanding of the endocrinology of the prostate and in the treatment of carcinoma of the prostate. The papers of the symposium critically review the present state of knowledge of the subject and provide a sound basis for future advances.

We are indebted to Professor Etienne-Emile Baulieu (France), Professor Bertil Högberg (Sweden), Professor Börje Uvnäs (Sweden), and Professor Klaus-Dieter Voigt (Germany), who joined two of the Editors (E. D. and P. L. M.) to constitute the Organizing Committee for the symposium, and to Dr. Jonas Müntzing (Sweden), who served as Secretary of the Committee. We express our gratitude to Leo Research Foundation of Helsingborg, Sweden, for generously supporting the symposium and for underwriting the extra cost of publication of the proceedings. We also wish to express our appreciation to the officers and staff of Leo Research Foundation who were responsible for the local arrangements for the symposium and for the warm hospitality enjoyed by all participants.

The second section of this volume comprises five chapters reviewing thiaminases (Evans), amino acid imbalance in pellagra (Gopalan and Jaya Rao), myo-inositol lipids (Hawthorne and White), hormonal regulation of cartilage (Lebovitz and Eisenbarth), and steroid hormone receptors (Baulieu *et al.*)

Volume **33** is the first volume of this distinguished serial publication in which Professor Robert S. Harris has not served as a principal editor. Although Professor Harris's retirement from the board of coeditors had been anticipated and was announced a year ago, the full impact of his absence from this position was first realized in the preparation of the present volume. We miss him enormously and are grateful to him for continuing with the enterprise as a Consulting Editor.

The present volume is also the first in which, as previously announced, Robert E. Olson, Professor of Biochemistry and Head of the Department at St. Louis University School of Medicine, serves as a coeditor. Professor Olson replaces Professor Harris, with special responsibility—along with Professor Glover—for reviews in the vitamin field, in which he is a notable investigator and a respected authority.

Egon Diczfalusy
Paul L. Munson

Endocrine Control of the Prostate

An International Symposium in Honor of Dr. Charles Huggins

Organized by the Leo Research Foundation in Collaboration with *Vitamins and Hormones* and held in Helsingborg, Sweden, on June 2–4, 1975

Organizing Committee

Chairman
Dr. Egon Diczfalusy, Sweden

Dr. Etienne-Emile Baulieu, France
Dr. Bertil Högberg, Sweden
Dr. Paul L. Munson, U.S.A.
Dr. Börje Uvnäs, Sweden
Dr. Klaus-Dieter Voigt, Germany

Secretary
Dr. Jonas Müntzing, Sweden

Morphological and Biochemical Parameters of Androgen Effects on Rat Ventral Prostate in Organ Culture

E. E. BAULIEU, C. LE GOASCOGNE, A. GROYER,
T. FEYEL-CABANES, AND P. ROBEL

*Unité Recherches sur le Métabolisme Moléculaire et la Physio-Pathologie
des Stéroïdes de l'Institut National de la Santé et de la Recherche Médicale
(Inserm) and ER 125 Cnrs, Département de Chimie Biologique,
Faculté de Médecine Paris-Sud, Bicêtre, France**

* Postal address: Lab Hormones, 94270 Bicêtre, France.

1

I. Introduction

The rat ventral prostate is a typical target organ for androgens. Detailed histological effects of these hormones as they occur *in vivo* were published in 1930 by Moore, Price, and Gallagher, a group from Chicago, and Harkin performed electron microscopic studies in 1957. Lasnitzki (1965), in the Strangeways Laboratories at Cambridge, reported the action of testosterone* on the maintenance in organ culture of ventral prostate explants. This observation has allowed further studies since, in culture, the hormonal milieu can be fully defined and systemic effects that might interfere *in vivo* are eliminated. Then the activities of various testosterone 5α-metabolites in prostatic tissue *in vitro* were described (Baulieu *et al.*, 1967, 1968a), and on the basis of joint histological and steroid metabolism studies, it was proposed that, in this system, testosterone action is mediated at least partly by its transformation into metabolites, the latter having different activities adding up to the overall effect. Therefore, the concept of "prehormone" (see discussion in Baird *et al.*, 1968; Baulieu *et al.*, 1965) may possibly apply in part to testosterone acting on one of its target organs. The significance, the general character, and the possible pathopharmacological interest of this eventuality have been discussed since 1968 on many occasions, and the matter is not yet definitely settled.

Besides the effects they have in culture, testosterone metabolites have been extensively studied otherwise. It has been known, from the work of several authors, in particular Farnsworth, Kochakian, Ofner, and Pearlman (see reviews by Williams-Ashman and Reddi, 1971; Liao and Fang, 1969; Baulieu *et al.*, 1971), that testosterone metabolites, especially of the 5α-series, are present in the rat ventral prostate. A significant role for the most important of these metabolites, 5α-androstan-17β-ol-3-one or androstanolone (Aolone) or (5α) dihydrotestosterone (DHT), was strongly suggested when it was shown that it has a preferential nuclear localization in prostatic cells, as demonstrated *in vivo* (Bruchovsky and

---

* Abbreviations and trivial names: testosterone, 17β-hydroxy-4-androsten-3-one; androstanolone (dihydrotestosterone), 17β-hydroxy-5α-androstan-3-one (Aolone); 3β-androstanediol, 5α-androstane-3β,17β-diol (3β-Diol); 3α-Androstanediol,5α-androstane-3α,17β-diol; androstenedione, 4-androstene-3,17-dione; Androstanedione, 5α-androstane-3,17-dione; Estradiol, 1,3,5(10)-estratriene-3,17β-diol; progesterone, 4-pregnene-3,20-dione; cortisol, 11β,17,21-trihydroxy-4-pregnene-3,20-dione; Corticosterone,11β,21-dihydroxy-4-pregnene-3,20-dione; cyproterone acetate,1,2α-methylene-6-chloro-17α-yl-acetoxy-4,6-pregnadiene-3,20-dione; R 2956, 17β-hydroxy-2α,2β,17α-trimethyl-4,9,11-estratrien-3-one; R 4414, 17β-ethynyl-4-estren-3-one; BSA, bovine serum albumin; SDS, sodium dodecyl sulfate; TCA, trichloracetic acid; PCA, perchloric acid; NCS, Nuclear Chicago solubilizer.

Wilson, 1968) and *in vitro* (Anderson and Liao, 1968). Since androsta-nolone is the first compound on the "17-hydroxy metabolic pathway" of testosterone (Baulieu and Mauvais-Jarvis, 1964) and had been known as a potent androgen for a long time (Dorfman and Shipley, 1956), it was also the first to be studied in organ culture (Baulieu *et al.*, 1967, 1968a). It is the convergence of the two lines of research, on metabolism and action, which was critical in designating androstanolone as an androgen playing an important physiological role in the rat ventral prostate. This conclusion became even more acceptable when ventral prostate androgen *receptors* were described and found to bind androstanolone with greater affinity than testosterone (Fang *et al.*, 1969; Mainwaring, 1969; Baulieu and Jung, 1970; Unhjem *et al.*, 1969). It has also become clear that, at different developmental stages of the male genital tract (Jost, 1970; Wilson and Lasnitzki, 1971), androstanolone is the major androgen responsible for the differentiation and growth of the prostate (Wilson and Gloyna, 1970; Siiteri and Wilson, 1974), including that of man, as recently again suggested by the studies of individuals lacking genetically the 5α-reductase enzyme (Imperato-McGinley *et al.*, 1974; Walsh *et al.*, 1974).

In this paper, we are not reviewing the field of testosterone metabolism vs. androgen action in rat ventral prostate or the interference of other hormones with testosterone effects. We are not even reproducing in any detail the published results obtained in culture (Baulieu *et al.*, 1968a,b; Robel, 1971; Roy *et al.*, 1972a,b). New data are being presented that deal specifically with (1) differential effects of testosterone, androstano-lone, and 3β-androstanediol; (2) a new method clearly improving organ culture and called "constant-flow" organ culture, in which hormones and nutrients are renewed and the metabolites are eliminated continuously; (3) morphological studies, especially by electron microscopy and radioautography; (4) protein and RNA synthesis; and (5) the demonstration that in organ culture the regressed ventral prostate of the 2-week castrated rat can be stimulated by androgen, whereas previous reports had only shown that intact structures can be maintained. It is hence proposed that organ culture is an interesting tool for studying hormone and antihormone effects on the different cellular components of rat ventral prostate.

Remarkable reviews have been written which should be consulted: the text of Price and Williams-Ashman (1961) is basic for understanding the biology and the physiology of male accessory glands of mammals; Jost (1961) has described the role of androgens in development; and Wilson and Gloyna (1970), Williams-Ashman and Reddi (1971), and Liao and Fang (1969) have emphasized hormones, 5α-reductase, and *receptors*. This laboratory has contributed several review papers on the subject (Baulieu *et al.*, 1971, this volume, p. 649; Baulieu, 1974).

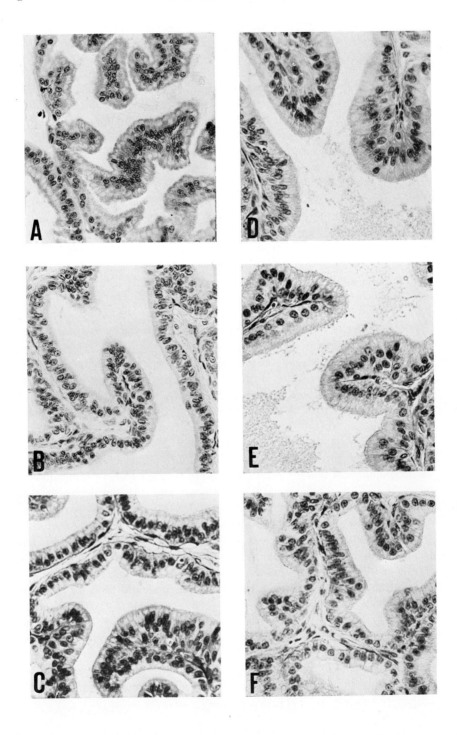

II. Morphological Studies in Static and Constant-Flow Culture

A. Maintenance Effects of Androgens

The aim is to keep young adult (7–9 weeks) ventral prostate explants in culture, morphologically maintained and responding normally to hormones. The ventral prostate gland of the adult rat (Fig. 1A) consists of ducts and alveoli separated by thin strands of fibromuscular stroma and lined with cuboidal or mostly columnar secretory epithelium, which often projects in folds into the lumen of alveoli. The columnar cells exhibit a well defined supranuclear clear zone corresponding essentially to the Golgi apparatus. Occasionally, basal cells can be seen wedged between the superficial tall cells and the basal lamina. In the young adult gland used in these experiments, secretory activity is still weak.

The predominant columnar cells have an apical pole, a Golgi zone, and supranuclear, nuclear, and basal regions (see Fig. 3G). At the apical pole, membrane-bound secretory granules accumulate. The luminal plasma membrane shows minute cytoplasmic projections (microvilli). The Golgi apparatus is formed of stacks of cisternae and vesicles. Lysosomes are scarce. Numerous concentric cisternae of rough endoplasmic reticulum are seen in the supra- and perinuclear region, oriented in the long axis of the cell. Endoplasmic reticulum is also present in the basal region. Mitochondria are distributed everywhere, particularly at the apical pole. In the nucleus, the nucleolus is composed of intermingled fibrillar and granular components. Perichromatin granules are easily visible at the frontier between condensed and clear chromatin (see Fig. 7). Grains similar to these perichromatin granules have been detected in the cisternae of the endoplasmic reticulum in the paranuclear region (Le Goascogne, 1973). The basal lamina is easily observed as a band between the epithelial cells and the ground substance of the interstitial tissue. Fibroblasts, collagen fibers, and smooth muscles are disposed concentrically, forming narrow strands around the alveoli.

1. "Static" Culture

a. Technique. The ventral prostate glands obtained from 7-week-old Wistar rats are used for the experiments and grown in organ culture by

FIG. 1. Intact rat ventral prostate explants in static and constant-flow culture. (A) No culture. (B and C) Static culture (7 days); testosterone 4.1 and 530 nM, respectively. (D, E, and F) Constant-flow culture (6 days). Androstanolone, 0.4 nM; testosterone, 4.1 nM; and 3β-androstanediol, 530 nM, respectively. All cultures were performed as indicated in Section II, A, 1 and 2. $\times$300.

a method previously described (Lasnitzki, 1964, 1965). The glands are removed under aseptic conditions, washed with Tyrode solution containing penicillin, and freed from the surrounding fat, connective tissue, and capsule. They are then transferred to a glass plate and the tissue is divided gently into fragments, approximately $2 \times 3 \times 3$ mm in size, by cutting the stroma separating the small lobules with a sharp Swann–Morton No. 10 blade. Four to 10 explants are mounted with cataract knives onto a strip of moistened lens paper, and two such strips are arranged on a grid of stainless steel. The grid is placed in a culture chamber of borosilicate glass, which is filled with medium up to the level of the grid, usually 4 ml. Two chambers rest in a petri dish carpeted with several layers of dampened filter paper to avoid evaporation. The petri dishes are stacked in a Lwoff incubator, which is perfused with a mixture of 93% O_2 and 7% CO_2 for 31 minutes at a flow rate of 345 ml/min. This results in a concentration of $62 \pm 2\%$ oxygen inside the incubator. It remains constant unless the incubator is opened and is renewed after each transfer of the cultures to fresh medium. The medium consists of Morton and Parker's medium 199 based on Earle's solution with 10% serum obtained from the Pasteur Institute, containing antibiotics. Usually there is a first 24-hour culture only with medium, and then steroids are eventually introduced as reported elsewhere (Robel et al., 1971), with new medium. Then, explants are cultured for two 3-day periods, with one change of the (hormone-containing) medium after 3 days.

Fixation, coloration, preparation for electron microscopy, and finally labeling with radioactive amino acid or nucleoside are as described in Robel et al. (1971) or below.

b. No Hormone. When cultivated without hormone (see Fig. 4D and E), the overall alveolar organization persists, but if nothing is visible optically after 1 day, already after $1 + 3$ days the supranucleolar region of epithelial cells has markedly regressed and the cells are mostly cuboidal. However, the changes are not fully reproducible, but continuing the culture for another 3 days gives constant criteria of regression. At $1 + 3 + 3$ days, the epithelium is composed almost exclusively of flat cells. Sometimes, it takes on pseudostratified aspects (possibly because of shrinking of the alveoli).

The fibromuscular stroma is apparently increased. The muscular cells are thicker and more visible than in intact animals, forming "basketlike investments" (Flickinger, 1972). They lie between fibroblasts, and the collagen appears to be abundant. The alveoli are generally less folded, and their diameter has decreased (from normal 240 μm to 140 μm, approximate mean values).

In order to establish semiquantitatively the maintenance effect of steroids, an "epithelial index" was calculated as the ratio of the number of alveoli having columnar and/or cuboidal cells over the number of alveoli showing only flat cells; 200–800 acini were counted per experimental point. In normal ventral prostate, the index was never <6, and usually it was between 6 and 8 (mean 7.3), while the $1 + 3 + 3$ day culture without hormone always led to a value <0.2 (mean 0.1) (Table IA).

At the subcellular level, there is marked involution of the components of the Golgi apparatus, and they are reduced to groups of collapsed cisternae and very few tiny vesicles. Secretory granules have disappeared. Microvilli become shorter and sparse. The rough endoplasmic reticulum undergoes a significant regression and is restricted also to a few scattered small cisternae. Ribosomes have decreased in number and tend to become isolated instead of being associated in polyribosomes. The nucleus is shrunken, becoming irregular with deep invaginations, and the nucleolus is smaller, mainly because its granular component is reduced (as in Fig. 6E). Perichromatin granules are less numerous (see Fig. 7).

 c. *Hormonal Effects.* Results obtained between 0.4 nM and 2.1 μM of hormones are reported in Table IA and Fig. 1B and C. It is seen that for the epithelial index androstanolone is as active as testosterone, or more so, whereas 3β-androstanediol is equal to testosterone only at the 1 μM level. Testosterone activity may be explained by its conversion to androstanolone, because the yield of steroid metabolism is large under these conditions. However, it has been shown, as far as ^{3}H-labeled 3β-androstanediol 3 μM is concerned, that incubation for 22 hours does not lead to detectable amounts of ^{3}H-labeled androstanolone in nuclei, and less than 0.5% transformation has been detected in analyzing the medium and cytosol (Robel *et al.*, 1971). Therefore, the radiochemical method does not allow one to rule out the formation of very small, but nevertheless active, amounts of androstanolone. In any case, one does not reach full maintenance of the index with 2.1 μM testosterone. In Fig. 1B and C, two concentrations of testosterone are compared, 4.1 nM, where the epithelium is partially maintained, and 530 nM, which is more satisfactory. It has been noted also that although approximately 1 μM testosterone or 3β-androstanediol can keep the stroma at its minimum, as in intact animals, surprisingly androstanolone is not as active on connective tissue; this leads to peculiar images where well developed periacinar stroma is seen among alveoli with well maintained epithelial cells (see also in Fig. 4B the same phenomenon observed with castrated rat ventral prostate exposed to steroids).

At the subcellular level, testosterone or androstanolone at 100–500 nM, which seem maximally effective by optical criteria in maintaining the

TABLE I

HISTOLOGICAL INDICES OF ANDROGEN EFFECTS ON RAT VENTRAL
PROSTATE EXPLANTS IN CULTURE

Part A: Epithelial Index of Intact Rat Ventral Prostate[a]

Intact normal Culture 1 + 3 + 3 days: (Steroids nM)	"Static" culture Control 7.3 No steroid 0.2			"Constant-flow" culture Control 7.3 No steroid 0.2		
	Testo-sterone	Aolone	3β-Diol	Testo-sterone	Aolone	3β-Diol
0.004	—	—	—	—	0.8	—
0.04	—	—	—	—	2.1	—
0.4	0.2	0.8	—	2.1	2.7	—
2	1.1	—	—	—	2.3	—
4.1	1.3	1.5	—	2.3	2.2	0.2
8.2	1.4	—	—	—	3.0	0.5
16.5	1.0	—	—	2.9	—	0.4
33.1	1.3	—	—	—	—	—
134	2.1	2.4	—	—	—	—
269	—	4.3	—	—	—	—
538	2.7	—	—	2.5	—	2.4
1070	3.4	—	3.3	3.0	—	—
2150	2.9	—	—	—	—	—

Part B: Epithelial Index, Alveolar Diameter, and Stroma/Alveoli Surface Ratio of Castrated Rat Ventral Prostate[b]

	Epithelial index	Alveolar diameter (μm)	Stroma/alveoli[c]
Control (no culture):	0.2	90	2.9
Control (culture, no hormone):	0.1	70	5.7
Steroids (nM)			
Testosterone			
8	0.9	87	3.3
80	2.5	135	0.9
800	3.0	130	1.3
Androstanolone			
8	1.3	97	2.3
80	1.6	103	2.3
800	3.0	125	1.5

[a] The epithelial index is defined in Section II, A. All values are means of at least three experiments. Techniques of cultures are indicated in Sections II, A, 1 and 2.

[b] Seven-week-old rats, castrated 14 days previously, were used for static culture of explants. The epithelial index is defined in footnote a. The mean value of alveolar diameter is calculated from the weight of histological photographs after cutting out the stroma zones. The ratio of the surfaces of alveoli and stroma is also deduced from weighed photographic zones.

[c] In intact rat ventral prostate, this ratio is approximately 0.7.

epithelium, preserve also microvilli, the Golgi apparatus, and the endoplasmic reticulum. However, the secretory granules remain almost completely absent. There are still a few lysosomes. 3β-Androstanediol seems very weakly active, but at the 1 μM level the epithelial index is 3.3 and the microvilli, Golgi apparatus, and endoplasmic reticulum are rather well maintained.

2. Constant-Flow Culture

In view of the fact that even 1 μM testosterone or 500 nM androstanolone in "static" culture could not maintain completely the epithelial index and that grains were almost absent, further studies were conducted. It was shown that the concentration of active steroid decreases rapidly in the culture medium, as far as testosterone and androstanolone are concerned (Robel *et al.*, 1971), and, therefore, that tissues may be exposed successively to the highest and to lower hormone concentrations during the two times 3-day culture.

It was then decided to build a chamber that could be continuously perfused for several days under the proper conditions of culture, including sterility (Robel and Baulieu, 1972).

a. Technique. The main apparatus for constant-flow organ culture is a Teflon dish, represented in Fig. 2. The central culture chamber has a hole in the bottom, receiving the input tubing by connectors with Luerlok bore and core, and a hole on the side wall, 5 mm above the bottom, similarly connected to the output tubing. The volume of culture medium contained in the chamber is 1.2 ml. The outer circular space of the culture dish can be filled with sterile water. It is covered with a borosilicate glass plate. Two such dishes with their Teflon tubing and stainless steel connections are put in a Lwoff chamber. The tubings come out of the side wall of the chamber through tight airproof junctions. The tubings are connected to 5- or 50-ml syringes (ref. 72,205 and 72,195 Braun Melsungen). These syringes are mounted on a Perfusor IIa pump (Braun Melsungen), which has been modified to hold 4 syringes at the same time to superfuse both culture dishes. The prostate explants, approximately $1 \times 1 \times 2$ mm in size, are laid on a specially cleaned and siliconized lens paper, which floats at the surface of the culture medium. The flow of medium 199 containing 10% calf serum is 0.375 ml/hour. The $O_2 + CO_2$ atmosphere in the Lwoff incubator is the same as for the "static" cultures and is renewed every 24 hours.

b. Hormonal Effects. With the constant-flow system, the epithelial index (Table IA) is already above its nonhormone control values at 4 pM androstanolone, and is approximately 2 with 0.4 nM testosterone and 0.04 nM androstanolone, respectively. However, it did not yield a value

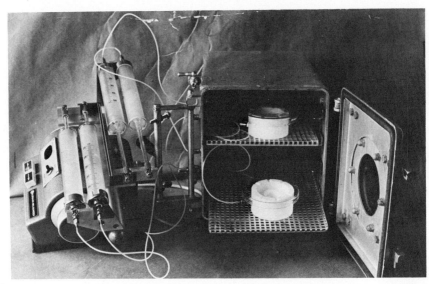

A

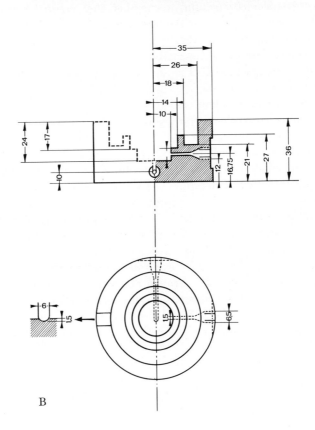

B

higher than 3 with as much as 10 nM androstanolone or 1 μM testosterone. 3β-Androstanediol gives a visible slight response at 8 nM and reaches 2.4 at 500 nM. Histological results are reported in Fig. 1D, E and F, and one can see the better result obtained here with testosterone at 4.1 nM, when compared to the static culture, as well as the result with androstanolone at 0.4 nM.

Representative results obtained with constant-flow culture are given in Fig. 3. Summarizing a large series of observations, one can say that a definite normalization of microvilli is obtained already with 10 nM testosterone or 2 nM androstanolone. Endoplasmic reticulum and Golgi apparatus are satisfactorily maintained from the lowest concentrations of testosterone (4 nM) and androstanolone (0.03 nM) and fully maintained with 10 times more of either steroid. However, secretory granules remain scarce, a result that does not necessarily mean that there is not secretory activity. In fact, vacuoles originating in the Golgi region are observed, but without dense content. Since, as demonstrated by the endoplasmic reticulum images and the biochemical analyses, protein synthesis is still active, it may be envisaged that the culture conditions preclude the condensation in secretory granules.

The low dose of 3β-androstanediol at 4 nM does not maintain the cellular ultrastructure. However, already at 17 nM, contrasting with the poor endoplasmic reticulum and the nearly absent microvilli (Fig. 3F), the Golgi apparatus is relatively well preserved (Fig. 3D). This striking effect of 3β-androstanediol on the Golgi apparatus at relatively low concentration is remarkable, and it may point to a still unsuspected selective action of this steroid. However, when a large concentration of 3β-androstanediol (500 nM) is used and maintains somewhat the overall structure, the result is possibly explained by some conversion to androstanolone, as suggested before in the static culture system. An experiment was performed that was specially devised to test quantitatively this conversion; explants were superfused with ³H-labeled 3β-androstanediol, 10 nM, and androstanolone recovery was checked with ¹⁴C-labeled tracer (Table II). The results, confirming previous enzymic studies (Levy *et al.*, 1974), indicated again that the formation of the 5α-dihydro-derivative of testosterone is a possible mechanism for the 3β-androstanediol effect; the distribution of this metabolic androstanolone was not studied in the explants.

Fig. 2. Constant-flow organ culture dish. (A) (top) Two constant-flow dishes in a Lwoff chamber on the right side (door open). They are connected to syringes mounted on a modified Perfusor IIa Braun pump on the left side. See details in Section II, A, 2, a. (B) Scheme of the constant-flow dish. All numbers indicate millimeters.

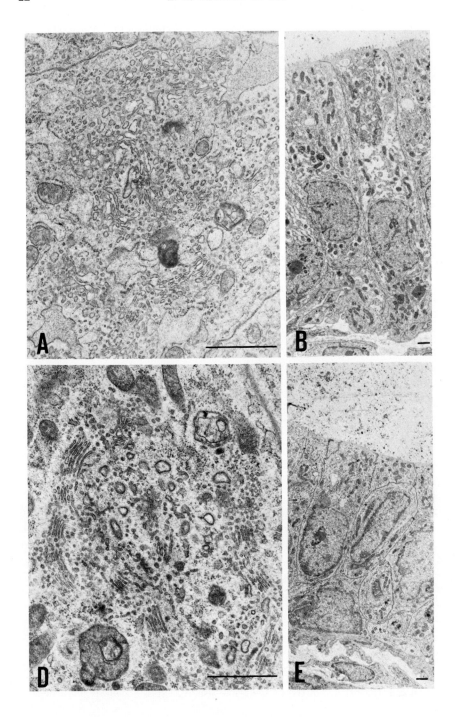

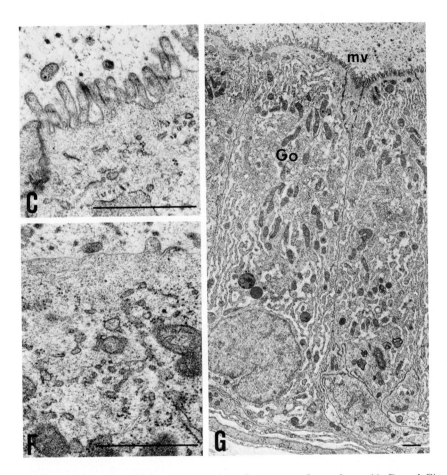

FIG. 3. Intact rat ventral prostate explants in constant-flow culture. (A, B, and C) Androstanolone, 0.8 nM.(D, E, and F) 3β-Androstanediol, 17 nM. (G) Testosterone, 17 nM. (A) and (D), $\times$19,000; (B) and (E), $\times$2900; (C) and (F), $\times$28,000; (G) $\times$4800. The scale line corresponds to 1μm; mv, microvilli; Go, Golgi apparatus. The technique of constant-flow culture is described in Section II, A, 2. Note that intact rat ventral prostate epithelial cells are very similar to the one seen in (G), with numerous secretory granules at the apical pole.

B. STIMULATION OF CASTRATED RAT VENTRAL PROSTATE BY ANDROGENS

Both the standard and the constant-flow culture techniques have been used. Seven-week-old Wistar rats are castrated, left for an additional 2 weeks, and then the ventral prostate is studied. The regression of the alveoli and their epithelial cells is obvious (Figs. 4D and 6E), with a

TABLE II

ANDROSTANOLONE IN RAT VENTRAL PROSTATE EXPLANTS IN CONSTANT-FLOW
CULTURE WITH 10 nM TESTOSTERONE-^{3}H, ANDROSTANOLONE-^{3}H, AND
3β-ANDROSTANEDIOL-^{3}H

Steroid	Explants (mg)	Androstanolone	
		Dpm	Fmoles/mg
Testosterone-^{3}H	40	34,441	8.67
Androstanolone-^{3}H	60	44,370	7.15
3β-Androstanediol-^{3}H	50	1,245	0.24

[a] A 24-hour constant-flow organ culture of intact rat ventral prostate explants with medium 199, calf serum 10% (0.2 ml/hour). Testosterone-^{3}H (SA 45 Ci/mmole), androstanolone-^{3}H (SA 47 Ci/mmole) or 3β-androstanediol-^{3}H (SA 47 Ci/mmole) were dissolved in the corresponding culture medium. At the end of the superfusion, explants were quickly rinsed with 0.5 ml of chilled distilled water, then homogenized and extracted with dichloromethane after addition of 9000 dpm of androstanolone-^{14}C (SA 50 mCi/mmole) and of 10 μg of testosterone.

Androstanolone-^{3}H-^{14}C was separated by thin-layer chromatography (TLC) on silica gel GF plates in the system benzene–acetone 85:15, located by a radiochromatogram scanner, eluted, and submitted to repeated crystallizations after addition of 20 mg of reference steroid, until constant specific activity of crystals and mother liquors. From the final ^{3}H/^{14}C ratio, the dpm of androstanolone present in the corresponding homogenate were calculated and expressed in femtomoles per milligram of tissue.

large stroma and visible muscular cells (see in Table IB a semiquantitative estimation). The epithelial index is <0.2.

After 7-day static culture without hormone, the picture is even more accentuated, with an epithelial index of <0.1. The diameter of alveoli regresses from an approximate mean value of 90 μm to 70 μm. Figures 4E and F, are explicit in showing particularly the profound regression of the Golgi apparatus and the endoplasmic reticulum and the disorganization of polyribosomes.

It is therefore remarkable that the culture conditions allow an effective hormonal stimulation leading to an overall restructuring of the tissue and its epithelial cells (Feyel-Cabanes et al., 1974). The improvement over all published attempts and our previous experiments is attributable to the use of a mixture of Waymouth 752 and 1066 media, 1:1, v/v. The mixture contains more cysteine, glucose, and vitamins than the Parker 199. The presence of calf serum has not been found necessary. The only addition of androgen to the static or flow culture stimulates definitely the explanted tissue. Alveoli become bigger, and the epithelial index with 8 nM testosterone in static culture without serum (Fig. 4C) is already approximately 1. The mean diameter after testosterone at 0.8 μM is 130 μm (Table IB). It may be seen again that testosterone and androstanolone (0.8 μM in static medium) are very efficient (Fig. 3A and B). However, whereas testosterone restores well the overall organization, including the rather thin strands of interstitial tissue, with androstanolone a larger surface of connective tissue remains, with very visible muscular cells. At the subcellular level, the normalization of the nucleolus (Fig. 6F), of the endoplasmic reticulum with polyribosomes and of mitochondrias (Fig. 4C) is impressive. The Golgi apparatus is also very much improved, but microvilli and grains remain absent.

Biochemical studies described in Section III confirm these observations.

C. Other Hormones

1. *Glucocorticosteroids*

Lasnitzki (1964) has observed that cortisol (10–40 μM) can maintain rat ventral prostate in culture. Similar observations were obtained in static culture, with the epithelium partially maintained by cortisol 3–25 μM. With lower doses, 0.3–1 μM, maintenance can be also obtained in serum-free medium, even it seems that the stroma does not regress as it does with an active dose of testosterone. Cortisol, 14 μM, does not potentiate the stimulation of castrated rat ventral prostate by testosterone, 16 nM, in static culture. Finally, using corticosterone, 4 nM, in constant-flow maintenance experiments with serum-containing medium, a minimal effect on both epithelium and stroma cells has been observed. More studies are obviously needed in this important area.

2. *Estradiol*

Not much work has been done with estrogens in organ culture. Laznitzki (1964) has shown an antimaintenance effect. In the static system, working with intact rat ventral prostate, estradiol up to 1 μM has not shown any maintenance effect, and at the high doses necrosis has been observed quite often. By means of the constant-flow system, estradiol 4 nM has been superfused for 6 days; it did not maintain prostatic explants, showing thus a great difference from the testosterone effect.

3. *Progesterone*

Introduced in the constant-flow system at the same concentration of 4 nM, progesterone too showed no maintenance effect (even though at 100 nM, in the static medium, a slight maintenance effect has been occasionally observed).

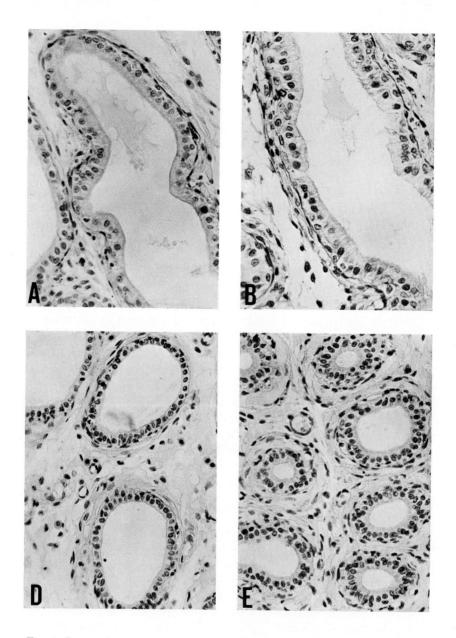

Fig. 4. Castrated rat ventral prostate explants in "static" culture. (A) Testosterone, 0.8 μM. (B) Androstanolone, 0.8 μM. (C) Testosterone, 8 μM. (D) Control, no culture. (E and F) No hormone in the culture. (A), (B), (D), and (E), $\times 300$; (C) and (F), $\times 28{,}000$. Scale line corresponds to 1 μm. ER, rough endoplasmic reticulum; M, mitochondria; N, nucleus. Seven-day cultures are performed as described in Section II, A, 1. Note that regressed prostate from intact rat after static culture without hormone gives a picture very similar to (D) (same size of alveoli) and (E) (same stroma).

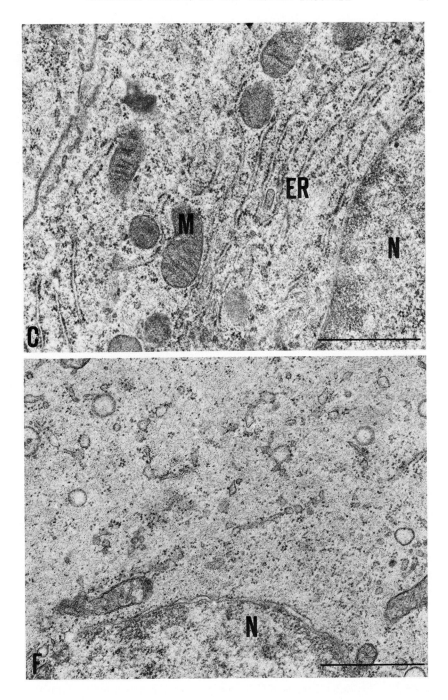

4. *Antiandrogens*

Cyproterone acetate, an active antiandrogen, was tested by Lasnitzki and Robel (1968) and shown to antagonize the testosterone maintenance effect; Santi and Johansson (1973) have also counteracted testosterone at 0.1 μM by cyproterone acetate at 10 μM. Preliminary experiments using 0.5 and 1 μM cyproterone and cyproterone acetate have demonstrated some weak androgenic effects of these compounds, corroborating the observations of Mowszowicz *et al.* (1975). The use of R 2956 at 0.5 μM, an antiandrogen of the 19-nor series, indicated that it is practically devoid of androgenic effect, but that it may counteract partly the testosterone 5 nM effect in the static system used for maintenance experiments. Bonne (1975) has also observed an antiandrogenic effect of this compound in static culture for 3 days by measuring alkaline phosphatase activity.

Incidentally, in order to block 5α-reductase activity in ventral prostate explants with a compound which, unlike progesterone, is not bound to the androgen *receptor*, the steroid R 4414 was used at a concentration of 0.5 μM. Its activity was demonstrated since the amount of androstanolone derived from testosterone decreased in the medium by 61%; however, in these experiments performed with a constant-flow of testosterone-^{3}H 1 nM, androstanolone did not decrease in the explants themselves, suggesting that, to be active, an anti 5α-reductase agent should be practically 100% effective. If not, enough androstanolone will be available for binding to the *receptor*.

5. *Insulin*

Some biochemical effects of insulin are reported in Section III, B. However, the histological or ultrastructural evaluation of maintenance effects of insulin at 0.4–2 μM in the static system indicated no change vs control, nor any potentiating effect on the maintenance effect of testosterone. In regressed prostatic tissue from castrated rat, insulin at 1μM, alone or added to testosterone in static culture, did not exhibit any morphologically demonstrable activity. However, at the very high doses of 10 μM (50 μg/ml), a slight testosterone-like effect on epithelial and stroma cells was observed.

III. BIOCHEMICAL STUDIES OF PROTEIN AND RNA SYNTHESIS IN CULTURED EXPLANTS

A. TECHNIQUES

Eighty explants are used for each experimental point, and only the static culture is performed. The medium is Parker 199 in intact rat culture and Waymouth 752–1066, 1:1 (v/v) for castrated rat prostate. It is not complemented with serum. Most experiments last 48 hours. In cases of longer culture, the medium is changed after 24 hours and then every 48 hours (up to 192 hours). When incorporation of l-leucine-^{3}H radioactivity into protein and uridine-^{3}H radioactivity into RNA is determined, explants from each grid are divided into two parts, respectively, for further 60-minute incubations at 37°C in the presence of the radioactive precursor. Specific activity of l-leucine-^{3}H is calculated from the concentration of the tracer and of the content of the medium in dl-leucine; it is 11 mCi/mmole, and the uridine-^{3}H is 54 Ci/mmole and used at 0.1 nM concentration.

Homogenization and centrifugation at 3600 g for 10 minutes yield a supernatant and a pellet in the protein studies. After addition of BSA to the supernatant, precipitation is obtained by TCA, 10%; after three washes with TCA, the final precipitate is dissolved in NCS and counted. The pellet is used for measuring DNA according to Burton. When determining radioactive RNA, the extracts are treated with PCA, 0.5 N at 0°C, homogenized, and centrifuged. The supernatant (actually after a second round of precipitation and centrifugation and ethanol washing of the pellet) serves to measure the acid-soluble radioactivity. The pellet is treated by KOH, 0.3 N at 37°C, for hydrolyzing RNA, and proteins and DNA are eliminated by PCA precipitation. Radioactivity and OD at 260/280 nm are determined.

Electrophoretic studies of proteins have been also undertaken. The TCA precipitate is treated with SDS and submitted to SDS polyacrylamide electrophoresis as reported elsewhere (Pennequin et al., 1975; Weber and Osborn, 1969). Double-label experiments are performed using ^{3}H- and ^{14}C-labeled l-leucine (SA 11 and 4 mCi/mmole, respectively).

B. Maintenance of Intact Rat Ventral Prostate

As indicated in Table III, insulin at 42 nM (as in Calame and Lostroh, 1964; Santti and Johansson, 1973) and testosterone at 10 nM, separately, can increase above control both the incorporation of radioactivity of l-leucine-^{3}H into protein and the concentration of protein per explant or DNA content of tissue maintained in culture. The measurement of the acid-soluble radioactivity suggests that the changes are not explained by an increased uptake of the radioactive amino acid by the explants. The effects of testosterone and insulin introduced at the same time are not completely additive, but they are also not mutually exclusive, and a significant further increase is observed in comparison with the effect with one hormone. With the assumption that insulin effects are "nutritional" more than specific for prostate, most experiments reported below include insulin in the control.

TABLE III

EFFECTS OF INSULIN AND TESTOSTERONE ON PROTEIN OF INTACT RAT
VENTRAL PROSTATE EXPLANTS IN CULTURE[a]

Treatment	^{3}H-protein /mg protein	^{3}H-acid soluble /mg protein	Protein (μg/10 explants)	Protein (μg/μg DNA)
Control	100[b]	100[c]	100[d]	100[e]
Insulin	166	40	250	226
Testosterone	169	58	201	226
Insulin + testosterone	188	55	303	244

[a] Explants from intact rats are grown for 48 hours in medium 199 and then incubated for 60 minutes at 37°C in l-leucine-^{3}H (SA 11 mCi/mmole calculated from tracer and l-leucine in the medium). Insulin, 42 nM; testosterone, 10 nM.
[b] 21,852 dpm ± 2049 (mean ± SEM). All results are significant vs appropriate controls ($p < 0.01$).
[c] 13,466 dpm ± 604.
[d] 100.0 μg ± 2.7. All results are significant vs appropriate controls ($p < 0.01$).
[e] 3.38 μg ± 0.06. All results are significant vs appropriate controls ($p < 0.01$).

TABLE IV

EFFECTS OF TESTOSTERONE ON THE INCORPORATION OF RADIOACTIVITY FROM
LEUCINE-^{3}H INTO PROTEIN AND FROM URIDINE-^{3}H INTO RNA OF NORMAL
RAT VENTRAL PROSTATE EXPLANTS IN CULTURE[a]

	Time zero	24 Hours	48 Hours	96 Hours	192 Hours
Control	100[b]	37	20	47	47
Testosterone		48	28	75	47
Treated/control × 100		129	136	158	101[d]
Control	100[c]	98	55	115	150
Testosterone		118	58	202	234
Treated/control × 100		121	104	175	155

[a] Explants from intact rats were grown for 24, 48, 96, or 192 hours in medium 199 containing insulin at 42 nM and then (upper part) incubated for 60 minutes at 37°C in l-leucine-^{3}H at 5 μM (SA 11 mCi/mmole calculated from tracer and l-leucine in the medium), or (lower part) in uridine-^{3}H (SA 54 Ci/mmole), 0.1 nM. Testosterone, 10 nM, when indicated.
[b] 925,884 Dpm ± 9646 (mean ± SEM).
[c] 618,024 Dpm ± 7,664.
[d] All results except this are significant vs appropriate control.

A time-course study (Table IV) investigates the action of testosterone added to insulin-containing medium. It shows that, in the surviving explants kept in the absence of androgen, protein synthesis decreases for 2 days and then increases. However, it is not restored completely even when testosterone is present. Similar studies with radioactive uridine show a better restoration of the radioactive RNA formation. The responses to the androgen vary with time (the day 8 failure for protein is not understood), and the 2-day schedule has been chosen for other experiments because the control values (no testosterone) are lowest. In fact, it may have been the wrong choice, since, *in vivo*, after deprivation of hormone, it is also the time of decrease of the *receptor* (Baulieu and Jung, 1970; Blondeau *et al.*, this volume, p. 319).

Comparative morphological studies having been performed with testosterone, androstanolone, and 3β-androstanediol, it has been of interest to obtain also some parallel biochemical parameters: 48-hour organ culture in the presence of insulin is used (Table V). Clear responses are obtained for 1 μM and 100 nM for both testosterone and androstanolone and for androstanolone, 10 nM, in terms of increase of ^{3}H-labeled protein and ^{3}H-labeled RNA. Results are also positive, even at the limit of the significance, for testosterone, 10 nM, and 3β-androstanediol, 1 μM and 100

TABLE V

EFFECTS OF DIFFERENT CONCENTRATIONS OF TESTOSTERONE, ANDROSTANOLONE, AND 3β-ANDROSTANEDIOL ON INCORPORATION OF RADIOACTIVITY FROM LEUCINE-^{3}H INTO PROTEIN AND URIDINE-^{3}H INTO RNA IN NORMAL RAT VENTRAL PROSTATE EXPLANTS IN CULTURE[a]

Treatment	Testosterone	Androstanolone	3β-Androstanediol
Control (no steroid)	100[b]	100[b]	100[c]
1 μM	114	151	109
100 nM	106	129	114
10 nM	101	121	94[d]
Control (no steroid)	100[e]	100[f]	100[g]
1 μM	191	269	124
100 nM	181	386	121
10 nM	126	162	92[d]

[a] Explants from intact rat ventral prostate were grown for 48 hours in medium 199 containing insulin at 42 nM, and then (upper part) incubated for 60 minutes at 37°C in l-leucine-^{3}H at 5 μM (SA 11 mCi/mmole calculated from tracer and l-leucine in the medium), or (lower part) in uridine-^{3}H (SA 54 Ci/mmole) 0.1 nM. Results are expressed as treated/control $\times$ 100.

[b] 391,854 Dpm $\pm$ 1750 (5 experiments with testosterone, 4 experiments with androstanolone) (mean $\pm$ SEM).

[c] 258,342 Dpm $\pm$ 5103 (2 experiments).

[d] All results except those marked [d] are significant vs control values ($p < 0.01$).

[e] 225,696 Dpm $\pm$ 7660 (5 experiments).

[f] 83,755 Dpm $\pm$ 8941 (4 experiments).

[g] 1,111,151 Dpm $\pm$ 21,018 (2 experiments).

nM. No response is observed with 3β-androstanediol, 10 nM. The magnitude of the effects is roughly a function of the concentrations, even if the RNA effect of androstanolone, 100 nM, is curiously high.

An electrophoretic analysis of leucine-^{3}H-labeled proteins of the culture medium after 6 days shows a series of bands similar to the tissue ^{3}H-labeled proteins (not shown). However, if those proteins in the medium may be secreted proteins, the presence of components accidentally released by mechanical disruption of cells, necrosis, etc. cannot be excluded.

Double-label experiments for the study of explants proteins have also been performed. Controls are obtained by labeling both (insulin-containing) controls or testosterone-treated explants by either ^{3}H- or ^{14}C-labeled leucine and running ^{3}H-control/^{14}C-control and ^{3}H-treated/^{14}C-treated mixtures through electrophoresis: in these cases the ^{3}H/^{14}C ratio is the same in all proteins and a horizontal line is obtained (data not shown; a similar experiment with castrated rats is shown in Fig. 5). However, when ^{3}H-treated vs. ^{14}C-control proteins are coelectrophoresed, the profile is very irregular. In most of the 60 fractions, the tritiated proteins are above the corresponding ^{14}C values (and exceptions are mainly in the region where degraded products migrate), but the relative augmentation varies very much along the gel. As expected after 2-day culture, several

TABLE VI

EFFECTS OF TESTOSTERONE ON INCORPORATION OF RADIOACTIVITY FROM LEUCINE-^{3}H INTO PROTEIN AND FROM URIDINE-^{3}H INTO RNA IN 14-DAY CASTRATED RAT VENTRAL PROSTATE EXPLANTS IN CULTURE[a]

Treatment[b]	^{3}H-Protein /mg-protein	^{3}H-Acid-soluble /mg protein	^{3}H-RNA /mg RNA
No steroid (control)	100[c]	100[d]	100[e]
1 μM (1)	170	132	191
100 nM (2)	148	114	164
10 nM (5)	135	102	136
1 nM (3)	123	94	118
0.1 nM (3)	130	92	115

[a] Explants were grown for 6 days in Waymouth 752–1066 1:1 (v/v) containing insulin 42 nM, and antibiotics. They were then incubated for 60 minutes at 37°C, in l-leucine-^{3}H (5 μM) (SA 11 mCi/mmole after correction for l-leucine content of the medium) (columns 2 and 3) or in uridine-^{3}H (SA 54 Ci/mmole), 0.1 nM (column 4). Results are expressed as treated/control $\times$ 100. Values for 1 μM, 100 nM, and 10 nM are significant above controls ($p < 0.01$).

[b] Number of experiments is given in parentheses.

[c] 284,354 Dpm $\pm$ 7983 (mean $\pm$ SEM).

[d] 98,982 Dpm $\pm$ 11,904.

[e] 658,658 Dpm $\pm$ 26,279.

types of proteins appear then to have increased under the testosterone treatment.

C. Hormonal Stimulation of Castrated Rat Ventral Prostate

Biochemical studies confirm the possibility, already seen histologically, that one can stimulate *in vitro* castrated rat regressed prostatic tissue.

Ventral prostate explants from 14-day castrated rats are grown for 6 days in the insulin-containing medium, then labeled with l-leucine-^{3}H or uridine-^{3}H. The magnitude of the response to testosterone, from 1 μM down to 0.1 nM, is largely dependent on the concentration (Table VI). Moreover, again in insulin-containing medium, the proper effects of 10% fetal calf serum, as directly obtained or after charcoal treatment, are similar to the action of testosterone, 10 nM (Table VII). There is no further increase when the androgen and the serum are added together. The S1 factor (Hoffman *et al.*, 1973) has no effect, as also confirmed histologically. Another series of 6-day culture experiments was performed

TABLE VII

Effects of Testosterone and Various Serum Preparations on Radio-
activity Incorporation from Leucine-^{3}H into Protein and from
Uridine-^{3}H into RNA in 14-Day Castrated Rat Ventral Prostate
Explants in Culture[a]

Treatment[b]	^{3}H-Protein /mg protein	^{3}H-RNA /mg RNA
Control (4)	100[c]	100[d]
Serum (2)	152	192
Charcoal-treated serum (2)	149	150
S1 factor (1)	122	112
Testosterone (1)	207	185
Serum and testosterone (2)	196	206
Charcoal-treated serum and testosterone (2)	195	204
S1 factor and testosterone (1)	185	189

[a] Explants were grown for 6 days in medium 752–1066 1:1 (v/v) containing insulin at 42 nM and various serum preparations: fetal calf serum, 10%, or charcoal-treated fetal calf serum, 10%, or S1 purified according to Hoffman *et al.* (1973), 25 μg/ml, and then incubated for 60 minutes at 37°C in l-leucine-^{3}H (SA 11 mCi/mmole), or in uridine-^{3}H (SA 54 Ci/mmole), 0.1 nM. Testosterone at 10 nM, when indicated. All results are significant vs control.

[b] Number of experiments in this series is given in parentheses

[c] 331,612 Dpm ± 6109 (mean ± SEM).

[d] 871,807 Dpm ± 2008.

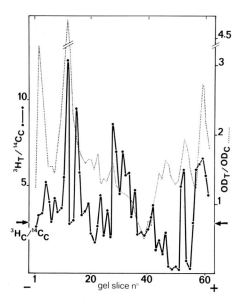

FIG. 5. Ventral prostate explants in culture: effects of testosterone on the labeled protein electrophoretic pattern. Castrated-rat ventral prostate explants have been cultivated, as described in Section III, C, for 2 days in the static system, without or with testosterone at 10 nM. Treated explants have been labeled with *l*-leucine-³H and control explants with either leucine-³H or *l*-leucine-¹⁴C. Double-labeled proteins were prepared from mixtures of ³H-treated and ¹⁴C-control and of ³H-control and ¹⁴C-control explants, and submitted to sodium dodecyl sulfate polyacrylamide electrophoresis. Technical references are indicated under Section III, A. The level of the linear pattern of ³H/¹⁴C for the control/control experiment is indicated by the two arrows. Dotted line: the profile of 280 nm adsorption of the treated/control experiment.

in medium without insulin (data not shown). It was observed, as for maintenance experiments (Table III), that the addition of testosterone, 10 nM, or insulin, 42 nM, increases equally the incorporation of leucine-³H into proteins, while their combination gives higher (not fully additive) results. All these findings are difficult to interpret in terms of partial agonism and/or antagonism, and the maximum response does not reach the level obtained with intact rat explants.

The SDS electrophoresis of proteins from a double-label experiment is shown in Fig. 5. The considerations reported for the maintenance experiments (Section III, B) apply here too. Moreover, when the effects of insulin and testosterone and their association were tested as indicated in the preceding paragraph, the protein profiles were very similar.

Double-label experiments have also been performed to evaluate the possibility that testosterone increases the incorporation of leucine-³H into protein by increasing the specific activity of the leucine pool in explants. The $^3H/^{14}C$ ratio in the free amino acid fraction of the cytosol (7.2) is lower than the mean $^3H/^{14}C$ ratio of protein (10.3, certain proteins higher than 14), suggesting that there is in fact an increased rate of protein synthesis. However, the ratio of the amino acid fraction is greater in the explants than in the incubation medium (3.7), a result suggesting an increased entry of amino acid into testosterone-treated explants. Finally, increased protein synthesis and amino acid entry may well operate simultaneously.

In conclusion, the effects of insulin and testosterone initially observed in maintenance experiments with total protein and RNA are confirmed in various ways. The results of electrophoretic analyses indicate that the increased incorporation of radioactivity into protein is certainly not only a matter of amino acid pool, which could not produce such uneven changes of the different proteins as those observed. Hormonal effects are also visible on the very regressed tissue of castrated animals. The complexity of the response should be emphasized, and also that these studies are very primitive: the apparent pattern of the response is influenced by the proper rates of synthesis and degradation of each protein, the possible transfers between cellular compartments (operationally defined in soluble and pellet fractions), etc.

IV. The RNA Synthesizing Machinery in Prostatic Epithelial Cells

The early and profound changes provoked by either castration or administration of androgens to the rat on prostatic RNA synthesis are well known (Liao and Fang, 1969; Williams-Ashman and Reddi, 1971). The regression of the rough-surfaced endoplasmic reticulum in the absence of hormone can be observed also in culture (Fig. 4F), as well as its restoration under androgenic stimulation (Fig. 4C) and also the effects of various hormones on RNA synthesis (Tables IV–VII). Two classes of organelles implicated in RNA metabolism can be studied morphologically at the nuclear level, the nucleolus and the perichromatin granules. The nucleolus is engaged in the synthesis of ribosomal RNA precursors. The granules are ribonucleoprotein particles that might be related to the transport and processing of messenger RNAs.

A. Nucleolus of Epithelial Cells

After castration and 7-day static culture without hormone (Fig. 6E), the nucleolus has decreased in size and lost most of its granular compo-

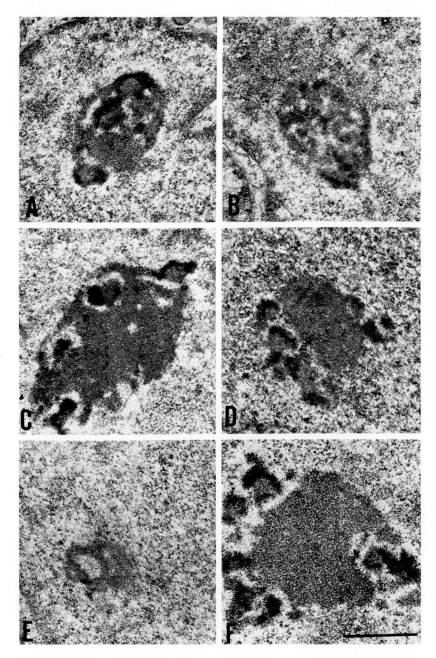

Fig. 6. Ventral prostate explants in culture: effects of androgens on the nucleolus of epithelial cells. All explants were kept for 7 days in static culture, as indicated in Section II, A, 1. (A, B, C, and D) Results of maintenance experiments from intact rats, with, respectively, testosterone, 0.6 μM; 3β-androstanediol, 1.1 μM; 4-androstenedione, 0.6 μM; and androstanolone, 4 nM. (E and F) From 14-day castrated rats, no culture and 6-day culture, respectively, with testosterone at 0.6 μM. $\times$20,000; scale line represents 1 μm.

nent. If androstanolone, 0.6 μM is added to the medium, a remarkable stimulation is observed (Fig. 6F) ; the difference is particularly striking in the case of the granular component.

In maintenance experiments with intact rat ventral prostate for 7 days in static culture, testosterone at 0.6 μM keeps the architecture of the nucleolus (Fig. 6A) normal; the result is almost the same with 3β-andro-stanediol at 1.1 μM (Fig. 6B). If androstenedione at 0.6 μM or andro-stanolone at 4 nM is present, the nucleolus is even more stimulated (Fig. 6C and D). The distribution of the granular and fibrillar components is modified, and the prominent granular part segregates in the center, whereas in normal rat prostate and in explants maintained in culture with testosterone and 3β-androstanediol, the two parts of the nucleoli are intermingled. The low active concentration of androstanolone clearly indicates its potency. The differences observed in the granular and fibrillar distribution may evoke a possible selectivity in the effects of the different androgens on ribosomal RNA production.

B. Perichromatin Granules of Epithelial Cells

As seen in the inset of Fig. 7, perichromatin granules are located at the periphery of condensed chromatin (heterochromatin). They are sur-

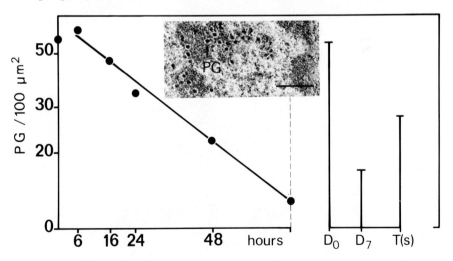

FIG. 7. Perichromatin granules (PG) of ventral prostate epithelial cells. The left part of the graph shows the postcastration regression (in hours) of the number of perichromatin granules/100 μm^2 of ultrathin sections of nuclei as determined on electron micrographs. The right part reports an experiment with control D_0 (intact rat), D_7 after 7 days static culture without hormone, and T(s) after 7-day static culture with 0.5 μM testosterone. Inset: electron micrograph of intact rat ventral prostate epithelial cell nucleus. $\times 10,000$; scale line represents 1 μm.

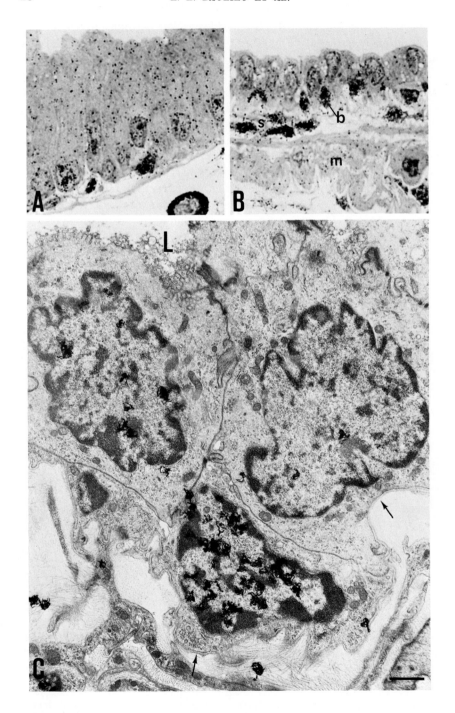

rounded by a clear halo, and their mean size is approximately 40 nm. They may be identical to the "informofers" of Samarina *et al.* (1973), a possibility already discussed by Le Goascogne (1973). The number of perichromatin granules has been evaluated by a counting method and expressed per surface unit of ultrathin section micrographs.

As reported in Fig. 7, a correlation with hormonal status can be established. After castration, the number of perichromatin granules decreases regularly, reaching a minimum level on the third day with an apparent half-life of approximately 1 day. When intact rat prostate explants are cultivated (static method, 7 days) without hormone, the diminution of perichromatin granules is similar to that observed after castration. It is possible to prevent partially this regression with hormones, as indicated here with testosterone at 0.5 μM.

C. RNA Radioautography

Biochemical studies as reported in Section III cannot distinguish which cells undergo hormone-induced changes of RNA metabolism.

In Fig. 8A and B are compared the pictures of intact and 8-day castrated rat ventral prostate epithelium, as obtained after incubation of explants in uridine-^{3}H. The interesting feature is the high labeling of some cells in the castrated rat epithelium. They have been identified by electron microscopy as basal cells (Fig. 8C), which are known to proliferate on day 4 of castration (Secchi and Bonne, 1973). Labeling of fibroblasts does not seem to be influenced by the change of hormonal status. It is concluded that in the biochemical studies of RNA synthesis in ventral prostate under different hormonal conditions the changes in cell population should be taken into account.

V. Discussion and Conclusions

Previous experiments have been performed with rather high concentrations of androgens (Robel *et al.*, 1971; Gittinger and Lasnitzki, 1972),

---

Fig. 8. Rat ventral prostate: uridine-^{3}H radioautography. (A) Intact rat. (B and C) 8-Day castrated rat. Labeling was performed by adding uridine-^{3}H (SA 54 Ci/mmole), 0.37 nM, to Eagle's medium. The explants were incubated for 20 minutes at 37°C under O_2 95%–CO_2 5%, quickly washed at 0°C in uridine (10 mg/ml), fixed in osmic acid, and included into Epon. Ilford L4 emulsion was used, and exposure was for 3 weeks. (A) and (B) Semithin section, 1 μm; ×1000. (C) Electron micrograph; ×10,000; the scale line represents 1 μm. b, Basal cells; m, muscular cells; →, basal lamina.

and the test was the maintenance in culture for several days of young adult rat ventral prostate explants. Satisfactory morphological and biochemical criteria were met, and the general organization of the rat ventral prostate with its tubuloalveolar structure and fibromuscular stroma was always preserved, in the presence or in the absence of hormones.

A. Maintenance Effects of Physiological Concentrations of Androgens

Young adult rat ventral prostate explants can be maximally maintained in the static culture system for a week by 100 nM concentrations of testosterone and androstanolone. With as low as 10 nM testosterone, the physiological concentration in the rat plasma (Robel et al., 1973), definite morphological maintenance and stimulation (vs culture without hormone) of protein and RNA syntheses are obtained; recently Johansson and Niemi (1975) have also observed an effect on protein and DNA syntheses with 10 nM steroid. The presence of serum in the medium is not necessary to obtain these results and, even in the static as well as in the constant-flow culture, greater effects are obtained in absence of serum for the same hormone concentration, confirming Lasnitzki and Franklin (1975). The constant-flow culture gives better results in the range of lower concentrations, and a significant maintenance of intact adult prostate is obtained with 1 nM androstanolone or even less. The theoretical basis for the superiority of the constant-flow culture is not quite clear. It is expected that the changes of hormone concentration due to local metabolism, and eventually of other limiting factors in the culture medium, are obviated by the continuous supply of medium, and that steroid and organic metabolites which may be harmful to the tissue are eliminated.

B. Stimulation of Castrated Rat Prostate in Static Culture

Until now no stimulation of fully regressed prostate, as obtained from animals castrated 2 weeks previously, has been observed in culture. Lostroh (1968), working with castrated mice ventral prostate explants, could not get an effect of testosterone in static organ culture unless the animals were pretreated with testosterone or insulin was added to the medium. Indeed no effect of testosterone was obtained in this laboratory with medium 199, whatever the experimental conditions, and positive results were obtained only with the 1:1 (v/v) mixture of media 752 + 1066.

However, it must be stressed that with either intact or castrated rats, whatever the culture medium or the hormones are, and even with the use of the constant-flow culture, the rat prostate explants are never completely maintained or fully stimulated. For example, the epithelial index is seldom above 3 and never above 4, and secretory granules remain sparse in the best conditions. Therefore, it may be that the constituents of the culture medium are still not optimal, that certain hormones, such as glucocorticosteroids and prolactin or growth factors, are not present or are present in inappropriate concentrations, that the dynamics of the constant-flow culture are not representative of physiological conditions, etc.

C. Differences between Androgens

1. *Quantitative Aspects*

With the use of low concentrations of androstanolone, testosterone, and 3β-androstanediol, the clear-cut distinction between androstanolone giving epithelial hyperplasia and 3β-androstanediol stimulating only epithelial hypertrophy and secretion is no longer observed. Concerning the optical criteria of epithelial cell maintenance, a semiquantitative comparison is possible between the three androgens, especially when low concentrations are used in constant-flow culture. Androstanolone is slightly more active than testosterone, a result that may be related to a large but incomplete conversion of testosterone into androstanolone (Robel *et al.*, 1975) and/or the higher affinity of androstanolone for the androgen *receptor*. Androstenedione activity is very similar to that of testosterone; it is converted into androstanolone to the same extent, testosterone formation appearing to be negligible (Roy *et al.*, 1972a). Androstenedione is not bound to specific plasma proteins (unlike testosterone in man and rabbit). It follows that, despite its low concentration in blood, it becomes a potential active steroid of importance in man, and studies with human prostate seem necessary. 3β-Androstanediol is not effective at low concentrations, whereas 0.5–1 μM concentrations of testosterone, androstanolone, and 3β-androstanediol give rather similar results. It cannot be excluded that a small metabolic conversion of 3β-androstanediol into androstanolone might, at least in part, explain the latter result.

2. *Qualitative Aspects*

In addition to the above-mentioned quantitative differences between androgens used at low or moderate concentrations, discrete qualitative differences may be reported, bearing on the epithelium-stroma relationships and the subcellular structures.

a. Epithelium–Stroma Relationships. When ventral prostate explants of intact rats are maintained, or explants of castrated rats are stimulated by testosterone, coordinated effects take place, monitoring the epithelial cell height and the alveolar diameter on one side, and the regression of the stroma on the other side. Such coordination is similar to that observed after administration of testosterone *in vivo* to castrated rats. The 3β-androstanediol has the same activity as testosterone in this respect. With androstanolone, it was repeatedly observed, mainly in static culture and with castrated rats, that whereas the stimulation of alveolar components is more marked than with testosterone, the perialveolar strands of fibroblasts and smooth muscular cells remain prominent, so that the rat ventral prostate resembles more the dog or human prostate. These differences between androgens are difficult to interpret, since the hormonal control of the stromal elements is not known. In particular, radioautography experiments performed after administration of testosterone-³H or androstanolone-³H *in vivo* showed almost no labeling of fibroblast or smooth muscle nuclei, suggesting that the androgen *receptor* was localized in the epithelial cells (Tveter and Attramadal, 1969; Sar *et al.*, 1970).

b. Subcellular Components. It has been observed that, at low concentrations which do not have an overall maintenance effect, 3β-androstanediol has a significant maintenance effect on the Golgi apparatus, evoking a possible selective effect on secretory processes. Moreover, studies at the nucleolar level have also shown differences between androgens. At concentrations that elicit similar epithelial cell maintenance, the nucleoli from cultures with testosterone and 3β-androstanediol display the normal intermingled structure characteristics of the intact rat, while androstanolone, even at very low concentration, and androstenedione tend to provoke a segregation between the granular and fibrillar components which may indicate a selective effect on the ribosomal RNA processing mechanism.

D. ANDROGEN EFFECTS ARE SPECIFIC

A major characteristic of the prostate organ culture is its hormonal specificity. At steroid concentrations below 10 nM in constant-flow culture, only testosterone and androstanolone have a significant maintenance effect. Although not carefully investigated, such a conclusion can be extended to other androgens which are readily converted into androstanolone (androstenedione, androstanedione, 3α-androstanediol). Negative results were obtained with the same low concentrations of estradiol, progesterone, and corticosterone. The presence of specific *receptors* for these steroids is still not certain in the rat ventral prostate, but both estradiol and progesterone compete for androstanolone binding to the androgen *receptor*.

E. Prostate Culture, State of the Art, Limitations, and Future

Physiological concentrations of androgens can maintain normal ventral prostate in constant-flow organ culture, and the regressed prostate of castrated animals can be partially stimulated. These conclusions have been substantiated at the biochemical and at the morphological levels. Moreover, differences between testosterone, androstanolone, and 3β-androstanediol have been observed bearing on alveolar–stromal relationships and some subcellular structures. This may contradict the simple hypothesis that androstanolone formation is the only parameter of importance for androgen activity, even if it is realized that the rate of formation of androstanolone from different precursors may play an important role.

A series of limitations preclude the drawing of definitive conclusions. Indeed, measuring overall protein and RNA synthesis and even with the use of SDS polyacrylamide gel electrophoresis of proteins, the effect of testosterone is biochemically mimicked by insulin, as seen also by Santi and Johansson (1973), who showed, moreover, the same effect on CO_2 production from glucose. Much work also remains to be done for understanding the role of glucocorticosteroids, insulin, and other protein hormones and factors on the system, as well as the possible effects of the compounds, which are candidates for being antiandrogenic and may have also other activities, for example, estradiol and progesterone. The complexity of the situation *in vivo* has already been considered for estradiol and cortisone (Tisell, 1971) or for the potentiation of androgen in culture by glucocorticosteroid and insulin (Santi and Johansson, 1972, 1973).

To progress in the understanding of hormone action on the ventral prostate gland in culture, one should use physiological concentrations of unbound hormones and more sophisticated techniques to analyze products of the steroid and the organic metabolism. It remains that the complex tissue modifications may hide the early molecular changes that occur after formation of the hormone–*receptor* complex. Studies should also investigate more carefully the role of hormones in the stroma and the possible interactions between the cells of the connective tissue and the epithelial cells. Finally, it is not at all clear that results obtained for a given lobe at a given age in a given animal species can be easily generalized.

ACKNOWLEDGMENTS

We would like to thank Brigitte Brismontier, Monique Gouezou, and Marie-Thérèse Picard-Groyer for skillful technical assistance. We thank also Mrs. Holback and Christiane Barrier for the photographs. Dr. Maria Marchut (Cracow, Poland) performed the experiment reported in Table II. The editorial assistance of Anne Atger and Daniele Prod'homme is gratefully acknowledged.

REFERENCES

Anderson, K. M., and Liao, S. (1968). *Nature (London)* **219**, 277.

Baird, D., Horton, R., Longcope, C., and Tait, J. F. (1968). *Perspect. Biol. Med.* **2**, 384.

Baulieu, E. E. (1974). *In* "Physiology and Genetics of Reproduction" (E. M. Coutinho and F. Fuchs, ed.), Vol. 4, Part A, p. 113. Plenum, New York.

Baulieu, E. E., and Jung, I. (1970). *Biochem. Biophys. Res. Commun.* **38**, 599.

Baulieu, E. E., and Mauvais-Jarvis, P. (1964). *J. Biol. Chem.* **239**, 1569.

Baulieu, E. E., Corpéchot, C., Dray, F., Emiliozzi, R., Lebeau, M. C., Mauvais-Jarvis P., and Robel, P. (1965). *Recent Progr. Horm. Res.* **21**, 411.

Baulieu, E. E., Robel, P., Mercier, C., and Lasnitzki, I. (1967). *Res. Steroids* **3**, 65.

Baulieu, E. E., Lasnitzki, I., and Robel, P. (1968a). *Nature (London)* **219**, 1155.

Baulieu, E. E., Lasnitzki, I., and Robel, P. (1968b). *Biochem. Biophys. Res. Commun.* **32**, 575.

Baulieu, E. E., Alberga, A., Jung, I., Lebeau, M. C., Mercier-Bodard, C., Milgrom, E., Raynaud, J. P,. Raynaud-Jammet, C., Rochefort, H., Truong, H., and Robel, P. (1971). *Recent Progr. Horm. Res.* **27**, 351.

Bonne, C. (1975). Ph.D. Dissertation, University Rene Descartes of Paris, Paris, France.

Bruchovsky, N., and Wilson, J. D. (1968). *J. Biol. Chem.* **243**, 2012.

Calame, S. S., and Lostroh, A. J. (1964). *Endocrinology* **75**, 451.

Dorfman, R. I., and Shipley, R. A., eds. (1956). "Androgens." Wiley, New York.

Fang, S., Anderson, K. M., and Liao, S. (1969). *J. Biol. Chem.* **244**, 6584.

Feyel-Cabanes, T., Pennequin, P., Baulieu, E. E., and Robel, P. (1974). *C. R. Acad. Sci.* **278**, 2181.

Flickinger, C. J. (1972). *Amer. J. Anat.* **134**, 107.

Gittinger, J. W., and Lasnitzki, I. (1972). *J. Endocrinol.* **52**, 459.

Harkin, J. C. (1957). *Endocrinology* **60**, 185.

Hoffman, R., Rislow, H. J., Veser, J., and Frank, W. (1973). *Exp. Cell Res.* **85**, 275.

Imperato-McGinley, J., Guerrero, L., Gautier, T., and Peterson, R. E. (1974). *Science* **186**, 1213.

Johansson, R., and Niemi, M. (1975). *Acta Endocrinol. (Copenhagen)* **78**, 766.

Jost, A. (1961). *Harvey Lect.* **55**, 201.

Jost, A. (1970). *Phil. Trans. Roy. Soc. London, Ser. B* **25**, 119.

Lasnitzki, I. (1964). *J. Endocrinol.* **30**, 225.

Lasnitzki, I. (1965). *J. Nat. Cancer Inst.* **35**, 339.

Lasnitzki, I., and Franklin, H. R. (1975). *J. Endocrinol.* **64**, 289.

Lasnitzki, I., and Robel, P. (1968). *Advan. Biosci.* **3**, 175.

Le Goascogne, C. (1973). *Acta Endocrinol. (Copenhagen), Suppl.* **180**, 160.

Levy, C., Marchut, M., Baulieu, E. E., and Robel, P. (1974). *Steroids* **23**, 291.

Liao, S., and Fang, S. (1969). *Vitam. Horm. (New York)* **27**, 17.

Lostroh, A. J. (1968). *Proc. Nat. Acad. Sci. U.S.* **60**, 1312.

Mainwaring, W. I. P. (1969). *J. Endocrinol.* **45**, 531.

Moore, C. R., Price, D., and Gallagher, T. F. (1930). *J. Anat.* **45**, 71.

Mowszowicz, I., Bieber, D. E., Chung, K. W., Bullock, L. P., and Bardin, C. W. (1975). *Endocrinology* **95**, 1589.

Pennequin, P., Robel, P., and Baulieu, E. E. (1975). *Eur. J. Biochem.* (in press).

Price, D., and Williams-Ashman, H. G. (1961). *In* "Sex and Internal Secretions" (W. G. Young, ed.), 3rd ed., p. 366. Williams & Wilkins, Baltimore, Maryland.

Robel, P. (1971). *Acta Endocrinol (Copenhagen), Suppl.* **153**, 279.

Robel, P., and Baulieu, E. E. (1972). *C. R. Acad. Sci.* **274**, 3295.

Robel, P., Lasnitzki, I., and Baulieu, E. E. (1971). *Biochimie* **53**, 81.

Robel, P., Roy, A. K., Levy, C., and Baulieu, E. E. (1975). *In* "Normal and Abnormal Growth of the Prostate" (M. Goland, ed.), p. 144. Thomas, Springfield, Illinois.

Roy, A. K., Baulieu, E. E., Feyel-Cabanes, T., Le Goascogne, C., and Robel, P. (1972a). *Endocrinology* **91**, 396.

Roy, A. K., Robel, P., and Baulieu, E. E. (1972b). *Endocrinology* **91**, 404.

Samarina, O. P., Lukanidin, E. M., and Georgiev, G. P. (1973). *Acta Endocrinol. (Copenhagen)*, **74**, *Suppl.* 180, 130.

Santi, R. S., and Johansson, R. (1972). *Gynecol. Invest.* **2**, 276.

Santi, R. S., and Johansson, R. (1973). *Exp. Cell Res.* **77**, 111.

Sar, M., Liao, S., and Stumpf, W. E. (1970). *Endocrinology* **86**, 1008.

Secchi, J., and Bonne, C. (1973). *C. R. Soc. Biol.* **167**, 1331.

Siiteri, P. K., and Wilson, J. D. (1974). *J. Clin. Endocrinol. Metab.* **38**, 113.

Tisell, L. E. (1971). *Acta Endocrinol. (Copenhagen)* **68**, 485.

Tveter, K. J., and Attramadal, A. (1969). *Endocrinology* **85**, 350.

Unhjem, O., Tveter, K. J., and Aakvaag, A. (1969). *Acta Endocrinol. (Copenhagen)* **62**, 153.

Walsh, P. C., Madden, J. D., Hamrod, M. J., Goldstein, J. C., McDonald, P. C., and Wilson, J. D. (1974). *N. Engl. J. Med.* **291**, 944.

Weber, K., and Osborn, M. (1969). *J. Biol. Chem.* **244**, 4406.

Williams-Ashman, H. G., and Reddi, A. H. (1971). *Annu. Rev. Physiol.* **33**, 31.

Wilson, J. D., and Gloyna, R. E. (1970). *Recent Progr. Horm. Res.* **26**, 309.

Wilson, J. D., and Lasnitzki, I. (1971). *Endocrinology* **89**, 659.

DISCUSSION

E. Diczfalusy: We are very grateful to Drs. Baulieu and Robel for making morphology so exciting to endocrinologists. I have two questions: (1) How does the effect of 5α-androstane-3α,17β-diol compare with those of 5α-dihydrotestosterone and 5α-androstane-3β,17β-diol in your system? (2) Has Δ^5-androstene-3β,17β-diol any comparable effects?

E. E. Baulieu: Besides the original work with Ilse Lasnitzki [E. E. Baulieu, I. Lasnitzki, and P. Robel, *Nature (London)* **219**, 1155 (1968)], which shows interconvertibility of 3α-androstanediol with androstanolone and its very potent overall androgenic activity, we have not devoted more efforts to analyzing in detail 3α-androstanediol. It would be interesting to do it since unsuspected effects may come up, as we have observed with Δ^4-androstenedione. Moreover, we have not studied the Δ^5-androstene-3β,17β-diol specifically, but some work with dehydroisoandrosterone [A. K. Roy, P. Robel, and E. E. Baulieu, *Endocrinology* **97**, 404 (1972)] has shown that 3β-hydroxy compounds are not very active "constitutively"; this does not mean that there is nothing specific with them.

I. Lasnitzki: Androgen withdrawal causes labilization of lysosomal membranes, resulting in a release of acid proteases that are involved in the degradation of cytoplasmic organelles and possibly of receptor proteins. The function of the 3β-diol may be to stabilize lysosomal membranes and thereby prevent the degenerative changes.

K. Griffiths: Analysis of human benign prostatic tumors by high-resolution mass fragmentography has shown a higher concentration of 5α-androstane-3α,17β-diol than of 5α-androstane-3β,17β-diol.

E. E. Baulieu: The studies with mass spectrometry indicating that there is more 3α-androstanediol than 3β-androstanediol lead to similar results as those observed in the rat with conventional radiochromatographic technology.

I. Lasnitzki: In our hands, testosterone and 3β-diol always maintained the integrity of the endoplasmic reticulum, the Golgi apparatus, and microvilli.

E. E. Baulieu: We have not investigated the effects of hormones, and eventually 3β-androstanediol, on lysosome stability. We see in culture that the number of lysosomes increases when androgen effect is weak. As far as the effects of 3β-diol are concerned, it seems to us that 3β-diol is particularly effective on the Golgi apparatus. Finally, it is also seen in our work that the absence of serum proteins seems to allow a greater effect of the same dose of testosterone or androstanolone, probably because of the deficient extracellular protein binding.

M. B. Lipsett: In view of the interest in prolactin, two abstracts for the Endocrine Society Meeting of June 1975 show that testosterone increases the number of prolactin receptors in the prostate.

E. E. Baulieu: The interplay between steroid effects and protein hormone receptors becomes an interesting story in various systems, including the prostate and the ovaries.

I. Lasnitzki: In organ cultures of rat ventral prostate, prolactin augments the effects of subthreshold doses of testosterone.

K. Griffiths: In Cardiff, we have been particularly concerned with the possible effects of prolactin on the prostate. Have you studied, in your perfusion system, the effects of prolactin in association with testosterone?

E. E. Baulieu: We have not worked on prolactin effects in our culture system.

I. Lasnitzki: Testosterone and dihydrotestosterone are bound to serum albumin, and more specifically to testosterone-estradiol binding globulin (TEBG). We have demonstrated in organ cultures of rat ventral prostate that the uptake and biological action of testosterone is inversely related to the amounts of TEBG present, i.e., that only the free form of the hormone is available for the target organ.

H. G. Williams-Ashman: I would like to point out a potential difficulty in the use of serum from ruminants in media used for organ cultures of rat ventral prostate. This is one of the very few organs in the body whose secretions contain large amounts of spermidine and spermine extracellularly in the lumens of the acini, these polyamines being secreted by the epithelial cells. Now the serum of ruminants and a few related species, such as the hippopotamus, contains a very active oxidizing enzyme, absent from the blood serum of other mammalian species, that oxidizes spermine and spermidine to very toxic aldehyde products. It therefore seems quite possible that addition of a ruminant serum to the culture medium for rat ventral prostate organ cultures would produce outside the cells some very toxic substances that could get into and damage the prostate cells, but which would not be formed in organ cultures of most other tissues. It seems to me that if a serum is to be used in such studies, it should be obtained from a nonruminant species whose blood plasma is devoid of polyamine oxidizing enzymes.

E. E. Baulieu: It is a very good suggestion to try other serum preparations. However, maybe the perfusion system is a good way to get rid rapidly of oxidation products, and in any case we have obtained effects by steroid hormones in the absence of serum.

B. Uvnäs: How do you explain the beneficial effect of your perfusion system in comparison with a static incubation system?

E. E. Baulieu: The beneficial effect of the constant-flow system may be attributable to the following reasons: (1) The establishment of a fixed concentration of hormone; when you perform ordinary "static" culture and change the medium, for instance every 3 days, you have successively highest and very low levels of hormone, both being possibly damaging by "toxic" and "deprivation" effects, respectively. With the perfused system, we feel that we are more "physiological." (2) The perfusion system probably removes steroid metabolites and organic metabolites that could be harmful to the tissues and then mimics *in vitro* some mechanical benefits of the blood circulation. (3) We may even, following Dr. Williams-Ashman's remarks on the possible degradation of prostatic polyamines by calf serum, remove some "toxic" components coming from the serum introduced into the medium.

M. B. Lipsett: What is the role of estrogen-binding proteins and other serum factors in the perfused system?

E. E. Baulieu: We have not studied estrogens with the constant-flow system. However, in the calf serum that we have used, we have not found that charcoal pretreatment changes its properties (see text Table II). Moreover, as far as binding proteins and other serum factors are concerned, as indicated in the same table, it can be seen that there is an effect of "total" serum, but not of the isolated factor. The overall story is far from being complete and clear, but definitely we can observe a response to testosterone in the absence of other hormones (including insulin) and in the absence of serum. I firmly believe that testosterone can be active on its own.

K.-D. Voigt: With reference to the demonstrated conversion of 3β- and 3α-diol to 5α-DHT under *in vivo* conditions in rat [M. Krieg, H. J. Horst, and M. L. Sterba, *J. Endocrinol.* **64,** 529 (1975)], my question is whether Dr. Baulieu in his investigations compared uptake and conversion of testosterone under *in vivo* conditions with the data obtained under organ culture conditions.

E. E. Baulieu: In the prostatic explants *in vitro*, we see, as indicated in the paper, a slight conversion of 3β-androstanediol into androstanolone. We do not know whether this feeble conversion, which does not lead to detectable amounts of androstanolone in nuclei at the concentrations of 3β-androstanediol used, is the mechanism by which 3β-androstanediol acts, or whether there is only a direct effect, as indicated by the series of differences between 3β-androstanediol and androstanolone effects which we summarize in the Conclusion Chapter. In the *in vivo* situation, we cannot decide whether or not androstanolone coming from 3β-androstanediol has been produced in the liver or elsewhere in the body, or in the prostatic tissue itself, but whatever is the metabolic pattern for the formation of androstanolone, it may still have some importance for evaluating the whole situation *in vivo*.

A. Mittelman: Can you determine qualitative differences in protein synthesis with variation of hormonal stimuli? Does the effluent promote a mean of studying this?

E. E. Baulieu: With the technique we have used, we have not studied in more detail than total synthesis and sodium dodecyl sulfate electrophoretic profiles of the explant proteins. In a few cases, the proteins found in the medium have been analyzed, and the changes were very similar to those observed in explant homogenates. However, I feel that the present technology, and the fact that we are investigating, in this system, the effects of hormones after several hours or several days, does not allow us to see a possible early specific effect on protein synthesis. With another biological material, we are investigating specific proteins and their specific messenger RNA's but to my knowledge there is no way to do such work in prostate and even less in small explants in culture.

J.-A. Gustafsson: I was interested to hear that you have found a biological activity of 4-androstene-3,17-dione in prostate. We have shown the presence in rat liver cytosol of a protein that binds 4-androstene-3,17-dione with high affinity and low capacity. Furthermore, ^{3}H-labeled 4-androstene-3,17-dione is specifically accumulated in liver nuclei after injection of 1,2,6,7-^{3}H-labeled testosterone into castrated rats. We have speculated that 4-androstene-3,17-dione may be involved in the mechanism of action of androgens in the liver. Would you care to expand a little on the question of 4-androstene-3,17-dione activity in the prostate?

E. E. Baulieu: I am aware of the work on Δ^4-androstenedione binding in liver nuclei. We have seen a sort of special nucleolar effect. Whether or not this effect is a specific direct effect of androstenedione on some step implicated in RNA synthesis and/or processing, or is indirectly due to metabolites of androstenedione (incidentally, there is no testosterone detectable in the tissue from androstenedione [A. K. Roy, E. E. Baulieu, T. Feyel-Cabanes, C. LeGoascogne, and P. Robel, *Endocrinology* **91**, 396 (1972)]) cannot be determined at the present time.

Polynucleotide Polymerizations and Prostate Proliferation*

H. G. WILLIAMS-ASHMAN, B. TADOLINI, J. WILSON,
AND A. CORTI†

*The Ben May Laboratory for Cancer Research,
Departments of Biochemistry and Pharmacological and Physiological Sciences,
University of Chicago, Chicago, Illinois*

I. DNA Replication and Rat Prostate Growth

This contribution outlines some recent studies, still largely unpublished, on DNA polymerizing enzymes in relation to the hyperplastic element of androgen-induced growth of the rat prostate.

A model system for study of biochemical correlates of cell division during prostate growth was devised by Coffey et al. (1968). Elderly rats were orchiectomized, and their male genital glands were allowed to regress extensively over a period of 7 days. Daily treatments with large amounts of androgen were then inaugurated, so as to promote the size and total DNA content of the ventral prostate to converge toward maximal values that were somewhat larger, although not enormously so, than those of normal control animals with intact testicles. As determined by ^{3}H-labeled thymidine incorporation either *in vivo,* or *in vitro* by isolated prostate minces, DNA synthesis in either normal adult prostate or in the glands of untreated castrates is exceptionally low. After commencement of androgen injections in saturation doses into 1-week castrates, marked increases in the RNA/DNA ratio as well as in the activity of a variety of enzymes are manifest within 1 day, but with no corresponding enhancement of total prostate DNA, thymidine incorporation, or of the activity of "replicative DNA polymerase" activity. Enzyme(s) cata-

* These investigations were supported in part by a research grant (HD-04592) from the U.S. Public Health Service.
† Present address: Istituto di Chimica Biologica, University of Bologna, Italy.

lyzing the latter reaction were found mainly in soluble ultracentrifuged extracts of ventral prostate homogenates prepared in dilute buffered salt solutions containing thiols; the polymerizations of a single labeled deoxyribonucleoside triphosphate (dNTP) were enhanced by addition of the three complementary dNTPs, and heat-denatured DNA was a better template-primer than double-stranded DNA in the presence of Mg^{2+}. The entry of labeled thymidine into DNA, as measured either *in vivo* or *in vitro*, was tremendously enhanced by the second day after starting treatment with testosterone propionate and reached a zenith at 3 days, after which time the thymidine incorporations gradually declined toward the levels observed with prostates from untreated castrates by 10 days of continuous androgen administration. The soluble "replicative" DNA polymerase activity did not rise greatly before the third day after commencement of daily androgen treatment, reached a maximum on day 4, and thereafter fell markedly, despite the continuous hyperphysiological androgenic stimulus. These findings are summarized in Fig. 1.

Such experimental systems have been extended, and also exploited as a tool for study of the actions of antiandrogens and cancer chemotherapeutic agents on prostate growth, by Sufrin and Coffey (1973) and Sloan *et al.* (1975). And similar observations on the latent period of androgen enhancement of the accumulation and thymidine labeling of rat prostate nuclear DNA were reported by Lesser and Bruchovsky (1973) and Doeg *et al.* (1972). It was found by Lesser and Bruchovsky (1973) that the growth response in this rat ventral prostate system to testosterone was somewhat slower than that induced by 5α-dihydrotestosterone (DHT). Similar more rapid and extensive responses to DHT as compared with testosterone were noticed by Tuohimaa and Niemi (1968) in their radioautographic examination of thymidine labeling of epithelial cells in the ventral prostates of adult castrated rats. A cytokinetic analysis of the proliferative response to androgen of the prostates of castrated mice by Morley *et al.* (1972) hinted that the hormone markedly affected movement of cells into, and subsequently out of, the G_0 phase of the cell cycle.

On the basis of measurements of thymidine incorporation into prostatic nuclei that were fractionated according to their position in the cell cycle by velocity sedimentation under unit gravity, Lesser and Bruchovsky (1974b) concluded that the hyperplastic phase of rat ventral prostate growth induced by DHT in 7-day castrates involved the cell population undergoing 1.8 doublings with a doubling time of 40 hours. The process seemed to entail almost four rounds of cell division with a cell-generation time of 20 hours. All cells present at the start of DHT-induced prostate growth appeared eventually to undergo at least one division although individual cells could multiply from one to four times. Although secretory

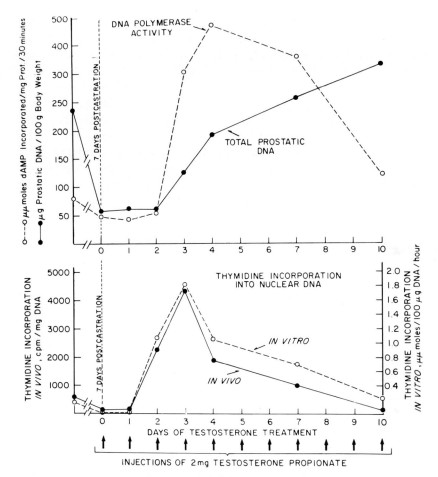

Fɪɢ. 1. "Replicative" DNA polymerase activity (top), and incorporation of thymidine into DNA *in vivo* and *in vitro* (bottom), during androgen-induced growth of rat ventral prostate. Data from Coffey *et al.* (1968).

epithelial cells predominate in the normal adult rat prostate, the organ is also comprised of different cell types in the lamina propria and the fibromuscular stroma, plus the endothelial cells of blood vessels. This obviously complicates interpretation of analyses of cell cycles based on the techniques of the sort used by Lesser and Bruchovsky (1974b). Androgen-dependent epithelial or other discrete types of cells from normal prostate have not been grown as pure cell lines in tissue culture under conditions where hormonal effects on their replication can be analyzed experimentally. Smith and King (1972) reported that addition of androgens approximately doubled the growth rate of Shionogi carcinoma 115 cells grown in culture, but it is debatable whether investigations with such androgen-dependent malignant cells are very pertinent to the steroid hormonal regulation of normal prostate cell replication.

A careful analysis of androgenic enhancement of growth, and thymidine incorporation into DNA, in the ventral prostates of rats that were treated with DHT beginning at various intervals after orchiectomy, was undertaken by Lesser and Bruchovsky (1974a). They noted that whether increase in secretion rather than in cell proliferation occurred predominantly in the first few days after commencement of daily injections of DHT depended on the length of time between castration and initiation of hormone treatment. In animals castrated less than 3 days previously, largely secretory activity but hardly any DNA synthesis or cell division was evoked, in contrast to the intense increase in cell proliferation in the prostates of rats that had been castrated for a week or longer. Lesser and Bruchovsky (1974a) rightly emphasized that any androgen-induced biochemical changes determined during the active phase of adult rat ventral prostate involution between about 2 and 6 days after orchiectomy are extremely difficult to interpret because of variations between cells in their proliferative versus secretory responses, at least in the epithelium.

II. Multiplicity of DNA Polymerizing Enzymes

Many enzymes in animal tissues are involved in DNA replication and in the related processes of DNA repair and genetic recombination. The monomeric building blocks are invariably the deoxyribonucleoside triphosphates dATP, dCTP, dGTP, and dTTP. Nothing is known about fluctuations in intracellular deoxyribonucleotide pools, or in the activity of their biosynthetic enzymes, in the prostate gland. The synthesis of DNA in animal cells seems to occur by a discontinuous mechanism involving the joining of intermediate short deoxyribopolynucleotide chains by DNA ligases that have been demonstrated and characterized in some animal cells, but not in the prostate or other male genital glands. Certain intracellular deoxyribonucleases may play a role *in vivo* in DNA synthesis as well as in DNA degradation, but any possible relationship of prostatic DNases to DNA synthesis in this organ does not seem to have been examined. There are also no available data on DNA methylating enzymes in the prostate, which in certain tissues may conceivably be involved in termination of the biosynthesis of DNA or its maturation. Thymidine kinase certainly is active in prostate tissue since labeled thymidine is readily incorporated into its DNA; but thymidine kinase is not on the main biosynthetic route for dTTP formation in animal tissues and probably represents part of a "salvage" pathway. It would undoubtedly be profitable to examine all the aforementioned groups of enzymes related to DNA synthesis vis-à-vis androgenic influences on prostate growth and differentiation.

As discussed in some recent reviews (Keir and Craig, 1974; Kornberg, 1974; Loeb, 1974), mammalian cell extracts catalyze a host of reactions that result in the entry of nucleotides from dNTP precursors into polydeoxyribonucleotide chains. Terminal deoxynucleotidyltransferases that add single nucleotides to the free 3'-hydroxyl ends of single-stranded oligo- or polynucleotide initiators, and which do not require a DNA template, seem to be confined to the thymus and bone marrow among nonmalignant mammalian cells. A wide variety of DNA polymerases that require both an initiator (primer) and a template have been demonstrated in many types of animal cells. These reactions vary, among other things, in their requirements for (1) templates and initiators, (2) metal ions, and (3) various dNTPs, as well as in many other properties, including optimal pH and salt concentrations; affinities for various dNTPs, initiators, and templates; and responses to all sorts of inhibitors. All animal cells seem to contain both large (6–8 S) and small (3–4 S) forms of DNA polymerase that are found to some extent in both nuclear and cytoplasmic fractions, together with a distinct mitochondrial DNA polymerase.* However, the precise multiplicity of constitutive animal cell DNA polymerases, and their relationships to one another, remains far from settled, especially with regard to the nature of the polypeptide chain subunits of which some of these enzymes may be comprised. Some animal cells may additionally harbor DNA-directed or RNA-directed DNA polymerases that are encoded for by various viral genomes, and which may be involved in the replication of viral nucleic acids.

Several characteristics of the "replicative" DNA polymerase reactions that are greatly increased during the hyperplastic phase of rat ventral prostate growth (Coffey et al., 1968) are similar to those of some of the forms of the large (6–8 S) DNA polymerases that exist predominantly in the cytoplasm of animal cells (Chang et al., 1973; Lewis et al., 1974; Spadari and Weissbach, 1974a; Craig and Keir, 1975a,b; Craig et al., 1975; Hecht, 1975; Smith et al., 1975). However, insufficient evidence is at hand to decide whether the previously studied deoxyribonucleotide polymerizations by soluble prostate extracts are catalyzed by one or more discrete enzymes, and what contributions these enzyme(s) make to the replication or repair of DNA in various intracellular compartments in

---

* See *Note Added in Proof* at the end of this article.

intact prostate cells. Accordingly, we began to examine ventral prostate extracts from rats of differing androgenic status to promote DNA synthesis as directed by a number of different templates.

III. New Explorations of Prostatic Polynucleotide Polymerase Reactions

The following types of deoxyribonucleotide polymerizations were found to be readily catalyzed by soluble extracts of rat ventral prostate:

1. Mg^{2+}-stimulated synthesis of DNA using heat-denatured DNA as template-initiator in reactions requiring all 4 dNTPs. These *"D-DNA polymerase"* reactions were determined with either dATP or dTTP as labeled substrate(s), and many of their properties have already been described by Coffey et al. (1968).

2. Mn^{2+}-dependent polymerization of labeled dTTP with poly(rA)·oligo $d(pT)_{12-18}$ as template-initiator (*"R-DNA polymerase"* activity).

3. Polymerization in the presence of Mn^{2+} of labeled dTTP with poly(dA)·oligo $d(pT)_{12-18}$ as template-initiator.

In addition, a fourth reaction was studied:

4. Addition of polyadenylate tracts to a poly (A) initiator (primer) in Mn^{2+}-stimulated reactions that do not require any template (*"poly(A) polymerase"*) and with rATP as substrate. These reactions are not involved in DNA synthesis, but are related to the addition of polyadenylate tracts in the nuclear processing of messenger and perhaps other types of RNA molecule, and also possibly to the maintenance of poly(A) tracts attached to the 3′-termini of cytoplasmic mRNA molecules, which might play a role in the stability and/or translation of mRNA molecules outside the cell nucleus (Giron and Huppert, 1974; Tsiapalis et al., 1973; Winters and Edmonds, 1973; Burkard and Keller, 1974; Mans and Stein, 1974).

The characteristics of reactions (1) to (4) as catalyzed by prostate extracts were examined in considerable detail so as to establish optimal assay conditions, which are described in Tables I and II. Only a few key features of the properties of these reactions will be described here.

Reactions (1) to (3), utilizing dNTP substrates, proceeded at maximal rates only if ATP plus a high-energy phosphate-generating system (phosphoenolpyruvate and pyruvate kinase) were added to the reaction mixtures, as was observed in earlier studies on rat prostate D-DNA polymerase (Coffey et al., 1968). The optimal concentration of ATP varied with the particular reaction studied and whether or not the phosphate generating system was also added. High (>5 mM) levels of ATP were inhibitory. A variety of factors probably contribute to this diphasic effect of ATP, including competition between ATP and dNTPs for binding sites on the deoxyribonucleotide polymerizing enzymes, the substantial contribution of large amounts of ATP to the total ionic strengths of the reactions mixtures, and metal chelation (especially in those reactions where Mn^{2+} rather than Mg^{2+} proved to be the superior activator). The stimulatory effects of ATP in lower and optimal concentrations are almost certainly due in part to prevention of destruction of dNTPs by the prostate extracts. In the absence of pyruvate kinase plus phosphoenolpyruvate, the stimulatory effect of ATP could not be replaced by 5'-AMP. Also noteworthy was the lack of effect in either the D- or the R-DNA polymerase reactions of addition of 3',5'-cyclic AMP (cAMP) in concentrations as high as 2 mM. The poly(A) polymerase (reaction 4) was also uninfluenced by cAMP under a variety of conditions.

Kosto et al. (1967) reported that when various adult rat organs were homogenized in dilute thiol-containing buffers and then ultracentrifuged, high D-DNA polymerase activities were observed only with soluble extracts of tissues, such as spleen and testis, that contained large numbers of dividing cells. This is confirmed by the new experiments shown in Table I, which also illustrates that, in comparison with D-DNA polymerase, the R-DNA polymerase activities measured with poly(A) as template and oligo d(pT)$_{12-18}$ as initiator were strikingly high in normal resting rat ventral prostate, less so in testis, and extremely low in spleen. In contrast, poly(A) polymerase reactions, in which rAMP residues derived from the rATP substrate are polymerized by stepwise addition to the ends of poly(rA) primers (initiators) that serve no template function, proceed most rapidly with comparable soluble extracts of testis, the activities of the ventral and other lobes of the prostate being low in rank among the fairly large number of normal rat tissues examined in the experiments summarized in Table II.

The unexpectedly vigorous R-DNA polymerase activities in resting rat ventral prostate prompted experiments aimed at gaining insight into the nature of the enzyme(s) catalyzing these reactions and their functional significance. Unlike the prostate D-DNA polymerase reactions for which Mg^{2+} is the superior activator, the R-DNA polymerizations were only feebly enhanced by Mg^{2+} over the concentration range of 0.5–10 mM, but were strongly activated by Mn^{2+}. The optimal concentration of Mn^{2+} was 1.5 mM with inhibition at higher levels of this metal ion. In the assay system for R-DNA polymerase (see Table I), only negligible polymerization of dTTP was observed when either the poly(rA) template or the oligo d(pT)$_{12-18}$ initiator were singly omitted; when both the template and initiator were present there was no polymerization of labeled dATP added in place of the usual dTTP substrate. Under the conditions

TABLE I

R-DNA AND D-DNA POLYMERASE ACTIVITIES IN SOLUBLE EXTRACTS OF
VARIOUS NORMAL ADULT RAT TISSUES[a]

Tissue	Polymerase activity (pmoles dTMP incorporated/mg protein/hr)		
	R-DNA polymerase	D-DNA polymerase	R-DNA/D-DNA
Ventral prostate	539	21.5	25.1
Anterior prostate (coagulating gland)	40	6.5	6.1
Seminal vesicle	49	14.6	3.4
Testis	375	155	2.4
Liver	27	16	1.7
Brain	354	50	7.1
Kidney	228	48	4.8
Spleen	18	463	0.04

[a] Tissues from male Sprague-Dawley rats (greater than 350 gm in body weight) were homogenized at 0°C with 50 mM Tris-HCl of pH 7.5 at 4°C containing 1 mM dithiothreitol (DTT). After centrifugation at 35,000 g for 10 minutes, the precipitate was washed with the homogenizing medium and centrifuged again. The combined supernatant fluids were then centrifuged at 100,000 g for 1 hour, and the resulting soluble extracts were used for the enzyme assays. The standard R-DNA polymerase assay system contained 50 mM Tris-HCl of pH 7.5 at 37°C; 1 mM DTT; 1 mM ATP; 1.7 M glycerol; 5 mM sodium phospho(enol) pyruvate; 4 μg of crystalline pyruvate kinase per milliliter; 1.5 mM MnCl$_2$; 100 mM KCl; 0.06 mM ^{14}C-dTTP; 0.1 A_{260} units of oligo d(pT)$_{12-18}$ per milliliter; 5 μg of poly(rA) per milliliter; and enzyme extract added to initiate the reaction. The standard D-DNA polymerase assay system contained 50 mM Tris-HCl of pH 7.5 at 37°C; 1 mM DTT; 1.7 M glycerol; 0.5 mM ATP; 5 mM MgCl$_2$; 5 mM sodium phospho(enol) pyruvate; 4 μg of crystalline pyruvate kinase per milliliter; 0.2 mM each of dGTP, dCTP, and dATP; 0.06 mM ^{14}C-dTTP; 100 μg of heat-denatured calf thymus DNA per milliliter; and enzyme extract added to initiate the reaction. In both polymerase systems, the termination of the reactions and the processing of the acid-insoluble material for measurement of incorporation of radioisotope into DNA was performed essentially according to Coffey et al. (1968). It is noteworthy that homogenates and ultracentrifuged soluble extracts of rat ventral prostate tissue have a powerful ability to degrade oligodeoxyribonucleotides such as oligo(dT)$_{12-18}$. For this reason, the amounts of oligo(dT)$_{12-18}$ required for maximal rates of the "R-DNA polymerase" activities under the conditions shown in this table and in Table III must be established by separate titration experiments with each batch of this oligodeoxyribonucleotide initiator, and with respect to the particular levels of prostate enzyme preparations added to the reaction mixtures.

shown in Table I, lowering of the incubation temperature from 37°C to 25°C decreased the R-DNA polymerase by only 18% whereas the D-DNA polymerase declined by 84%, so that at 25°C, the R-DNA/D-DNA polymerase ratio was more than 3 times greater than the already high value seen at 37°C.

TABLE II

Mn²⁺-STIMULATED AND POLY(A)-PRIMED SYNTHESIS OF POLYADENYLATE BY
SOLUBLE EXTRACTS OF VARIOUS ADULT RAT TISSUES[a]

Tissue	Nanomoles of AMP incorporated/mg protein/30 min	
	Male	Female
Testis	49.2	—
Uterus	—	10.0
Thymus	9.9	9.1
Spleen	9.2	8.5
Small intestine	7.8	—
Kidney	9.0	13.0
Epididymis	3.2	—
Liver	3.2	3.0
Brain	3.1	—
Ovary	—	1.9
Ventral prostate	4.6	—
Anterior prostate (coagulating gland)	1.0	—
Dorsal prostate	0.8	—
Seminal vesicle	0.2	—
Spermatozoa[b]	0	—
Mammary tumor[c]	—	23

[a] The assays were performed with crude soluble centrifuged tissue extracts. Pooled tissues were obtained from male (c. 300 gm body weight) and female (c. 250 gm body weight) animals. The test system contained 100 mM Tris-HCl, pH 8.2; 5 mM dithiothreitol; 1.5 mM MnCl$_2$; poly(A) (2 mg/ml); 1 mM ¹⁴C-ATP. Incubated at 37°C.

[b] The preparation consisted of dialyzed soluble proteins from sonicated epididymal spermatozoa.

[c] 7,12-Dimethylbenz[a]anthracene-induced mammary carcinomas.

Another remarkable difference between the two deoxyribonucleotide polymerizations catalyzed by soluble prostate extracts is that the R-DNA polymerase reaction was much more inhibited by the direct addition of low concentrations of ethidium bromide than was the D-DNA polymerase. This is illustrated in Fig. 2, which also shows that, with normal resting ventral prostate extracts, if the poly(rA) template in the R-DNA polymerase assay was replaced with poly(dA), then (1) the polymerization of dTTP was considerably faster with poly(dA) than with poly(rA) as template (control experiments indicated that the oligo d(pT)$_{12-18}$ initiator was essential in both instances), and (2) ethidium bromide is considerably less inhibitory for polymerization of dTTP with poly(dA) as compared with poly(rA) as template under these conditions. Concentrations

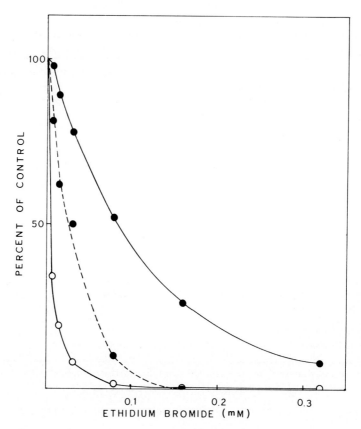

Fig. 2. Influence of ethidium bromide on D-DNA and R-DNA polymerase reactions catalyzed by soluble extracts of normal rat ventral prostate. The experimental conditions are the same as in Table I. ○——○: R-DNA polymerase (100% value: 265 pmoles per milligram of protein per hour). ●---●: the R-DNA polymerase assay in which the poly(rA) was replaced with poly(dA) at a final concentration of 5 μg/ml (100% value: 1034 pmoles per milligram of protein per hour). ●——●: D-DNA polymerase with heat-denatured calf thymus DNA as template-initiator (100% value: 26 pmoles per milligram of protein per hour).

of ethidium bromide that obliterate the prostate R-DNA and D-DNA polymerase reactions are without effect on the poly(A) polymerase with rATP as substrate as determined in soluble extracts of various rat tissues (Corti *et al.*, 1975).

Enzymes catalyzing R-DNA polymerase reactions similar to those in Table I have been demonstrated in both cytoplasmic and nuclear fractions of Hela (Spadari and Weissbach, 1974a) and other animal cells (Craig and Keir, 1975a,b; Craig *et al.*, 1975; Smith *et al.*,

1975). The multiplicity of *constitutive* animal-cell enzymes that form complementary polydeoxyribonucleotides with homopolyribonucleotides as templates (see also Kornberg, 1974), and the relationships of these enzymes to any of the various multiple forms of animal DNA-directed DNA polymerases, remains far from settled (Keir and Craig, 1974). Yet regardless of these considerations, it is well known that the "true" reverse transcriptases of animal oncogenic RNA viruses can not only synthesize complementary DNA copies of appropriate oncogenic viral RNA molecules, but also catalyze polymerization of dTTP with poly (rA) · oligo d (pT)$_{12-18}$ as template-initiator (Kornberg, 1974; Smith *et al.*, 1975). This raises the question whether the R-DNA polymerase activity we found to be intense in normal rat prostate extracts might, at least in part, reflect the presence of viral reverse transcriptase(s). This seems unlikely on the following grounds. First, the same prostate extracts failed to polymerize dGTP when poly (rC) · oligo (dG) was added as template-initiator in the presence of Mn^{2+} (compare Dion *et al.*, 1974). Second, acid-insoluble products were not formed when prostate soluble extracts were incubated with labeled dNTPs and oligo d (pT)$_{12-18}$ under the conditions of the R-DNA polymerase assay but with replacement of the usual poly (rA) template with a variety of natural tRNA and ribosomal RNA preparations as potential templates. However, oncogenic viral RNAs were not tested as templates and, as Spadari and Weissbach (1974a) and others have pointed out, attempts to distinguish constitutive cellular R-DNA polymerases from genuine viral reverse transcriptases on the basis of differential capacities to copy homoribopolynucleotide templates are fraught with difficulties. Germane to our results with rat prostate is the report of Arya *et al.* (1975) of their chromatographic separations of at least two enzyme fractions from human prostate tissue that catalyze D-DNA polymerase reactions and also R-DNA reactions with poly (rA) · oligo d (pT)$_{12-18}$ as template-initiator; their experiments indicated, however, that these polymerizations in human prostate did not seem to be promoted by enzymes resembling the reverse transcriptases of oncogenic viruses.

Our experiments involving (a) differential centrifugation of rat prostate homogenates prepared in sucrose-Mg^{2+} or in dilute buffered salt solutions, and (b) extraction of nuclear and other cell particulate fractions by sonication or treatment with detergents bolstered previous conclusions (Coffey *et al.*, 1968) that most of the prostate D-DNA polymerase activity was solubilized by the standard tissue extraction procedures summarized in Table I. However, as much as 30% of the total R-DNA polymerase activity may remain rather firmly associated with nuclear material under these extraction conditions. It proved impossible to gauge any gross differences in the sedimentation characteristics of the enzyme(s) catalyzing the prostatic D-DNA and R-DNA polymerase reactions by centrifugation of the soluble extracts through sucrose gradients because addition of sucrose in relatively low concentrations substantially inhibited the R-DNA polymerase system, even though the 1.7 M glycerol routinely added to the assay mixture was not inhibitory. The small (3–4 S) DNA polymerase of some animal tissues that Chang (1973, 1974) observed to copy poly(rA) templates was reported to be much less sensitive to inhibition by ethanol than are the larger (6–8 S) forms of animal DNA polymerases. In this connection we noticed that direct addition of ethanol in increasing concentrations over the range of 2–10% (v/v) progressively inhibited both the D-DNA and R-DNA polymerase reactions of soluble prostate extracts with only slight selective depression of the two activities. Since certain animal cells contain a variety of R-DNA polymerases that vary in their sensitivity to ethanol, and which in at least some instances seem to be distinct from D-DNA polymerases (Spadari and Weissbach, 1974a), our studies on ethanol inhibition did not clarify the relationships between the soluble rat ventral prostate enzymes that promte the D-DNA and R-DNA polymerizations.

IV. Effects of Androgens

The representative experiments in Table III show that the rat prostate soluble D-DNA and R-DNA polymerase reactions exhibit very different patterns of changes in response to alterations in the androgenic status of the animals. There was a relatively greater decline in the R-DNA activity in the regressed prostates 1 week after orchiectomy, and this parameter reattained normal values only after 5 subsequent daily injections of testosterone propionate. More strikingly, there was no tremendous "overshoot" in the R-DNA polymerase reactions over the period of 3–7 days following the onset of androgen treatment of castrates, as always occurs with the D-DNA polymerase activities during this transient period of intense cell proliferation in the androgenic repair of involuted rat ventral prostates.

When expressed in terms of comparable molar units, the nontemplated poly(A) polymerase activity of normal rat ventral prostate extracts is more than an order of magnitude greater than that of the R-DNA polymerase and more than two orders of magnitude higher than that of the D-DNA polymerase activities (Tables I–III). In the involuted ventral prostates at 1 week after orchiectomy, there occurred a marked decline in poly(A) polymerase activity that returned to normal within 2 days after beginning of continual androgen treatments, the enzyme levels rising further to 150% of normal after 7 days, but not increasing beyond this value after an additional week of daily testosterone injections. This behavior of the nontemplated poly (A) polymerase in response to castration-induced involution of rat ventral prostate and subsequent androgenic repair stands in contrast to (a) the smaller and more sluggish changes in R-DNA polymerase, and (b) reports of swifter enhancement by androgens *in vivo* of RNA polymerase reactions directed by endogenous DNA, and measured at low ionic strengths, in prostate cell nuclei from castrated rats (Liao *et al.*, 1965; Liao and Fang, 1969; Williams-Ashman and Reddi, 1972).

V. Remarks on Polyamines

The rat ventral prostate resembles the human gland inasmuch as their cells and secretions contain unusually large amounts of aliphatic polyamines. Recently there has been a great upsurge of interest in the chemical physiology of the polyamines spermidine and spermine, especially from the standpoint of their regulation of the production, turnover, and posttranscriptional modification of RNA molecules, of protein biosynthetic reactions, and of various phases of DNA replication. This is not the place to discuss details of this very broad and active field, which has entailed many studies on prostate glands and their secretions, and that has been amply reviewed (Pegg *et al.*, 1970; Cohen, 1971; Williams-Ashman *et al.*, 1969, 1972; Bachrach, 1973). But a few brief remarks may be in order in the context of the aforementioned experimental findings and of other published correlations between the accumulation of RNA and/or DNA and polyamine levels during the growth and differentiation of many animal tissues.

Some measurements by Pegg *et al.* (1970) of the concentrations of putrescine, spermidine, and spermine, and of the activities of their two biosynthetic decarboxylases, during different phases of the testosterone-induced growth of involuted rat ventral prostate—obtained under virtually the same biological conditions as those used in our studies on DNA polymerizing reactions—are included in Table III for comparative purposes. During the hyperplastic phase of prostate enlargement, alterations in RNA rather than in DNA accumulation correlate fairly well with increases in total spermidine concentrations whereas spermine levels fluctuate in a different fashion. (It is noteworthy that under these circumstances, it was not ascertained how far the increased accumulation of polyamines occurs extracellularly in secretions in the glandular lumens as well as within epithelial and other cells.) Manyfold increases in the polyamine biosynthetic enzymes ornithine decarboxylase and putrescine-

TABLE III

Androgen-Dependent Changes in Polyamines and Enzymes during Prostatic Hyperplasia[a]

Total days castrated	Cumulative days of TP treatment	Total prostate DNA	Total prostate RNA	Polyamines			Enzyme activities				
				Put	Spd	Sp	ODC	ADC	D-DNA	R-RNA	Poly(A)
0	—	233	558	0.36	6.2	6.9	0.34	0.72	0.018	0.39	7.5
7	0	59	34	0.11	1.3	2.6	0.06	0.06	0.019	0.25	3.4
9	2	50	161	0.28	2.5	2.5	0.20	0.46	0.023	0.17	7.2
12	5	—	—	0.45	4.5	2.5	—	—	0.168	0.36	9.6
14	7	252	590	0.45	5.8	3.6	0.30	0.66	0.121	—	11.2
21	14	—	—	—	—	—	0.36	0.74	0.030	0.37	9.2

[a] The values for total ventral prostate RNA and DNA contents (in microgram, normalized to that equivalent to 100 gm of body weight) are taken from Coffey et al. (1968). The levels of the polyamines putrescine (Put), spermidine (Spd), and spermine (Sp) expressed as micromoles per gram fresh weight, and also the values for ornithine decarboxylase (ODC) and putrescine-activated S-adenosylmethionine decarboxylase (ADC), are recalculated from the data of Pegg et al. (1970). These previously published data are shown for comparative purposes. The D-DNA polymerase (D-DNA), R-DNA polymerase (R-DNA), and poly(A) polymerase [Poly(A)] were newly determined using the assay conditions described in Tables I and II, employing rats of the same strain and approximately the same age as those stated in the aforementioned publications, and using the same control and hormone injection schedules and dietary regimen. All enzyme activities are calculated in terms of nmoles product formed per hour per milligram of protein at 37°C in the soluble ventral prostate extracts. The standard errors never exceeded 8% of the values depicted, which are the means of at least four groups that usually were each comprised of tissues pooled from a number of animals. The enzyme reactions were determined under conditions where their rates were proportional to the amount of prostate extracts added and to the times of incubation. TP in the second column refers to injection of 2 mg of testosterone propionate per day.

activated S-adenosylmethionine decarboxylase occur within less than a day after commencing continual treatment of 7-day castrates with hyperphysiological doses of testosterone, and precede the first upswings in spermidine concentrations (Pegg et al., 1970). It is well known that low concentrations of spermidine and/or spermine can directly enhance various DNA-directed RNA polymerase reactions catalyzed by isolated cell nuclei or chromatin preparations from many types of animal cells (Williams-Ashman et al., 1969; Cohen, 1971; Bachrach, 1973; Moruzzi et al., 1975).

Interactions of polyamines with isolated animal DNA synthetic enzymes have been studied much less extensively. Chiu and Sung (1971, 1972) observed that one of the two forms of DNA-dependent DNA polymerase they isolated from rat brain was strongly enhanced by 0.05–0.1 mM spermine and by 0.5–2 mM spermidine, possibly because of stabilization by the polyamines of complexes between DNA and various combinations of subunits of the polymerase. However, as shown in Fig. 3, we could not detect any significant activation of the D-DNA or R-DNA polymerase reactions promoted by soluble ventral prostate extracts by addition of spermidine or spermine, which were inhibitory at the higher concentrations. Nevertheless, the relationships of polyamines to the induction and eventual limitation of DNA replication during androgen-stimulated prostate growth obviouly merits much more intensive scrutiny, especially in view of recent reports that spermidine profoundly affects a "DNA-unwinding" protein that is of central importance in bacterial multienzyme systems responsible for the replication of single-stranded viral DNA templates (Schekman et al., 1974).

Nobody seems to have looked for interactions of polyamines with the many other enzymes besides DNA polymerases that are involved in mammalian DNA synthesis or dNTP production, including RNA-dependent processes that may be required for initiation of deoxyribonucleotide polymerizations. Of interest to the regulation of DNA polymerases in rat ventral prostate—which manufactures and secretes much spermidine and spermine—are some comparable studies on the rat anterior prostate (coagulating) gland which contains only small amounts of polyamines and does not secrete them. Brasel et al. (1968) observed that the time course and magnitude of changes in RNA and DNA content, and of immense but transient elevations of soluble "replicative" DNA polymerase activity, were during the hyperplastic phase of anterior prostate growth even larger than those reported by Coffey et al. (1968) in the ventral lobe of the gland.

That spermidine may specifically regulate DNA synthesis in certain higher animal cells seems likely from some recent experiments of Morris

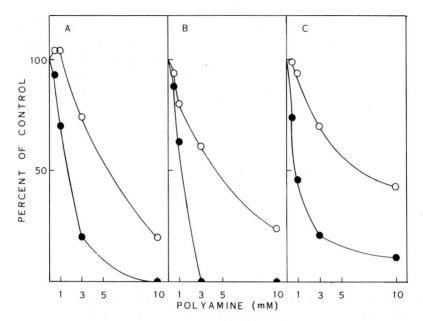

FIG. 3. Effects of spermine (●—●) and spermidine (○—○) on various DNA polymerase reactions catalyzed by soluble extracts of normal rat ventral prostate. D-DNA polymerase reactions were determined with 150 μg per milliliter of either heat-denatured (panel A) or native (panel B) calf thymus DNA. The other ingredients of the reaction mixtures for D-DNA polymerase were 50 mM Tris-HCl of pH 7.5; 5 mM MgCl$_2$; 5 mM DTT; 1.7 M glycerol; 2.5 mM ATP; 5 mM sodium phospho(enol) pyruvate; 4 μg of crystalline pyruvate kinase per milliliter; 0.075 mM each of dGTP, dCTP, and dTTP; and 0.04 mM ³H-dATP. The R-DNA polymerase reactions shown in panel C were measured under the same conditions as recorded in the footnote to Table I except that the ATP concentration was 2 mM rather than 1 mM. The 100% values were: D-DNA polymerase: with heat-denatured DNA (panel A): 70 pmoles per milligram of protein per hour; with native DNA (panel B): 49 pmoles per milligram of protein per hour; and in the R-DNA polymerase reaction (panel C): 611 pmoles per milligram of protein per hour.

(1974). He showed that the anticancer drug, methylglyoxal bis(guanylhydrazone) (MGBG), which is a very specific and potent inhibitor of the putrescine-activated S-adenosylmethionine decarboxylase that is a key and rate-limiting reaction in polyamine biosynthesis (Williams-Ashman *et al.*, 1972), blocks the increases in spermidine and spermine evoked by addition of concanavalin A to lymphocytes. When the cells are transformed by the lectin in the presence of MGBG, the enhanced synthesis and processing of RNA and the increased protein synthesis are not impaired despite the shutdown of spermidine and spermine production.

Nevertheless, lectin-induced DNA synthesis is strongly depressed by MGBG, the inhibitory effects of which are reversed by exogenous spermidine. There was no inhibition of DNA synthesis if MGBG was later added to cells that had been allowed to accumulate their maximum complement of polyamines following exposure to concanavalin A.

Physiological concentrations of spermidine and spermine can enhance the RNA polymerase activities of rat ventral prostate cell nuclei (Caldarera et al., 1968; Barbiroli et al., 1971; Moruzzi et al., 1971). Nevertheless, there is no evidence that the well known rapid stimulation of prostate nuclear RNA polymerase reactions by androgens in vivo is primarily related to increases in the intracellular polyamine concentrations in prostate cells. Rather, the available evidence (Pegg et al., 1970) is more consonant with the view that during the early phases of testosterone action on the regressed prostates of castrated rats, there occurs a close coupling between cytoplasmic (largely ribosomal) RNA accumulation and increases in intracellular spermidine. Spermine levels in rat ventral prostate increase more sluggishly than do spermidine concentrations in response to androgenic stimulation (cf. Table III), but the alterations in spermine by no means exactly parallel the transient increases in DNA synthesis that begin only after 48 hours after initiation of continual testosterone treatment. Here it must also be remembered that many other biochemical processes known to be profoundly and directly affected by polyamines—such as stabilization of ribosomes, inhibition of certain nucleolytic enzymes, and increase of tRNA methylation—have yet to be examined in relation to various phases of androgen-induced prostatic growth and differentiation. Williams-Ashman and Tadolini (1975) have discussed the eventuality that reactive aldehyde enzymic oxidation products of spermidine and/or spermine might conceivably perturb normal DNA synthetic mechanisms in the prostate.

Polyamines are present in large amounts in the prostatic secretions of some species (Williams-Ashman et al., 1972), which contrasts with the presence of only traces of these bases in normal blood serum and other body fluids. Although the functions of spermine and spermidine in prostatic fluid are obscure (Williams-Ashman and Lockwood, 1970), some of the early increases in these polyamines in the prostate gland of castrates in response to androgens may represent a marker of secretion by the epithelial cells.

VI. Prospectives

The overall growth of the involuted prostates of adult mammalian castrates in response to androgens entails, on the one hand, multiplication of elements of the epithelium, lamina propria, fibromusclar stroma, and blood vessels, and, on the other hand, hypertrophy of epithelial cells with the resulting formation of extracellular secretory products. As is the case with respect to the growth of so many other organs, the interrelationships between these processes of cell replication and cell differentiation remain very poorly understood.

The majority of contemporary investigations on molecular and cellular aspects of androgen action on the prostate have centered around two biochemical areas. The first of these are the transformations of the principal circulating androgen, testosterone, into unconjugated DHT and related 5α-androstanes, and the tight association of DHT with cytoplasmic forms of specific androgen–receptor proteins that are required for the nuclear sequestration and retention of DHT (Liao, 1975). And, second, there are the early androgen-evoked increases in nuclear RNA synthesis and processing which seem to be germane to many of the later androgen-induced alterations in the abundance of cytoplasmic polyribosomes and mRNAs (Williams-Ashman and Reddi, 1972). However, it is by no means certain that all the effects of androgens on prostatic protein biosynthesis are dependent on prior increases in nuclear RNA production. This is underscored by the recent report of Liang and Liao (1975) that extremely soon (10 minutes) after injection of DHT into androgen-deficient rats, there is marked enhancement in the binding to a cytoplasmic factor of methionyl-tRNA$_f$, the initiator of protein synthesis, via processes that are apparently unrelated to any changes in RNA synthesis. These features of androgen action on the prostate are obviously pertinent to the functional differentiation of the epithelial cells, but their immediate relevance to the hyperplastic element of prostate growth is foggy.

Androgens are mandatory triggers for the initial morphogenesis, during restricted and critical periods of embryonic life, of the prostate and some other male secondary sexual organs that differentiate from the urogenital sinus or the Wolffian duct. As discussed by Williams-Ashman and Reddi (1972), it is conceivable that the degree of androgenic stimulation of anlage of certain male genital structures during fetal or early neonatal existence may be pertinent to limitations of growth of these organs that occur during normal puberty and adulthood, or after administration of even hyperphysiological amounts of androgens to normal or castrated adults, provided that frank neoplasia does not ensue.

Synergisms between certain anterior pituitary hormones and androgens on the growth of certain lobes of the prostate have been observed in some species (Williams-Ashman and Reddi, 1972). It seems unlikely, however, that hypophyseal hormones are major determinants of the patterns of increases in DNA synthesis, and in the major D-DNA polymerase, in the ventral prostate of castrated rats after androgen treatment, since similar testosterone-induced changes were found in hypophysectomized animals (Kosto *et al.*, 1967).

Many enzymes of DNA synthesis appear to be elaborated and maintained in large amounts only at periods close to the S (synthetic) phase of the cell cycle in higher animals. It is interesting in this regard that the very active R-DNA polymerase activity of normal rat ventral prostate does not undergo an immense transitory enhancement that is comparable to the increases in the major cytoplasmic D-DNA polymerase during the hyperplasia of this organ that occurs transitorily following administration of testosterone to adult castrates. The functions of the R-DNA polymerase(s) in the prostate—which as mentioned above seem to be a constitutive enzyme(s) unrelated to any true reverse transcriptases of the type elaborated by oncogenic RNA viruses—merit further investigation.

Future research on the biochemistry of restrictions on unlimited cell division in the normal prostate should take into consideration many other factors that have been implicated in the size limitation of other mammalian organs. These include: (1) the possibility of tissue-specific chalones; (2) effects of constituents of prostatic secretions on the formation and functions of enzymes involved in DNA synthesis and mitosis; (3) cAMP/cGMP ratios; (4) cholinergic and adrenergic stimuli to secretory processes in prostate epithelial cells; (5) postreplicative modifications of nuclear DNA, including the extent of formation of 5-methylcytidine; (6) specific aging changes unrelated to neoplastic transformations; and (7) selective alterations in macromolecules associated with the outer surfaces of prostate cell plasma membranes.

Note Added in Proof

Since this paper was submitted for publication, wider consensus has been reached in the literature concerning the classification of deoxyribonucleotide polymerizing enzymes from animal tissues. This subject has been very clearly reviewed by Weissbach (1975). Our investigations are consistent with the view that the activity designated above as R-DNA polymerase (i.e., Mn^{2+}-stimulated polymerization of dTTP with poly(rA) as template and oligo(dT) as initiator) in rat ventral prostate is catalyzed, to a substantial degree, by enzymes of the "DNA polymerase-γ" variety according to the terminology considered by Weissbach (1975).

REFERENCES

Arya, S. K., Carter, W. A., Zeigel, R. F., and Horoszewicz, J. S. (1975). *Cancer Chemother. Rep.* **59**, 39.

Bachrach, U. (1973). "Function of Naturally Occurring Polyamines." Academic Press, New York.

Barbiroli, B., Corti, A., and Caldarera, C. M. (1971). *FEBS (Fed. Eur. Biochem. Soc.) Lett.* **13**, 169.
Brasel, J. A., Coffey, D. S., and Williams-Ashman, H. G. (1968). *Med. Exp.* **18**, 321.
Burkard, G., and Keller, E. B. (1974). *Proc. Nat. Acad. Sci. U.S.* **71**, 389.
Caldarera, C. M., Moruzzi, M. S., Barbiroli, B., and Moruzzi, G. (1968). *Biochem. Biophys. Res. Commun.* **33**, 266.
Chang, L. M. S. (1973). *J. Biol. Chem.* **248**, 6983.
Chang, M. L. S. (1974). *J. Biol. Chem.* **249**, 7441.
Chang, L. M. S., Brown, M., and Bollum, F. J. (1973). *J. Mol. Biol.* **74**, 1.
Chiu, J.-F., and Sung, S. C. (1971). *Biochim. Biophys. Acta* **246**, 44.
Chiu, J. F., and Sung, S. C. (1972). *Biochim. Biophys. Acta* **281**, 535.
Coffey, D. S., Shimazaki, J., and Williams-Ashman, H. G. (1968). *Arch. Biochem. Biophys.* **124**, 184.
Cohen, S. S. (1971). "Introduction to the Polyamines." Prentice-Hall, Englewood Cliffs, New Jersey.
Corti, A., Williams-Ashman, H. G., and Wilson, J. (1975). *Boll. Soc. Ital. Biol. Sper.* (in press).
Craig, R. K., and Keir, H. M. (1975a). *Biochem. J.* **145**, 215.
Craig, R. K., and Keir, H. M. (1975b). *Biochem J.* **145**, 225.
Craig, R. K., Costello, P. A., and Keir, H. M. (1975). *Biochem. J.* **145**, 233.
Dion, A. S., Vaidya, A. B., and Fout, G. S. (1974). *Cancer Res.* **34**, 3509.
Doeg, K. A., Polomski, L. L., and Doeg, L. H. (1972). *Endocrinology* **90**, 1633.
Giron, M. L., and Huppert, J. (1974). *Biochim. Biophys. Acta* **287**, 448.
Hecht, N. B. (1975). *Biochim. Biophys. Acta* **383**, 388.
Keir, H., and Craig, R. K. (1974). *Biochem. Soc. Trans.* **1**, 1073.
Kornberg, A. (1974). "DNA Synthesis." Freeman, San Francisco, California.
Kosto, B., Calvin, H. I., and Williams-Ashman, H. G. (1967). *Advan. Enzyme Regul.* **5**, 25.
Lesser, B., and Bruchovsky, N. (1973). *Biochim. Biophys. Acta* **308**, 426.
Lesser, B., and Bruchovksy, N. (1974a). *Biochem. J.* **142**, 429.
Lesser, B., and Bruchovsky, N. (1974b). *Biochem. J.* **142**, 483.
Lewis, B. J., Abrell, J. W., Smith, R. G., and Gallo, R. C. (1974). *Biochim. Biophys. Acta* **349**, 148.
Liang, T., and Liao, S. (1975). *Proc. Nat. Acad. Sci. U.S.* **72**, 706.
Liao, S. (1975). *Int. Rev. Cytol.* **41**, 87.
Liao, S., and Fang, S. (1969). *Vitam. Horm. (New York)* **27**, 17.
Liao, S., Leininger, K. R., Sagher, D., and Barton, R. W. (1965). *Endocrinology* **77**, 763.
Loeb, L. (1974). *In* "The Enzymes" (P. D. Boyer, ed.), 3rd ed., Vol. 10, p. 173. Academic Press, New York.
Mans, R., and Stein, G. (1974). *Life Sci.* **14**, 437.
Morley, A., Wright, N., Appleton, D., and Alison, M. (1973). *Trans. Biochem. Soc.* **1**, 1081.
Morris, D. R. (1974). *Abstr. FEBS Meet., 9th 1974* Abstract s364, p. 139.
Moruzzi, G., Barbiroli, B., Corti, A., and Caldarera, C. M. (1971). *Ital. J. Biochem.* **20**, 6.
Moruzzi, G., Barbiroli, B., Moruzzi, M. S., and Tadolini, B. (1975). *Biochem. J.* **146**, 697.
Pegg, A. E., Lockwood, D. H., and Williams-Ashman, H. G. (1970). *Biochem. J.* **117**, 17.

Schekman, R., Weiner, A., and Kornberg, A. (1974). *Science* **186**, 987.
Sloan, W. R., Heston, W. D. W., and Coffey, D. S. (1975). *Cancer Chemother. Rep.,* Part 1 **59**, 185.
Smith, J. A., and King, R. J. B. (1972). *Exp. Cell Res.* **167**, 80.
Smith, R. G., Abrell, J. W., Lewis, B. J., and Gallo, R. C. (1975). *J. Biol. Chem.* **250**, 1702.
Spadari, S., and Weissbach, A. (1974a). *J. Biol. Chem.* **248**, 5809.
Spadari, S., and Weissbach, A. (1974b). *J. Mol. Biol.* **86**, 11.
Sufrin, G., and Coffey, D. S. (1973). *Invest. Urol.* **11**, 45.
Tsiapalis, C. M., Dorson, J. W., DeSante, D. M., and Bollum, F. J. (1973). *Biochem. Biophys. Res. Commun.* **51**, 704.
Tuohimaa, P., and Niemi, M. (1968). *Acta Endocrinol. (Copenhagen)* **58**, 696.
Weissbach, A. (1975). *Cell* **5**, 101.
Williams-Ashman, H. G., and Lockwood, D. H. (1970). *Ann. N.Y. Acad. Sci.* **171**, 882.
Williams-Ashman, H. G., and Reddi, A. H. (1972). *In* "Biochemical Actions of Hormones" (G. Litwack, ed.), Vol. 2, pp. 257–294. Academic Press, New York.
Williams-Ashman, H. G., and Tadolini, B. (1975). "Workshop on Benign Prostatic Hyperplasia" (in press).
Williams-Ashman, H. G., Pegg, A. E., and Lockwood, D. H. (1969). *Advan. Enzyme Regul.* **7**, 291.
Williams-Ashman, H. G., Janne, J., Coppoc, G. L., Geroch, M. E., and Schenone, A. (1972). *Advan. Enzyme Regul.* **10**, 225.
Winters, M. A., and Edmonds, M. (1973). *J. Biol. Chem.* **248**, 4756.

DISCUSSION

W. I. P. Mainwaring: I want to comment on the presence of a DNA-unwinding protein in rat ventral prostate. In experiments in collaboration with Paul Rennie and Elisabeth Symes, we assayed unwinding activity by a technique based on the fact that ^{3}H-labeled *native* prostate DNA is not retained on nitrocellulose filters. We fractionated the DNA-unwinding protein by DNA-cellulose chromatography. When testosterone is administered to castrated male rats, DNA-unwinding activity is strongly enhanced in the ventral prostate, but not in spleen, during the period of intense cell multiplication in the growth of the prostate.

I. Lasnitzki: I was very interested in your observation on the limitation of cell replication after prolonged testosterone treatment. We had similar results in organ cultures of rat ventral prostate: dihydrotestosterone in concentrations of 10^{-5} M stimulates epithelial cell proliferation, leading to marked hyperplasia of the alveolar epithelium after 6–10 days of treatment. If the treatment is prolonged, however, the hyperplastic epithelium is shed and replaced by one row of cells lining the alveoli, and it seems that the mechanism limiting cell replication may be similar *in vivo* and *in vitro*.

E. E. Baulieu: Referring to your work on DNA-polymerase, let me tell you that working with estrogen-sensitive chicken issues, and mainly chicken oviduct, Drs. P. H. Schmelke and M. Cl. Lebeau in our group have recently made the observation that estrogen can promote the increase of the nuclear "small" DNA-polymerase very rapidly (6 hours), as it can be tested in a cellular preparation with an exogenous template. The results have been checked as far as specificity of the nuclear polymerase, recovery, absence of DNase activity, etc., are concerned. It is rather satisfactory to see a nuclear enzyme in charge of some DNA synthesis increasing when the hormone promotes DNA synthesis and increases cell division. Moreover, progesterone is antiestrogenic in this respect. Interestingly enough, progesterone is synergistic with estrogen as far as protein (ovalbumin) synthesis is concerned. This then means that in chicken oviduct one sees at the same time two different effects of progesterone on two different proteins, namely DNA-polymerase and ovalbumin. Preliminary investigations with radioautography indicate that these two phenomena do not take place in the same cells at the same time.

Speaking again of connective tissue, to which I alluded very much during my presentation, I think that it would indeed be worthwhile to study cellular components of this connective tissue in terms of their hormonal sensitivity. As a matter of fact, working recently with mouse fibroblasts (L cells) coming from the periareolar region of the mammary gland, we find androgen and estrogen receptors, and we are studying hormone effects in these cells in culture.

Hormonal Effects on Cell Proliferation in Rat Prostate

N. BRUCHOVSKY, B. LESSER, E. VAN DOORN,
AND S. CRAVEN

Department of Medicine, University of Alberta, Edmonton, Alberta, Canada

I. Introduction

The growth and function of male accessory sex glands are under the direct control of androgens, and consequently these tissues can potentially serve as an excellent model system for the study of the regulation of cell proliferation by steroid hormones. In this review, a number of aspects of the proliferative response of rat ventral prostate to androgens will be discussed, including the possibility that organ growth, homeostasis with respect to cell number, and involution of differentiated tissue represent the expression of genetic constraint mechanisms which govern hormonal responsiveness.

Three phases can be distinguished in the response of rat prostate to changes in the hormonal status of the animal, and these are summarized in Fig. 1. First, if the number of cells in the gland is below normal, deoxyribonucleic acid (DNA) synthesis and cell proliferation are initiated by the administration of androgen. Second, when the number of cells is restored to normal, DNA synthesis is curtailed and cell proliferation is markedly reduced although secretion continues to be stimulated by androgen. This phase is characterized by a "wearing-off" effect where an increase in the number of mitoses in prostate under the influence of hormone is followed by a decrease of mitotic activity despite the excess of hormone in the animal. Discussions by Swann (1957, 1958) and Kosto

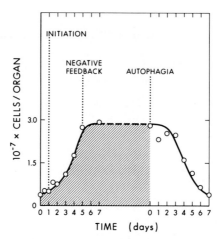

FIG. 1. Growth phases of rat ventral prostate. Groups of 3–7 rats castrated 7 days previously were treated with daily doses of 400 μg of dihydrotestosterone per 100 gm body weight, and at various times the number of cells per prostate was determined by measuring the number of nuclei in the glandular tissue as described by Lesser and Bruchovsky (1973). The shaded area under the curve indicates the period of hormone treatment. Withdrawal of hormone, as by castration, is followed by a reduction in the number of cells per prostate to the basal level. The three phases of growth are initiation of DNA synthesis and cell proliferation, negative feedback, and autophagia.

et al. (1967) have stressed the importance of this constraint mechanism in organ homeostasis, and Epifanova (1971) stated that negative feedback not only is a form of regulation which applies to the synthesis of steroid hormones in endocrine glands, but also is manifested in the case of homonal regulation of cell division in the adult organism. Hence, the term negative feedback is used throughout this review to denote the period when proliferative growth of prostate becomes refractory to androgenic stimulation. Third, withdrawal of androgens, as by orchiectomy, is followed by involution of prostate, an effect that depends on the activation of autophagic processes resulting in autolysis of cells and loss of functional performance. Since androgenic effects on cell proliferation are most conveniently understood within the framework of the aforementioned phases of hormonal responsiveness, a description of the action of androgens pertaining to each of the three phases follows. Use of the term "homeostatic constraint mechanisms" is intended to convey the impression that the separate phases of glandular response to hormones in reality are a tightly coordinated set of anabolic and catabolic processes, which are either activated or potentiated by steroid hormones. To avoid confusion that might arise from nuances of meaning, no distinction is made between hormonal dependence and hormonal responsiveness in this review.

II. HOMEOSTATIC CONSTRAINT MECHANISMS

A. INITIATION OF DNA SYNTHESIS AND CELL PROLIFERATION

The first direct attempt to study the regulation of cell proliferation in an androgen-dependent organ was made by Burkhart (1942), who measured the mitotic activity in prostate and seminal vesicles of castrated rats following the injection of different doses of testosterone propionate. A wave of mitotic activity was induced in prostate of rats castrated 40 days previously by as little as 0.013 mg of androgen administered in a single injection, while the latent period which precedes mitotic activity in response to 0.1 mg of androgen was shortened significantly by the administration of 0.3 mg of testosterone propionate. Later studies by Cavazos and Melampy (1954) confirmed these results, but not until the last decade was a description available of the stimulatory action of androgens on actual DNA synthesis in rat prostate. Sheppard *et al.* (1965) examined the effects of methandrostenolone on DNA replication in prostate and seminal vesicles of castrated rats and noted that the enhanced incorporation of radioactive thymidine into DNA seen after 2 days of treatment almost disappeared after 7 days of treatment. The stimulation and the "wearing-off" effect received more detailed attention in the studies of Kosto *et al.* (1967) and of Coffey *et al.* (1968); these investigators found that treatment of castrated rats with testosterone propionate produced a massive but transitory increase in the incorporation of radioactive thymidine into DNA of prostate both *in vitro* and *in vivo*, which was paralleled by an elevation and decline in DNA polymerase activity. DNA content increased to a maximal level within 2 weeks and could not be augmented by further treatment for as long as 25 days; in contrast, prostatic weight continued to increase over the duration of the experiment owing to excessive secretion by overstimulated epithelial cells.

The reports of Bruchovsky and Wilson (1968a) and of Anderson and Liao (1968) that 5α-androstan-17β-ol-3-one (dihydrotestosterone) is selectively concentrated in nuclei of prostatic cells after administration of testosterone to castrated rats highlighted the possibility that this metabolite of testosterone might be responsible for certain androgenic actions at the cellular level. Robel *et al.* (1971) found that dihydrotestosterone is not only more potent than testosterone in maintaining epithelial height and secretory activity in prostatic explants in culture, but is also more effective in stimulating epithelial hyperplasia. Schmidt *et al.* (1972) reported that dihydrotestosterone has a greater effect than testosterone on the wet weight and DNA content of prostate and seminal vesicles of immature castrated rats. Lesser and Bruchovsky (1973) compared the effects of testosterone and of dihydrotestosterone on the proliferative growth of prostate in rats castrated 7 days previously, and found that dihydrotestosterone induces a rate of proliferation that is about twice as great as that stimulated by testosterone. These observations, taken together with analogous findings in other systems (King and Mainwaring, 1973), provided a basis for the view that the function of dihydrotestosterone is concerned with initiation of DNA synthesis and cell proliferation.

Although dihydrotestosterone may be essential for inducing mitotic activity, another factor that must be considered in this response is the degree of sensitivity of the prostate to androgens. The decisive nature of this condition was demonstrated by Lesser and Bruchovsky (1974a), who measured the response of involuted prostate to androgen administration at various times following castration, when the size of the prostate ranged from normal to less than 15% of normal. The parameters of wet weight and number of nuclei were used as indicators of functional status of the prostate, and the rate of incorporation of radioactive thymidine by prostatic minces *in vitro*, along with changes in number of nuclei were taken as indices of proliferative activity. In all cases, animals received daily injections of 400 μg of dihydrotestosterone per 100 gm body weight which was the dose determined to have maximal effects on the prostate (Lesser and Bruchovsky, 1973). As shown in Fig. 2A, dihydrotestosterone stimulates DNA synthesis in prostates of 4-day or 7-day castrates, which contain fewer than the normal number of nuclei, but has no significant effects on prostates of normal animals or 1-day castrates, in which the number of nuclei has not yet fallen below the normal level. The onset of DNA synthesis in prostates of 7-day castrates is very precisely defined with respect to time; a lag period of 24–36 hours is observed before DNA synthesis begins followed by an increase to 100-fold the control rates by 72 hours. Paralleling the change in rate of DNA synthesis, the number of nuclei per prostate (Fig. 2B) is stimulated to increase in 4-day and 7-day castrates, but no significant changes are observed in normal or 1-day castrate animals. Furthermore, the stimulation of cell proliferation that is observed is transitory despite continued administration of hormone, as demonstrated by the decrease in rate of DNA synthesis (Fig. 2A) and in production of nuclei (Fig. 2B). The switch in rate of proliferation is correlated with attainment of the normal number of cells by the growing tissue; although proliferation is curtailed, wet weight of tissue

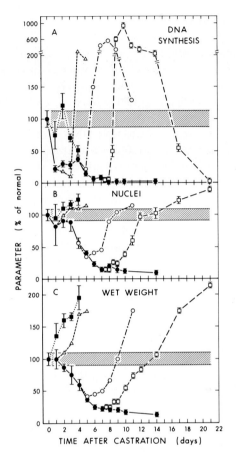

FIG. 2. Response of prostate to dihydrotestosterone. Groups of 3–7 rats were castrated on day 0. Animals were left untreated (●), or treatment with daily doses of 400 μg of dihydrotestosterone per 100 gm body weight was commenced immediately (■), or 1 day (△), 4 days (○), or 7 days (□) after castration. Values for normal rats are shown as zero-time points. At the appropriate time the animals were killed and prostates were removed and weighed. Rate of DNA synthesis was assayed *in vitro* and nuclei were isolated and counted as described by Lesser and Bruchovsky (1973). Error bars where shown indicate the mean ±SEM for at least 3 separate determinations; otherwise each point represents a single experiment. All values are expressed as percentages of the corresponding value for normal animals. (A) Rate of incorporation of [Me-^{3}H]thymidine (measured as dpm/μg DNA per 20 minutes. (B) Number of nuclei per prostate. (C) Prostatic wet weight. From Lesser and Bruchovsky (1974a), with permission.

continues to increase under the influence of hormone (Fig. 2C). The occurrence of an overshoot phenomenon in the production of nuclei with continuing maximal stimulation of prostate by large doses of dihydrotestosterone (Fig. 2B, 7-day castrates) is of interest in connection with the potential causative role of dihydrotestosterone in benign prostatic hyperplasia (Siiteri and Wilson, 1970; Gloyna et al., 1970; Bruchovsky and Lesser, 1975).

The preceding results demonstrate that DNA synthesis and cell division in prostate are refractory to stimulation unless sensitized by declining cell number. The results also demonstrate how the prostate can regulate its size by rapidly curtailing DNA synthesis and the cell proliferation through a negative feedback effect (Epifanova, 1971) when the number of cells is brought to normal. Therefore, organ homeostasis seems to be achieved in part by balanced function of two cellular constraint mechanisms, one responsible for initiating DNA synthesis and cell proliferation, the other responsible for suppressing these processes. That the two constraint mechanisms represent separate levels of control is suggested by the dissociation of their phenotypic expression in hormone-responsive tumors (Bruchovsky et al., 1975a).

B. Negative Feedback

The results presented in Fig. 2 indicate that a vital factor determining the magnitude of the proliferative response of prostate to androgens is the number of cells in the gland relative to normal. When this number is normal, as in short-term castrates, a proliferative response to androgen is not observed, although androgen is able to induce a large increase in tissue weight due to stimulation of secretory activity. Tissues that contain fewer than the normal number of cells respond to hormone administration by proliferating rapidly, but once the number of cells has returned to normal the rate of proliferation declines sharply.

In order to gain further insight into negative feedback control, Lesser and Bruchovsky (1974b) studied the division potential of individual cells during regeneration of prostate. Prostatic nuclei were separated according to their position in the cell cycle, and their progress was followed through successive divisions thus enabling the determination of a number of kinetic parameters of growth. The method used was based on the observation of McBride and Peterson (1970) that nuclei of mammalian cells can be fractionated on the basis of size, and hence of position in the cell cycle, by the technique of velocity sedimentation under unit gravity (Miller and Phillips, 1969). In this approach isolated nuclei are allowed to settle through a shallow gradient of bovine serum albumin for 8 hours and the gradient is then fractionated. The resultant resolution of cell cycle phases is depicted in Fig. 3. Nuclei are distributed as a peak sedimenting at a rate of 2 mm/hour, skewed toward larger sedimentation velocities. The slowly sedimenting peak consists solely of debris. After a 1-hour pulse of radioactive thymidine *in vivo* prior to removal of the prostate, radioactivity is found in a peak heavier than that of the majority of the nuclei. The main peak of nuclei contains the diploid amount of DNA per nucleus; nuclei that incorporated radioactive thymidine contain amounts of DNA intermediate between diploid and tetraploid, and the nuclei sedimenting most rapidly contain the tetraploid amount of DNA. Therefore, prostatic nuclei can be fractionated into G_1-phase, S-phase, and G_2-phase nuclei based on increasing size during the cell cycle, and hence increasing sedimentation velocity.

Sequential analysis of regenerating prostate by this procedure yields an estimate of the rate of progression of cells through the division cycle. In experiments performed for this purpose by Lesser and Bruchovsky (1974b), rats castrated 7 days previously were treated with daily injections of dihydrotestosterone; as shown by the results in Fig. 4, the effect

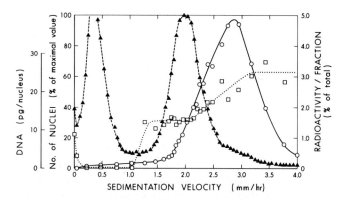

FIG. 3. Fractionation of nuclei according to phases of the cell cycle. Rats castrated 7 days previously were injected subcutaneously with 800 μg of dihydrotestosterone per 100 gm body weight daily for 3 days. At the time shown by the arrow in Fig. 4, the rats were injected intraperitoneally with 5 μCi of [Me-^{3}H]thymidine (specific radioactivity 50–55 Ci/mmole) per 100 gm body weight and 1 hour later were killed. A total of 1.2×10^8 isolated nuclei was applied to the gradient in a volume of 40 ml. The distribution of particles after 8 hours is shown for each fraction as a percentage of the value of the peak at 2 mm/hour. The distribution of radioactivity is expressed for each fraction as a percentage of the total radioactivity recovered, and DNA is shown as picograms per nucleus. Fractions that contained a small number of nuclei were pooled to obtain sufficient DNA. Material recovered: nuclei (▲), radioactivity (○), DNA (□). From Lesser and Bruchovsky (1974b), with permission.

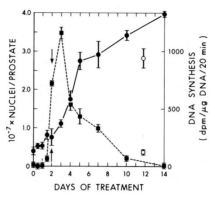

FIG. 4. Cell cycle parameters during response of prostate to dihydrotestosterone. On day 7 after orchiectomy, animals were injected subcutaneously with 400 μg of dihydrotestosterone per 100 gm body weight; the injection was repeated every 24 hours. After various periods of treatment, groups of 3–5 animals were killed and prostates were pooled. The tissue was weighed, and then minced and incubated with [Me-³H]thymidine (specific radioactivity 50–55 Ci/mmole) *in vitro* for 20 minutes. Nuclei were isolated and counted, and incorporation of radioactivity into nuclear DNA was determined. Results are expressed as mean ± SEM for at least three separate experiments. Incorporation of [Me-³H]thymidine (■); number of nuclei recovered per prostate (●). Values of [Me-³H]thymidine incorporation and nuclear content of prostates of normal rats (□) and (○), respectively. The arrow indicates the time of administration of [Me-³H]thymidine to label nuclei in preparation for sequential sedimentation-velocity analysis. From Lesser and Bruchovksy (1973), with permission.

of this treatment is to stimulate increases in the rate of DNA synthesis and the number of nuclei per prostate, first detectable 48 hours after treatment is started. During the next 3 days rapid growth occurs, and by Day 5 the number of nuclei per prostate has returned to normal. At this time the rate of production of nuclei declines to 25% of the maximal rate and the rate of DNA synthesis falls to a negligible value. During the 3 days when the growth rate is at a maximum, the cell population undergoes about 1.8 doublings and the time required for one doubling is approximately 40 hours.

At 48 hours after the start of therapy the animals received a single intraperitoneal injection of radioactive thymidine (the time of this injection is indicated by the arrow in Fig. 4, and is equated to zero time in the following discussion), and the fate of radioactively labeled nuclei was then followed for the next 48 hours by sequential velocity-sedimentation analysis. The results obtained during the first 12 hours are shown in Fig. 5. After 1 hour (Fig. 5B), radioactive nuclei are in the S-phase region of the gradient, and after 2 hours the radioactivity has shifted to heavier regions. By 4 hours (Fig. 5C) some radioactive label has ap-

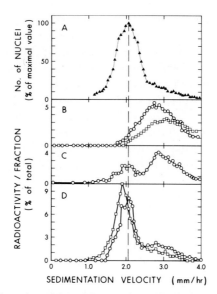

FIG. 5. Fractionation of nuclei 1–12 hours after the administration of [Me-³H]thymidine. Rats castrated 7 days previously were injected subcutaneously with 800 μg of dihydrotestosterone per 100 gm body weight at 24-hour intervals. Along with the third injection at 48 hours, the animals were injected with 5 μCi of [Me-³H]thymidine per 100 gm body weight. The time of the latter injection is shown by the arrow in Fig. 4. At 1, 2, 4, 8, and 12 hours after the injection of radioactive nucleoside, the rats were killed and prostatic nuclei were fractionated as described in Fig. 3. The distribution of nuclei is indicated in terms of the number of nuclei recovered in each fraction calculated as a percentage of the peak value. The distribution of radioactivity is similarly expressed in terms of the amount recovered in each fraction as a percentage of the total amount recovered. Distribution of nuclei: (A) distribution of radioactivity: (B) at 1 (○) or 2 (□) hours; (C) at 4 hours (○); (D) at 8 (○) or 12 (□) hours as shown. From Lesser and Bruchovsky (1974b), with permission.

peared in the G_1-phase region, representing nuclei that have completed their first division, and the major peak occurs in the late S-phase and G_2-phase regions. After 8 hours (Fig. 5D) most of the radioactivity is in the G_1-phase area, and by 12 hours the shift is almost complete and little radioactivity remains in the S-phase and G_2-phase regions. Reappearance of radioactive nuclei in the S-phase region is detected at 20 hours (data not shown) and indicates that the minimum duration of the cell cycle is about 20 hours. From the results presented in Fig. 5 it can be deduced that the 20-hour cycle consists of a G_1 phase of approximately 10 hours, an S phase of 7–8 hours, and a G_2 phase of 2–3 hours.

Velocity-sedimentation analysis was also used to measure the proportion of the labeled population of cells that undergoes a second round of division by measuring the fraction of radioactivity that reappears in the S + G$_2$-phase regions of the gradient during the second 20-hour period following injection of radioactive thymidine. This fraction is approximately 50%, compatible with the possibility that one daughter cell resulting from each division differentiates while the other continues to divide.

It was determined from the results shown in Fig. 3 that during regeneration of prostate in the 7-day castrate animal, the number of nuclei per prostate increases from about 27% of normal to the normal value, during the 72-hour period of most rapid proliferation between 48 hours and 120 hours after the initiation of hormone therapy. Since the division cycle time is 20 hours, 3.6 rounds of cell division can occur during prostatic regeneration. At the beginning of the 72-hour period of rapid proliferation, the labeling and mitotic indices were determined by radioautography to be 16% and 2.1%, respectively. During this period these indices increase to a maximal value 24 hours later (coincident with the peak rate of DNA synthesis in Fig. 4) and then decline.

Knowledge of the foregoing cell cycle parameters is essential for calculating the fraction of cells involved in the prostatic growth process and the number of divisions completed by an individual cell. For the sake of simplicity in the following discussion the average values of the labeling and mitotic indices during proliferation will be taken as those measured at the beginning of the period, namely 16% and 2.1%, respectively. While this introduces an error when one considers a particular time during the proliferative period, the error is small when analysis is integrated over the entire proliferative period so as not to affect the conclusions reached below.

Assuming constant labeling and mitotic indices, the fraction of cells involved in the prostatic growth process (growth fraction, GF) will also be constant. Therefore the kinetics of cell proliferation can best be described mathematically by modifying the derivation of Cleaver (1967) such that after one cell cycle time the number of cells is equal to $(1 + GF) N_0$, where N_0 is the number originally present, rather than $2N_0$ as would be the case if the growth fraction were 1.0. By comparison, the analysis of Cleaver (1967) assumes that all daughter cells remain in the proliferative cycle; hence the size of the proliferating subpopulation would increase exponentially and the growth fraction would increase with time. Using the former assumption the equation describing the kinetics of cell production becomes:

$$N_t = N_0 e[t/T \ln (1 + GF)] \tag{1}$$

or

$$N_t = N_0 (1 + GF)^{t/T} \tag{2}$$

where N_t is the number of cells at time t, N_0 is the number of cells at time 0, and T is the cell cycle time. Hence, by following the analysis of Cleaver (1967) the mitotic index (MI) and the labeling index (LI) can be described by the equations:

$$MI = (1 + GF)^{t_m/T} - 1 \qquad (3)$$

and

$$LI = (1 + GF)^{t_g/T}[(1 + GF)^{t_s/T} - 1] \qquad (4)$$

where t_m, t_g, and t_s are the durations of mitosis, G_2-phase $+ \frac{1}{2}$ mitosis, and S- phase, respectively. Using the values determined for the various parameters, the average growth fraction during proliferation is calculated to be 0.51 or 0.50 if mitotic index or labeling index data, respectively, are used. It is of interest to note that a population doubling time of 40 hours and a cell cycle time of 20 hours requires a minimal growth fraction of 0.41, assuming a constant growth fraction. This value is in reasonable agreement with the value of 0.5 determined from cell cycle analysis, indicating that assumption of a constant average growth fraction during proliferation does not introduce major errors.

The results of the preceding studies on the kinetics of proliferation in regenerating prostate can be summarized as follows: the population undergoes 1.8 doublings with a doubling time of 40 hours; the durations of the cell cycle phases are 10 hours for G_1 phase, 7–8 hours for S phase, 2–3 hours for G_2 phase, and 20 hours for the total cell cycle; of the cells involved in the first round of division, about half do not undergo a second division during the next round; and assuming a constant labeling index of 16% and mitotic index of 2.1%, the average growth fraction during proliferation is 0.5. Since half the daughter cells produced by mitosis do not reenter the proliferative cycle, in order to explain how the growth fraction is maintained at its average value of 0.5, one is forced to conclude that previously nonproliferating cells are recruited into the cycle. Furthermore, over the period of cell proliferation the majority of the cells present in the prostates at the start of proliferation must divide at least once, but at most only 4–5 times. The observation that negative feedback can be specified in terms of a numerical limit on cell division may eventually bring the definition of negative feedback into better perspective.

It is clear that negative feedback is not a result of loss of ability to respond to hormone, since hormone can stimulate secretory activity even in the absence of cell division (Fig. 2C). This observation touches upon the more general and vexatious question of the relationship between proliferation and differentiation. In the context of negative feedback, is differentiation the stimulus that inhibits proliferation, or is proliferation completed before differentiation starts? Stoll (1974) has presented arguments in favor of the latter point of view, which, if correct, has important implications in the therapy of hormone-responsive cancers. For example, therapy might be aimed at inducing negative feedback in undifferentiated tumors which on morphological grounds would be classified as autonomous. Experimental evidence for the idea that proliferation and differentiation are under separate and reciprocal control is not lacking (Malamud, 1971), and the work of Schmid *et al.* (1973) suggests that in prostate these processes are indeed mutually exclusive, although DNA synthesis is a prerequisite for differentiation. However, such studies properly require a specific biochemical marker for prostatic function, such as the aldolase messenger RNA described by Mainwaring *et al.* (1974). A complicating factor in this approach might be the simultaneous existence of proliferating and secretory populations in the prostate, although this may not be a serious problem because of the high growth fractions in the regenerating prostate. Until more precise knowledge is available, the idea that negative feedback is independent of differentiation should be regarded at least as a strong theoretical possibility.

A second type of regulatory mechanism that can be eliminated as a basis for negative feedback is the existence of a small stem cell population in the prostate that is able to undergo a limited number of divisions before losing the capacity to proliferate. Rather, the kinetic studies described in this section indicate that the majority of cells in the prostate of the 7-day castrate animal contribute to the proliferative response; moreover, the cells proliferating initially do not comprise a continuously cycling pool. Indeed, if a pool of stem cells did exist, and the cells in this pool were able to divide the same number of times equally well in prostates of 4-day and 7 day castrates, the gland of the 4-day castrate would be expected to overshoot the normal size, since proliferation in the gland commences with almost four times as many cells. However, the absence of significant overshoot suggests that glandular size is not governed by the division potential of individual cells; on the contrary, division potential is apparently preordained by the total number of cells in the gland at the start of proliferation.

An attractive alternative possibility to explain negative feedback is that regulation of proliferative growth might depend on the production of substances like chalones (Bullough *et al.*, 1967), which inhibit cell proliferation. If functional prostatic cells produced an inhibitor such that the amount produced by the normal number of cells was just sufficient to shut off proliferation, then proliferation would occur only when the number of cells had fallen below the normal level, and would then be shut off in regenerating prostate once the normal number of cells had been restored, in accordance with the experimental observations. In effect, there would be two superimposed mechanisms regulating prostatic size, one internal (negative feedback) and one external (androgen). Androgens would be necessary but not sufficient for the overall effect on proliferative activity, but might be the sole requirement for stimulation of secretory activity.

In light of the above considerations, it can be visualized that the internal negative feedback mechanism might be defective in certain types of carcinoma, and that it might become reset at a level permitting increased numbers of cells in conditions such as benign prostatic hyperplasia.

C. Autophagia

During the growth response of prostate, each new cell is capacitated with the power to destroy itself but the process of self-destruction is suppressed in the presence of adequate concentrations of hormone. Activation of the autophagic mechanism results when the supply of hormone falls below normal and is followed by a marked reduction in tissue mass. Ironically, the importance of this homeostatic constraint mechanism is underlined by the ominous significance of its absence from tumors that arise from endocrine responsive organs.

The nature of the involutionary response in adult rat prostate has been documented in considerable detail beginning with the observation of Moore et al. (1930) of breakdown of cellular structure, as seen under the light microscope, following castration. The changes, which are confined mainly to epithelial elements (MacKenzie et al., 1963), have been studied extensively by electron microscopy (Harkin, 1957; Brandes and Groth, 1963). The appearance of large numbers of lysosomes (Brandes, 1966; Harkin, 1957, 1963) is believed to be responsible for degradation of cellular material (de Duve, 1959) largely through the formation of autophagic vacuoles (Brandes, 1974; Paris and Brandes, 1974). Biochemical processes that decline after castration include production of prostatic secretion (Brandes and Bourne, 1963; Huggins, 1947; Kirchheim and Scott, 1965; Mann, 1964), ribonucleic acid (RNA) and protein synthesis (Brandes and Bourne, 1963; Mangan et al., 1967; Butler and Schade, 1958; Williams-Ashman et al., 1964), and respiration rate (Butler and Schade, 1958; Nyden and Williams-Ashman, 1953).

Prostatic involution has also been characterized in terms of effect on DNA synthesis and cell number (Lesser and Bruchovsky, 1973). The results shown in Fig. 6 indicate that rate of DNA synthesis declines dramatically within 24 hours after castration, followed within 3 days by a decrease in wet weight and number of nuclei. By day 7 all parameters have fallen to a small fraction of their normal value; after this time

N. BRUCHOVSKY ET AL.

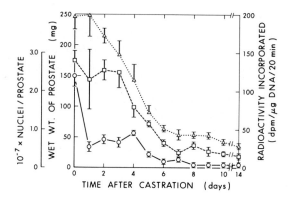

Fig. 6. Regression of prostate following orchiectomy. Male rats weighing 250–300 gm were castrated at day 0. At daily intervals for 10 days and then at 14 days after castration animals were sacrificed and 3–7 prostates were pooled, weighed, and incubated *in vitro* with [Me-³H]thymidine for 20 minutes. Nuclei were then isolated and counted, and incorporation of radioactivity into nuclear DNA was determined. Results are expressed as mean ±SEM for at least 3 determinations. Values obtained for normal animals are shown as the zero time points on the ordinate. Incorporation of [Me-³H]thymidine (○), nuclei isolated per prostate (□), wet weight of prostate (△). From Lesser and Bruchovsky (1973), with permission.

little further decrease occurs. By day 14, the longest time studied, prostatic weight has decreased to 36 mg as compared to the normal weight of approximately 250 mg. Burkhart (1942) reported that after 40 days, prostatic weight declines further to 14 mg (correcting for body weight of animals), a rate of about 3% per day between day 14 and day 40 as compared to 25–30% per day during the period of rapid atrophy between days 3 and 6. Therefore, castration of an adult rat is followed within a week by extensive diminution of prostatic tissue.

Another approach to the study of tissue involution is to induce growth of prostate in a castrated animal with a single injection of androgen, and then follow the regression of tissue as the effects of the hormone begin to wane. Lesser and Bruchovsky (1973) administered a single dose of dihydrotestosterone to rats castrated 7 days previously, and then measured the rate of DNA synthesis, number of nuclei per prostate, and wet weight of prostate for several days after. As shown in Fig. 7, all three parameters are stimulated to increase, but only transiently; the wet weight and number of nuclei each about half their normal values, shown in Fig. 2, before starting to decline. Thus, continued hormonal stimulation is required for the involuted rat prostate to reach and maintain its normal size and function. It is noteworthy that the effects of a single injection of hormone are apparent up to 7 days, indicating either that androgens

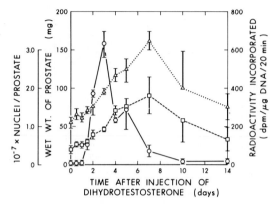

Fig. 7. Effect of a single dose of dihydrotestosterone on prostatic growth. Male rats were castrated 7 days prior to the beginning of the experiment. On day 0 the rats were given an injection of 400 μg of dihydrotestosterone per 100 gm body weight. At various times thereafter, 3–7 prostates were pooled, weighed, and incubated *in vitro* with [Me-³H]thymidine for 20 minutes. Nuclei were then isolated and counted, and incorporation of label into nuclear DNA was determined. Results are expressed as mean ± SEM for at least 3 separate experiments. Incorporation of [Me-³H]thymidine (○), number of nuclei isolated per prostate (□), wet weight of prostate (△). From Lesser and Bruchovsky (1973), with permission.

are very long lived in the prostate or that proliferation, once initiated, can continue for some time independent of further hormonal stimulation. The latter possibility has been suggested by Coffey (1974).

An interesting question to consider is the nature of the prostatic cells that can survive castration since, even long afterward, a small number of the original group of cells remains to regenerate the organ if androgen is restored. One possible explanation of this phenomenon is that the prostate contains a small pool of undifferentiated cells which is perpetuated in the absence of hormone. In the normal prostate there is a slow rate of DNA synthesis, presumably to replace cell loss due to functional turnover. Lesser (1974) examined the possibility that the cells which multiply in the normal prostate are those which preferentially survive castration; adult male rats were labeled continuously with radioactive thymidine for 72 hours and then, after a period of time to allow elimination of unincorporated isotope, the animals were castrated. At various times after castration, the amount of radioactivity present in the prostate and the labeling index (the percentage of labeled nuclei) were determined. The results in Fig. 8 show that both parameters remain essentially constant during prostatic regression, indicating no selective retention of labeled cells. Thus, if there exists a pool of cells in the normal prostate that preferentially survives castration, the cells in this pool cannot be distin-

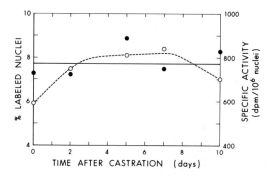

Fig. 8. Survival of labeled cells following orchiectomy. Adult male rats were injected intraperitoneally every 8 hours with 25 μCi of [Me-^{3}H]thymidine (specific radioactivity 50–55 Ci/mmole) per 100 gm body weight for a total of 9 injections. At 32 hours after the last injection, the animals were castrated. At various times after castration groups of rats were killed and prostatic nuclei were isolated. Nuclear radioactivity was determined by scintillation counting, and labeling index by radioautography. Labeling index (●), specific activity (○). From Lesser (1974).

guished on the basis of ability to incorporate radioactive thymidine. This does not eliminate the existence of such a pool which might be distinguished in other ways, such as by the presence of androgen receptors. Because of the lack of methods of permanently labeling or distinguishing cells *in vivo* other than with radioactive thymidine, such studies would be confined to measuring changes in particular functions of the cell. For example, if cells containing a certain protein were able to survive androgen depletion while those lacking the protein could not, then the concentration of this protein measured on a per cell basis would be expected to increase during atrophy. However, interpretation of such studies would be complicated by possible changes in the level of the substances in question within individual cells.

If loss of cells during prostatic involution is indeed random, then the survival of a small fraction of cells might be explained by a mechanism dependent on total cell number, similar to the one postulated in Section II, B to limit cell proliferation. Although cell production does stop immediately after castration, the subsequent loss of cells is much more rapid than is accounted for by normal turnover, based on the rate of accumulation of labeled nuclei during continuous labeling of normal animals (only 8% in 3 days, Fig. 8). Thus prostatic atrophy is an active process; presumably autolysis of cells is caused by the action of degradative enzymes, such as nucleases and proteases, normally confined to the lysosomes (de Duve, 1959), which apparently are released when the level of androgens declines following castration. It follows that one of the effects of androgens on the prostate might be to inhibit the synthesis or the activation of lysosomal enzymes. Since protein synthesis stops after castration, it is possible that survival of some of the prostatic cells may simply be accounted for by depletion of lysosomes before the cells are fully destroyed. Alternatively, a diffusible lysosome-activating factor secreted by a small number of prostatic cells might be responsible for inducing catabolic changes in the whole tissue, but its action would be antagonized by androgens. After castration, declining levels of androgens would result in lysosome activation and autolysis of cells, but, as the number of cells declined, less activating factor would be produced and autolysis would stop.

III. Factors Affecting the Function of Homeostatic Constraint Mechanisms

A. Androgen Concentration

Much evidence has accumulated suggesting that the multiplication of prostatic epithelial cells is dependent on the formation of dihydrotestosterone in the cytoplasm and on the subsequent incorporation of dihydrotestosterone into the cell nucleus (Anderson and Liao, 1968; Bruchovsky and Wilson, 1968a; Gloyna et al., 1970; Siiteri and Wilson, 1970; Bruchovsky, 1971; Robel et al., 1971; Lesser and Bruchovsky, 1973). The important effect of dose of dihydrotestosterone on DNA synthesis and cell proliferation is shown in Fig. 9. In experiments performed by Lesser and Bruchovsky (1973), increasing doses of dihydrotestosterone were injected daily into rats castrated 7 days previously and the rate of incorporation of labeled thymidine into DNA was measured after 48 hours of treatment, at which time the rate of incorporation of thymidine is increasing linearly. Whereas maximal responses are obtained with doses in the range of 400–800 μg per 100 gm body weight corresponding to optimal doses reported by other investigators for either DNA synthesis (Coffey et al., 1968) or restoration of weight (Tuohimaa et al., 1973), the precise concentration of androgen required within the cell to obtain this response is not known. Neither is much known about factors that regulate the assimilation and retention of dihydrotestosterone by the cell nucleus, although evidence has accumulated suggesting that the magnitude of the response of target tissues to testosterone and a number of other androgenic compounds is determined by the concentration of dihydrotestosterone within this structure (Bruchovsky, 1971; Bruchovsky et al., 1975b). Since the upward change in rate of DNA synthesis with dose of dihydro-

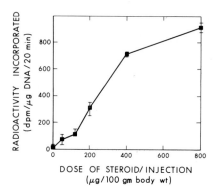

Fɪɢ. 9. The effect of dose of dihydrotestosterone on the incorporation of [Me-³H]thymidine. Male rats castrated 7 days previously were given a subcutaneous injection of various doses of dihydrotestosterone in 10% ethanol and 10% Tween 40 and the injection was repeated 24 hours later; 48 hours after the first injection, incorporation of [Me-³H]thymidine by prostatic minces *in vitro* was determined. Results are shown as the mean ±SEM for at least 3 separate determinations. From Lesser and Bruchovsky (1973), with permission.

testosterone (Fig. 9) is caused by the entry of increasing numbers of cells into S phase of the division cycle (Lesser and Bruchovsky, 1973), it seems that a critical concentration of dihydrotestosterone must be attained within the cell or the cell nucleus before DNA synthesis can begin. However, once started DNA synthesis is probably completed at the same rate in all cells that enter the S phase, even though hormone levels may fall during the interval of replication. Evidence compatible with the idea that the initiation of DNA synthesis is an irreversible event is discussed in Section II, C.

In order to clarify aspects of the relationship between the concentrations of androgen in the cytoplasmic and nuclear compartments, Bruchovsky *et al.* (1975b) measured the molar concentration of androgens in the nucleus as a function of the molar concentration of androgens in the cytoplasm. An estimate of the physiological concentration of testosterone is body fluids and tissues was obtained on the basis of published results. For example it is known that the concentration of testosterone in male plasma is about 10–20 nM (Robinson and Thomas, 1971; Lucas and Abraham, 1972; Coyotupa *et al.*, 1973) corresponding to the concentration in prostatic tissue (Siiteri and Wilson, 1970; Gloyna *et al.*, 1970; Robel *et al.*, 1973). The relation is probably explained by the passive diffusion process which accounts for the exchange of steroidal compounds between the circulation and the cytoplasmic compartment of the cell (Bruchovsky *et al.*, 1975b).

Thus to compare the relative concentrations of androgens in cytoplasm and nuclei under conditions that are approximately physiological, the effect of increasing doses of radioactive testosterone on the amount of radioactive androgens incorporated into cytoplasm and nuclear fractions of rat prostate during an interval of 1 hour was investigated. In a parallel study dihydrotestosterone was injected instead of testosterone in order to determine whether androgen transfer into the nucleus is enhanced when the enzymic conversion of testosterone to dihydrotestosterone is circumvented by the direct administration of dihydrotestosterone. The results of these experiments are shown in Fig. 10. It is evident that incorporation of both dihydrotestosterone and testosterone into cytoplasm (Fig. 10A) increases as a linear function of dose. In contrast, the radioactivity incorporated into nuclei, as shown in Fig. 10B, increases as a linear function of dose until a level of 1200×10^3 dpm/gm (8 pmoles per milligram of DNA) is attained; no more than this amount appears to be incorporated, and the results are similar whether testosterone or dihydrotestosterone is injected.

The results presented in Fig. 10 indicate that the total amount of androgens in nuclei is exceeded by the amount in cytoplasm; this difference is particularly evident when the dose of androgen is 200 μCi (4.6 nmoles) or greater. However, when the experimental data are calculated on the

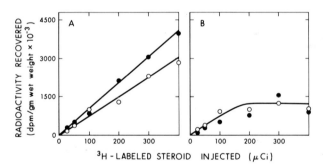

FIG. 10. Effect of dose on the concentration of androgens in cytoplasm and nuclei. Groups or 2 or 3 male rats (250–300 gm) castrated 24 hours previously were functionally hepatectomized and eviscerated and immediately afterward were injected intravenously with doses of [1,2-³H]testosterone or [1,2-³H]dihydrotestosterone (specific radioactivity 40–44 Ci/mmole) ranging from 25 μCi (0.57 nmole) to 400 μCi (9.2 nmole). After 60 minutes the rats were killed, and the appropriate cytoplasmic and nuclear fractions were prepared and assayed for radioactivity. In addition the metabolites of [1,2-³H]testosterone were identified in each fraction by thin-layer chromatography, and recovery of [1,2-³H]dihydrotestosterone was measured. Radioactivity recovered in (A) cytoplasm, (B) nucleus. Radioactive androgen injected: [1,2-³H]Dihydrotestosterone (●); [1,2-³H]testosterone (○). From Bruchovsky *et al.* (1975b), with permission.

basis of molar concentration of androgens in cytoplasm and nuclei, thus taking into account the different volumes of each compartment, the results shown in Fig. 11 are obtained (Bruchovsky *et al.*, 1975b). In Fig. 11 the actual concentration of total radioactive androgens in nuclei and cytoplasm is plotted as a function of dose of testosterone injected. Whereas the final concentration in nuclei is in the vicinity of 250 n*M*, the maximal concentration in cytoplasm is 100 n*M*. The curves in Fig. 11B show the relative concentrations of dihydrotestosterone recovered in cytoplasm and nuclei in this experiment. A cytoplasmic concentration of dihydrotestosterone as low as 10 n*M* produces a nuclear concentration of about 125 n*M*. These relationships are summarized more clearly in Fig. 12. Identification of the metabolites in cytoplasm and nuclei following the injection of radioactive dihydrotestosterone was not carried out; however, on the basis of previous analytical data (Bruchovsky, 1971) and the results presented in Fig. 10, it can be estimated that a cytoplasmic concentration of dihydrotestosterone of approximately 20 n*M*, in the absence of testosterone, will produce a nuclear concentration of dihydrotestosterone in the vicinity of 250 n*M*. Thus *in vivo* testosterone effectively competes with dihydrotestosterone in transport; this competition may explain why testosterone is biologically less potent than dihydrotestosterone in stimulating proliferative growth (Lesser and Bruchovsky, 1973).

Three further points merit emphasis in connection with the observations presented in Figs. 10–12. First, the kinetics of androgen transport across the plasma and nuclear membranes are clearly different in that transport into the nucleus appears to be a limited process compared to

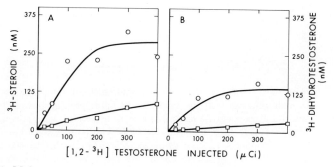

[1,2-³H] TESTOSTERONE INJECTED (μCi)

Fɪɢ. 11. Molar concentration of androgens in cytoplasm and nuclei. The experimental procedure was identical to that described in the legend to Fig. 10. However, the results are expressed in terms of molar concentrations of androgens recovered in cytoplasm and nuclei, calculated as described by Bruchovsky *et al.* (1975b). Molar concentration: (A) total ³H-labeled androgens; (B) [1,2-³H]dihydrotestosterone. Cytoplasm (□); nucleus (○). From Bruchovsky *et al.* (1975b), with permission.

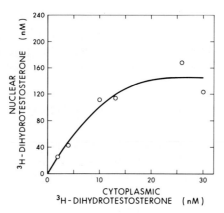

Fig. 12. Relationship between nuclear and cytoplasmic concentrations of dihydro-testosterone. The data in Fig. 11 is replotted to show the nuclear concentration of dihydrotestosterone as a function of the cytoplasmic concentration. From Bruchovsky and Lesser (1975), with permission of University Park Press.

transport into the cytoplasm (Fig. 10, and Bruchovsky *et al.*, 1975b). One might expect that the inducibility of a variety of cellular and molecular biosynthetic processes would be limited by this restriction on transport. Second, the metabolic conversion of testosterone to dihydrotestosterone which takes place in cytoplasm does not reduce transport and very likely, therefore, only affects the ratio of testosterone and dihydrotestosterone transferred into the nucleus. Third, and perhaps most important, the results presented in Fig. 12 suggest that small changes in the cytoplasmic concentration of dihydrotestosterone, within the physiological range of 0–10 nM, will produce much greater changes in the nuclear concentration of dihydrotestosterone—spanning the range of 0–120 nM with a ceiling of 250 nM in the absence of testosterone. Orchiectomy reduces circulating levels of testosterone to 10% or less of normal (Robinson and Thomas, 1971; Lucas and Abraham, 1972; Coyotupa *et al.*, 1973) and would not sustain a cytoplasmic concentration of dihydrotestosterone greater than 1–2 nM. This decline would be accompanied by a fall in the concentration of nuclear dihydrotestosterone to below 25 nM, a concentration probably insufficient to maintain the cell in a state of full differentiation.

It is of interest that if the plasma concentration of dihydrotestosterone were very much higher than 10–20 nM, the prostatic cell would be unresponsive to small fluctuations in circulating levels of testosterone, and if the adrenal glands were capable of secreting threshold levels of testosterone, orchiectomy would have little effect on prostatic size.

The presence of a concentrative mechanism to regulate the nuclear concentration of dihydrotestosterone may be expained by the observation that for many steps in differentiation the full range of induction may require substrate changes greater than 100-fold (Lin and Riggs, 1975). It is clear that the prostatic cell is well adapted to provide this flexibility of supply.

1. Effect of Androgen Metabolism on the Concentration and Distribution of Dihydrotestosterone

Since the amount of dihydrotestosterone in the nucleus is related to the amount in the cytoplasm, processes that change the cytoplasmic concentration may also affect the intranuclear concentration. In this regard, the concentration of dihydrotestosterone in the cytoplasm is increased by enzymes that metabolize natural androgens through one or more steps to dihydrotestosterone; conversely, its concentration is reduced by enzymes that convert dihydrotestosterone to other metabolites, chiefly 3α-androstanediol (Bruchovsky, 1971). The demonstration of the relative formation of dihydrotestosterone from a number of possible androgenic precursors was accomplished by identifying the androgens localized in prostate following the injection of approximately 2 nmoles of each androgen listed in Table I into castrated adult male rats (Bruchovsky, 1971).

TABLE I

FORMATION OF DIHYDROTESTOSTERONE FROM NATURAL ANDROGENS[a,b]

| | ^{3}H-Labeled steroids recovered ($10^3 \times$ nmoles/gm wet weight of prostate) | | | |
| | Total | | Dihydrotestosterone | |
[3]H-Steroid injected	Cytoplasm	Nuclei	Cytoplasm	Nuclei
Testosterone	7.8	3.9	2.9	2.6
Dihydrotestosterone	3.9	2.2	1.6	2.0
3α-Androstanediol	4.1	3.0	2.0	2.8
Androstenedione	3.9	1.1	0.5	0.8
Androsterone	4.0	0.8	1.0	0.7
Androstanedione	4.0	0.5	0.6	0.5
3β-Androstanediol	4.9	0.3	0.8	0.2
Dehydroepiandrosterone	8.2	0.1	0.7	0.1

[a] Recovery of radioactive androgens in cytoplasm and nuclei of rat prostate. Each of 8 natural androgens was injected by the intravenous route into 2 or 3 castrated, eviscerated, functionally hepatectomized rats. After 1 hour the rats were killed and the prostatic tissue was separated into cytoplasmic and nuclear fractions. The radioactivity in each sample was measured by liquid scintillation counting. [1,2-^{3}H]Dihydrotestosterone was identified by thin-layer and gas–liquid chromatography, and in some instances by recrystallization to constant specific activity.

[b] From Bruchovsky and Lesser (1975), with permisson of University Park Press.

Except after the administration of testosterone and dehydroepiandrosterone, the total amounts of steroid recovered from cytoplasm were almost equal. In contrast, the amounts recovered from nuclei varied from 3.9×10^{-3} nmoles/gm after the administration of testosterone to 0.1×10^{-3} nmoles/gm after the administration of dehydroepiandrosterone.

Identification of the metabolites in the cytoplasm and nuclear fractions indicated that dihydrotestosterone was present in both fractions after administration of each of the androgens tested. The amounts of dihydrotestosterone recovered from cytoplasm varied from 2.9×10^{-3} nmoles/gm after the administration of testosterone to 0.5×10^{-3} nmoles/gm after the administration of androstenedione. The amounts of dihydrotestosterone recovered from nuclei varied from 2.8×10^{-3} nmoles/gm after the administration of 3α-androstanediol to 0.1×10^{-3} nmoles/gm after the administration of dehydroepiandrosterone.

On the basis of these and other studies (Bruchovsky, 1971) a scheme of pathways leading to the formation of dihydrotestosterone can be derived as shown in Fig. 13. Dihydrotestosterone is formed directly from testosterone by the action of 3-oxo-5α-steroid Δ^4-dehydrogenase (EC 1.3.99.5) (5α-reductase), from androstanedione by the action of 17β-hydroxysteroid dehydrogenase (EC 1.1.1.51), and from 3α- and 3β-andro-

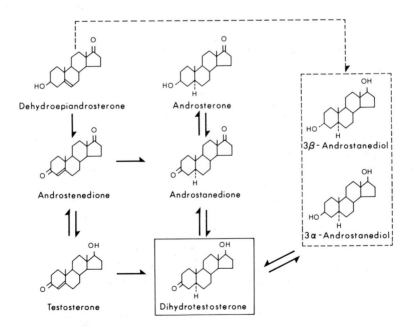

FIG. 13. Formation of dihydrotestosterone from natural androgens. From Bruchovsky and Lesser (1975), with permission of University Park Press.

stanediols by the action of 3α-hydroxysteroid dehydrogenase (EC 1.1.1.50) and the 3β-enzyme (EC 1.1.1.51), respectively. Other precursor androgens are converted to dihydrotestosterone through the intermediate formation of testosterone, androstanedione, and androstanediols. Therefore, on the one hand, the 5α-reductase, 17β-hydroxysteroid dehydrogenase, and 3α- and 3β-hydroxysteroid dehydrogenases raise the intracellular concentration of dihydrotestosterone: on the other hand, because of the irreversible nature of the 5α-reductase reaction, only the 17β-hydroxysteroid dehydrogenase and the 3α- and 3β-hydroxysteroid dehydrogenase lower the intracellular concentration of dihydrotestosterone. The available data also suggest that the 3α- and 3β-hydroxysteroid dehydrogenases are more active than the 17β-hydroxysteroid dehydrogenase in forming or metabolizing dihydrotestosterone (Bruchovsky, 1971).

Thus, if the proliferative response of prostate should indeed vary with intranuclear concentration of dihydrotestosterone, it is evident that prostatic enzymes which promote the formation or metabolism of dihydrotestosterone may strongly influence the size of the growth response to an androgen. This conclusion is supported by the evidence in Table I, showing that the amount of dihydrotestosterone incorporated into the prostatic nucleus following the administration of several natural androgens is generally correlated with the relative potency of each compound (Bruchovsky, 1971).

2. Effect of Androgen Receptors on the Concentration and Distribution of Dihydrotestosterone

The observation that the transfer of androgens into the nucleus appears to depend on the formation of androgen–receptor complexes in the cytoplasm (Rennie and Bruchovsky, 1973; King and Mainwaring, 1973; Liao et al., 1974) suggests a second way in which the nuclear concentration of dihydrotestosterone might be regulated. Although the cytoplasm of prostate contains a number of androgens, only those that form androgen–receptor complexes, notably testosterone and dihydrotestosterone, are incorporated into the nucleus. Other intracellular androgens, such as 3α- and 3β-androstanediol, androsterone, androstanedione, androstenedione, and dehydroepiandrosterone, as a rule do not enter the nucleus; as discussed in Section III, A, 1, these androgens are first converted to dihydrotestosterone in the cytoplasm and the active metabolite is then transported across the nuclear membrane. Thus, since the binding of testosterone and dihydrotestosterone to cytoplasmic receptors and the subsequent transfer of androgen–receptor complex into the nucleus seems to be an obligatory step in the transport process, the level of androgens in the nucleus may depend on the number of receptors in the cytoplasm. Despite the attractiveness of this assumption, it remains unverified principally because of the difficulty of proving that cytoplasmic and nuclear receptors which are characterized by different physical properties (King and Mainwaring, 1973; Rennie and Bruchovsky, 1972, 1973; Liao et al., 1974; Bruchovsky et al., 1975b) are indeed related molecules.

Experiments on the incorporation of androgens and androgen receptors into nuclei have generally been performed with cell-free systems, but some doubts have arisen as to whether the results obtained with this experimental approach can be extrapolated to the in vivo situation. The properties of the nuclear membrane are quite different in the whole cell, and unique properties which characterize this membrane in vivo vanish when the cell is fractionated (Bruchovsky et al., 1975b). Whereas the transfer of dihydrotestosterone into the nucleus is a concentrative process in vivo (Fig. 12), this process changes to resemble passive diffusion when the nucleus is isolated (N. Bruchovsky, unpublished).

To circumvent the question of the validity of cell-free experiments and yet clarify some of the poorly understood aspects of the relationship between cytoplasmic receptors and the concentration of androgens and androgen receptors within the nucleus, Bruchovsky et al. (1975b), and Bruchovsky and Craven (1975) examined the transport of androgens in cells depleted of cytoplasmic receptors. Recent reports by Jung and Baulieu (1971), Mainwaring and Mangan (1973), and Sullivan and Strott (1973) have drawn attention to the apparent lost of cytoplasmic receptor with increasing time after orchiectomy. By taking advantage of this effect, it appeared feasible to determine, first, whether the depletion of cytoplasmic receptor is accompanied by a reduction in the incorporation of androgens into nuclei of prostatic cells, and, second, whether prostatic cells retain the competence to form nuclear receptor in the absence of detectable cytoplasmic receptor. The results in Fig. 14 compare the presence of cytoplasmic receptor in prostatic tissue 1 day and 7 days after castration. Analysis of androgen binding by gel-exclusion chromatography (Fig. 14A) yields a peak of radioactivity in fractions 30–45 which represents binding of radioactive dihydrotestosterone to a cytoplasmic receptor processing a Stokes radius of 48 Å and a sedimentation coefficient of 4.4 S measured in 0.6 M NaCl (Bruchovsky et al., 1975b). From the results shown in Fig. 14B it is clear that this receptor is not detected in prostate of animals orchiectomized 7 days previously. The estimated concentration of cytoplasmic receptor 1 day after castration is 174 ± 24 fmoles per milligram of protein, and it falls to near zero (i.e., less than 30 fmoles/mg) 7 days after castration.

Assuming that nuclear receptor is derived from cytoplasmic receptor, the loss of cytoplasmic receptor should be paralleled by a reduction in the capacity of the cell to transfer both androgens and androgen receptors into the nucleus. Bruchovsky and Craven (1975) tested this prediction

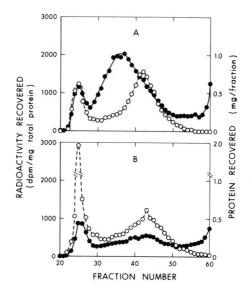

Fig. 14. Androgen receptor in the cytoplasm. Prostatic tissue was minced and incubated with 750 nM [1,2-³H]dihydrotestosterone (specific radioactivity 40 Ci/mmole) for 2 minutes at 37°C. Protein recovered from cytosol was analyzed by gel-exclusion chromatography with Sephadex G-200 (dual-column method). Fraction size was 1.4 ml. Radioactivity (●); protein (○). (A) At 1 day after orchiectomy; (B) 7 days after orchiectomy. From Bruchovsky and Craven (1975), with permission of Academic Press, Inc.

by comparing the incorporation of radioactive androgens into nuclei of prostatic cells at 1 day and 7 days after castration under conditions that promote maximal incorporation of androgens and androgen receptors into nuclei of prostatic cells. From the results presented in Table II, it is evident that the incorporation of androgens into cytoplasm is virtually the same at 1 day and 7 days after castration whether *in vivo* or *in vitro* labeling techniques are used. In contrast, the *in vivo* incorporation of androgens into nuclei is reduced approximately 70% whereas the *in vitro* incorporation is reduced approximately 40%. But, despite the apparent lack of cytoplasmic receptor, the cell clearly retains significant capacity to transfer androgens into the nucleus.

Since the potential for intracellular androgen transport is partially sustained in regressing cells, Bruchovsky and Craven (1975) also tested these cells for competence to form nuclear receptor. Extracts of nuclei recovered in experiments described in Table II were analyzed by gel-exclusion chromatography, and the results are shown in Fig. 15. In prostatic nuclei obtained 1 day after castration, radioactivity is recovered in 3 peaks (Fig. 15A); the first peak is eluted in a volume of 20–30 ml,

TABLE II
INCORPORATION OF ANDROGENS[a]

| Experiment | Days after orchiectomy | Radioactivity recovered | |
		Cytoplasm (dpm/gm $\times 10^{-5}$)	Nucleus (dpm/nucleus $\times 10^4$)
In vivo	1	20.3 ± 1.3 (3)	115.6 ± 15.9 (3)
	7	17.6 ± 0.8 (3)	35.3 ± 10.0 (3)
In vitro	1	336.4 ± 18.2 (6)	26.0 ± 3.9 (5)
	7	334.0 (2)	16.5 ± 4.2 (3)

[a] *In vivo:* Groups of 3–14 rats (250–300 gm) orchiectomized 1 and 7 days previously received intravenous injections of 300 μCi (6.9 nmoles) of [1,2-³H]testosterone. After 60 minutes the animals were killed and the radioactivity in cytoplasmic and nuclear fractions of prostate was measured. At both 1 day and 7 days after orchiectomy, dihydrotestosterone is the principal intracellular metabolite of testosterone. *In vitro:* Prostatic tissue (1 gm) was minced and incubated with [1,2-³H]dihydrotestosterone (750 nM) for 10 minutes at 37°C. The tissue was extensively washed and then separated into cytoplasmic and nuclear fractions which were analyzed for content of radioactivity. The results are expressed as the mean ±SEM of the number of experiments shown in parentheses. From Bruchovsky and Craven (1975), with permission of Academic Press, Inc.

corresponding to the excluded fractions, and represents binding to a large molecular weight component of the nucleus presumed to be chromatin (Bruchovsky and Wilson, 1968b); the second peak is eluted in a volume of 30–50 ml and represents binding to nuclear receptor possessing a sedimentation coefficient of 3.3 S (Bruchovsky et al., 1975b); the third peak is eluted in a volume of 55–65 ml and represents free androgen. In prostatic nuclei obtained 7 days after castration (Fig. 15B) the distribution of radioactivity is similar but the elution of receptor is delayed. It was estimated by chromatographic methods that the Stokes radius of nuclear receptor observed 1 day after orchiectomy is 24–25 Å, while that of the receptor observed 7 days after orchiectomy is only 19–20 Å (Bruchovsky and Craven, 1975).

Certain deductions based on the foregoing results underline the difficulty of proving that the cytoplasmic receptor is an exclusive determinant of the presence of androgens and androgen receptors in the prostatic nucleus. For example, from the data in Table II, it is calculated that 70,000 androgen molecules are transferred into the nucleus *in vivo*; of these about one-third, or 23,000, are bound to receptor 1 day after orchiectomy (Fig. 15A). In the same tissue the maximal concentration of cytoplasmic receptor at 174 fmoles/mg protein is equivalent to only 8000 receptor molecules per cell corresponding to the level determined for a num-

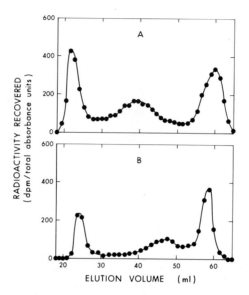

Fig. 15. Androgen receptor in the nucleus. Extracts of nuclei recovered in experiments described in Table I were analyzed by gel-exclusion chromatography with Sephadex G-200 (single-column method). The radioactivity in each fraction was divided by the total absorbance units at 260 nm. Radioactivity recovered: (A) 1 day after orchiectomy; (B) 7 days after orchiectomy. From Bruchovsky and Craven (1975), with permission of Academic Press, Inc.

ber of hormone-responsive organs (Wittliff *et al.*, 1971; Clark and Gorski, 1970; Limpaphayom *et al.*, 1971; Ballard and Ballard, 1972; Millgrom *et al.*, 1973; Funder *et al.*, 1972; Spaeren *et al.*, 1973; McGuire *et al.*, 1974), including prostate (Sullivan and Strott, 1973; Shain *et al.*, 1975). A similar discrepancy appears 7 days after orchiectomy when the nucleus contains 22,000 androgen molecules and 7000 nuclear receptors under conditions that mitigate against the existence of any cytoplasmic receptor. Thus, in both cases, it seems that the quantity of cytoplasmic receptor is insufficient to account for the total influx of androgens and androgen receptors into the nucleus if a mole-to-mole relationship is assumed.

Since the regressing prostate contains factors, presumed to be proteolytic enzymes, which destroy the binding of dihydrotestosterone to cytoplasmic receptor (Bruchovsky and Craven, 1975), it is possible that the concentration of cytoplasmic receptor may be underestimated because of the inactivation of receptor during analytical procedures. On the other hand, the detection of nuclear receptor in cells that contain little or no cytoplasmic receptor raises the possibility that nuclear receptor may arise from a source other than cytoplasmic receptor. This impression is supported by the observation that the nuclear receptor observed 7 days after orchiectomy is smaller than the one observed 1 day after orchiectomy. Such a result is unexpected if it is assumed that nuclear receptor is derived directly from the same cytoplasmic source at both times after orchiectomy.

These results when viewed in light of the different physical properties of cytoplasmic and nuclear receptors are compatible with the idea that cytoplasmic receptor functions independently to increase the permeability of the nuclear membrane to the passage of androgens and in this sense behaves as a permease. Thus, in undifferentiated cells such as those surviving long-term castration, which have little requirement for androgen, there is only a small amount of cytoplasmic receptor, and the nuclear membrane is relatively impermeable. Differentiated cells such as those in prostate 1 day after orchiectomy have a greater requirement of androgen; and cytoplasmic receptor, by increasing the permeability of the nuclear membrane to the passage of androgens, may function to maintain levels of nuclear androgen high enough to support the full range of differentiation. One might expect that differentiation itself produces an increased requirement for androgens in order to sustain continuous transcriptional activity, and it is not unreasonable to think that cytoplasmic receptor is produced in response to the pressures of differentiation, rather than being responsible itself for initiating such cellular responses. For discussions of the potential direct effect of cytoplasmic receptor on transcriptional processes, the reader is referred to the reviews by King and Mainwaring (1973), Liao et al. (1974), and Mainwaring et al. (1974).

Evidence for the hypothesis that nuclear and cytoplasmic receptors are related remains equivocal, and the precise function of nuclear receptor awaits clarification. The question whether nuclear receptor can affect DNA synthesis and cell proliferation is discussed in Section III, C in relation to experiments designed to measure the concentration of this molecule during active and quiescent phases of prostatic growth. However, the absence of nuclear receptor in Shionogi carcinoma cells, which are dependent on androgens for growth (Bruchovsky et al., 1975a), suggests that this receptor is not involved in the initiation of growth but may be important in negative feedback or autophagia (Bruchovsky and Lesser, 1975).

The evidence reviewed in this section supports the view that cytoplasmic receptors and the capacity to transport androgens into the nucleus are closely linked pheontypic markers of intracellular steroid hormone action. However, it seems likely that the control of androgen concentration in the nucleus is achieved in a more subtle fashion than simply through a dependence on the translocation of 4.4 S androgen receptor complex into the nucleus, if indeed the latter event takes place. The presence of cytoplasmic receptor is associated with enhanced ability of the cell to incorporate androgens into the nucleus, but whether nuclear receptor is related to cytoplasmic receptor remains equivocal.

B. Adenosine 3′,5′-Cyclic Monophosphate

In view of the evidence in several experimental systems that cell proliferation is inhibited by adenosine 3′,5′-cyclic monophosphate (cAMP) (Ryan and Heidrick, 1968; Otten *et al.*, 1971, 1972; Sheppard, 1971; Froehlich and Rachmeler, 1972; Thomas *et al.*, 1973; Abell and Monahan, 1973; Eker, 1974), and that there is an inverse relationship between the intracellular concentration of cAMP and DNA synthesis (Otten *et al.*, 1972; Froechlich and Rachmeler, 1972; Macmanus *et al.*, 1972) the need to examine the possibility that cAMP is a significant factor in promoting or inhibiting prostatic growth understandably followed.

Craven *et al.* (1974) measured the level of cAMP during a period of tissue involution induced by castration and during a period of tissue regeneration induced by administration of dihydrotestosterone as depicted in Fig. 16A. The effects of castration and androgen replacement therapy with dihydrotestosterone on the level of cAMP in prostate are shown in Fig. 16B. No significant change is observed in cAMP concentration at any time compared to the day 0 control value ($p < 0.05$ for all experimental results shown) when the amount of cAMP is calculated on the basis of DNA content. This evidence indicates that androgens do not alter gross intracellular levels of cAMP; furthermore, no relationship appears to exist between cyclic AMP and DNA synthesis nor between cAMP and cell proliferation.

In order to determine whether the growth-promoting effects of androgens are produced or modified by cAMP, Craven *et al.* (1974) administered cAMP, dibutyryl cAMP, dihydrotestosterone or dihydrotestosterone plus dibutyryl cAMP, in multiple successive doses to rats 7 days after orchiectomy. Cyclic nucleotides were injected concomitantly with theophylline. No direct effects of cAMP or dibutyryl cAMP were observed on growth, and dibutyryl cAMP neither enhanced nor inhibited the increase in prostatic weight and number of nuclei induced by the administration of dihydrotestosterone.

Taken together these results affirm the impression that the role of cAMP in mediating the action of androgens is probably confined to a circumscribed effect on cell metabolism (Mangan *et al.*, 1973; Robinson *et al.*, 1974).

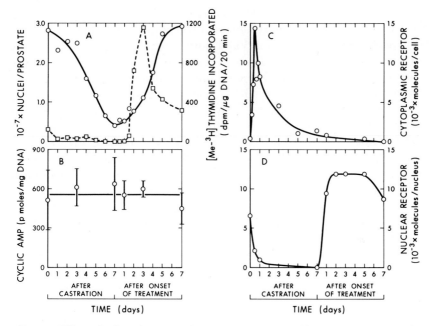

FIG. 16. Effect of adenosine 3,5-cyclic monophosphate (cAMP) cytoplasmic andro-gen receptor, and nuclear androgen receptor on prostatic growth and homeostasis. Groups of 3–12 male rats weighing 250–300 gm were castrated under ether anesthesia. At daily intervals for 7 days prostatic tissue was analyzed for content of nuclei, capacity to synthesize DNA, levels of cAMP, cytoplasmic receptor, and nuclear receptor. cAMP was measured by a competitive protein-binding technique utilizing a protein obtained from bovine cardiac muscle (Craven *et al.*, 1974). Cytoplasmic receptor was measured as described in the legend to Fig. 14. Nuclear receptor was measured by incubating extracts of nuclei, prepared as described by Rennie and Bruchovsky (1972, 1973) in the presence of [1,2-^{3}H]dihydrotestosterone (specific radioactivity 40 Ci/mmole) at a concentration of 20 nM for 18 hours at 20°C. To calculate the number of molecules of receptor in the cytoplasm and nucleus, it was assumed that 1 molecule of androgen is bound to 1 molecule of receptor. At 7 days after castration, groups of rats were treated with subcutaneous injections of dihydrotestosterone for a second interval of 7 days. During this time, tissue was analyzed as before. (A) Number of nuclei per prostate (○); rate of incorporation of [Me-^{3}H]thymidine (□). (B) Concentration of cAMP. (C) Number of molecules of cytoplasmic receptor. (D) Number of molecules of nuclear receptor. The results shown in panel B are expressed as the mean ±SEM of at least 3 separate experiments.

C. ANDROGEN RECEPTORS

Since the regulation of DNA synthesis and cell proliferation probably depends on the intranuclear concentration of dihydrotestosterone, it was suggested in Section III, A, 2 that androgen receptors could influence these processes indirectly by altering the level of dihydrotestosterone in the nucleus. A direct effect of androgen receptors is also conceivable and this premise was tested by E. J. Van Doorn, S. Craven, and N. Bruchovsky (unpublished) by measuring the concentration of cytoplasmic and nuclear receptors during active and quiescent phases of prostatic growth. The results presented in Fig. 16C indicate that the number of detectable cytoplasmic receptors increases sharply from 500 per cell to 14,000 per cell during the 12-hour period immediately following castration, and then declines rapidly to less than 1000 per cell by 5–7 days. Treatment of animals castrated 7 days previously with dihydrotestosterone fails to provoke the appearance of cytoplasmic receptor during the phase of prostatic growth which brings the number of cells per prostate back to normal. A number of tissue mixing experiments were performed in which prostate from rats castrated 1 day previously was mixed in equal proportions with prostate either from normal uncastrated rats, or from rats castrated 7 days previously, or from rats castrated 7 days previously and treated with dihydrotestosterone for 7 days, and the results indicate that in both the long-term castrates and treated castrates, the prostate contains factors that eradicate the binding of dihydrotestosterone to cytoplasmic receptor. Therefore the failure to detect cytoplasmic receptor in regenerating prostate is not entirely due to the occupation of receptor sites by nonradioactive dihydrotestosterone. This finding indicates that even though the number of cells per prostate can be returned to normal, the tissue does not simultaneously revert to its precastration state. Suppression of receptor inactivating factors may represent a differentiated trait acquired by the cell sometime after cell division is arrested. Should this be the case, the increase in the number of cytoplasmic receptors immediately after castration probably results from the unmasking of binding sites as the concentration of endogenous androgen falls. Since the subsequent decline in cytoplasmic receptor is not in synchrony either with the fall in the rate of DNA synthesis after castration or with the decrease in the number of cells per prostate, and, since the receptor is not detected in regenerating prostate, it is unlikely that the function of cytoplasmic receptor is directly concerned with DNA synthesis and cell proliferation.

The number of detectable nuclear receptors (Fig. 16D) as measured by an *in vitro* isotope exchange method, decreases from a normal level of 6500 per cell to 900 per cell 1 day after castration, and no receptors are detected 7 days after castration. Treatment of 7-day castrates with dihydrotestosterone is followed by a rapid elevation in the number of nuclear receptors to 9400 per cell after 1 day of treatment, and to 12,000 per cell after 2 days of treatment. This number remains unchanged after 3 and 5 days of treatment but then declines slightly to 8700 per cell after

7 days. Three observations suggest that the control of DNA synthesis is unrelated to the concentration of nuclear receptor. First, in normal cells, the number of nuclear receptors is relatively high when the rate of DNA synthesis and cell turnover is very low. Second, the number of nuclear receptors is also high in prostate of 7-day castrates treated with dihydrotestosterone for 1 day, when DNA synthesis is not yet stimulated. Third, no change in the number of nuclear receptors is observed between the third and fifth days of treatment when the rate of DNA synthesis is markedly inhibited. Therefore, both initiation of DNA synthesis and negative feed-back are manifested in the absence of coincident changes in the concentration of nuclear receptor. While these observations tend to negate the possibility that nuclear receptor is directly responsible for switching DNA synthesis on or off, they do not exclude a potential role for this receptor in the regulation of the autophagic process. Indeed, it is conceivable that the nuclear receptor is the mechanism through which autophagia is induced in the differentiated cell when androgen levels fall below normal. Androgen would stimulate the formation of receptor, but receptor would not function as long as conditions favorable to the formation of androgen–receptor complex prevailed. In other words, the androgen–receptor complex is equated to an inactive form of nuclear receptor. The absence of nuclear receptor in Shionogi mammary carcinoma cells, which are dependent on androgens for growth (Bruchovsky et al., 1975a), suggests similarly that nuclear receptor is not involved in the initiation of growth but may be important in negative feedback or autophagia.

IV. Hypothesis: Initiator, Nullifier, and Autophage Genes

We have outlined how the growth of an androgen-responsive organ can be divided into three phases, each of which may depend on the function of a cellular constraint mechanism. Furthermore, it has been suggested that for the complete expression of growth-regulating constraint mechanisms, several properties underlying hormonal responsiveness must be manifested by the cell, including the ability to metabolize testosterone to dihydrotestosterone, the presence of cytoplasmic receptor, the ability to transfer androgens into the nucleus, and the competence to form nuclear receptor. Without doubt, the manner in which the action of these mechanisms is controlled will prove to be complex; nevertheless with our present level of understanding one can account for most of the actions of androgens, broadly speaking, by invoking the existence of only three regulatory elements which, for purposes of discussion, are assumed to be components of the cellular genome. A scheme to explain the overall

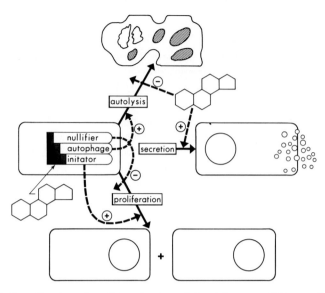

FIG. 17. Coordination of proliferative growth by initiator, nullifier, and autophage genes. From Bruchovsky and Lesser (1975), with permission of University Park Press.

coordination of proliferative growth by a hypothetical set of genes is depicted in Fig. 17. First, the initiator is responsible for switching on DNA synthesis and cell proliferation in the presence of an adequate concentration of androgen. Second, the nullifier is responsible for switching off DNA synthesis and cell proliferation when the prostate teaches a normal size, and accounts for negative feedback. Third, the autophage programs a cell for its own eventual destruction by capacitating the autophagic mechanism, this process being inhibited by androgen. A fall in the concentration of androgen below threshold levels required for the maintenance of a differentiated cell thus stimulates autolysis and removal of cells.

The vertical bars suggest that the initiator, autophage, and nullifier are activated or potentiated when androgen concentrations in the nucleus reach specific levels, but nonsteroidal factors may also contribute to achieve homeostasis. In addition to affecting these particular genes and inhibiting cellular autolysis, androgens promote secretory activity by stimulating transcriptional or posttranscriptional processes (Mainwaring et al., 1974; Ichii et al., 1974; Liang and Liao, 1975). Cyclic AMP also takes part in the secretory response (Singhal et al., 1971; Mangan et al., 1973; Singhal and Sutherland, 1974).

It follows that if the growth of a normal target organ is indeed ordered by the function of genetically determined constraint mechanisms, the failure of any one of these mechanisms may lead to an abnormal pattern of growth. For example, deletion of the nullifier gene and the resultant absence of negative feedback might produce a growth pattern similar to the one that distinguishes the growth of rat mammary carcinoma induced by 7,12-dimethylbenz[a]anthracene where the negative feedback process is clearly lacking (McGuire and Julian, 1971). Further loss of functional genes or relaxation of their control over growth would bring the cell closer to an autonomous state.

The possibility that relaxation of genetic control occurs in neoplastic growth and that genetic control can be restored by endocrine therapy is suggested by a number of observations on the behavior of human mammary and prostatic cancers. Administration of estrogen may either stimulate or inhibit the growth of breast cancer in young women according to the dose level utilized. It has therefore been suggested that there is an optimal dose level of estrogen which effects tumor growth while either higher or lower concentrations may depress tumor growth (Segaloff, 1966).

Tumor regression in breast cancer is commonly seen following the administration of estrogens in postmenopausal women (Stoll, 1969), and such a response is seen occasionally also in premenopausal women with breast cancer given massive doses of estrogen (Nathanson and Kelly, 1952; Kennedy, 1962). Kaufman and Escher (1961) observed that most patients whose tumor has regressed under estrogen therapy will experience tumor reactivation, but some will benefit from subsequent withdrawal of the steroid because further tumor regression is induced by this change. In a related observation, Band et al. (1973) found that some patients with metastatic prostatic cancer, no longer responsive to conventional doses of estrogens, showed objective improvement when switched to high doses of estrogens.

These observations can be accommodated by the model proposed in Fig. 17 as follows. Regulation by the nullifier is restored in the postmenopausal woman with small doses of estrogen and with large doses in the premenopausal woman whose cancer presumably is unable to concentrate estrogens in the nucleus in the usual way. If carcinostasis only is achieved, reduction of tumor mass follows slowly as a result of cell turnover without regeneration. A carcinocidal effect is explained by the failure of estrogens to inhibit an activated autophage, but conversely, regression of an apparently autonomous tumor after withdrawal of estrogens entails the activation of an estrogen-inhibited autophagic process. A similar rationale might be adduced to explain the behavior of prostatic cancers in which high doses of estrogens may stimulate the nullifier and autophage to respond.

In the absence of a satisfactory explanation for the paradoxical behavior of many hormone-responsive cancers, the foregoing speculations are useful if only to emphasize the potential importance of the intranuclear concentration of steroidal hormones in the achievement of homeostasis.

V. SUMMARY

Growth of prostate is divided into three phases. First, the phase of initiation is induced if the number of cells in the gland is below normal. During this response, DNA synthesis and cell proliferation are stimulated by administration of androgen. Second, the phase of negative feedback occurs when the number of cells is restored to normal; DNA synthesis is curtailed and cell proliferation is markedly reduced although secretion continues to be stimulated by the administration of androgen. Third, the phase of autophagia commences after the withdrawal of androgens as by orchiectomy and is characterized by extensive autolysis of cells and loss of functional performance.

During the phase of initiation, dihydrotestosterone may be essential for inducing mitotic activity, but DNA synthesis and cell division are refractory to stimulation except in those tissues containing fewer than the normal number of cells. If regeneration begins and goes to completion, as in the prostate of the 7-day castrate animal, the cell population undergoes 1.8 doublings with a doubling time of 40 hours and a division cycle time of 20 hours. Half the daughter cells produced by mitosis do not reenter the proliferative cycle, and to maintain the growth fraction at an average value of 0.5, previously nondividing cells are recruited into the cycle. Over the period of cell proliferation the majority of the cells at the start of proliferation must divide at least once but at most only 4–5 times.

Although negative feedback can be specified in terms of a numerical limit on cell division, it is not governed by the division potential of individual cells; rather, division potential is preordained by the total number of cells in the gland at the start of proliferation.

Autophagia results in the elimination of a large number of prostatic cells, but a few of the original group persist to regenerate the gland if androgen is restored. This residual pool of cells is not one that survives the autophagic process preferentially; on the contrary, it is likely that the loss of cells during prostatic involution is stochastic.

The phases of prostatic growth may represent the expression of genetically determined homeostatic constraint mechanisms which are sensitive to the intranuclear concentration of dihydrotestosterone. Since the concentration of dihydrotestosterone in the nucleus is affected by enzymes that form or metabolize dihydrotestosterone and also by cytoplasmic receptors, the magnitude of the growth response of prostate may be influenced by these means. Although cytoplasmic receptors and the capacity to transport androgens into the nucleus are closely linked phenotypic markers of intracellular steroid hormone action, it appears that the control of androgen concentration in the nucleus is achieved in a more intricate fashion than simply through a dependence on the translocation of 4.4 S androgen–receptor complex into the nucleus. The presence of cytoplasmic receptor is associated with enhanced ability of the cell to incorporate androgens into the nucleus but whether nuclear receptor is related to cytoplasmic receptor remains equivocal.

Sequential analysis of the concentrations of cAMP, cytoplasmic receptor, and nuclear receptor during phases of prostatic involution and growth shows that changes in rates of DNA synthesis and cell proliferation are not attended by coincident changes in the foregoing biochemical parameters. These observations imply that cAMP and androgen receptors are not directly responsible for switching DNA synthesis and cell proliferation on and off. It remains possible that androgens alone are required for the initiation of DNA synthesis and cell proliferation and that the function of nuclear receptor is concerned with the regulation of the autophagic process.

Finally, it is proposed that the expression of homeostatic constraint mechanisms is dependent on the presence of initiator, nullifier, and autophage genes and that loss of functional genes or relaxation of their control over growth is associated with the emergence of neoplasia.

ACKNOWLEDGMENTS

We wish to express our appreciation to Drs. P. Band, T. Nihei, and T. Shnitka for many hours of discussion and time spent in critical evaluation of the ideas presented in this review. We also express our thanks to Sheila Wilson and Carol Dann for painstaking care in assembling and typing the manuscript.

The preparation of this review was aided by grants from the Medical Research Council of Canada (MT 3729) and the National Cancer Institute of Canada (NCI BRU). Dr. N. Bruchovsky is a Scholar of the Medical Research Council of Canada. Drs. B. Lesser and E. Van Doorn are Fellows of the Medical Research Council of Canada.

REFERENCES

Abell, C. W., and Monahan, T. M. (1973). *J. Cell Biol.* **59,** 549.
Anderson, K. M., and Liao, S. (1968). *Nature (London)* **219,** 227.
Ballard, P. L., and Ballard, R. A. (1972). *Proc. Nat. Acad. Sci. U.S.* **69,** 2668.
Band, P. R., Banerjee, T. K., Patwardhan, V. C., and Eid, T. C. (1973). *Can. Med. Ass., J.* **109,** 697.
Brandes, D. (1966). *Int. Rev. Cytol.* **20,** 207.
Brandes, D. (1974). *In* "Structure and Function of Male Accessory Sex Organs" (D. Brandes, ed.), pp. 184. Academic Press, New York.

Brandes, D., and Bourne, G. H. (1963). *Nat. Cancer Inst., Monogr.* **12**, 29.

Brandes, D., and Groth, D. P. (1963). *Nat. Cancer Inst., Monogr.* **12**, 47.

Bruchovsky, N. (1971). *Endocrinology* **89**, 1212.

Bruchovsky, N., and Craven, S. (1975). *Biochem. Biophys. Res. Commun.* **4**, 837.

Bruchovsky, N., and Lesser, B. (1975). *Advan. Sex. Horm. Res.* (in press).

Bruchovsky, N., and Wilson, J. D. (1968a). *J. Biol. Chem.* **243**, 2012.

Bruchovsky, N., and Wilson, J. D. (1968b). *J. Biol. Chem.* **243**, 5953.

Bruchovsky, N., Sutherland, D. J. A., Meakin, J. W., and Minesita, T. (1975a). *Biochim. Biophys. Acta* **381**, 61.

Bruchovsky, N., Rennie, P. S., and Vanson, A. (1975b). *Biochim. Biophys. Acta* **394**, 248.

Bullough, W. S., Laurence, E. B., Iverson, O. H., and Elgjo, K. (1967). *Nature (London)* **214**, 578.

Burkhart, E. Z. (1942). *J. Exp. Zool.* **89**, 132.

Butler, W. W. S., and Schade, A. L. (1958). *Endocrinology* **63**, 271.

Cavazos, L. F., and Melampy, R. M. (1954). *Endocrinology* **54**, 640.

Clark, J., and Gorski, J. (1970). *Science* **169**, 76.

Cleaver, J. E. (1967). *In* "Thymidine Metabolism and Cell Kinetics" (J. E. Cleaver, ed.), p. 247. North-Holland Publ., Amsterdam.

Coffey, D. S. (1974). *In* "Structure and Function of Male Accessory Sex Organs" (D. Brandes ed.), p. 307. Academic Press, New York.

Coffey, D. S., Shimazaki, J., and Williams-Ashman, H. G. (1968). *Arch. Biochem. Biophys.* **124**, 184.

Coyotupa, J., Parlow, A. F., and Kovacic, N. (1973). *Endocrinology* **92**, 1579.

Craven, S., Lesser, B., and Bruchovsky, N. (1974). *Endocrinology* **95**, 1177.

de Duve, C. (1959). *Exp. Cell Res., Suppl.* **7**, 169.

Eker, P. (1974). *J. Cell Sci.* **16**, 301.

Epifanova, O. (1971). *In* "The Cell Cycle and Cancer" (R. Baserga, ed.), p. 145. Dekker, New York.

Froehlich, J. E., and Rachmeler, M. (1972). *J. Cell Biol.* **55**, 19.

Funder, J. W., Feldman, D., and Edelman, I. S. (1972). *J. Steroid Biochem.* **3**, 209.

Gloyna, R. E., Siiteri, P. K., and Wilson, J. D. (1970). *J. Clin. Invest.* **49**, 1746.

Harkin, J. C. (1957). *Endocrinology* **60**, 185.

Harkin, J. C. (1963). *Nat. Cancer Inst., Monogr.* **12**, 85.

Huggins, C. (1947). *Harvey Lect.* **42**, 148.

Ichii, S., Izawa, M., and Murakami, N. (1974). *Endocrinol. Jap.* **21**, 267.

Jung, I., and Baulieu, E. E. (1971). *Biochimie* **53**, 807.

Kaufman, R. J., and Escher, G. C. (1961). *Surg., Gynecol. Obstet.* **113**, 635.

Kennedy, B. J. (1962). *Cancer* **15**, 641.

King, R. J. B., and Mainwaring, W. I. P. (1973). *In* "Steroid-Cell Interactions," p. 41. Univ. Park Press, Baltimore, Maryland.

Kircheim, D., and Scott, W. W. (1965). *Invest. Urol.* **2**, 393.

Kosto, B., Calvin, H. I., and Williams-Ashman, H. G. (1967). *Advan. Enzyme Regul.* **5**, 25.

Lesser, B. (1974). Ph.D. Thesis, University of Alberta, Edmonton, Alberta.

Lesser, B., and Bruchovsky, N. (1973). *Biochim. Biophys. Acta* **308**, 426.

Lesser, B., and Bruchovsky, N. (1974a). *Biochem. J.* **142**, 429.

Lesser, B., and Bruchovsky, N. (1974b). *Biochem. J.* **142**, 483.

Liang, T., and Liao, S. (1975). *Proc. Nat. Acad. Sci. U.S.* **72**, 706.

Liao, S., Fang, S., Tymoczko, J. L., and Liang, T. (1974). *In* "Structure and Function of Male Accessory Sex Organs" (D. Brandes, ed.), p. 237. Academic Press, New York.

Limpaphayom, K., Lee, C., Jacobson, H. I., and King, T. M. (1971). *Amer. J. Obstet. Gynecol.* **111**, 1064.

Lin, S., and Riggs, A. (1975). *Cell* **4**, 107.

Lucas, L. A., and Abraham, G. E. (1972). *Anal. Lett.* **5**, 773.

McBride, O. W., and Peterson, E. A. (1970). *J. Cell Biol.* **47**, 132.

McGuire, W. L., and Julian, J. A. (1971). *Cancer Res.* **31**, 1440.

McGuire, W. L., Chamness, G. C., Costlow, M. E., and Shepherd, R. E. (1974). *Metab., Clin. Exp.* **23**, 75.

MacKenzie, A. R., Hall, T., Lo, M. C., and Whitmore, W. F. (1963). *J. Urol.* **89**, 864.

Macmanus, J. P., Franks, D. I., Youdale, T., and Braceland, B. M. (1972). *Biochem. Biophys. Res. Commun.* **49**, 1201.

Mainwaring, W. I. P., and Mangan, F. R. (1973). *J. Endocrinol.* **59**, 121.

Mainwaring, W. I. P., Mangan, F. R., Irving, R. A., and Jones, D. A. (1974). *Biochem. J.* **144**, 413.

Malamud, D. (1971). *In* "The Cell Cycle and Cancer" (R. Baserga, ed.), p. 145. Dekker, New York.

Mangan, F. R., Neal, G. E., and Williams, D. C. (1967). *Biochem. J.* **104**, 1075.

Mangan, F. R., Pegg, A. E., and Mainwaring, W. I. P. (1973). *Biochem. J.* **134**, 129.

Mann, T. (1964). *In* "The Biochemistry of Semen and the Male Reproductive Tract" (T. Mann, ed.), p. 161. Methuen, London.

Milgrom, E., Thi, L., Atger, M., and Baulieu, E. E. (1973). *J. Biol. Chem.* **248**, 6366.

Miller, R. G., and Phillips, R. A. (1969). *J. Cell. Physiol.* **73**, 191.

Moore, C. R., Price, D., and Gallagher, D. F. (1930). *Amer. J. Anat.* **45**, 71.

Nathanson, I. T., and Kelly, R. M. (1952). *N. Engl. J. Med.* **246**, 135.

Nyden, S. J., and Williams-Ashman, H. G. (1953). *Amer. J. Physiol.* **172**, 588.

Otten, J., Johnson, G. S., and Pastan, I. (1971). *Biochem, Biophys. Res. Commun.* **44**, 1192.

Otten, J., Johnson, G. S., and Pastan, I. (1972). *J. Biol. Chem.* **247**, 7082.

Paris, J. E., and Brandes, D. (1974). *In* "Structure and Function of Male Accessory Sex Organs," (D. Brandes, ed.), p. 223. Academic Press, New York.

Rennie, P., and Bruchovksy, N. (1972). *J. Biol. Chem.* **247**, 1546.

Rennie, P., and Bruchovsky, N. (1973). *J. Biol. Chem.* **248**, 3288.

Robel, P., Lasnitzki, I., and Baulieu, E. E. (1971). *Biochimie* **53**, 81.

Robel, P., Corpechot, C., and Baulieu, E. E. (1973). *FEBS (Fed. Eur. Biochem. Soc.) Lett* **33**, 218.

Robinson, J. H., Smith, J. A., and King, R. J. B. (1974). *Cell* **3**, 361.

Robinson, M. R. G., and Thomas, B. S. (1971). *Brit. Med. J.* **4**, 391.

Ryan, W. L., and Heidrick, M. L. (1968). *Science* **162**, 1484.

Schmid, G. H., Schell, G. H., and Heyder, N. (1973). *Virchows Arch. B* **15**, 65.

Schmidt, H., Noack, I., and Voigt, K. D. (1972). *Acta Endocrinol. (Copenhagen)* **69**, 165.

Segaloff, A. (1966). *Recent. Progr. Horm. Res.* **22**, 351.

Shain, S. A., Boesel, R. W., and Axelrod, L. R. (1975). *Arch. Biochem. Biophys.* **167**, 247.

Sheppard, H., Tsien, W. H., Mayer, P., and Howie, N. (1965). *Biochem. Pharmacol.* **14,** 41.

Sheppard, J. R. (1971). *Proc. Nat. Acad. Sci. U.S.* **68,** 1316.

Siiteri, P. K., and Wilson, J. D. (1970). *J. Clin. Invest.* **49,** 1737.

Singhal, R. L., and Sutherland, D. J. B. (1974). *Advan. Sex Horm. Res.* **1,** 226.

Singhal, R. L., Parulekar, M. R., Vijayvargiya, R., and Robison, G. A. (1971). *Biochem. J.* **125,** 329.

Spaeren, U., Olsnes, S., Brennhovd, I., Efskind, J., and Phil, A. (1973). *Eur. J. Cancer* **9,** 353.

Stoll, B. A. (1969). *In* "Hormone Management in Breast Cancer," p. 54. Lippincott, Philadelphia, Pennsylvania.

Stoll, B. A. (1974). *In* "Mammary Cancer and Neuroendocrine Therapy" (B. A. Stoll, ed.), p. 57. Butterworth, London.

Sullivan, J. N., and Strott, C. A. (1973). *J. Biol. Chem.* **248,** 3202.

Swann, M. M. (1957). *Cancer Res.* **17,** 727.

Swann, M. M. (1958). *Cancer Res.* **18,** 1118.

Thomas, D. B., Medley, G., and Longwood, C. A. (1973). *J. Cell Biol.* **57,** 397.

Tuohimaa, P., Oksanen, A., and Niemi, M. (1973). *Acta Endocrinol. (Copenhagen)* **74,** 379.

Williams-Ashman, H. G., Liao, S., Hancock, R. L., Jurkowitz, L., and Silverman, D. A. (1964). *Recent Progr. Horm. Res.* **20,** 247.

Wittliff, J. L., Hilf, R., Brooks, W. F., Jr., Savlov, E. D., Hall, T. C., and Orlando, R. A. (1971). *Cancer Res.* **32,** 1983.

DISCUSSION

B. Uvnäs: Would you comment on how the use of animal models like the rat prostate has helped in the elucidation of human disease?

N. Bruchovsky: I think it is clear that animal model systems contribute to the development of concepts which often have relevance to human disease and thereby help to stimulate interest in such conditions. For example, the recognition of the metabolism of testosterone in the rat prostate was a prelude to the important observation of dihydrotestosterone accumulation in benign prostatic hyperplasia. The possibility that certain developmental abnormalities, namely male pseudohermaphroditism, may arise because of lack of dihydrotestosterone formation has also been suggested.

D. S. Coffey: In answer to the question of Dr. Uvnäs, we are all aware of the vast physiological and functional differences that are observed in the male reproductive tract in various species. In addition, our knowledge of the development and function of the normal human prostate is very limited. One should be cautious, therefore, in extrapolating studies on rat prostate to predictions of the effects on human normal and abnormal prostatic tissue. However, there are similarities. To my knowledge, there are no estrogens, androgens, or antiandrogens that affect the human prostate and do not also affect the rodent prostate. The reverse, however, has not been established. In addition, both human and rodent prostates have androgen receptors that have similar properties. If one wishes to understand the molecular basis of hormone action, it would certainly be easier to establish this in rodents than in man. Once this is established, it would be important to test these systems in human prostatic tissue.

It may also be incorrect to state that rats do not develop prostatic adenocarcinoma. Dr. Pollard and his colleagues at Notre Dame have observed spontaneous prostatic adenocarcinoma in very old rodents.

M. B. Lipsett: In response to Professor Uvnäs-question, it is important to realize that hormones act as cocarcinogens or promoters of carcinogenesis. There is little evidence that hormones are the direct carcinogens. The carcinogenic event, be it chemical, radiation, or viral, acts on a target tissue that has been stimulated by hormone.

P. Davies: Concerning the relationship between cytoplasmic and nuclear receptors, we have shown that both receptors stimulate rat prostatic nuclear RNA polymerase B equivalently, owing to a conversion of the cytoplasmic receptor complex to a form similar to that of the nuclear receptor complex. A similar conversion of the human cytoplasmic receptor complex can be observed. This suggests functional or physical similarities between the two forms.

N. Bruchovsky: The finding is very interesting and certainly represents one of the first indications that functionally these two forms of binding protein are similar. More of this type of evidence would build a convincing base for the similarity of the cytoplasmic and nuclear receptors.

B. Uvnäs: Can the cytoplasmic receptor seen to occur after castration originate from the nucleus?

N. Bruchovsky: The possibility that the increase in cytoplasmic receptor following castration is explained by the discharge of nuclear receptor into cytoplasm has not been settled. Three points seem to argue against this possibility. First, the increase in the number of cytoplasmic receptors does not appear to be inversely proportional to the decrease in the number of nuclear receptors, although the correlation is close. Second, the rate of increase in the number of cytoplasmic receptors does not correspond to the reciprocal of the rate of decrease of the number of nuclear receptors, at least not exactly. Finally, the cytoplasmic receptor observed has a different configuration than the nuclear receptor.

I. Mainwaring: Would you please comment on the number of nuclear receptor sites? Your estimate of approximately 23,000 per nucleus is considerably higher than the 4000–6000 reported by other investigators. Can this difference in findings be attributed to methodological differences?

N. Bruchovsky: There is no doubt that the difference in the estimates is explained by the use of different methodologies. In our experience, the *in vivo* labeling techniques are far more efficient than the *in vitro* labeling techniques with whole cells or cell-free systems using isolated nuclei. This, I suspect, may account for the varying observations.

E. E. Baulieu: Are there any differences in the types of cells labeled in your velocity sedimentation experiments?

N. Bruchovsky: The cells labeled by radioactive thymidine when administered by a pulse dose under the conditions described are epithelial cells. This has been monitored by radioautography.

E. E. Baulieu: I am not sure that the sort of thymidine labeling index which is constant in terms of proportion of labeled cells in prostatic tissue after castration may mean that you have a uniform pool in which cells are randomly sensitive to hormones. In fact, different cells may react differently to the changes of hormonal conditions, and you should probably take into account the complexity of the cell populations. Moreover, what I discussed after Dr. Williams-Ashman's presentation in terms of gene polymerase and ovalbumin synthesis indicates that it is difficult for me to see, in your overall scheme, two positive actions on cell division and protein synthesis taking place in the same cells at the same time, and I would wish that you introduce into your model a further dimension—time.

Another remark deals with receptor, androstanolone, and their presence in the nuclei. I do not believe in free androstanolone in prostatic nuclei besides the amount released from the high-affinity receptor in virtue of the law of mass action or because of inactivation of the receptor. Moreover, considering the possibility of a nuclear receptor in the absence of cytoplasmic receptor, it is a situation that we have seen, for instance, in chicken liver [M. C. Lebeau *et al., Eur. J. Biochem.* **36,** 294 (1973)]. From a series of considerations, I may state that most likely the cytosol receptor is rapidly transferred into the nucleus when it has bound the hormone, and there remains no "reserve" of receptor in the cytoplasm.

Is any steroid of the nucleus truly free?

N. Bruchovsky: I agree that there may not be any free steroid in the nucleus and that the material appearing in the free peak with chromatographic analysis of nuclear extracts is really loosely bound. However, it should be remembered that free and bound forms of steroid and steroid–receptor complex are in some form of equilibrium within the nucleus.

S. Liao: In some steroid-sensitive tissues, steroids can indeed bind directly to the specific nuclear (receptor) protein. For example, Δ^5-3β,-17β-androstenediol may act in the vaginal cell in this manner. In the rat ventral prostate we still believe that the cytoplasmic receptor is related to the nuclear receptor. The difference between your data and mine may be due to differences in the techniques we are using, as Dr. Mainwaring has pointed out. A definite answer may come from the labeling of the receptor itself, and as I understand, Dr. Tamaoli is working on this.

N. Bruchovsky: Dr. Liao is correct in pointing out that different techniques have been used to label cytoplasmic receptors. While these different techniques may label similar binding sites, the configuration of the protein responsible for the binding is probably determined to some extent by the method of labeling, and therefore I think it is reasonable to predict that heterogeneity of receptor forms might be observed.

Animal Models in the Study of Antiprostatic Drugs

F. NEUMANN,* K.-D. RICHTER,† AND TH. SENGE‡

I. INTRODUCTION

There are very few organs which exhibit such marked species-specific differences as the prostate, and this is true not only for morphological structure, but also for function. Because of this, the extrapolation of animal results to conditions occurring in man are subject to great restrictions.

Unlike in man, spontaneous prostatic tumors are relatively rare in most animal species. This explains why there is not just one animal model in prostatic tumor research, but many models. The animal models currently being used to study drugs active in diseases of the prostate yield only limited information about the suitability of various substances in the therapy of prostatic adenoma or carcinoma.

* *Research Laboratories of Schering AG, Department of Endocrinpharmacology, Berlin, Germany.*

† *Experimental Animal Department, University of Münster, Münster, Germany.*

‡ *Department of Urology, Klinikum, Essen, Germany.*

II. Morphology and Hormonal Regulation of the Prostate of Various Species

A. Morphology of the Prostate in Various Species

The size of the prostate is species-specific being related to that of the testis as it compares to the body size of the respective species (Ellenberger, 1943). In domestic species the prostate is largest in the dog, and it is only in this species that it attains the same degree of compactness as found in man. Hence, by reason of gross anatomy alone, only the dog is suitable for comparative studies. In other domestic animals, such as the bull, the pig, the sheep, and the goat, the prostate is only rudimentary.

The prostates of all the laboratory species are characterized by their pronounced lobulation and differ markedly from the human prostate.

Figure 1 shows a comparison of the histological pictures of the normal rat and dog prostates. The appearance of the latter indicates that the human and canine prostates are rather similar. Depending on the secretory cycle and functional condition, the epithelium is either highly cylindrical with basally situated nuclei (high activity) or cubically shallow (low activity). In contrast to that of the small laboratory animals, the fibromuscular stroma of the dog and human prostate is relatively highly developed. This is the reason for the compactness of the canine and human prostate. In the normal prostate the parenchyma (glandular tissue) predominates throughout all phases of life (for details on species differences of the prostate, see also Bloom, 1954; Franks, 1954; Gerber, 1961; Price, 1962).

B. Hormonal Regulation of the Prostate

The growth and function of the normal prostate are androgen dependent. The prostate atrophies in the absence of androgens (for review, see Huggins, 1945; Price and Williams-Ashman, 1961). Even the rudimentary development of the prostate is androgen dependent. The prostate fails to develop if castration is performed before somatic sexual differentiation (for reveiw, see Jost, 1965). The same effect can be achieved by treating the pregnant mothers with an antiandrogen (for review, see Neumann et al., 1970a, b).

Which other hormones apart from androgens are or could be of significance for prostatic function? First of all, there are the estrogens and prolactin. As far back as 1939, Korenchevsky and Dennison (1939) attributed physiological importance to the estrogens stating that estrogens exert their main effect on the stroma, that is, on the fibromuscular section of the prostate.

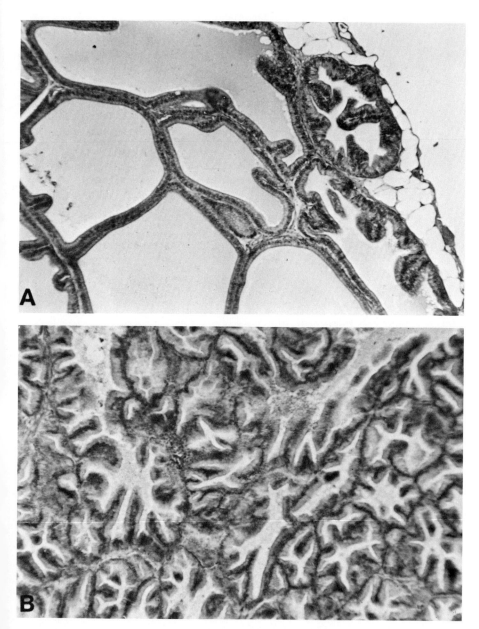

FIG. 1. Normal prostate histology. (A) Rat. (B) Dog. Hematoxylin and eosin; ×100.

To quote Korenchevsky and Dennison (1939): "Two effects produced by estrone in castrated rats appear to be physiological and were seen in the seminal vesicles and coagulating gland and to a lesser degree in the prostate: (a) stimulation of the development of smooth muscle (b) enhancement of the effect produced by testicular hormone." The observation that involution of the prostate is more pronounced after hypophysectomy than after castration indicates that the pituitary hormones can also have a direct influence on the prostate. This observation was made by Huggins and Russel in 1946, and we quote: "After hypophysectomy, the prostatic epithelium undergoes profound atrophy, being reduced to the prepuberal state. Prostatic acid phosphatase is decreased below the castrate level to values comparable with those found in juvenile animals. Alkaline phosphatase is decreased to prepuberal levels after hypophysectomy."

Attention was immediately centered on prolactin as a matter of course, partly for the simple reason that, at that time, nothing was known about the function of prolactin in male individuals. There are now a great number of studies on the role of prolactin in prostatic function (Chase et al., 1957; Grayhack, 1963; Grayhack et al., 1955; Reddi, 1969; Segaloff et al., 1956; von Berswordt-Wallrabe et al., 1969). There is no room here for more than a telegram-style account of some of the findings.

Prolactin increases the accumulation of zinc in the prostate (Moger and Geschwind, 1972). It potentiates generally the effects of androgens on the prostate. It should also be mentioned that the prostate binds prolactin to a much greater extent than any other organ. Asano (1965) even found some indication that a negative feedback mechanism exists between prostatic activity and prolactin secretion. The secretion of prolactin diminished after treatment of rats with prostatic fluid.

Other hormones said to have a positive influence on the prostate are progesterone (von Berswordt-Wallrabe et al., 1970, 1971), growth hormone (Lostroh, 1962), ACTH (Tisell and Angervall, 1969), and glucocorticoids (Harper et al., 1974; Lloyd, 1965; Mobbs et al., 1973; Roland et al., 1975).

III. EFFECT OF EXOGENOUSLY ADMINISTERED HORMONES ON THE FUNCTION OF THE NORMAL PROSTATE

Since prostate function is androgen dependent, it naturally becomes drastically reduced after hypophysectomy, castration, treatment with fairly potent antigonadotropic substances, such as estrogens, and treatment with antiandrogens.

Atrophy of the organ and loss of enzymes that are specific for active prostatic function occur. This is true for all species.

A number of models are available in which can be studied the action of hormones or drugs in general on the function of the normal prostate. Intact animals are sometimes used as models, but more often castrated, androgen-substituted animals are used.

A. Effect of Androgens

Tesar and Scott (1964), who have tested a large number of hormones and other drugs for their effect on the rat prostate, have thoroughly analyzed the varying effects that weak and strong androgens have in intact animals and in castrated animals undergoing androgen replacement (cf. Fig. 2).

The situation in the intact animals is shown in the left half of Fig. 2. The normal feedback mechanism is shown on the far left, and the effect of a weak androgen can be seen in the middle. A weak androgen suppresses the pituitary gonadotropins, probably only interstitial cell-stimulating hormone (ICSH) or luteinizing hormone (LH), thus diminishing the testicular secretion of androgens. A relative androgen deficiency must

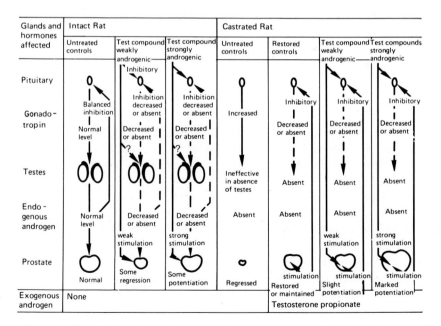

Fig. 2. Influence of weak and strong androgens on prostate weight in intact and castrated androgen-substituted rats. From Tesar and Scott (1964).

exist at the level of the prostate, since a weak androgen is not strong enough to compensate fully for the decrease of testicular androgens. Thus, slight regression of the prostate can be observed. Although the administration of a strong androgen also inhibits the testicular biosynthesis of androgens, the direct stimulating effect of the administered androgen is strong enough to compensate for the absence of testicular androgens. If the dose administered is high enough, even hyperstimulation is possible, as we have already shown. The situation is simple in castrated animals undergoing replacement therapy with testosterone propionate. The effect of both weak and strong androgens is, so to speak, added to the effect of the replaced androgen (right half of Fig. 2).

B. Effect of Estrogens

In intact animals, estrogens affect the accessory sex glands, and thus the prostate as well, in two ways: (1) indirectly—via inhibition of gonadotropin secretion and thus suppression of testicular androgen synthesis; (2) directly.

Very great species-specific differences have been observed with regard to the direct effect of estrogens on the prostate (for reviews, see Huggins, 1945; Price and Williams-Ashman, 1961).

The indirect effect of estrogens on the prostate, that is, the inhibition of testicular androgen biosynthesis, causes regressive changes similar in part to those that occur after castration. The weight decreases, there is involution of the epithelium, and the prostate ceases its secretory activity.

The direct effect of estrogens manifests itself (a) as a stimulation of the fibromuscular tissue (Korenchevsky and Dennison, 1939); (b) during prolonged treatment as the induction of squamous hyperplasia and metaplasia of the epithelium (Korenchevsky and Dennison, 1939).

Keratinization has also been described, although it has not yet been observed in man.

In intact animals, the direct and indirect effects of estrogens overlap each other. If, for instance, we consider only the fibromuscular tissue, then we observe synergism between estrogens and androgens. Conversely, if we take a look at the epithelium or measure the secretory activity as a parameter for the functional condition of the organ, then we find that antagonism exists. These situations have been excellently reviewed in a paper by Tesar and Scott (1964).

In Fig. 3 (left), the normal feedback mechanism can again be seen, next to it is a picture of what happens when an intact animal is treated with estrogens. The testicular secretion of androgens decreases via an inhibition of gonadotropin secretion and regression of the prostate occurs.

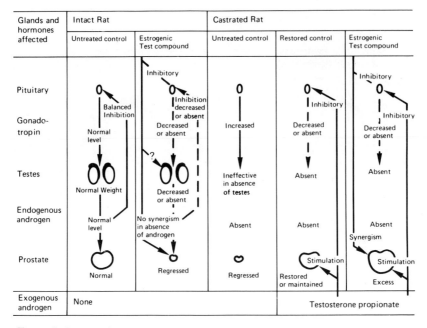

FIG. 3. Influence of estrogens on prostate weight in intact and castrated androgen-substituted rats. From Tesar and Scott (1964).

Since no androgens are available, no synergism can be observed at the level of the prostate. If, however, castrated animals under androgen replacement are treated with estrogens, then synergism is observed in this organ.

The issue of estrogen/androgen antagonism is confused, and the findings of various investigators differ markedly. The results apparently depend also on the species being studied. It is clear that in intact animals—and naturally in man as well—estrogens bring about involution of the prostate via an inhibition of gonadotropin secretion. It is surprising that a direct antagonism apparently also exists in some species, for example, in the dog (Huggins and Clark, 1940; Goodwin et al., 1961).

The secretory activity of the prostate can be maintained by androgen replacement in castrated and hypophysectomized dogs. If such animals are treated with diethylstilbestrol, prostatic secretion decreases and finally ceases altogether (Fig. 4). The mechanism by which this effect occurs is not known. However, whatever the actual mechanism, it must be a direct one in the prostate itself. We ourselves have been unable to demonstrate a direct estrogen/androgen antagonism in rats (Neumann et al., 1967).

The metaplasia-inducing effect is a very specific estrogen effect, and

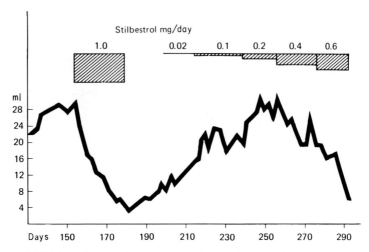

Fɪɢ. 4. Inhibition of prostatic secretion in the fistula dog. Testosterone propionate, 10 mg/day. Note the direct androgen/estrogen antagonism. From Huggins and Clark (1940).

apparently all organs or tissues that originate embryologically from the epithelium of the urogenital sinus react to the administration of estrogens with squamous metaplasia or even cornification. The prostate is one such organ. Zuckerman (1940), who conducted a great deal of research into the effects of estrogens on the accessory sex glands, wrote as follows on this subject: "Stratified squamous proliferation of metaplasia is usually a primary response of tissue in whose development oestrogen sensitive entodermal sinus epithelium has played a part."

It has also been found possible to induce epithelial metaplasia in almost all accessory sex glands in rats by means of neonatal estrogen treatment (Arai, 1968).

The direct effects of estrogens on the prostate have been described very clearly by Korenchevsky and Dennison (1939). However, they wrote about the pathological effects, and we quote: "Of the pathological effects of oestrone the most important are the fibrosis and epithelial metaplasia produced in some of the secondary sex organs in castrated rats. In particular the following changes in the prostate of castrated rats are produced: in all lobes a slight increase in the size of the epithelial tubules and in the amount of secretion; in the dorsal lobe a hyper- and metaplasia of the epithelial cells converting a number of tubules into nearly solid chords; in the dorsal lobe a hyper- and metaplasia of the epithelial cells converting a number of tubules into nearly solid chords; chiefly in the dorsal and central lobes an increase of smooth muscle and to a greater extent of fibrous tissue. The administration of testicular hormones simultaneously with oestrone into castrated rats almost completely prevented these changes in the secondary sex organs, nor were these changes present to a significant extent in normal rats possessing natural testicular hormone, when these rats were injected with oestrone."

C. Effect of Antiandrogens

Following administration of effective antiandrogens, atrophy of the prostate occurs and the secretory activity ceases both in rodents and in

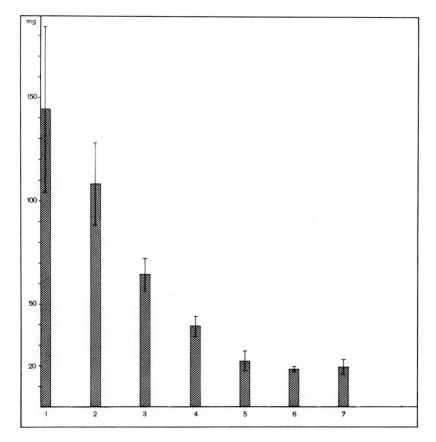

Fig. 5. Inhibition of the effect of testosterone propionate (TP) by cyproterone acetate (CA) in castrated rats (100 gm body weight). Parameter: prostate weight; duration of treatment: 7 days. Daily dose per animal given subcutaneously: group 1: TP, 0.1 mg; group 2: TP, 0.1 mg + CA, 0.1 mg; group 3: TP, 0.1 mg + CA, 0.3 mg; group 4: TP, 0.1 mg + CA, 1.0 mg; group 5: TP, 0.1 mg + CA, 3.0 mg; group 6: TP, 0.1 mg + CA, 10.0 mg; group 7 is castrated control.

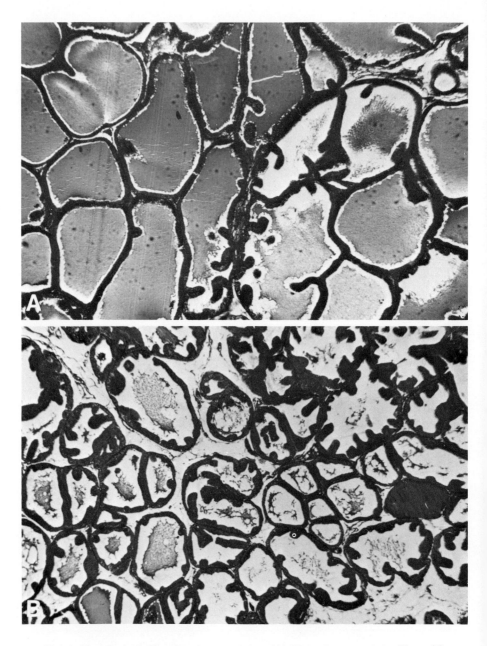

FIG. 6. Hostological slices from rat prostates. (A) Normal rat prostate. The epithe-lium is cuboidal or cylindrical. The glandular lumina are filled with secretion. (B) Rat prostate after 4 weeks of subcutaneous implantation with five silicone-rubber devices containing cyproterone actate. The acini are small in comparison to those of controls and the epithelium is reduced in height. There is little, or hardly any, secretion left in the lumina. The prostate is atrophied. Release rate: ∼300–400 μg/day. Azan stain; ×64.

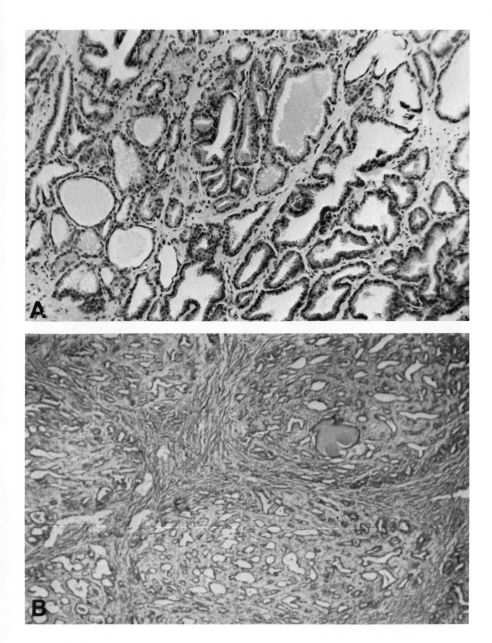

Fig. 7. Canine prostate. (A) Untreated control. (B) After treatment with a daily intramuscular dose of 10 mg of cyproterone acetate per kilogram for 32 days. Hematoxylin and eosin; ×160.

dog and man. It has been shown in rats and mice that antiandrogens are therefore active both in intact and in castrated androgen-substituted animals (for review, see Neumann and Steinbeck, 1974).

A few examples of this are presented below: Figure 5 shows the dose-dependent decrease of prostatic weight of rats following treatment with an antiandrogen, cyproterone acetate. Histologically, there is atrophy of the glandular alveoli, the epithelial cells are shallow, and the lumina of the alveoli are no longer filled with secretion (see Fig. 6).

Dogs react with even greater sensitivity than rodents to antiandrogens, or at least to treatment with cyproterone acetate. Pronounced signs of prostatic regression occurred after only 32 days of treatment with 10 mg/kg intramuscularly per day (see Fig. 7). The effects were even more pronounced after 55 weeks of oral treatment with 100 mg/kg daily. It

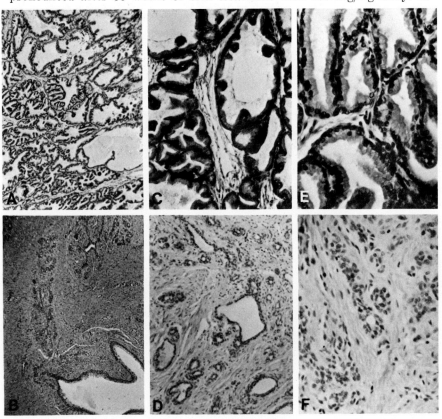

FIG. 8. Canine prostate. (A, C, E) Untreated control. (B, D, F) After treatment with a daily peroral dose of 100 mg of cyproterone acetate per kilogram for 55 weeks. Note complete atrophy of the glandular epithelium. Hematoxylin and eosin; (A), (B), ×40; (C), (D), ×160; (E), (F), ×400.

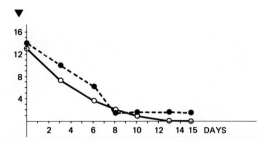

Fig. 9. Prompt reduction in the volume of prostatic secretion (ordinate milli-liters of prostatic fluid) in two prostatic fistula dogs (dog 4.11, ●---● ; dog 4.20, ○—○) the daily intramuscular administration of 10.0 mg of cyproterone acetate. From Bridge and Scott, (1964).

was even difficult to recognize the prostate as an organ. The epithelial section had almost completely disappeared, and the stroma was apparently increased—I say "apparently" because, after long-term treatment with cyproterone acetate, the atrophy occurs almost exclusively at the expense of the parenchyma. I shall return to this aspect. Figure 8 shows the regressive changes in the canine prostate following 55 weeks of treatment with cyproterone acetate. Using the Huggins fistula dog (Huggins and Sommer (1953), Bridge and Scott (1964) were able to show that the secretory function of the prostate ceases completely within 14 days after the administration of 10 mg of cyproterone acetate per kilogram daily (see Fig. 9).

It is known from the study of the ejaculate in men treated with daily doses of 50 mg and more cyproterone acetate that the normal human prostate reacts to antiandrogens in the same way (for review, see (Mothes *et al.*, 1972; Ott, 1968; Ott and Hoffet, 1968).

IV. Spontaneous Tumors of the Prostate in Animals and the Influence of Hormones

Benign prostatic hypertrophy has been observed only in dogs (see Fig. 10). In contrast to prostatic adenoma in man, it occurs diffusely throughout the whole organ (in man, prostatic adenoma originates in the periurethral glands, the so-called inner prostate). Thus, prostatic adenoma in man and prostatic hypertrophy in the dog are not comparable with one another (Brendler, 1962; Moore, 1943).

In contrast to prostatic adenoma in man, prostatic hypertrophy in the dog can be cured by eliminating the source of androgens. It is known from the early studies of Huggins (1945) that the benign hypertrophy of the canine prostate regresses after castration. This observation has

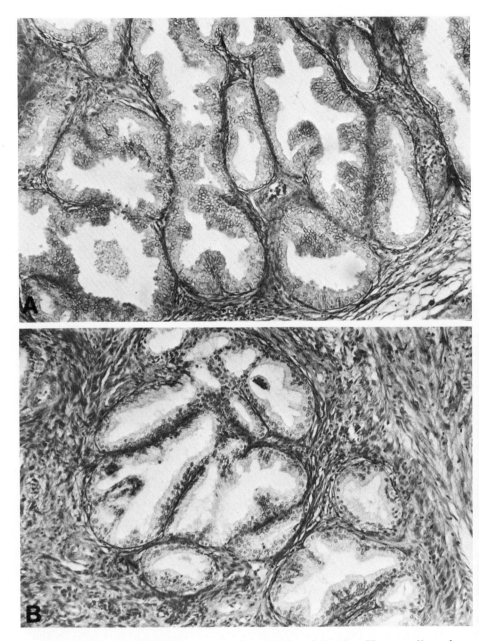

FIG. 10. (A) and (B) Benign prostate hypertrophy of the dog. Hematoxylin and eosin; ×100.

been confirmed following the use of cyproterone acetate in curative veterinary medicine. The dogs became free of all symptoms within 14 days.
The daily dose administered was 0.5 to 0.75 mg/kg (Schmidtke and
Schmidtke, 1968). Furthermore, prostatitis in the dog was also recommended as an indication for the antiandrogen. It has also been established
that cyproterone acetate has a favorable influence on anal and preputial
epitheliomata in the dog (Schmidtke and Schmidtke, 1968).

Neri and co-workers (Neri, 1971; Neri et al., 1968; Neri and Monahan,
1972) investigated three antiandrogens, cyproterone acetate, 16-methyl-
enechlormadinone acetate and the nonsteroidal antiandrogen, flutamide,
using benign prostatic hypertrophy of the dog as a model. All three substances proved to be effective, as demonstrated by parameters such as
the size of the organ, the height of the epithelium, and histochemically
by the disappearance of the acid phosphatases. Two examples of this
study group are shown in Fig. 11 and Table I.

Thus, benign prostatic hypertrophy in the dog reacts to hormones just
as does the healthy prostate. Unfortunately, this is not true for human
prostatic adenoma, so the results gained with this model have only very
little relevance to human medicine.

Spontaneously occurring prostatic carcinomas, and more rarely sar-
comas, are likewise occasionally observed in the dog (Dixon and Moore,
1952). However, the frequency of prostatic carcinoma in the dog is far
too low for the experimental testing of hormones or drugs, and all the
more so since almost all the observations are made by chance.

Mastomys might be a suitable model for the investigation of substances
in respect of their effect in prostatic carcinoma. These as yet little domes-
ticated South African rodents present us with a peculiarity inasmuch as
the female animals also have a well developed ventral prostate even without previous androgen stimulation (Brambell and Davis, 1940) (see Figs.
12 and 13). There is even a report on the spontaneous occurrence of
adenocarcinomas in the prostate of female *Mastomys* (Snell and Stewart,
1965). Otherwise, the occurrence of prostatic adenocarcinoma has only
been reported in the Syrian golden hamster (Fortner et al., 1962).

V. EXPERIMENTAL INDUCTION OF PROSTATIC TUMORS

A. *In Vivo*

Since in the usual laboratory animals prostatic tumors do not occur
at all, or only exceptionally, there have been numerous attempts at inducing such tumors in the hope of finding a useful model for the testing
of hormones and other drugs. Indeed, tumors have been induced in the

TABLE I

EFFECTS OF CYPROTERONE ACETATE (CA), ORCHIECTOMY, AND TESTOSTERONE PROPIONATE (TP) ON CANINE PROSTATE HYPERTROPHY[a]

No. of dogs	Condition of prostate	Treatment and daily dose	Prostate volume[b] (cm³ ± SE)	Diameter of glands (μm ± SE)	Epithelial cell height (μm ± SE)	Ratio of smooth muscle to fibrous tissue
4	Hyperplastic	CA, 10 mg	B 43.6 ± 8.3	201.0 ± 27.4	26.4 + 4.1	3:1
			T 11.6 ± 2.7**	83.1 ± 18.4**	7.5 ± 1.5**	1:5
2	Hyperplastic	Orchiectomy	B 34.9 ± 6.3	148.6 ± 1.8	21.0 ± 2.4	3:1
			T 8.5 ± 1.5**	45.5 ± 4.2**	5.4 ± 0.3**	1:6
4	Hyperplastic	Controls	B 27.4 ± 3.9	157.4 ± 13.5	23.2 ± 1.2	3:1
			T 28.7 ± 3.2	183.4 ± 15.5	24.6 ± 0.3	4:1
3	Normal	TP, 25 mg	B 12.7 ± 1.6	97.2 ± 2.4	12.0 ± 0.3	1:1
			T 32.4 ± 4.5*	210.6 ± 1.4**	35.1 ± 1.0**	3:1

[a] From Neri et al. (1968).
[b] B = beginning; T = terminal autopsy.
* Significantly different from beginning biopsy, $p < 0.05$.
** Significantly different from beginning biopsy, $p < 0.01$.

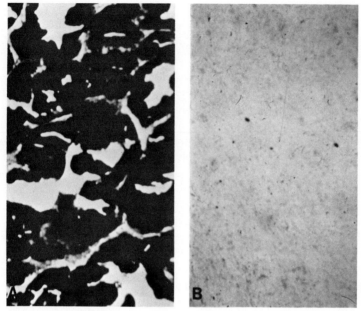

FIG. 11. Canine prostate hypertrophy. Gomori's acid phosphatase reaction. (A) Untreated control. (B) Six weeks after treatment with cyproterone acetate, 10 mg/day intramuscularly. Note lack of acid phosphatase activity. ×100 From Neri *et al.,* (1968).

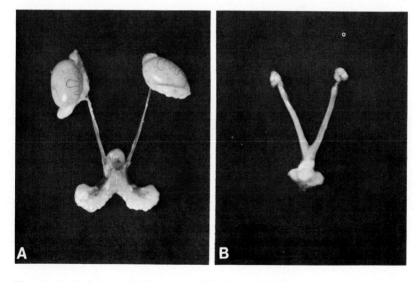

FIG. 12. Genital tract of *Mastomys*. (A) Male. (B) Female. Note the prostate in the female. ×5.

prostates of rats or mice by the local application of carcinigenic hydrocarbons in the form of crystals (Bonzoni *et al.*, 1968), pellets (Dunning,
1962; Dunning *et al.*, 1946; Segaloff, 1962), or impregnated threads
(Schirmer, 1962).

Attempts at induction were also successful on homologous prostatic
transplants of the mouse, using methylcholanthrene (Horning, 1946).
Squamous cell carcinoma was induced in most cases (Horning and
Dmochowski, 1947; Moore and Melchiona, 1937), and more rarely adenocarcinoma (Gupta *et al.*, 1971; Mirand and Stubitz, 1956). Metastatic
spread was observed extremely rarely.

Unfortunately, all these models proved to be of little value because
there was no hormone dependency. Paradoxically, even stimulation of
the tumor tissue was occasionally observed under estrogens (Kazuta,
1967).

In their chapter in "Sex and Internal Secretion" on the subject of the
accessory sex glands, Price and Williams-Ashman (1961) expressed in
one sentence everything that can be said about these models: "Such investigations have contributed to an understanding of early neoplastic
changes in the rodent prostate, but have had limited applicability to the
problem of hormonal control of prostatic cancer in men."

B. *In Vitro*

In vitro attempts to induce degeneration of prostatic cells with the
help of carcinogenic hydrocarbons have also been successful (Lasnitzki,
1962). For instance, after the addition of 20-methylcholanthrene to cultures, anaplastic areas with focal mitoses were found in addition to metaplastic and hyperplastic areas.

Multilayer cultures, with cells showing anaplastic changes and abnormal mitoses, developed from monolayer cultures after the addition of
carcinogenic hydrocarbons (Chen and Heidelberger, 1969). Even the re-
transplantation of *in vitro* malignantly degenerated cells has been partially successful; the result was the development of fibrosarcomas. However, also these models have proved to be of little use in applied research
for the same reasons obtaining for the corresponding *in vivo* models—
either because of a lack of response to hormones or because of paradoxical
hormone effects.

VI. Tissue Culture of Prostatic Tumors

Both carcinoma and adenoma tissue can be cultivated. There are two
basic techniques for this—suspension cultures and organ cultures. In the

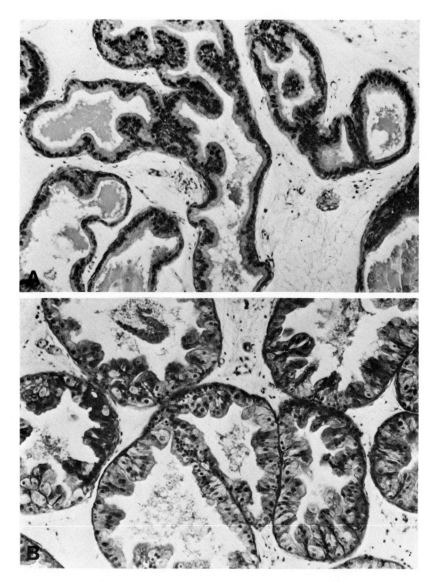

FIG. 13. Histological appearance of the prostate in the male and female *Mastomys*. (A) Male. (B) Female. Hematoxylin and eosin; ×160.

suspension culture method, the prostatic cells are separated from the cell unit by means of proteases (trypsin) and then grow on the bottom of a petri dish. In the organ culture method, small pieces of tissue are embedded in a petri dish and then covered with the medium. Cells then

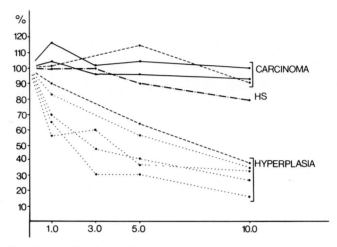

F_IG. 14. Monolayer cell culture of prostate carcinoma and prostate adenoma cells. Effect of testosterone (μg/ml, abscissa) on relative plating efficiency. - · · - · ·, cutis. From Brehmer and Madsen (1973).

bud out of the tissue specimens. Such cultures can be kept alive for weeks and even months.

However, for various reasons the value of the information gained from these models is also low. Tissue cultures are inhomogeneous, in addition to epithelial cells there are also fibroblasts and muscle cells and also epithelium-like cells that do not originate from the prostatic glandular epithelium (Brehmer et al., 1972; Riemann et al., 1973; Schröder, 1973; Wojewski, 1965). One particular type of cell can predominate and over-grow all other types. The culture medium does not correspond to the physiological milieu, the cells lose properties which are specific for the prostate, to be replaced by new properties which are not usually present. It has also been demonstrated that it is primarily the prostatic carcinoma cell which dies and the metaplastic epithelial cell which survives.

From what has just been said it is obvious that the results on the hormone dependency of prostatic carcinoma or adenoma tissue cultures are very contradictory. Generally speaking, estrogens have a growth-inhibiting effect (Brehmer and Madsen, 1973), which is not really surprising since it is known that, at unphysiologically high concentrations, estrogens possess antimitotic properties. On the other hand, testosterone also has a growth-inhibiting effect in some cultures (Brehmer and Madsen, 1973), or at least no androgen withdrawal syndrome could be observed in the cultures (Schröder, 1973; Wojewski, 1965) (see also Figs. 14 and 15).

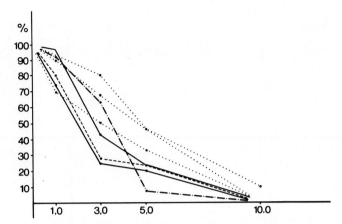

FIG. 15. Monolayer cell culture of prostate carcinoma and prostate adenoma cells. Effect of diethylstilbestrol (μg/ml, abscissa) on plating efficiency. —, Prostate carcinoma; · · ·, prostate hyperplasia; ·---, cutis. From Brehmer and Madsen (1973).

It can be concluded that extrapolation from such studies *in vivo* conditions is hardly justified.

After reimplantation of a cell strain of a prostatic carcinoma (EB 33) (Okada and Schröder, 1974) into the nude mouse, mainly dedifferentiated tumors developed. These fast growing carcinomas had no similarities with the original tumor (see Fig. 16). Hormone dependence was not shown (Okada *et al.*, 1975). Thus, the present cell culture methods are hardly suitable for the testing of antiprostatic cancer drugs.

VII. HETEROLOGOUS TRANSPLANTATION OF PROSTATIC TUMORS AND THE INFLUENCE OF HORMONES

This method, developed by Senge and co-workers (1973), was based on the technique of heterotransplantation of human cervical epithelium into newborn rats, which was described by Forsberg and Ingemanson (1967). The modified method involves the implantation of human prostatic adenoma tissue from the lateral lobe into the femoral muscles of newborn rats. Immunosuppression is assured by subcutaneous injection of antilymphocyte serum. The study takes 3 weeks. Histological and histochemical enzyme reactions are regarded as the criteria for the viability of the transplanted adenoma tissue (Richter *et al.*, 1971). Another proof of tissue viability is active DNS synthesis (Senge *et al.*, 1972).

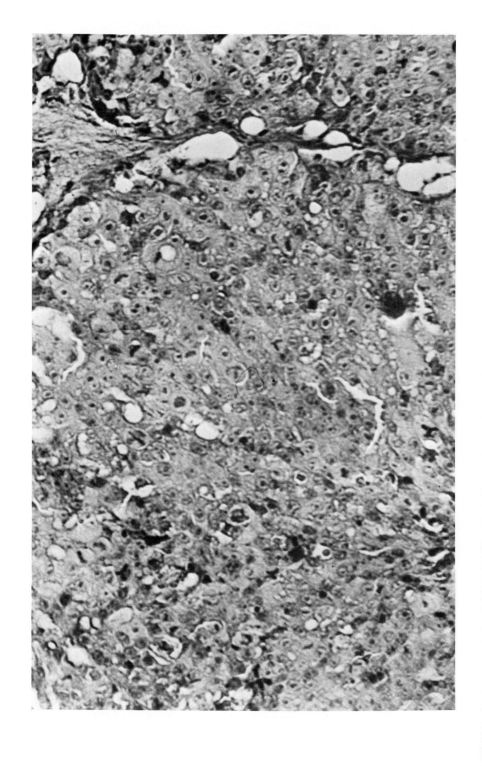

Some of the findings obtained by the use of this model are indicated in Fig. 17.

Without androgen replacement the transplant develops well, although the rate of progress is reduced and the secretory activity is low. Following androgen replacement, the transplants showed the typical differentiation of prostatic hyperplasia. They consist of stroma and parenchyma and show secretory activity—as evidenced by positive acid phosphatase—and Hale reactions. The presence of succinodehydrogenase activity shows that the energy exchange is undisturbed (Fig. 17). However, the stimulating effect of androgen replacement is already recognizable in the histological picture. The glandular epithelium becomes highly cylindrical, pseudo-papilli develop, and the mitosis rate in the epithelium is increased, which is also recognizable by the increased uptake of ^{3}H-labeled thymidine (Lunglmayr et al., 1973a,b).

Since the increased amount of prostatic fluid cannot be drained off, epithelial atrophy is sometimes observed in the glandular alveoli because of fluid congestion (secondary epithelial atrophy). Very frequently, metaplastic changes of the glandular epithelium can be observed in the transplants. This is squamous cell metaplasia, which displays an altered biological quality (Fig. 17).

We presume that this metaplasia develops as a result of nutritional disturbances. The metaplastic epithelium has lost a number of properties that are specific for the prostate. The reaction to acid phosphatase becomes negative, and secretory activity can now be observed only in the unchanged epithelium lining the residual lumina of the glandular alveoli, as indicated in Fig. 17.

Studies on the hormone dependency or, even better, suppressibility of adenoma tissue have produced some interesting results. The adenoma tissue was influenced neither by estrogens nor by treatment with anti-androgens (cyproterone acetate). However, the metaplastically changed epithelium behaved differently. Both estrogen and cyproterone acetate treatment led to hydropic vacuolar degeneration (Fig. 17).

It can be concluded from these results that (1) estrogens exert their effect directly, not only via inhibition of the endogenous testosterone synthesis; (2) antiandrogens exert their effect in a similar way to estrogens—that is, likewise directly.

FIG. 16. Histology of a prostatic tumor grown in the "nude" mouse, 35 days after sucutaneous injection of 1.0×10^6 cells of the EB 33 strain derived from a human prostatic carcinoma (mouse treated with 25 mg of testosterone enanthate subcutaneously every 3 weeks). The solid carcinoma shows extreme nuclear pleomorphism and many mitotic cells. This fast growing carcinoma has no similarities to the original tumor. Hormone dependence was not shown. Hematoxylin and eosin; ×250. From Okada et al. (1975).

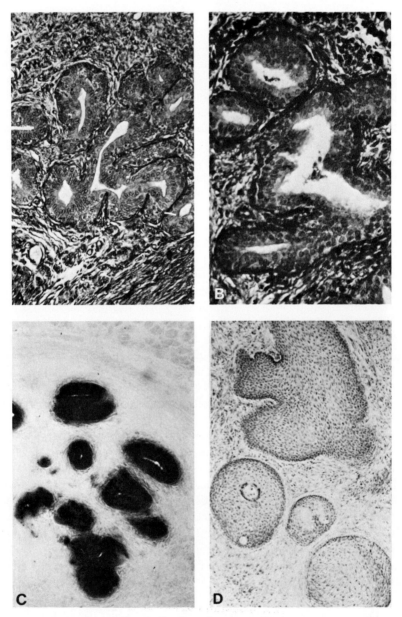

FIG. 17. For legend see page 128.

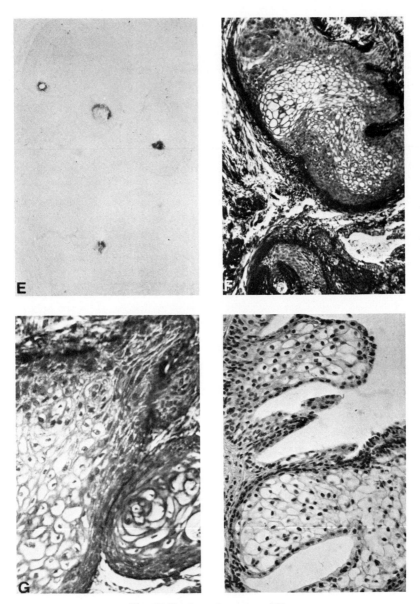

FIG. 17. For legend see page 128.

Using this model, it has not been possible so far to transplant carcinoma tissue. Rejection of the implanted tissue always occurs. Nevertheless, certain tentative conclusions about the effectiveness of antiandrogens in the treatment of prostatic carcinoma can be drawn from the results of heterotranplantation of adenoma tissue. For instance, it is known that following estrogen treatment degenerative changes of the cells occur in the metaplastic areas of the carcinoma tissue that are similar to those that occur in the metaplastic areas of the adenoma transplants (Faul et al., 1971; Franks, 1960; Fergusson, 1972; Huggins et al., 1941; Kahle et al., 1943; Ruppert, 1953). Since cyproterone acetate brings about the same changes in these areas as estrogens, it can be cautiously concluded by analogy that cyproterone acetate will have the same effect in prostatic carcinoma. However, the proof of this is still outstanding.

FIG. 17. (A–E) Prostate heterotransplant under androgen treatment. Prostate adenoma tissue was grafted immediately after prostatectomy into newborn female Sprague-Dawley rats. Twenty-four hours after the operation, 0.07 ml of antilymphocyte serum was injected subcutaneously into the neckfolds of the rats. From the third day on, the dose was increased to 0.1 ml of antilymphocyte serum once every second day until day 17 after transplantation. Testosterone propionate, 1.2 mg, was given subcutaneously to the host animal in a 1:5 mixture of benzyl benzoate and castor oil between day 6 and day 18 of the experiment, divided into three injections each.

(A, B) Note fully developed glandular epithelium, which is clearly active and has pseudopapillary proliferations. (A) Azan, ×150; (B) Goldner; ×250.

(C) Acid phosphatase reaction. Note strong positive reaction of the acid phosphatase in the active glandular epithelium of typical alveoli. ×250.

(D) Note proliferation and metaplastic transformation of the glandular epithelium. Hematoxylin and eosin; ×100.

(E) Acid phosphatase reaction. Note absence of reaction of the acid phosphatase in the metaplastic epithelium, positive reaction restricted to the rest of the secretory epithelium. ×100.

(F) Prostate heterotransplant under simultaneous treatment of estradiol benzoate plus testosterone propionate. Transplantation techniques the same as for (A)–(E). Estradiol benzoate, 0.8 mg, plus 0.6 mg of testosterone propionate as given subcutaneously to the host animals in a 1:5 mixture of benzyl benzoate and castor oil between day 6 and day 18 of the experiment, divided into three equal injections. Note bloated type of degeneration and pycnosis in the metaplastic epithelium. Azan; ×100.

(G) Prostate heterotransplant under combined treatment of testosterone propionate plus cyproterone acetate. Transplantation techniques the same as for (A)–(E). Cyproterone acetate, 36 mg, plus 0.6 mg of testosterone propionate was given. Note bloated type of degeneration of the metaplastic epithelium. Azan; ×250.

(H) Human prostate carcinoma tissue after estrogen treatment (biopsy) provided by courtesy of Dr. Haberich of the Pathologisches Institut der Krankenanstalten Neuss, West Germany. Note bloated type of degeneration and pycnosis in carcinoma tissue. Hematoxylin and eosin; ×250.

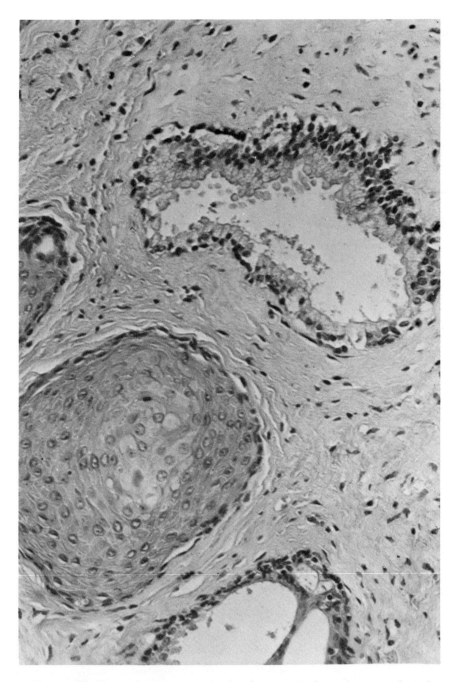

FIG. 18. Histology of a human prostatic adenoma, 82 days after transplantation into the "nude" mouse (mouse treated with 25 mg of testosterone enanthate subcutaneously every 3 weeks). High columnar and secretory active epithelial cells can be seen in the acini on the right side. The acinus on the left is completely filled with metaplastic epithelial cells. Hematoxylin and eosin; ×~400. From Okada *et al.* (1975).

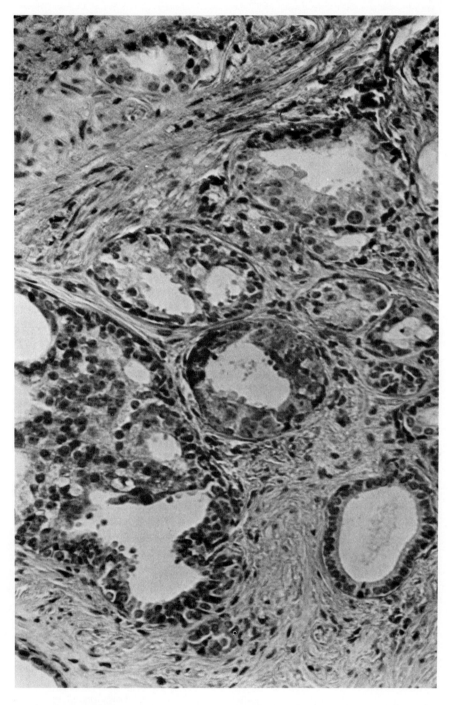

Fig. 19. Histology of a human prostatic carcinoma, 82 days after transplantation into a castrated male "nude" mouse without substitution of testosterone, excision after 40 days. Hematoxylin and eosin; ×~400. From Okada et al. (1975).

Schröder's study group (Schröder *et al.*, 1974) in Würzburg has now succeeded in transplanting human prostatic carcinoma and adenoma tissue into the nude mouse (absence of thymus) (see Figs. 18 and 19). It is possible that this model will provide more definite conclusions about the effect of antiandrogens and hormones or drugs generally on human prostatic carcinoma.

VIII. Summary and Conclusions

1. Since there are considerable species differences in the macroscopic and histological structure as well as in the function of the prostate, there is no perfect animal model for the study of antiprostatic drugs. The canine prostate is more comparable to the human prostate than that of any other species.

2. As regards the hormonal regulation of the normal prostate, all species behave identically or at least very similarly. To study the effect of antiprostatic drugs one can use intact or castrated animals, rodents or dogs. Of importance is the fact that a direct androgen–estrogen antagonism in a narrower sense exists only in the dog, but not in the rat—that is, not in the castrated rat under androgen replacement therapy.

3. With the exception of benign prostatic hypertrophy in the dog, spontaneous tumors of the prostate are rare in animals. However, prostatic hypertrophy in the dog is poorly comparable to that in man. In contrast to prostatic adenoma in man, prostatic hypertrophy in the dog is just as hormone (androgen) dependent as the normal prostate. This model (prostatic hypertrophy of the dog) therefore offers few advantages over normal canine prostate.

4. Studies on prostatic tumors induced experimentally by carcinogens (*in vivo* and *in vitro*) are of relatively little value because these tumors are not hormone dependent or because paradoxical reactions occur.

5. Tissue cultures as models to study antiprostatic drugs are likewise of limited value owing to the dedifferentiation of the cells, the inhomogeneity of the cellular material and the more or less unspecific reaction to hormones.

6. The most promising method currently available appears to be the heterologous transplantation of human prostatic adenoma and carcinoma tissue—principally because (a) it involves the use of human material; (b) the original structure of the adenoma or carcinoma tissue can be recognized quite clearly; (c) functional characteristics of the prostate are conserved to a great extent; and (d) a hormonal responsiveness in a manner expected appears to exist.

The disadvantage of this method consists in its great complexity. It is hardly possible to screen a large number of substances in a heterotransplantation model.

ACKNOWLEDGMENTS

We are grateful to Dr. Brehmer (Department of Urology, University of Essen) and Dr. Schröder (Department of Urology, University of Würzburg) for sending us unpublished material and for the permission to present it at this Symposium.

REFERENCES

Arai, Y. (1968). *Experientia* **24**, 180.

Asano, M. (1965). *J. Urol.* **98**, 87.

Bloom, F. (1954). "Pathology of the Dog and Cat." Evanston, Illinois.

Bonzoni, G., Alquati, P., Poba, P, and Alcini, E. (1968). *Chir. Patol. Sper.* **16**, 435.

Brambell, F. W. R., and Davis, D. H. S. (1940). *J. Anat.* **75**, 64.

Brehmer, B., and Madsen, P. O. (1973). *Verh. Deut. Ges. Urol.* **24**, 238.

Brehmer, B., Maquart, H., and Madsen, P. O. (1972). *J. Urol.* **108**, 890.

Brendler, H. (1962). *Nat. Cancer Inst., Monogr.* **12**, 343.

Bridge, R. W., and Scott, W. W. (1964). *Invest. Urol.* **2**, 99.

Chase, M. D., Geschwind, J. J., and Bern, H. A. (1957). *Proc. Soc. Exp. Biol. Med.* **94**, 680.

Chen, T. T., and Heidelberger, C. (1969). *Int. J. Cancer* **4**, 166.

Dixon, F. J., and Moore, R. A. (1952). "Atlas of Tumor Pathology," Sect. VIII, Fasc. 31b and 32. Armed Forces Inst. Pathol., Washington, D.C.

Dunning, W. F. (1962). *Nat. Cancer Inst., Monogr.* **12**, 351.

Dunning, W. F., Curtis, M. R., and Segaloff, A. (1946). *Cancer Res.* **6**, 256.

Ellenberger, W., ed. (1943). "Handbuch der vergleichenden Anatomie der Haustiere," 8th ed. Parey, Berlin.

Faul, P., Klosterhalfen, H., and Schmiedt, E. (1971). *Urologe* **10**, 120.

Fergusson, J. D. (1972). *In* "Endocrine Therapy in Malignant Disease" (B. Y. Stoll, ed.), pp. 237–246. Saunders, Philadelphia, Pennsylvania.

Forsberg, J. G., and Ingemanson, C. A. (1967). *Acta Obstet. Gynecol. Scand.* **46**, 581.

Fortner, J. G., Funkhauser, J. W., and Cullen, M. R. (1962). *Nat. Cancer Inst., Monogr.* **12**, 371.

Franks, L. M. (1954). *Ann. Roy. Coll. Surg. Engl.* **14**, 92.

Franks, L. M. (1960). *Cancer* **13**, 490.

Gerber, H. (1961). Inaugural-Dissertation, Art. Institut Füssli AG, Zürich.

Goodwin, D. A., Rasmussen-Taxdal, D. S., Ferreira, A. A., and Scott, W. W. (1961). *J. Urol.* **86**, 134.

Grayhack, J. T. (1963). *Nat. Cancer Inst., Monogr.* **12**, 189.

Grayhack, J. T., Bunce, P. L., Kearns, J. W., and Scott, W. W. (1955). *Bull. Johns Hopkins Hosp.* **96**, 154.

Gupta, S. K., Mthur, I. S., and Kar, A. B. (1971). *Indian J. Exp. Biol.* **9**, 296.

Harper, M. E., Pirke, A., Peeling, W. P., and Griffiths, K. (1974). *J. Endocrinol.* **60**, 117.

Horning, E. S. (1946). *Lancet* **2**, 829.

Horning, E. S., and Dmochowski, L. (1947). *Brit. J. Cancer* **1**, 59.

Huggins, C. (1945). *Physiol. Rev.* **25**, 281.

Huggins, C., and Clark, P. J. (1940). *J. Exp. Med.* **72**, 747.

Huggins, C., and Russel, P. S. (1946). *Endocrinology* **39**, 1.

Huggins, C., and Sommer, J. L. (1953). *J. Exp. Med.* **97**, 663.

Huggins, C., Scott, W. W., and Hodges, C. V. (1911). *J. Urol.* **46**, 997.

Jost, A. (1965). *In* "Organogenesis" (R. L. De Haan and H. Ursprung, eds.), Chap. 24. Holt, New York.

Kahle, P. I., Schenken, I. R., and Burns, E. L. (1943). *J. Urol.* **50**, 711.

Kazuta, M. (1967). *Acta Urol. Jap.* **13**, 3.

Korenchevsky, V., and Dennison, M. (1939). *J. Pathol. Bacteriol.* **41**, 323.

Lasnitzki, I. (1962). *Nat. Cancer Inst., Monogr.* **12**, 381.

Lloyd, C. W. (1965). *Proc. Int. Congr. Endocrinol., 2nd, 1964* Int. Congr. Ser. No. 83, p. 591.

Lostroh, C. W. (1962). *Endocrinology* **70**, 747.

Lunglmayr, G., Senge, T., Breitenecker, G., Richter, K. D., and Reis, H. E. (1973a) *Urologe A* **12**, 316.

Lunglmayr, G., Senge, T., Breitenecker, G., Richter, K. D., and Reis, H. E. (1973b). *Verh. Deut. Ges. Urol.* **24**, 235.

Mirand, E. A., and Stubitz, W. J. (1956). *Proc. Soc. Exp. Biol. Med.* **93**, 457.

Mobbs, B. G., Johnson, I. H. E., and Conolly, J. G. (1973). *J. Endocrinol.* **59**, 335.

Moger, W., and Geschwind, J. J. (1972). *Proc. Soc. Exp. Biol. Med.* **141**, 1017.

Moore, R. A. (1943). *J. Urol.* **50**, 680.

Moore, R. A., and Melchiona, R. H. (1937). *Amer. J. Cancer* **30**, 731.

Mothes, C., Lehnert, J., Samimi, F., and Ufer, J. (1972). *Life Sci., Monogr.* **2**, 65.

Neri, R. O. (1971). *Proc. Int. Congr. Horm. Steroids, 3rd, 1970* Int. Congr. Ser. No. 210, p. 1022.

Neri, R. O., and Monahan, M. (1972). *Invest. Urol.* **10**, 123.

Neri, R. O., Casmer, C., Zeman, W. V., Fielder, F., and Tabachnick, I. I. A. (1968). *Endocrinology* **82**, 311.

Neumann, F., and Steinbeck, H. (1974). *In* "Handbuch der experimentelen Pharmakologyie" (O. Eichler *et al.*, eds.), Vol. 35, Part 2, pp. 235–484. Springer-Verlag, Berlin and New York.

Neumann, F., Elger, W., Steinbeck, H., and von Berswordt-Wallrabe, R. (1967). *Symp. Deut. Ges. Endokrinol.* **13**, 78.

Neumann, F., Steinbeck, H., and Elger, W. (1970a). *Symp. Deut. Ges. Endokrinol.* **18**, 58.

Neumann, F., von Berswordt-Wallrabe, R., Elger, W., Steinbeck, H., Hahn, J. D., and Kramer, M. (1970b). *Recent Progr. Horm. Res.* **26**, 337.

Okada, K., and Schröder, F. H .(1974). *Urol. Res.* **2**, 111.

Okada, K., Schröder, F. H., Jellinghaus, W., and Wullstein, H. K. (1975). *Invest. Urol.* (in press).

Ott, F. (1968). *Praxis* **57**, 218.

Ott, F., and Hoffet, H. (1968). *Schweiz. Med. Wochenschr.* **98**, 1812.

Price, D. (1963). *Nat. Cancer Inst., Monogr.* **12**, 1.

Price, D., and Williams-Ashman, H. G. (1961). *In* "Sex and Internal Secretions" (W. C. Young, ed.), 3rd ed., Vol. 2, p. 366. Williams & Wilkins, Baltimore, Maryland.

Reddi, A. H. (1969). *Gen. Comp. Endocrinol., Suppl.* **2**, 81.

Richter, K. D., Senge, T., and Reis, H. E. (1971). *Z. Gesamte Exp. Med. Einschl. Exp. Chir.* **155**, 253.

Riemann, J. F., Brehmer, B., Madsen, P. O., and Bloodworth, J. M. B., Jr. (1973). *Verh. Deut. Ges. Urol.* **24**, 232.

Roland, H., Neumann, F., and Reinboth, R. (1975). *Endokrinologie* (submitted for publication).

Ruppert, H. (1953). *Z. Urol.* **46**, 443.

Schirmer, H. (1962). *Nat. Cancer Inst., Mongr.* **12**, 405.

Schmidtke, D., and Schmidtke, H.-O. (1968). *Kleintier-Prax.* **13**, 146.

Schröder, F. H. (1973). *Verh. Deut. Ges. Urol.* **24**, 229.

Schröder, F. H., Okada, K., and Wullstein, H. K. (1974). *Symp. Exp. Urol.* **2**, (abstr.).

Segaloff, A. (1962). *Nat. Cancer Inst., Monogr.* **12**, 407.

Segaloff, A., Steelman, S. L., and Flores, A. (1956). *Endocrinology* **59**, 233.

Senge, T., Richter, K. D., and Lunglmayr, G. (1972). *Invest. Urol.* **10**, 115.

Senge, T., Richter, K. D., and Reis, H. E. (1973). *Verh. Deut. Ges. Urol.* **24**, 234.

Snell, K. C., and Stewart, H. L. (1965). *J. Nat. Cancer Inst.* **35**, 7.

Tesar, C., and Scott, W. W. (1964). *Invest. Urol.* **1**, 482.

Tisell, L. E., and Angervall, L. (1969). *Acta Endocrinol. (Copenhagen)* **62**, 694.

von Berswordt-Wallrabe, R., Steinbeck, H., Hahn, J. D., and Elger, W. (1969). *Experientia* **25**, 533.

von Berswordt-Wallrabe, R., Bielitz, U., Elger, W., and Steinbeck, H. (1970). *J. Urol.* **103**, 180.

von Berswordt-Wallrabe, R., Scheuer, A., Dahnke, H. G., and Mosebach, K. O. (1971). *Acta Endocrinol. (Copenhagen), Suppl.* **152**, 7.

Wojewski, A (1965). *J. Urol.* **93**, 721.

Zuckerman, S. (1940). *Biol. Rev. Cambridge Phil. Soc.* **15**, 231.

DISCUSSION

R. O. Neri: You stated that cyproterone acetate given daily for one year to dogs sustained a marked reduction in prostate size. Have you had the opportunity to study cyproterone, the free alcohol, in the similar situation? I ask this knowing your experience in rats where the antiandrogenic effect of cyproterone is lost after a short period of time.

F. Neumann: No, we have not done any similar study with cyproterone (free alcohol), but because of the influence of cyproterone on the negative feedback system (increase in testosterone secretion), it can be assumed that the effects of cyproterone (free alcohol) will disappear after a certain time of treatment.

L. Röhl: You hinted that the metaplastic changes in the Senge model could be attributed to nutritional disturbances. Then you noted an effect of cyproterone acetate only on these changes. There is an extremely wide biological gap when it comes to xenotransplanting human prostatic cancer to the rat. The effect of ALS is very much unknown. Could the effect shown be influenced by transplantation biology as such?

Second, what is the fate of the Mrs. Dunning strain of marginate prostatic tumor? Is it still available and hormone dependent?

F. Neumann: To answer your second question first, we have no personal experience with this strain.

The conclusions concerning the effectiveness of antiandrogens on prostate carcinoma using this model have to be drawn very cautiously—so I agree in principle. But it is well known that under estrogen therapy especially those regions of the tumor show signs of degeneration which are metaplastic, whereas other parts of the tumor are not affected by the estrogen therapy.

The metaplastic regions in the heterotranplants of adenomatous tissue are similar to those seen in prostate carcinomas *in situ* and are affected by estrogen as well as by antiandrogens. Because of this similarity, I think that we may be allowed to speculate that antiandrogens might affect at least the metaplastic parts within the carcinoma.

I should add that degenerative changes of the metaplastic regions were never seen in untreated animals. So this is a very specific effect of estrogens and antiandrogens.

G. D. Chisholm: We have been interested in the South African mouse (*Mastomys*), and we have now characterized the hormone response by this female prostate. Using both labeled testosterone and estradiol, we have shown identical uptake by the female and male prostate [*Brit. J. Urol.* **47,** 77 (1975)].

I. Lasnitzki: MA 160 is a cell line derived from human benign prostatic hyperplasia; we found that cyproterone acetate induces a high incidence of cellular degeneration in this cell line.

E. Neumann: I wonder whether this is a specific effect or not.

P. Munson: Do you know of studies of incidence and nature of benign prostate hypertrophy and carcinoma of the prostate in large colonies of subhuman primates?

F. Neumann: To my knowledge, this has never been done.

E. Diczfalusy: I do not have any information on prostatic adenoma in subhuman primates; perhaps the Institute of Pathology of the Academy of the USSR in Sukhumi, Georgia, has. However, we have some information on circulating androgen levels in male baboons and rhesus monkeys (Aso, Gonchrov, Cekan, Pachaniya, and Diczfalusy, to be published). Both the baboon and the rhesus have higher circulating levels of 5α-dihydrotestosterone than the human, whereas the testosterone levels in baboons and humans are identical.

H. G. Williams-Ashman: In regard to attempts to obtain nonhuman primate models of human prostate neoplasms, I would like to make a plea for using marmosets as test animals, since they are now available readily from healthy colonies and are so much less expensive to maintain for long periods as compared with larger primate species.

Effects of Hormone-Cytostatic Complexes on the Rat Ventral Prostate *In Vivo* and *In Vitro*

J. G. FORSBERG AND P. A. HØISÆTER

The Institute of Anatomy and Department of General Surgery, Urology Section, University of Bergen, Bergen, Norway

I. Introduction

In the prostatic gland, testosterone is metabolized by the action of a 5α-reductase to 5α-dihydrotestosterone (DHT) which, bound to a receptor protein, is transferred into the nucleus (Bruchovsky and Wilson, 1968; Fang *et al.*, 1969; Mainwaring, 1969; Unhjem *et al.*, 1969; Mainwaring and Peterken, 1971; Jung and Baulieu, 1971; and several others). Since use of estrogen is the type of antiandrogenic therapy commonly used in the treatment of prostatic carcinomas the interference of estrogen with this intracellular androgen metabolism and the androgen receptor comes into focus. Estrogen inhibits 5α-reductase activity (Shimazaki *et al.*, 1965; Lee *et al.*, 1973a,b) and has a competitive effect on the binding of androgen to the DHT-receptor (Høisæter, 1974). There are also indications for the existence of a specific estradiol receptor in the prostate (Unhjem, 1970; van Beurden-Lamers *et al.*, 1974; Armstrong and Bashirelahi, 1974). Besides the mechanisms described here, there are also other possible alternatives for the favorable effect of estrogens in the treatment

137

of prostatic carcinomas (e.g., antigonadotropic effect, increasing the amount of androgen binding protein in serum, etc.). In some systems, high doses of estrogen have a direct mitosis-inhibiting effect (Forsberg, 1970; Forsberg and Lannerstad, 1970), in some cases similar to a colchicine effect (Agrell, 1954). The side effects caused by the high therapeutic doses of estrogen may sometimes lead to interruption of therapy.

Since combined treatment of mammary carcinomas with hormone and alkylating agents had a more promising effect than treatment with either substance alone (Watson and Turner, 1959; Wolff and Prahl, 1973), interest was soon directed to synthesis of steroid–cytostatic molecule complexes (Burstein and Ringold, 1961; Rao and Price, 1962). Comments on this early work and on the biological activity of the complexes synthesized were made by Wall et al. (1969). Provided such a hormone–cytostatic complex was taken up by the malignant cell and transferred by a receptor into the nucleus, the cytostatic part should be placed at its ideal point of action in a narrow range of different cell types. The complex between the steroid hormone and the cytostatic molecule may also be thought to reduce the side effects by either substance alone. However, there are several critical steps for this ideal action: metabolism, cellular uptake, presence or absence of receptor, etc. Some of the complexes had a favorable inhibiting effect on dimethylbenzanthracene (DMBA) induced mammary adenocarcinomas and rat leukemias. The steroidal esters, moreover, were less toxic than some pure nitrogen mustards.

A complex between estradiol and a cytostatic agent was synthesized at AB Leo Research Laboratories under the trade name Estracyt® (Leo 299, estramustine phosphate). The structural formula is shown in Fig. 1. Estramustine phosphate is phenolic bis(2-chloroethyl)carbamate of estradiol-17β-phosphate. In experimental systems, this complex has a very low toxicity on the hemopoietic system, it has a low uterotropic activity, it is antiestrogenic and antigonadotropic and it is nonandrogenic and nonanabolic (Jönsson and Högberg, 1971). In clinical trials, patients with advanced prostatic carcinomas, even cases earlier treated with conventional estrogen therapy, enjoy a good palliative effect from Estracyt in high doses (300 mg/day intravenously for 3 weeks), and this with only minor and reversible side effects (Jönsson, 1969; Alfthan and Rusk, 1969, Jönsson and Högberg, 1971; Lindberg, 1972; Nilsson and Müntzing, 1972, 1973; Klein, 1972; and others). Histological studies and studies of enzyme activity in the carcinomas (Nilsson and Müntzing, 1973) indicate a cytostatic or cytotoxic effect by Estracyt.

[131]γ-Labeled Estracyt accumulates in human prostatic cancerous tissue and hypertrophic prostatic nodules (Szendröi et al., 1973), but this does not mean that observed radioactivity reflects uptake of the whole com-

plex. In different species, Estracyt is more or less hydrolyzed before reaching the prostatic gland (Jönsson and Högberg, 1971; Kirdani *et al.*, 1974; Plym Forshell and Nilsson, 1974). In rat and dog, Estracyt has a definite antiprostatic effect: it decreases prostatic weight, prostatic secretion, and the activity of arginase and acid phosphatase. When these effects are compared to those of estradiol or other estrogens it is evident that the antiprostatic effect of Estracyt is complicated (Kirdani *et al.*, 1974). Estracyt interferes with the steroid uptake by both dog and rat castrate prostate (Kirdani *et al.*, 1974). A blockade of prostaglandin synthesis by Estracyt has been described in the bovine seminal vesicle (Perklev, 1973).

Thus, in conclusion, several studies have described a favorable clinical effect by Estracyt even in cases of estrogen-insensitive prostatic carcinomas. There is accumulating evidence that the mechanism of action of Estracyt is different from that of estradiol and the nitrogen mustard separately.

During the last years we have been interested in the intracellular mechanism of action of Estracyt (estramustine phosphate EMP) using the rat (Sprague-Dawley) ventral prostate as a test system. A short review of the results of our studies now follows.

II. Effects of Hormone-Cytostatic Complexes

A. Influence of Hormone-Cytostatic Complexes on the Rat Ventral Prostate in Organ Cultures

Explants from the ventral prostate were cultured as organ cultures for 3 days in 95% Parker medium 199 and 5% fetal bovine serum with antibiotics. Various hormones and test substances were added in a concentration of 4×10^{-5} M, control cultures were supplemented with the vehicle (distilled water or 96% ethanol) only. Methyl-^{3}H-labeled thymidine (TdR-^{3}H) was present for the last hour of the incubation. The amount of TdR-^{3}H incorporated was related to the DNA content of the explants and used as parameter for growth. Radioautograms showed a random distribution of labeled epithelial cells in the basal part of the alveoli (for details, see Høisæter, 1975a).

5α-Dihydrotestosterone (DHT) had no effect on TdR-^{3}H incorporation, which is the normal finding when the hormone is added to a serum-containing medium while a stimulating effect on DNA synthesis can be obtained in strictly defined media (Johansson and Santti, 1973; Johansson and Niemi, 1975). Nor had a DHT-cytostatic complex, with the same nitrogen mustard as in EMP, linked to carbon atom 17, any effect. Estra-

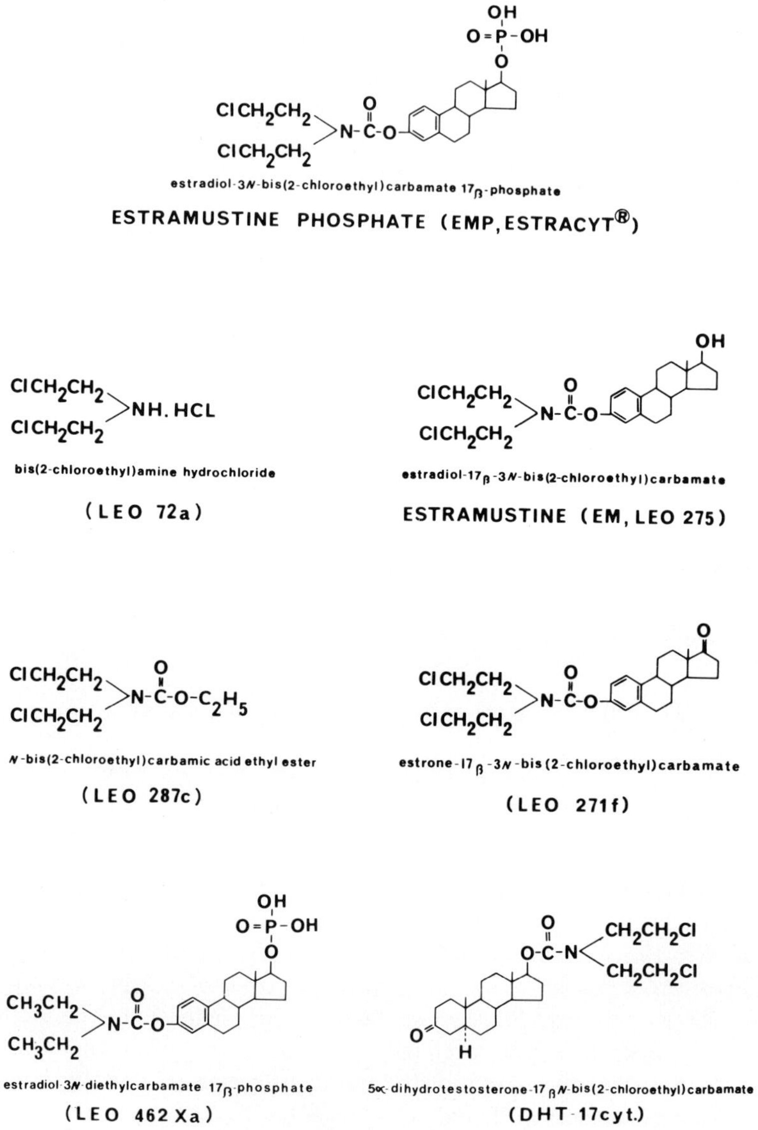

estradiol-3*N*-bis(2-chloroethyl)carbamate 17β-phosphate

ESTRAMUSTINE PHOSPHATE (EMP, ESTRACYT®)

bis(2-chloroethyl)amine hydrochloride

(LEO 72a)

estradiol-17β-3*N*-bis(2-chloroethyl)carbamate

ESTRAMUSTINE (EM, LEO 275)

N-bis(2-chloroethyl)carbamic acid ethyl ester

(LEO 287c)

estrone-17β-3*N*-bis(2-chloroethyl)carbamate

(LEO 271f)

estradiol-3*N*-diethylcarbamate 17β-phosphate

(LEO 462 Xa)

5α-dihydrotestosterone-17β*N*-bis(2-chloroethyl)carbamate

(DHT-17cyt.)

FIG. 1. Structural formulas for different test substances used.

diol (E_2) had a probably significant inhibiting effect and EMP a highly significant inhibiting effect. The mean reduction of TdR-^{3}H incorporation was for EMP to about 13% and for E_2 to about 54% of the values for the control cultures. This difference between EMP and E_2 is statistically significant.

The effect of addition of a small concentration of testosterone or DHT $(4 \times 10^{-6} \ M)$ to cultures containing the standard concentration of E_2 or EMP $(4 \times 10^{-5} \ M)$ was tested in two other series. The low dose of testosterone or DHT was in itself without effect. The E_2-induced inhibition was lost in the presence of testosterone. For EMP the addition of a low concentration of both androgens was without effect on the EMP-induced inhibition of TdR-^{3}H incorporation. The conclusion to be drawn from these experiments is that EMP has a profound inhibitory effect on prostatic TdR-^{3}H incorporation *in vitro*, far more than E_2, and this effect is not counteracted by a low amount of androgen.

We then tried to analyze which part of the EMP complex is the most important for the effect, or to establish if the complex has an action of its own. Thus we tested E_2, EMP, estradiol-17β-phosphate (E_2-P), Leo 462 Xa, Leo 72a, and Leo 275 (the structural formulas for these substances are shown in Fig. 1), all at the same molar concentration as used for EMP and E_2 in the earlier experiments $(4 \times 10^{-5} \ M)$. An inhibitory effect of about the same magnitude as that of EMP was seen by the nor-nitrogen mustard Leo 72a and the diethylcarbamate of estradiol-17β-phosphate, Leo 462 Xa. On the contrary, Leo 287c, a carbamic acid ethyl ester of the cytostatic, and E_2-P were both without an effect. The effect of E_2 was somewhat variable, in one series an effect was seen whereas in another series there was no effect. Overall, the effect by estradiol was small and questionable. The difference between the effect of EMP and E_2 was again pronounced and statistically significant.

It is crucial to know whether or not the EMP complex is hydrolyzed under the culture conditions. To study this, an ethyl acetate extract of the culture medium was analyzed, using thin-layer chromatography (TLC). In the presence of tissue explants in the culture medium, EMP was partially dephosphorylated and EM (Leo 275) was recovered from the medium besides EMP. A hydrolysis of the carbamic ester in EM or EMP could not be demonstrated, and the effect on TdR-^{3}H incorporation in this system thus seems to be dependent on the cytostatic part in the EM or EMP complexes. However, it must be stressed that the results refer to an *in vitro* system, and the results should be taken to represent a change in a biological parameter of this system, but do not justify any direct comparison to *in vivo* conditions.

Histological sections of explants grown in the presence of DHT or the DHT-cytostatic complex showed a somewhat better preserved epithelium than in the control cultures. This indicates that the cytostatic part of the DHT-cytostatic complex had no cytotoxic action, and this is in line with the results from TdR-^{3}H incorporation. With E_2 in the medium, regressive changes (flattening of the epithelial cells) were seen. The changes evoked by EMP were still more pronounced and widespread general necrosis occurred. The same conditions were found after adding Leo 72a, Leo 275, or Leo 462Xa to the medium. Those substances which were without effect on TdR-³H incorporation (Leo 287c and estradiol-17β-phosphate) did not evoke any histological changes.

In conclusion, EMP has a pronounced inhibitory effect on TdR-³H incorporation into the ventral prostate under *in vitro* conditions, and this effect is far more pronounced than for estradiol alone. The results argue for the nitrogen mustard part in the EMP (EM) complex being the factor responsible for the effect. The inhibition of TdR-³H incorporation is closely paralleled by regressive histological changes. A replacement of the chlorine atoms of the alkylating part in EMP and EM (Leo 275) with methyl groups (Leo 462Xa) does not exclude activity in this test system.

B. EFFECTS ON INCORPORATION OF THYMIDINE-³H AND ¹⁴C-LABELED
AMINO ACIDS INTO THE VENTRAL PROSTATE AFTER *in Vivo*
TREATMENT OF THE ANIMALS WITH ESTRAMUSTINE PHOSPHATE (EMP)
AND ITS ESTROGEN AND CYTOSTATIC MOIETIES

Sufrin and Coffey (1973) have presented a model for studying the growth inhibiting effect of different drugs on the ventral prostate *in vivo:* castration of adult male rats results in marked involution of the prostate after 7 days. Treatment with testosterone for the following 3 days stimulates prostate growth and drugs capable of inhibiting this hormone-induced growth reduced TdR-³H incorporation when compared to controls. This test system was adopted for studying the effects of EMP, Leo 72a, Estradurin® (polyestradiol phosphate, PEP) and estradiol-17β-phosphate (E₂-P). Each rat (7 days castrated) was given daily injections of 0.3 mg of testosterone propionate in olive oil for 3 days. At 3–4 hours after every testosterone injection, the test substance was injected intravenously into the femoral vein (with the exception of PEP, which was given intramuscularly). The dose of EMP was 10 or 100 mg/kg body weight, Leo 72a 34.3 mg/kg, E₂-P 67.6 mg/kg, and PEP 67.6 mg/kg. The EMP dose was chosen so as to correspond to the human therapeutic dose and to correspond approximately to a supposed difference in sensitivity to cytostatic agents between rat and man (cf. Freireich *et al.*, 1966). The other doses were calculated from the EMP dose. The effect of the different test substances was compared with the effect in control animals receiving saline only. The animals were killed 24 hours after the last testosterone injection (20–21 hours after the last injection of test substance or saline), and the ventral prostate was dissected out. After weighing, the tissue was minced into small fragments and incubated for 60 minutes in Parker medium 199, containing TdR-^{3}H or a mixture of ^{14}C-labeled amino acids (AA-^{14}C). The amount of incorporated TdR-^{3}H or AA-^{14}C was determined in a liquid scintillator and related to the DNA content of the fragments. Protein determinations were performed according to Klungsøyr (1969). For further details, see Høisæter (1975c).

EMP in a dose of 10 mg/kg body weight slightly augmented the testosterone-induced stimulation of TdR-^{3}H incorporation, but 100 mg EMP had a significant inhibitory effect (to about 26% of the control value). The latter effect was counteracted by increasing the testosterone dose 100-fold to 30 mg/kg. Leo 72a, E_2-P, and PEP were without effects. This may be due to rapid alkylation by the nitrogen mustard before reaching the prostatic gland, rapid excretion, rapid clearance of E_2-P, too little resorption of estradiol from the PEP depot, etc. Generally speaking, the same results were obtained when studying the AA-^{14}C incorporation.

The rats treated with 100 mg of EMP had a slight tendency to show body-weight reduction; this tendency also occurred in animals injected with E_2-P and Leo 72a, but not in those given PEP.

EMP was unique, as it was the only test substance resulting in a substantial fall in the number of white blood cells. In these experiments, of relatively short duration, the inhibitory effect on TdR-^{3}H and AA-^{14}C incorporation was not paralleled by any obvious histological changes in the ventral prostate. The inhibitory influence of EMP on the AA-^{14}C incorporation seems to be of a rather general nature because when related to the protein content no reduction was seen. With the high EMP dose used (100 mg) the inhibitory effect on AA-^{14}C incorporation was relatively more pronounced than that on TdR-^{3}H incorporation.

In conclusion, EMP in high doses has a growth-inhibiting effect on the ventral prostate *in vivo,* an effect that is not mimicked by corresponding doses of the main EMP components separately. A possible explanation for this difference between the complex and its components is that the effects are specific for the complex as a whole (Perklev, 1973). Thus far, however, an intracellular hydrolysis of the carbamic ester in EMP should not be excluded. The probably stimulatory effect by the low-dose EMP on TdR-^{3}H incorporation might seem to be a contradiction. Small doses of estradiol in a test system similar to ours (Karr *et al.,* 1974) enhance the stimulatory effect by estradiol. Provided that some hydrolysis of EMP takes place, this phenomenon explains our results whereas in the case of higher concentration of the complex relative to free estradiol the inhibitory effect may be the dominating one.

C. Effect of EMP on the 5α-Reductase Activity in the Rat Ventral Prostate

5α-Reductase converts testosterone to 5α-dihydrostestosterone (DHT) which, as discussed in the introduction, is a primary step in the androgen action at target cell level. Estradiol-17β, progesterone, and other steroids and steroidlike substances compete with testosterone as substrates for this enzyme (Lee *et al.*, 1973a,b; Massa and Martini, 1971/1972; Shimazaki *et al.*, 1972; and others).

Minced tissue from diaphragm, liver, and ventral prostate was incubated in Eagle L medium for 1 hour at 37°C in the presence of 3.5×10^{-10} M testosterone-^{3}H. Steroids were extracted with methanol/chloroform; after evaporation in N_2, the residue was dissolved in chloroform and subjected to TLC. Unlabeled testosterone, DHT, and androstanediol (5α-androstane-3β,17β-diol) were used as chromatographic markers. The percentage DHT-^{3}H formed out of the total amount of radioactive steroids extracted was taken as an indication of 5α-reductase activity. The effect on this activity was tested by adding 4×10^{-5} M unlabeled EMP, Leo 275 (EM), estradiol-17β (E_2) and estradiol-17β phosphate (E_2-P) to the incubates (for details, see Høisæter, 1975b).

In liver and diaphragm there was a very low activity of 5α-reductase, 2.8 and 3.8%, respectively, of DHT-^{3}H recovered, and this was in contrast to 49.3% for the ventral prostate. E_2 and E_2-P significantly depressed the reductase activity while EMP and EM were without effects in these *in vitro* incubations. The reduction by E_2 was about 31% and that by E_2-P about 16%.

In another experimental series, EMP in a dose of 100 mg/kg body weight was injected into male rats through the femoral vein. In "long-term" experiments the injections were made daily for 3 days and the animals were killed 24 hours after the last injection. In "short-term" experiments the animals were given one injection only and killed 35 minutes later. Thirty minutes before sacrifice all the animals were injected with 100 μCi of testosterone-^{3}H. The ventral prostate, diaphragm, and liver were removed and processed as described for the *in vitro* experiments.

In both the "short-term" and "long-term" experiments less than 10% of the total number of counts recovered from liver and diaphragm were DHT-^{3}H, and this amount was never influenced by EMP injections. The prostatic reductase activity was not influenced by EMP in "short-term" experiments but was significantly depressed (about 40%) in "long-term" experiments. The latter results are in line with those by Kirdani *et al.* (1974). The mechanism for this reductase inhibition is unknown.

D. Studies on the Metabolism of EMP in the Ventral Prostate
and Some Other Tissues of the Male Rat

The conversion of E_2-^{3}H (3.5×10^{-9} M) into estrone-^{3}H (E_1-^{3}H) was
studied in minced tissue from the liver and the ventral prostate. After
incubation in Eagle L medium, the radioactive metabolites were extracted
with chloroform/methanol. The solvent was evaporated in N_2, and the
residue was subjected to TLC. The radioactivity in the E_1 reference spot,
relative to the total amount extracted, was taken as a measure of 17β-
dehydrogenase activity (for details, see Høisæter, 1975d).

Both liver and ventral prostate had the capacity to convert E_2 into
E_1, but the liver was far more active. This is in line with earlier reports
(Unhjem, 1970).

An eventual inhibitory effect on the E_2–E_1 conversion was studied in
the same system, but after the addition of 1000-fold unlabeled E_2, EMP,
or Leo 275. For both liver and ventral prostate, addition of unlabeled
E_2 reduced the amount of E_1-^{3}H formed. EMP was without effect whereas
EM reduced the amount of E_1-^{3}H recovered from the liver tissue, but
not from the prostatic tissue.

These results were confirmed in an experimental series where tritiated
EM was added to incubations of the diaphragm, ventral prostate, liver,
and blood. Extractions took place with ethyl acetate, and the residue
after evaporation was subjected to TLC. The results demonstrate a conversion of the estradiol-cytostatic complex into an estrone-cytostatic
complex (Leo 271f) only for the liver tissue.

The next question was whether such a conversion also occurs *in vivo*
and whether the same difference between liver and ventral prostate can
be demonstrated after EMP injections. Male rats were injected with 100
mg of EMP per kilogram body weight into the femoral vein. Control
animals received saline only. The animals were divided into a "short-
term" group, which were killed 0.5 hour after the EMP injection, and
a "long-term" group, which received EMP injections for 3 days, then
were killed 24 hours after the last injection. Tissue from the ventral prostate, liver, diaphragm, and blood was extracted with ethyl acetate and
subjected to TLC.

For the "short-term" experiments the dominating spot on the TLC
plate in all the tissues studied was that for EM. Semiquantitatively, more
EM was extracted from liver and ventral prostate than from diaphragm
and blood. For the liver, but not for the prostate, there was a slightly
visible spot with the same R_f value as the Leo 271f. Extracts from the
spots taken to be representative for EM and Leo 271f gave mass spectra

identical to those of the reference standards. Taken together, the "short-term" experiments indicate that EMP is rapidly dephosphorylated after injection and that the liver has the capacity to convert the estradiol complex into an estrone-cytostatic complex. In "long-term" experiments, only faintly stained spots representing EM could be seen in extracts from liver and ventral prostate. The dominating spot from the ventral prostate was that one representing the estrone-cytostatic complex, whereas this was never seen in TLC from liver, diaphragm, and blood. Moreover, a slightly stained spot indicated the existence of free estrone in the ventral prostate. These results indicate a retention of the estrone-cytostatic metabolite from EMP in the prostate, and they are in accordance with those demonstrating a preferential localization of radioactivity to the prostate after injection of labeled Estracyt (Plym Forshell and Nilsson, 1974; Szendröi *et al.*, 1973).

The estrone-cytostatic complex might be related to the *in vivo* EMP effect in the ventral prostate because the *in vivo* effects, both on TdR-^{3}H and AA-^{14}C incorporation and on 5α-reductase activity, were seen at a time corresponding to that when we have been able to demonstrate the estrone-cytostatic complex. Since a small amount of estrone also was recovered at this time, it cannot be ruled out that one or both of the two main components after carbamic ester hydrolysis are more essential than the complex itself.

Even though liver and ventral prostate both have the capacity to convert estradiol into estrone, a conversion of the estradiol-cytostatic complex into an estrone-cytostatic complex seems to be preferentially restricted to the liver. It cannot be excluded that a low-grade conversion may also occur in the prostate. Different types of 17β-dehydrogenases responsible for the conversion may occur in the liver and ventral prostate. The ventral prostate has the capacity to retain the estrone-cytostatic complex and probably to hydrolyze the carbamic ester, to some extent at least, with the formation of free estrone and nitrogen mustard.

E. STUDIES ON THE BINDING OF EMP TO THE STEROID-BINDING
   MACROPROTEINS IN THE VENTRAL PROSTATE

Cytosol from the rat ventral prostate contains an 8 S androgen-binding macroprotein with high affinity and low capacity (androgen receptor, see Section I). This 8 S receptor was used to study the binding of DHT-^{3}H in the presence of unlabeled competitors (Høisæter, 1974). DHT-^{3}H was used in a concentration of 1.6×10^{-9} M and the competitors in a 500-fold concentration (8×10^{-7} M). The binding of the various test complexes and hormones (competitors) to the specific 8 S cytosol DHT receptor is reflected in the degree to which the unlabeled complexes are able to displace the DHT-^{3}H from the receptor peak. All animals used for studies of steroid-binding macroproteins were castrated 24 hours before they were killed.

Both estradiol-17β (E$_2$) and estradiol-17β-phosphate (E$_2$-P) depressed the 8 S peak representing protein-bound DHT-^{3}H in sucrose gradient centrifugation very strongly and to about the same degree, indicating that these substances in the concentration used can occupy binding sites on the DHT receptor. The same concentration of EMP had no influence on the DHT-^{3}H receptor peak. Nor was this the case when the nitrogen mustard was linked to carbon atom 17 of E$_2$ instead of carbon atom 3 as in EMP. On the other hand, DHT with the nitrogen mustard linked to carbon atom 17, or testosterone with the cytostatic agent in position 17, very strongly depressed the receptor peak. The conclusion is, therefore, that linkage of the nitrogen mustard to carbon atom 17 of DHT does not inhibit binding to the 8 S androgen receptor protein, but linkage of the nitrogen mustard to carbon atom 3 or 17 of E$_2$ inhibits the competitive effect exerted by E$_2$. Thus the EMP effect in the rat ventral prostate does not seem to be due to a competitive binding to the androgen receptor.

A clinical use of the DHT-cytostatic complex may be hazardous, because in case of hydrolysis of the carbamic ester, the net effect may be due to the relative activity of free steroid and cytostatic moiety. Then it cannot be excluded that free DHT may have an effect just contrary to that wanted. Such a reversed effect seems to be excluded using EMP. When the DHT complex was tested in organ cultures, the histological effect was the same as that seen by DHT (see Section II, A).

Results from different laboratories suggest the presence of a specific E$_2$ binding protein (E$_2$ receptor) in the rat prostate (Unhjem, 1970; van Beurden-Lamers et al., 1974; Armstrong and Bashirelahi, 1974). We have been able to confirm the existence of a specific, estradiol-binding protein with limited capacity in the 4 S region of sucrose gradients using the same technique as Armstrong and Bashirelahi (1974). In buffer of low ionic strength, an 100-fold unlabeled E$_2$ did not depress the 4 S peak representing protein-bound E$_2$-^{3}H whereas an 100-fold excess of unlabeled estradiol-cytostatic complex did. This may indicate a more pronounced affinity of the protein for the complex than for E$_2$.

Ventral prostate cytosol was incubated with 8×10^{-9} M E$_2$-^{3}H and used for gel filtration chromatography on Sephadex G-25 columns. The peak of protein-bound radioactivity was depressed by a 500-fold excess of unlabeled E$_2$ or E$_1$, but not by DHT. The same molar concentration (8×10^{-9} M) EM-^{3}H also resulted in a peak of protein-bound radioactivity but this peak was not depressed by a 500-fold excess unlabled

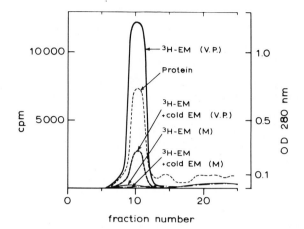

Fɪɢ. 2. Gel filtration of ventral prostate (V.P.) and skeletal muscle (M) cytosol fractions (0.8 ml) in 10 mM Tris-HCl (pH 8.5 at 4°C), containing 10 mM KCl, 1 mM EDTA, and 5 mM glutathione. Sephadex G-25 (fine) columns (1.6 × 20 cm), equilbrated with the same buffer as used for the cytosol. Fractions of 1 ml were collected; optical density at 280 nm. The cytosol was incubated with 1 × 10⁻⁶ M ³H-labeled estramustine (³H-EM) for 1 hour at 4°C or preincubated with 4 × 10⁻⁵ M unlabeled ("cold") EM for 5 minutes at 4°C, before addition of the ³H-labeled EM.

EM. Only a low amount of radioactivity was recovered in contrast to the conditions when using E_2-³H, a finding consistent with results from sucrose gradients. This may be due to a pronounced unspecific binding of the EM complex to glassware, gel material, etc. (B. Forsgren, G. Green, and R. Kant, personal communication 1975). To overcome this unspecific effect, the EM-³H concentration in the cytosol incubations was increased to 1 × 10⁻⁶ M. This resulted in a high peak of protein-bound radioactivity, which was now strongly depressed by a 40-fold excess of unlabeled EM (Fig. 2). In sucrose gradients using buffer of low ionic strength a peak of radioactivity appeared in the 4 S region, and this peak was again depressed by a 40-fold excess unlabeled EM.

Cytosol from skeletal muscle was used in control experiments and incubated with both the high and the low concentration of EM-³H. In neither case did we find any evidence for a peak of protein-bound EM-³H. Our experiments indicate that the estradiol-cytostatic complex definitely has a higher affinity for protein in ventral prostate cytosol than for proteins in muscle cytosol. The binding protein in ventral prostate cytosol occurs in the 4 S region of sucrose gradients. There are reasons to believe that this protein may be the same as the prostatic 4 S estradiol receptor, but the estradiol-cytostatic complex seems to be bound with higher affinity than estradiol.

F. Does the Estradiol-Cytostatic Complex Enter the Nuclei

Minced tissue from liver and ventral prostate was incubated in Eagle L medium at $37°$ in the presence of 1×10^{-6} M EM-^{3}H (sp. act. 80 Ci/mmole) and then washed in ice-cold Eagle L medium. After homogenization in 0.25 M sucrose containing 1 mM $MgCl_2$ and centrifugation at 600 g for 10 minutes, the pellet was resuspended in $2M$ sucrose containing 1 mM $MgCl_2$ and centrifugated at 50,000 g for 1 hour. The pellet was washed in 0.5% Triton-X-100 in 0.25 M sucrose + 1 mM $MgCl_2$. The final pellet after centrifugation at 600 g for 10 minutes contained nuclei which in the electron microscope were homogeneous and free from contaminating cytoplasmic material. Washing with Triton X-100 was included in order to remove the outer part of the nuclear membrane (cf. Anderson et $al.$, 1970), and thus excluded any nonspecific adherence of isotope to the nuclei. This wash resulted in a substantial decrease of radioactivity.

The radioactivity of the pure nuclear preparation was related to the DNA content and was found to be about 1000 cpm per milligram of DNA. In another experimental series, nuclei prepared in an identical way were extracted with ethyl acetate; after evaporation in a steam of N_2, the residue was dissolved in ethyl acetate and subjected to TLC. The radioactivity recovered emanated from EM-^{3}H, and no radioactive E_2 or E_1 could be demonstrated. Liver nuclei prepared in an identical way contained a less amount of radioactive material.

Our experiments indicate that the estradiol-cytostatic complex, under the experimental conditions used, enters the prostatic nuclei. Important effects may thus be exerted in both cytoplasm and nucleus.

To obtain an alkylating effect by the nitrogen mustard in EMP, a ring closure of the chloroethyl groups with the formation of an ethyleneimmonium ion is necessary (Wheeler, 1973). As long as the EMP complex is intact this ion formation does not take place, and the complex thus has no alkylating effect of its own. To investigate the possibility of a nonspecific interaction between EMP and DNA, the influence of the EMP complex on the DNA melting curve was studied. Calf thymus DNA (20 μg/ml) in 7×10^{-4} M phosphate buffer, pH 7.4, was used (T_m 63°C, melting range 51–75°C). No influence on the melting curve was observed by 4×10^{-5} M EMP, Leo 72a, or E_2. However, E_2 always provoked a higher OD value at 25°C than the other test substances, decreasing to control levels at 50°C (Fig. 3). This may indicate an intercalation on the DNA strands by the planar aromatic A ring of E_2 under the experimental conditions used. This E_2 effect was never seen when EMP was used. Thus there must be a difference between the EMP complex and E_2 in their interaction with DNA. The biological meaning of this finding is not clear. With a standard saline citrate buffer, the E_2 effect was never observed.

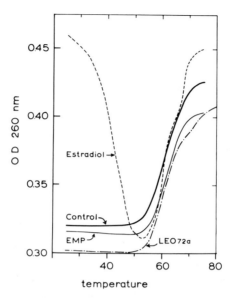

Fig. 3. Melting curves for calf thymus DNA (20 μg/ml) dissolved in 7×10^{-4} M phosphate buffer, pH 7.4 The test substances were added in a concentration of $4 \times 10^{-5} M$; the controls were added with the same amount of vehicle only.

III. Conclusions

From this review it is to be concluded that the estradiol-cytostatic complex used has effects different from those of the two components separately. Both in organ cultures and in *in vivo* experiments its inhibitory effect on TdR-^{3}H incorporation was far more pronounced than that by estradiol alone. As far as the clinical therapeutic situation is concerned, these results may reflect the favorable effect produced by the complex in the treatment of prostatic carcinomas, even in nonestrogen responders. For the *in vivo* experimental situation, the inhibitory effect of the complex on both TdR-^{3}H and ^{14}C-labeled amino acid incorporation was not imitated by either of its two main components when administered separately. After injection, the phosphorylated (17β-phosphorylation) complex is rapidly dephosphorylated and converted into an estrone-cytostatic complex, above all, in the liver. The estrone-cytostatic complex is retained in the ventral prostate. Since both the estradiol-cytostatic and the estrone-cytostatic complexes as well as low amounts of free estrone could be recovered from the ventral prostate, it is difficult to draw any definite conclusions about the relative importance of the three substances for the effects demonstrated. After injections of the estradiol-cytostatic complex, prostatic 5α-reductase activity decreased. A similar effect was not found *in vitro* and the reasons for this difference are discussed. The estradiol-cytostatic complex does not compete with the 8 S androgen cytosol receptor but is bound to a 4 S protein. A similar binding was not found in skeletal muscle. The complex entered the nuclei in *in vitro* experiments and could be extracted as the whole complex. Estradiol, but not the estradiol-cytostatic complex, had an interaction with calf DNA in studies on the DNA melting profile.

In recent years, another type of estradiol-cytostatic complex—a 3,17 diester of estradiol with the alkylating agent chlorphenacyl (NSC 112259)—has been tested in experimental systems. Like the complex used in our experiments, this diester has effects different from those of the components when given separately (Vollmer *et al.*, 1973). According to Everson *et al.* (1974), the diester inhibits the binding of estradiol-^{3}H to rat uterine cytosol at a diester concentration higher than 10^{-6} M. Such a competition was denied by Shepherd *et al.* (1974), using rat uterus or human breast cancer tissue. The discrepancy between the two studies may be at least to some extent due to the difference in concentration of unlabeled complex used to compete with estradiol-^{3}H. In this connection the effect of a pronounced stickiness to glassware, etc., as observed for our types of complex, should be taken into consideration.

Even though we have been able to demonstrate effects of an estradiol-cytostatic complex in the rat ventral prostate, this does not mean that the results are directly transferable to the human situation. This will be further analyzed. There are still fundamental questions to analyze: differences between estrogen and the estradiol-cytostatic complex with respect to cellular penetration and retention, different affinities for chromatin proteins, the importance of the inhibiting effect on prostaglandin synthetase (Perklev, 1973), etc. Moreover, the qualities of these types of complexes might be improved in different ways by varying the cytostatic part of the complex as well as the linkage to the steroid molecule.

ACKNOWLEDGMENTS

These studies were supported by grants from the Norwegian Research Council for Science and the Humanities, from the Norwegian Cancer Society (Landsforeningen mot Kreft) and from Leo Research Foundation. The test substances were kindly supplied by AB Leo, Helsingborg, Sweden.

REFERENCES

Agrell, I. (1954). *Nature (London)* **173,** 172.
Alfthan, O. S., and Rusk, J. (1969). *Ann. Chir. Gynaecol. Fenn.* **58,** 234.
Anderson, K. M., Lee, F. H., and Miyai, K. (1970). *Exp. Cell Res.* **61,** 371.
Armstrong, E. G., and Bashirelahi, N. (1974). *Biochem. Biophys. Res. Commun.* **61,** 628.
Bruchovsky, N., and Wilson, J. D. (1968). *J. Biol. Chem.* **243,** 2012.
Burstein, S. H., and Ringold, H. J. (1961). *J. Org. Chem.* **26,** 3084.

Everson, R. B., Turnell, R. W., Wittliff, J. L., and Hall, T. C. (1974). *Cancer Chemother. Rep., Part 1* 58, 353.
Fang, S., Andersson, K. M., and Liao, S. (1969). *J. Biol. Chem.* 244, 6584.
Forsberg, J.-G. (1970). *J. Exp. Zool.* 175, 369.
Forsberg, J.-G., and Lannerstad, B. (1970). *Acta Embryol. Morphol. Exp.,* 45.
Freireich, E. J., Gehan, E. A., Rall, D. P., Schmidt, L. H., and Skipper, H. E. (1966). *Cancer Chemother. Rep.* 50, 219.
Høisæter, P. Aa. (1973). *Biochim. Biophys. Acta* 317, 492.
Høisæter, P. Aa. (1974). *Invest. Urol.* 12, 33.
Høisæter, P. Aa. (1975a). *Invest. Urol.* 12, 479.
Høisæter, P. Aa. (1975b). *Acta Endocrinol. (Copenhagen)* 80, 188.
Høisæter, P. Aa. (1975c). *Invest. Urol.* (in press).
Høisæter, P. Aa. (1975d). Submitted for publication.
Johansson, R., and Niemi, M. (1975). *Acta Endocrinol. (Copenhagen)* 78, 766.
Johanson, R., and Santti, R. S. (1973). *Acta Endocrinol. (Copenhagen), Suppl.* 177, Abstract 61.
Jönsson, G. (1969). *Nord. Med.* 81, 618.
Jönsson, G., and Högberg, B. (1971). *Scand. J. Urol. Nephrol.* 5, 103.
Jung, I., and Baulieu, E.-E. (1971). *Biochimie* 53, 807.
Karr, J. P., Kirdani, R. Y., Murphy, G. P., and Sandberg, A. A. (1974). *Life Sci.* 15, 501.
Kirdani, R. Y., Müntzing, J., Varkarakis, M. J., Murphy, G. P., and Sandberg, A. A. (1974). *Cancer Res.* 34, 1031.
Klein, D. (1972). *Wien. Med. Wochenschr.* 122, 458.
Klungsøyr, L. (1969). *Anal. Biochem.* 27, 91.
Lee, D. K. H., Bird, C. E., and Clark, A. F. (1973a). *Steroids* 22, 677.
Lee, D. K. H., Young, J. C., Tamura, Y., Patterson, D. C., Bird, C. E., and Clark, A. F. (1973b). *Can. J. Biochem.* 51, 735.
Lindberg, B. (1972). *J. Urol.* 108, 303.
Mainwaring, W. I. P. (1969). *J. Endocrinol.* 45, 531.
Mainwaring, W. I. P., and Peterken, B. M. (1971). *Biochem. J.* 125, 285.
Massa, R., and Martini, L. (1971/1972). *Gynecol. Invest.* 2, 253.
Nilsson, T., and Müntzing, J. (1972). *Scand. J. Urol. Nephrol.* 6, 11.
Nilsson, T., and Müntzing, J. (1973). *Scand. J. Urol. Nephrol.* 7, 18.
Perklev, T. (1973). *In* "Prostaglandins and Cyclic AMP" (R. H. Kahn and W. E. M. Lands, eds.), pp. 219–221. Academic Press, New York.
Plym Forshell, G., and Nilsson, H. (1974). *Acta Pharmacol. (Copenhagen)* 35, Suppl. 1, 28.
Rao, G. V., and Price, C. C. (1962). *J. Org. Chem.* 27, 205.
Shepherd, R. E., Huff, K., and McGuire, W. L. (1974). *J. Nat. Cancer Inst.* 53, 895.
Shimazaki, J., Kurihara, H., Ito, Y., and Shida, K. (1965). *Gunma J. Med. Sci.* 14, 313.
Shimazaki, J., Ohki, Y., Koya, A., and Shida, K. (1972). *Endocrinol. Jap.* 19, 585.
Sufrin, G., and Coffey, D. S. (1973). *Invest. Urol.* 11, 45.
Szendröi, Z., Kocsár, L., Karika, Zs., Füzi, M., Tarján, Gy., Reischl, Gy., and Eckhardt, S. (1973). *Int. Urol. Nephrol.* 5, 311.
Unhjem, O. (1970). *Res. Steroids* 4, 139–143.
Unhjem, O., Tveter, K. J., and Aakvaag, A. (1969). *Acta Endocrinol. (Copenhagen)* 62, 153.

van Beurden-Lamers, W. M. O., Brinkmann, A. O., Mulder, E., and van der Molen, H. J. (1974). *Biochem. J.* **140**, 495.

Vollmer, E. P., Taylor, D. J., Masnyk, I. J., Cooney, D., Levine, B., and Piczak, C. (1973). *Cancer Chemother, Rep., Part 3* **4**, 121.

Wall, M. E. Abernathy, G. S., Carroll, F. I., and Taylor, D. J. (1969). *J. Med. Chem.* **12**, 810.

Watson, G. W., and Turner, R. L. (1959). *Brit. Med. J.* **2**, 1315.

Wheeler, G. P. (1973). *In* "Cancer Medicine" (J. F. Holland and E. Freii, eds.), p. 792. Lea & Febiger, Philadelphia, Pennsylvania.

Wolff, G., and Prahl, B. (1973). *Arch. Geschwultsforsch.* **41**, 363.

DISCUSSION

P. Robel: I do not think there is an estrogen receptor in rat ventral prostate. Have you demonstrated the selective uptake of estrogen cytostatic complex in rat ventral prostate compared to nontarget organs?

J.-G. Forsberg: Our results on the occurrence of an estrogen receptor in the ventral prostate are quite in line with those reported by other investigators [e.g., O. Unhjem, *Res. Steroids* **4**, 139 (1970); E. G. Armstrong and N. Bashirelahi, *Biochem. Biophys. Res. Commun.* **61**, 678 (1974)]. We found no retention of the estrone complex in the diaphragm and liver, only in the ventral prostate.

K. Griffiths: What was the effect of Estracyt on prostatic weight?

J.-G. Forsberg: We injected Estracyt for 3 days. A very small reduction in the wet weight of the ventral prostate was produced by the 100-mg dose, compared with controls, but not by the 10-mg dose.

D. S. Coffey: Dr. Warren Heston and I have tested the effects of Estracyt on the weight of the rat ventral prostate. If castrated rats are administered exogenous testosterone propionate for one week, the simultaneous administration of Estracyt has little effect on the wet weight of the gland.

K. Griffiths: We have studied a similar compound—diethylstilbestrol with 2 nitrogen mustard moieties attached to the phenolic hydroxyl groups. This compound displaces 5α-DHT from the 8 S-receptor with a 400 times excess.

M. B. Lipsett: We know that the alkylating agents act by reacting with DNA. Your finding that there was no Estracyt in liver nuclei implies that either Estracyt does not enter the liver cell or does not act as an alkylating agent. Do you have evidence about entry of Estracyt into other cells?

J.-G. Forsberg: Estracyt apparently entered liver cells since an estrone-cystostatic complex could be extracted from the liver half an hour after injection. At that time, the estrone complex was not recovered from blood, diaphragm, or ventral prostate. However, if the complex enters the cells, this does not necessarily mean that it enters the nuclei.

We do not believe that the estradiol-cytostatic complex or the extrone complex have any alkylating effect as long as the complex is intact. Our studies on prostatic nuclear preparations indicated that the complex was intact in prostatic nuclei. This does not exclude the possibility that it is later hydrolyzed slowly in the nuclei, and the nor-nitrogen mustard might then exert an alkylating effect on DNA or nuclear proteins. That the complex itself can have important inhibitory effects on nuclear activities should not be excluded.

I. Könyves: In your *in vivo* experiments you studied the retention of steroid cytostatic complex in the rat prostate after the hydrolysis of the 17-phosphate group. Have you any experimental data on the time of retention?

J.-G. Forsberg: No, not yet. What we want to stress is that in the "long-term" *in vivo* experiments the estrone-cytostatic complex could be recovered from the ventral prostate but not from liver and muscle tissue. Moreover, our results indicate that the conversion of the estradiol-cytostatic complex to the estrone-cytostatic complex was restricted to the liver, even though a low-grade conversion in the ventral prostate cannot be excluded.

A. Fritjofsson: You have been talking about "short-term" and "long-term" experiments. For me as a clinician, even your "long-term" experiments are very short. What would be the results if you followed your animals for a longer time?

J.-G. Forsberg: We have tried to define the "short-term" and the "long-term" experimental situations as clearly as possible. However, we agree that our "long-term" experiments are really short ones from a clinical point of view. As yet we have not followed the animals for a longer period than 3 days.

K. B. Eik-Nes: Estramustine phosphate (EMP) appeared to reduce prostatic 5α-reductase as measured by DHT production. Did EMP change prostatic 3-hydroxysteroid dehydrogenase activity—i.e., did more DHT go to the 5α-androstanediol with EMP?

J.-G. Forsberg: We did not observe any substantial change in the amount of 5α-androstanediols recovered after EMP treatment compared with controls.

W. Vahlensieck: What happens if you give EMP and there is a liver dysfunction? Did you study this situation?

J.-G. Forsberg: We have not studied this problem.

B. Uvnäs: Why do you need such a high dose as 100 mg/kg of EMP for significant recovery from the ventral prostate?

J.-G. Forsberg: The dose 100 mg/kg body weight was calculated so as to correspond to the human therapeutic dose after taking into consideration species differences in sensitivity to alkylating agents. It is possible that somewhat lower doses could be used, but we have no information on the critical dose level.

K. J. Tveter: What is the effect of EMP on the pituitary? Is it different from that of estradiol and other estrogens?

J.-G. Forsberg: We have not studied the effect of EMP on the pituitary gland. Nor are we aware of any information on this point.

H. J. Tagnon: I wish to report a clinical trial of Estracyt on 34 patients with mammary cancer who were treated by the daily intravenous injection of 160 mg of the compound. Two of 34 patients experienced remissions. This is less than what would be expected from estrogen alone. Details can be found in *Eur. J. Cancer* **5**, 1 (1969).

J.-G. Forsberg: We are quite aware of this study. However, our interest in Estracyt was initiated by several clinical reports indicating a favorable effect of Estracyt in the treatment of human prostatic carcinomas. One must be very careful when trying to extrapolate results from one species to another and note also that results from one organ may not be valid for another organ. Differences in uptake, retention, metabolism, etc. must be taken into consideration. Thus various types of carcinomas must be evaluated separately when the action of anticancer drugs is considered.

I. Könyves: The dosage was very low in the EORTC study (80–160 mg/day). The dosage of Estracyt for the treatment of prostatic carcinoma is 600–900 mg (in Europe) and 900–1200 mg in the United States.

Potential Test Systems for Chemotherapeutic Agents against Prostatic Cancer

A. A. SANDBERG

Roswell Park Memorial Institute, Buffalo, New York

I. INTRODUCTION

The testing of agents potentially useful in the therapy of prostatic cancer, as compared, for example, to those effective in leukemia, breast cancer, and lymphomas, is faced at present with at least one major shortcoming, i.e., the lack of an appropriate *in vivo* model system for cancer of the prostate in a suitable animal in which such drugs could be tested. Cancer of the prostate develops spontaneously only rarely in experimental animals, and chemically or virally induced prostatic cancers is a field, though dating back some years, that is still in its developing stages (see accompanying tabulation).

Nor is this the only problem with a test system for drugs against cancer of the prostate. Human prostatic cancer presents a variety of histological

156 A. A. SANDBERG

Experimentally Induced Tumors in the Prostate

Authors	Animal	Carcinogen	Type of tumor
Moore and Melchionna (1937)	Rat	1,2-Benzpyrene	Squamous cell carcinoma, sarcoma
Dunning et al. (1946)	Rat	20-Methylcholanthrene (pellets inserted in prostate)	Squamous cell carcinoma
Horning (1946)	Mice	20-Methylcholanthrene	Glandular carcinoma
Mirand and Staubitz (1956)	Rat	20-Methylcholanthrene (crystals inserted in gland)	Squamous cell carcinoma, adenocarcinoma, leiomyosarcoma
Higuchi et al. (1972)	Rat	20-Methylcholanthrene, 4-NWO	Leiomyoma

types, rates of growth, sensitivity to steroid hormones, and tendency for metastases (Györkey, 1973); thus, it may be necessary to develop a variety of such testing systems to parallel the clinical situation. A case in point is the R-3327 spontaneous prostatic tumor first observed in a Copenhagen rat in 1961 (Dunning, 1963), and classified as a papillary adenocarcinoma, apparently of a histological appearance corresponding to that of the dorsal gland of the rat. Recently, the tumor has been shown to be androgen sensitive and to have a receptor protein for dihydrotestosterone (DHT) (Voigt and Dunning, 1974). Admittedly, this tumor could serve as a very useful model for testing drugs against prostatic cancer. However, a serious obstacle to the widespread use of this tumor as a model for testing chemotherapeutic drugs is the inadequate number of inbred Copenhagen rats and the relatively slow growth rate of the tumor. It is hoped that in the future a variety of prostatic tumors in animals, either of spontaneous or induced origin, will become available for testing chemotherapeutic agents potentially effective against prostatic cancer.

Until the development of an animal tumor model system for testing drugs against prostatic cancer becomes a reality, several unique characteristics of the prostate gland seem to afford an opportunity for such testing. We chose three such unique features of the gland as targets for testing drugs possibly effective against human cancer of the prostate: (1) 5α-reductase activity, (2) arginase activity, and (3) steroid deposition in the prostate. This paper presents our experience with these test systems.

It is possible that these parameters of prostatic metabolism represent a rather narrow approach to cancer of the prostate and may, in fact, have little relevance to some forms of cancer of the prostate in the human, i.e., those cancers that do not have significant 5α-reductase or arginase activity or receptor proteins for androgens and/or estrogens. However, a certain percentage of cancers do have considerable enzyme activity (Jenkins and McCaffery, 1974; R. Y. Kirdani, and A. A. Sandberg, unpublished data, 1975), and evidence for the presence of intracellular receptor proteins for steroids has been demonstrated in some human prostatic cancers (Sinha et al., 1973; R. Y. Kirdani and A. A. Sandberg, unpublished data, 1975). Thus, drugs affecting these parameters could conceivably be of value in the treatment of at least those cancers characterized by the presence of 5α-reductase and arginase activities and steroid receptor proteins.

The introduction of hormonal therapy in cancer of the prostate not only represents a milestone in the therapy of this disease (Huggins and Hodges, 1941), but also in a number of other human cancerous conditions. Unfortunately, such hormonal therapy in prostatic cancer, even though of immense palliative and symptomatic relief to the patients, is not capable of curing the disease or affecting all forms of cancer of the prostate. Also, most patients ultimately become resistant to such therapy (Prout, 1973; Murphy, 1974). Thus, the development of chemotherapeutic agents against prostatic cancer assumes a crucial aspect in this disease, with full recognition and dependency on the value and implications of hormonal therapy in cancer of the prostate.

Undoubtedly, no single model system will prove to be universally useful in testing drugs against prostatic cancer. For example, drugs which affect DNA synthesis (Sloan et al., 1975) may not be effective in prostatic cancers which have a rather low mitotic index, i.e., slow turnover of DNA, but in which drugs affecting 5α-reductase or arginase activity may be effective, and vice versa.

II. The 5α-Reductase (5α-RA) Enzyme System

A. Background

This enzyme system (5α-reductase, reduced nicotinamide adenine dinucleotide phosphate: Δ^4-3-ketosteroid 5α-oxidoreductase) is present in a number of tissues, although the intracellular distribution and steroidal specificity of the enzyme system may differ from tissue to tissue (Roy, 1971; Wilson, 1972; Gustafsson and Pousette, 1974). In the prostate it appears to be primarily associated with the nuclear membrane

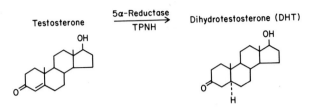

FIG. 1. The 5α-reductase reaction (5α-RA) in the prostate, showing the reduction of testosterone (T) to dihydrotestosterone (DHT).

(Bruchovsky and Wilson, 1968a,b; Shimazaki *et al.*, 1969a,b, 1972a,b, 1973b; Frederiksen and Wilson, 1971; Moore and Wilson, 1972, 1973), though also present in the microsomal fraction (Nozu and Tamaoki, 1974a,b), and to have the function of converting testosterone (T) to dihydrotestosterone (DHT, androstalolone, 5α-androstan-17β-ol-3-one) (Fig. 1). The latter steroid appears to be primarily responsible for the androgenic effects of T and is considered to be the active androgen in the prostate (Ofner, 1969; Wilson, 1972), (androstanediol, i.e., 5α-androstane-3α,17β-diol, may play the part of the active androgen in addition to DHT) (Baulieu, 1973), responsible for the maintenance of prostatic anatomy and function (e.g., protein and RNA synthesis in the gland) (Davies and Griffiths, 1974; Mainwaring *et al.*, 1974a; Isotalo and Santti, 1975) and has been implicated as the key androgen in some pathological states of the prostate in the human (Siiteri and Wilson, 1970; Wilson, 1972; Steins *et al.*, 1974). Interestingly, the level of 5α-RA in the prostate is preponderantly under the control of T and/or DHT (Wilson, 1972; Moore and Wilson, 1973); i.e., the administration of T or DHT to castrated animals restores prostatic weight to normal and the 5α-RA activity therein, with the enzyme activity in some cases exceeding that observed in normal glands (Karr *et al.*, 1974; Yamanaka *et al.*, 1975). The latter effect can be observed in intact rats to whom T or DHT has been administered.

The effects of estrogens on the 5α-RA are less clearly understood than those of androgens. The administration of estrogens to intact animals does decrease greatly the 5α-RA (Belham and Neal, 1971; Wilson, 1972), and this has been adduced to be primarily through interference with release of LH from the pituitary and consequent decreased secretion of T by the testes (Shearer *et al.*, 1973; Györkey, 1973; Boyns *et al.*, 1974). The low levels of circulating T are then reflected in the decreased 5α-RA in the prostate. Nevertheless, some workers have presented evidence that estrogens may have a direct effect on prostatic 5α-RA not requiring the intercession of pituitary and/or testicular effects (Farnsworth, 1969;

Bonne and Raynaud, 1973; Lee *et al.*, 1973; Giorgi *et al.*, 1972b, 1974), and in some cases an increased 5α-RA has been observed after the administration of estrogens to rats (Danutra *et al.*, 1973; Lee *et al.*, 1974).

Because of the efficacy of estrogens in remarkably alleviating the subjective and/or objective symptoms in a significant number of patients with cancer of the prostate and the key role played by 5α-RA in prostatic physiology, we felt that any drug affecting this enzymic parameter to a significant extent should be considered as a possible candidate for therapy against cancer of the prostate.

B. METHODS AND MATERIALS

Even though the rat prostatic gland (ventral and dorsolateral) is not entirely comparable to that of the human, the level of 5α-RA in the rat prostate is similar to that of the human and shows responses (to androgens, estrogens and castration) which make it a very suitable tissue for testing the effects on 5α-RA activity under various conditions, including the administration of chemotherapeutic agents (Sandberg *et al.*, 1975; Saroff *et al.*, 1975).

Male adult Wistar rats (weighing 330–450 gm) purchased from Charles River Breeding Laboratories, Wilmington, Massachusetts, were acclimated in our laboratory for about 1 week and then injected with various drugs. Each drug was injected intraperitoneally daily for 1 week, except for diglycolaldehyde, which was given for 5 days, and thiotepa and hydroxyurea, whose effects were tested over a period of 2 weeks. The rats were killed by ether anesthesia, and the ventral and dorsolateral prostates were removed.

The 5α-RA activity in prostatic tissue was determined by methods based on those used by Shimazaki *et al.* (1969a,b, 1792a,b) with modifications to fit our experimental conditions and design. A 50% homogenate of prostatic tissue was made by grinding the specimen by hand in a Potter-Elvehjem glass homogenizer at 4°C to which had been added an equal volume of 50 μM (pH 7.4) Tris-HCl buffer. The homogenate was filtered through gauze and the gauze squeezed by hand to drain out as much liquid as possible. Homogenate equivalent to 300 mg of tissue, wet weight, was taken for 5α-RA activity.

The homogenate was incubated in a total of 6 ml of medium at 37°C for 1 hour containing 1 mg of NADPH, 0.3 μCi of ^{14}C-testosterone (4-^{14}C) (specific activity 50 μCi/μmole) and 6 M fumarate. In more recent studies, we have added ^{3}H-labeled DHT (1,2-^{3}H) (48 μCi/μmole) to the incubation mixture to evaluate the possibility of further metabolic transformation of the ^{14}C-labeled DHT derived from the labeled T, and the calculations of the 5α-RA activity took these factors into consideration.

After incubation the reaction was stopped by the addition of ethanol to a minimal concentration of 70%. One hundred micrograms each of T, DHT, and androstenedione were added to the mixture and centrifuged. The resulting supernatant was evaporated to a small volume. Ten milliliters of water were added and extracted 3 times with equal volumes of ethyl acetate. The latter was washed with 0.1 volume of saturated Na_2HOC_3 and once with 0.1 volume of water. The ethyl acetate was reduced in volume and applied to paper strips for chromatography, and the paper was developed in the Bush-3 system. After scanning of the radioactivity on the paper, the conversion products were eluted and acetylated and the acetylated steroids then separated by chromatography in the Bush-A system. The DHT-acetate peak was eluted and together with the testosterone peak from the Bush-3 system quantitated for recovery by either gas chromatography (Kirdani et al., 1972), or by determining the UV absorption for T and androstenedione, or by the recovery of the DHT-^{3}H. The rate of 5α-RA activity toward T is expressed as μmoles of DHT formed during 1 hour per gram equivalent of the original prostatic tissue.

For the determination of the Michaelis constants, the concentration of T in the incubation medium varied from 0.17 to 1.02×10^{-9} M, at least 5 different concentrations being used for plotting the Lineweaver–Burk curves. The Michaelis constants (K_m and V_{max}) were established by Lineweaver–Burk reciprocal plots, and the results are expressed in terms of competitive, noncompetitive, and uncompetitive inhibition or activation (Dawes, 1967). Competitive inhibition was thought to exist when the V_{max} did not change, while the apparent K_m showed a definite increase; noncompetitive inhibition when there was a change in the V_{max} but no interference with the combination of the enzyme with the substrate; and uncompetitive inhibition when the slope of the linear plot essentially paralleled that of the control values. Activation took the same factors into consideration.

C. Drugs

The drug doses given to the rats (Table I) were established on the basis of comparable therapeutic doses in man and, in some cases, according to the effects observed in animal studies, particularly as described in the clinical brochures on the drugs supplied by the NCI. Further details on the drugs, including their NSC and CAS numbers and formulations, can be found in Sandberg et al. (1975).

TABLE I

CHEMOTHERAPEUTIC AGENTS TESTED AND DOSE
ADMINISTERED TO RATS[a]

Drug	Dose (mg/kg/day)
5-Fluorodeoxyuridine	30
Cyclophosphamide	50
Vincristine	50[b]
Procarbazine	5
Hexamethylmelamine	50
CCNU	40
Isophosphamide	100
Bleomycin	5
NSC-45388	5
Streptozotocin	15
Adriamycin	2.5
Diglycolaldehyde	50
Thiotepa	0.3 wk $\times$ 2[c]
Hydroxyurea	7/q.3 days $\times$ 5[c]

[a] Animals used were Wistar male rats (330–450 gm). All drugs except diglycolaldehyde, thiotepa, and hydroxyurea were injected intraperitoneally for 7 days; diglycolaldehyde was injected for 5 days. On day 8 rats were killed under ether anesthesia and prostates were removed.

[b] Micrograms per kilogram per day.

[c] Total milligrams injected—not per kilogram.

For some drugs, the doses ultimately used had to be decreased due to the death of the animals caused by the drugs. In such instances, we generally employed a dose that was 20–32% of the lethal dose. Usually, three drugs were tested concomitantly during each time period, with control animals accompanying each experimental group of rats. The control group consisted of 10 rats and each drug was administered to 18–30 animals. In deciding upon the length of time for the administration of drugs, it was felt that they should not be given for any period that would seriously affect total body weight or appetite or would produce other untoward toxic effects in the rats.

Prior to injection, hexamethylmelamine (obtained in capsules), cyclophosphamide powder and procarbazine (obtained as a crystalline powder) were dissolved in water. All other drugs were administered in the solution in which they were supplied either by the manufacturers or by the NCI.

D. RESULTS

Most drugs caused some decrease in body weight during administration

TABLE II

EFFECTS OF CHEMOTHERAPEUTIC AGENTS ON RAT BODY AND
PROSTATIC WEIGHTS

Drug	Decrease (%) in body weight compared to pretreatment weight	Prostatic weights (%) compared to controls[a]	
		Ventral	Dorsolateral
5-Fluorodeoxyuridine	−19	−26	−27
Cyclophosphamide	−23	−24	−20
Vincristine	−7	−1	−6
Procarbazine	−5	0	0
Hexamethylmelamine	−11	−16	−8
CCNU	−15	−28	−13
Isophosphamide	−22	−31	−18
Bleomycin	−23	−18	−35
NSC-45388	−2	−5	0
Streptozotocin	−13	−14	−20
Adriamycin	−10	−47	−31
Diglycolaldehyde	−15	−24	−17
Hydroxyurea	+5	+20%	+15%
Thiotepa	+2	+8%	+11%

[a] Control ventral prostatic weight: 402 ± 23–485 ± 24 gm. Control dorsolateral prostatic weight: 303 ± 15–344 ± 11 gm.

(Table II), ranging from 2% to 23% (mean, 13.8%) of the pretreatment weight, which compared with the 0–12% gain in body weight in the controlled rats. It is interesting that on the average the decrease in the prostatic weight tended to be higher (in the case of some drugs markedly so) than the decrease in body weight. The loss in prostatic weight, when the latter was compared to that of the controlled groups, ranged from 0 to 47% (mean, 19.5%) in the ventral gland and from 0 to 35% (mean, 16.5%) in the dorsolateral prostate. Cyclophosphamide, 5-FU, isophosphamide, adriamycin, diglycolaldehyde, bleomycin, and CCNU caused the largest decreases in prostatic weight. Hydroxyurea and thiotepa led to some gain in body weight and gains in prostatic weights.

Table III shows the K_m and V_{max} values for 5α-RA in the ventral and dorsolateral prostates of the rat. These results have also been graphically represented in Figs. 2–5 as Lineweaver–Burk plots. We interpret the significance of our findings to be that isophosphamide, bleomycin, and procarbazine produce a definite inhibition of 5α-RA, either noncompetitively or uncompetitively. This inhibition of the 5α-RA was manifested in the ventral and/or dorsolateral glands. On the other hand, 5-FU, vincristine, hexamethylmelamine, CCNU, streptozotocin, NSC-45388, and diglycolaldehyde actually produced either uncompetitive or noncom-

TABLE III

EFFECTS OF CHEMOTHERAPEUTIC DRUGS ON 5α-RA OF RAT
VENTRAL AND DORSOLATERAL PROSTATE

Drug	Ventral		Dorsolateral	
	$K_m \times 10^{-7}\ M$	V_{max} (10^{-9} mole/gm of tissue/hr)	$K_m \times 10^{-7}\ M$	V_{max} (10^{-9} mole/gm of tissue/hr)
5-Fluorodeoxyuridine	0.36	2.13	—	—
Cyclophosphamide	4.0	0.25	—	—
Vincristine[a]	0.90	3.94	—	—
Procarbazine	1.30	2.44	0.57	1.44
Hexamethylemel- amine	1.43	0.65	—	—
CCNU	1.73	4.17	0.95	4.72
Isophosphamide	1.56	0.62	0.25	0.67
Bleomycin	4.21	4.48	1.06	1.58
NSC-45388	0.84	1.57	1.75	4.06
Streptozotocin	1.04	4.02	3.76	8.27
Adriamycin	15.02	0.04	1.62	0.12
Diglycolaldehyde	2.56	5.49	—	—
Hydroxyurea	1.50	2.07	1.03	1.47
Thiotepa	2.38	1.69	7.20	0.68
Controls	1.00	3.42	0.50	2.60

[a] Values for combined dorsolateral and ventral glands.

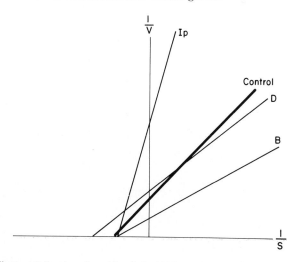

FIG. 2. Effects of isophosphamide (ip), NSC-45388 (D), and bleomycin (B) on
5α-RA in the rat ventral prostate as shown by Lineweaver–Burk reciprocal plots
and compared with plot of control values (Sandberg et al., 1975).

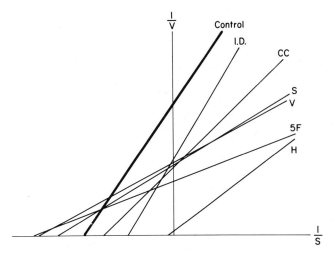

Fig. 3. Effects of diglycolaldehyde (I.D.), CCNU (CC), streptozotocin (S), vincristine (V), 5-fluorodeoxyuridine (5F), and hexamethylmelamine (H) on 5 α-RA in the rat ventral prostate as shown by Lineweaver–Burk reciprocal plots and compared with plot of control values (Sandberg *et al.*, 1975).

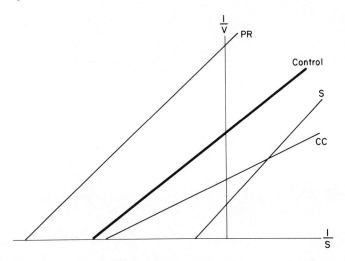

Fig. 4. Effects of procarbazine (PR), streptozotocin (S), and CCNU (CC) on 5α-RA in the rat dorsolateral prostate as shown by Lineweaver–Burk reciprocal plots and compared with plot of control values (Sandberg *et al.*, 1975).

petitive activation of 5α-RA in either or both glands of the rat. In more recent experiments we have shown that thiotepa and hydroxyurea also cause noncompetitive activation of 5α-RA in the dorsolateral and ventral glands of the rat (Table III).

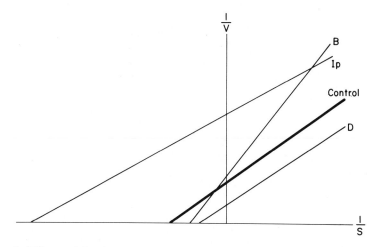

FIG. 5. Effects of isophosphamide (Ip), bleomycin (B), and NSC-45388 (D) on 5α-RA in the rat dorsolateral prostate as shown by Lineweaver-Burk reciprocal plots and compared with plots of control values (Sandberg *et al.*, 1975).

E. EFFECTS OF ESTRACYT

The effects on 5α-RA of the antiprostatic agent Estracyt [estradiol-3-bis(2-chloroethyl)-carbamate-17-dihydrogen phosphate] are shown for comparison. Estracyt has been used successfully in the treatment of cancer of the prostate (Mittelman *et al.*, 1975) although its exact mode of action remains unclear (Kirdani *et al.*, 1974). This agent is a chemical ester of a nitrogen mustard with estradiol-17β (E₂), and it is hoped that the latter, owing to its localization in the prostate, carries the mustard into the prostate "piggyback." In the gland hydrolysis of the molecule should yield both the mustard and E₂ in forms potentially effective intracellularly. Whether this occurs in every species is still a moot point.

The effects of various doses of Estracyt on rat prostatic 5α-RA were determined in groups of 7 animals each (Kirdani *et al.*, 1974). The drug was injected intraperitoneally for 4 days, and the weights and 5α-RA were measured in the ventral and dorsolateral glands and kidney. In Fig. 6 are shown the weight changes, which indicate substantially reduced weights of the prostatic glands with only minor changes in the kidney. In Fig. 7 are shown the alterations in 5α-RA. There is a definite effect on the 5α-RA of the ventral prostate, less than 50% of the control activity being induced by the higher doses of Estracyt. The effects were less consistent in the dorsolateral gland. The 5α-RA in the kidney was not decreased, and, if anything, some elevation in the activity was observed.

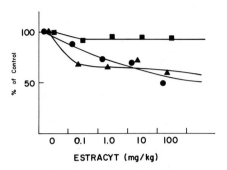

FIG. 6. Weight of prostate glands (●, ventral; ▲, dorsolateral) and kidney (■) in rats treated with various doses of Estracyt. The results are expressed as a percentage of control values. Each point consists of the average of the values obtained on 7 rat prostates. Only a slight decrease in the weight of the kidney was evident, whereas the 2 prostates showed significant decreases in weight, particularly the ventral gland (Kirdani *et al.*, 1974).

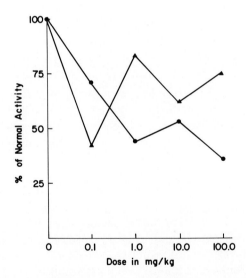

FIG. 7. The effects of various doses of Estracyt on 5α-reductase activity of rat prostates. The decrease in the activity of the ventral prostate (●) is profound, but is less so in the dorsolateral gland (▲). These values, taken in conjunction with the weight reduction of the glands (see Fig. 6), indicate very greatly decreased 5α-reductase activity in the prostates of the rat. The kidney did not show this decrease and, if anything, 5α-reductase activity was elevated by the administered Estracyt (Kirdani *et al.*, 1974).

III. PROSTATIC ARGINASE ACTIVITY

A. BACKGROUND

The enzyme arginase (EC 3.5.3.1, L-arginase ureohydrolase) is present in the liver and other tissues (brain, kidney, prostate, intestine) of ureotelic animals, as a member of the enzyme system involved in the urea cycle (Fig. 8). The function of arginase is the deamination of arginine to ornithine. The role of prostatic arginase is not as clearly understood as that of 5α-RA (Yamanaka *et al.*, 1971, 1972; Shimazaki *et al.*, 1973a), although it may play an important role in some facets related to the synthesis of polyamines (putrescine, spermidine, spermine), which are unique to the prostate and constitute an important moiety of the secretory element of this gland (Pegg *et al.*, 1970; Tabor and Tabor, 1972; Harik *et al.*, 1974). Similarly to 5α-RA, arginase activity in the prostate and the kidney is significantly under the control of androgens, though the activity of this enzyme after castration does not decrease to the same low levels in the prostate as those observed for 5α-RA. Therefore, it is probable that factors other than androgens also control the level of prostatic arginase, or that androgens control that moiety of the enzyme which is localized in specific prostatic cells (e.g., epithelial cells), whereas other substances control the enzyme activity in other cells (e.g., supporting cells).

B. METHODS

The prostatic tissue was homogenized with 10 volumes of 10 mM malic acid solution (pH 7.1) containing 30 μM manganese chloride in a glass homogenizer. An aliquot of the suspension to be assayed was incubated in a water bath at 55°C for 20 minutes and then 40 μM arginine-HCl

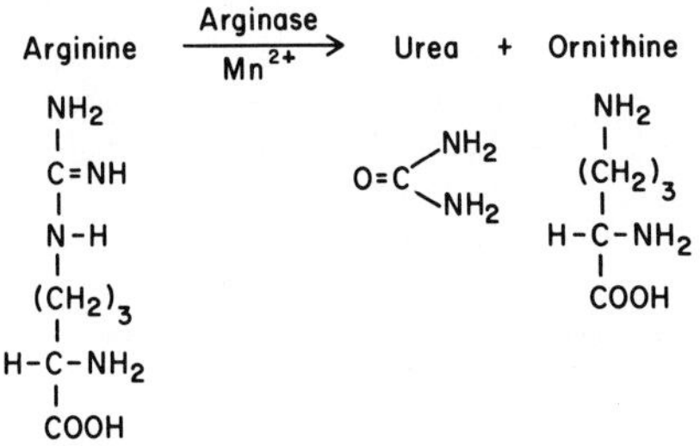

FIG. 8. The arginase reaction showing the deamination of arginase to ornithine and urea. Note requirement of Mn^{2+} for full activity of the enzyme.

solution (pH 9.7) was added to make a final volume of 0.5 ml, and this was then incubated at 37°C for 30 minutes. The reaction was stopped by adding 1 ml of ice-cold 10% trichloroacetic acid and the mixture was centrifuged. An aliquot of the supernatant was taken for urea determination by the α-isonitrosopropriophenone reaction (Schimke, 1964) and the enzyme activity was expressed as micromoles of urea formed per minute per 1 mg equivalent of tissue.

C. RESULTS

The effects of estrogens on prostatic and kidney arginase are shown in Table IV. There is a gradual decrease in arginase activity with increasing doses of E_2, the highest dose leading to an arginase activity only 60% that of the control animals. The decrease in the kidney was even more marked. On the other hand, testosterone administration to intact rats leads to a greatly increased enzyme activity, usually 200–300% of that of the controls.

The effects of the administration of various drugs on arginase activity are shown in Table V and Figs. 9 and 10. The calculation of the various constants and the protocol for the treatment of the animals (Table I) followed the same procedure as that described for 5α-RA. In contrast to the effects on 5α-RA, no activation of the enzymic activity was observed with any of the drugs used. The results indicated noncompetitive or competitive inhibition of arginase activity by the administration of

TABLE IV

EFFECTS OF ESTRADIOL-17β (E_2) ON RAT PROSTATIC (VENTRAL) AND KIDNEY ARGINASE ACTIVITY AND WEIGHT[a,b]

Conditions	Body weight (g)	Prostate weight (mg)	Prostate arginase		Kidney arginase[c]	
			(μmoles urea/min/gm)	%	(μmoles /urea/min/gm)	%
Control	457 ± 13	480 ± 13	1.86 ± 0.13	100	14.95 ± 1.13	100
E_2, 0.05 mg/day	425 ± 21	374 ± 18	1.48 ± 0.04	80	8.48 ± 0.14	57
E_2, 0.1 mg/day	409 ± 5	342 ± 9	1.41 ± 0.15	76	7.51 ± 1.07	50
E_2, 0.5 mg/day	417 ± 7	330 ± 38	1.02 ± 0.09	55	5.90 ± 0.70	40
E_2, 1.0 mg/day	412 ± 6	310 ± 21	1.15 ± 0.17	62	5.82 ± 0.15	39
E_2, 2.0 mg/day	415 ± 16	302 ± 24	1.12 ± 0.10	60	4.73 ± 0.14	32

[a] The studies were performed in normal adult Wistar rats injected intraperitoneally with estradiol valerate on four successive days; at the end of 96 hours the rats were sacrificed and the organ for study was removed.

[b] Expressed as mean ±S.E.

[c] No change in kidney weight occurred.

TABLE V

EFFECTS OF CHEMOTHERAPEUTIC DRUGS ON ARGINASE OF RAT
VENTRAL AND DORSOLATERAL PROSTATE

Drug	Ventral		Dorsolateral	
	$K_m \times 10^{-3} M$	V_{max} ($10^{-6} M$ urea/gm of tissue/min)	$K_m \times 10^{-3} M$	V_{max} ($10^{-6} M$ urea/gm of tissue/min)
5-Fluorodeoxyuridine	19.23	2.63	19.23	7.69
Cyclophosphamide	15.62	3.33	13.89	11.11
Vincristine	20.40	2.17	23.25	9.09
Procarbazine	21.28	2.50	18.52	6.67
Hexamethylmelamine	18.52	1.92	21.27	6.25
CCNU	10.00	2.50	11.62	6.25
Isophosphamide	11.76	3.33	11.11	6.25
Bleomycin	29.41	2.77	25.00	6.67
NSC-45388	13.89	1.67	11.49	5.56
Streptozotocin	10.53	2.08	13.34	6.25
Adriamycin	22.20	2.77	26.32	5.88
Diglycolaldehyde	18.50	3.23	12.66	6.67
Controls	13.33 ± 0.63	2.89 ± 0.15	11.50 ± 0.41	6.72 ± 0.43

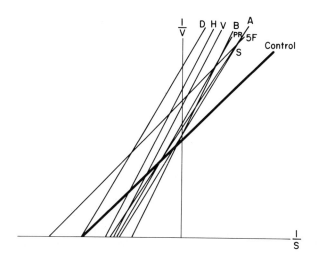

FIG. 9. Effects of NSC-45388 (D), hexamethylmelamine (H), vincristine (V), bleomycin (B), procarbazine (PR), adriamycin (A), 5-fluorodeoxyuridine (5F), and streptoxotocin (S) on arginase activity in the rat ventral prostate as shown by Lineweaver–Burk reciprocal plots and compared with plot of control values (Sandberg et al., 1975).

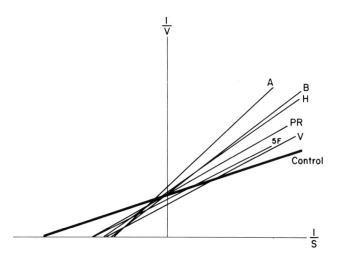

Fɪɢ. 10. Effects of adriamycin (A), bleomycin (B), hexamethylmelamine (H), procarbazine (PR), 5-fluorodeoxyuridine (5F), and vincristine (V) on arginase activity
in the rat dorsolateral prostate as shown by Lineweaver–Burk reciprocal plots and
compared with plot of control values (Sandberg *et al.,* 1975).

vincristine, bleomycin, procarbazine, adriamycin, and hexamethylmelamine, in both the ventral and dorsolateral prostates. On the other hand,
streptozotocin and NSC-45388 produced noncompetitive inhibition only
in the ventral gland. Bleomycin, hexamethylmelamine, procarbazine, and
possibly adriamycin produced competitive inhibition only in the dorsolateral gland. It appears that 5-FU led to uncompetitive inhibition of
arginase activity in both prostates. Cyclophosphamide, CCNU, isophosphamide, and diglycolaldehyde appeared to produce no effects on either
prostate. In more recent studies thiotepa and hydroxyurea produced
definite noncompetitive inhibition of the arginase activity in both ventral
and dorsolateral glands.

D. Effects of Estracyt and Flutamide

For comparison, the effects of two anti-prostatic agents (Kirdani *et
al.,* 1974; Varkarakis *et al.,* 1975b), i.e., Estracyt and Flutamide (SCH
13521, 4′-nitro-3′-trifluoromethylisobutyranilide), probably working
through different mechanisms, on prostatic arginase are shown for comparison. In Fig. 11 are shown the effects of various doses of Estracyt
(see section on 5α-RA for protocol and Fig. 6 for weight changes) on
the arginase activity of rat prostate and kidney. In general, the effects
on the ventral prostate are more marked and consistent than those on
the dorsolateral gland, i.e., with higher doses some activation of arginase

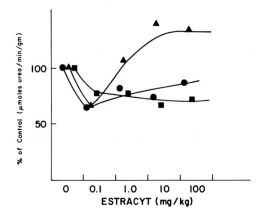

Fig. 11. Arginase activity, expressed per gram of tissue, in rat prostates and kidney following the administration of various doses of Estracyt. In the dorsolateral gland (▲), except for a decrease at the lowest dose, the arginase activity was increased with the higher doses. The decreased activities in the ventral gland (●) and kidney (■), although not very profound, were more consistent (Kirdani *et al.*, 1974).

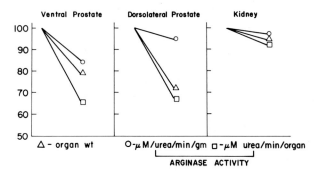

Fig. 12. Arginase activity (as percent of controls) in rat prostates and kidney before and after treatment of animals with Flutamide (SCH 13521) (10 mg per day orally for 4 days) (Varkarakis *et al.*, 1975b).

activity occurred in the dorsolateral gland. Flutamide (Fig. 12) caused a markedly decreased arginase activity in the ventral and dorsolateral glands, with only a small effect on kidney arginase. The weights of the prostatic glands were also substantially reduced. The inhibition of arginase in the prostate, but not in the kidney, indicates some specificity for the effects of Flutamide.

Since manganese ion (Mn^{2+}) is essential for full arginase activity (Schimke, 1964; Yamanaka *et al.*, 1971, 1972), we investigated the possibility that drugs may lead to a deficiency of this metal in the tissue

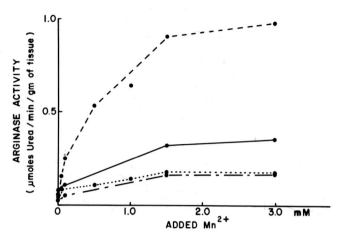

FIG. 13. Effect of Mn^{2+} concentrations on arginase activity of baboon prostates. The results indicate that Mn^{2+} is needed for optimal enzyme activity, as has been shown for human and rat prostates (Yamanaka *et al.*, 1972) ; and that the decreased levels of arginase activity caused by the administration of three drugs to baboons are real, not due to Mn^{2+} deficiency in the assay (Müntzing *et al.*, 1974). ●---●, Control; ●—●, Flutamide; ●⋯●, Estracyt; ●——-—●, stilbestrol.

test system. A representative study is shown in Fig. 13. The results shown were obtained with baboon prostate (Varkarakis *et al.*, 1975a), though similar data have been shown with prostatic tissue from other species, and indicate profound depression of arginase activity by Estracyt, Flutamide, and stilbestrol administered to baboons, regardless of the Mn^{2+} concentration in the medium.

IV. DEPOSITION OF LABELED STEROIDS IN THE DOG PROSTATE

A. BACKGROUND

The prostates of a number of species (dog, rat, baboon, man) have been shown to concentrate androgens (Harding and Samuels, 1962; Bruchovsky and Wilson, 1968a,b; Ghanadian and Fotherby, 1972; Kirdani *et al.*, 1972; Varkarakis *et al.*, 1971, 1973), and in some the presence of an intracellular protein (receptor) with high affinity and specificity for T and DHT has been demonstrated (Fang and Liao, 1969, 1971; Hansson *et al.*, 1972; Rennie and Bruchovsky, 1972; Mainwaring and Milroy, 1973; Baulieu, 1973). This receptor protein appears to behave like, and to have characteristics similar to, those present in other target tissues, e.g., uterus and breast, with affinity for estrogens (Jensen *et al.*, 1971; Jensen and de Sombre, 1972, 1973). Evidence is accumulating that the DHT–receptor complex is capable of stimulating prostatic RNA synthesis leading to the synthesis of proteins specific for the prostate. Of interest was the demonstration that the prostate in some species contained receptor proteins for estrogens (estradiol-17β, estriol) (Mangan *et al.*, 1967; McCann *et al.*, 1971; Jungblut *et al.*, 1971; Baulieu *et al.*, 1971; Armstrong and Bashirelahi, 1974). The presence of such receptor proteins in the prostate for both androgens and estrogens led us to believe that agents which interfered with the deposition of either or both steroid hormones in the prostate of the dog may be useful in the therapy of human prostatic cancer (Groom *et al.*, 1971). This was based not only on some similarities between the dog and the human and rat prostates (Kowarski *et al.*, 1969; Griffiths *et al.*, 1970; Gloyna *et al.*, 1970; Giorgi *et al.*, 1972a,b; Haltmeyer and Eik-Nes, 1972; Mawhinney *et al.*, 1974), but also on the theory that steroids associated with intracellular receptor proteins play a key role in the transcription of DNA and RNA synthesis necessary for protein synthesis in the prostate and are, therefore, important regulators of cellular function; and that an interference by drugs with the receptor–steroid association may be of value in treating cancer of the prostate.

We have shown that the adult dog prostate concentrates both androgens and estrogens (Figs. 14 and 15) and that the radioactivity in the gland following the injection of the labeled steroids consists more than 80% of the original or slightly modified steroid, e.g., testosterone and DHT, estradiol (E_2) and estrone (E_1), and estriol (E_3). The administration of unlabeled "cold" steroid definitely interferes with such deposition

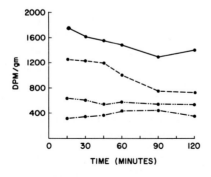

FIG. 14. Concentration of radioactivity in various dog tissues after single intravenous injection of 50 μCi of estriol-4-^{14}C (22×10^6 dpm). The prostate (●—●) contained 3.6 times the radioactivity present in muscle (●–·–·●) (Varkarakis *et al.*, 1973). ●—·—·●, Testes; ●---●, blood.

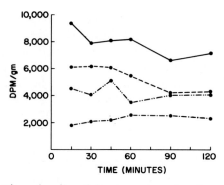

Fig. 15. Concentration of radioactivity in various dog tissues after single intravenous injection of 50 μCi of DHT-1,2-³H (110 × 10⁶ dpm). The prostate (●—●) contained 3 times the radioactivity present in muscle (●-·-·●) (Varkarakis *et al.*, 1973). ●-··-●, Testes; ●---●, blood.

in the gland, indicating competition between the labeled and unlabeled steroids for receptor sites in the prostatic cells (Varkarakis *et al.*, 1973).

B. Methods and Materials

Adult male mongrel dogs weighing 10–29 kg were used in the study. The radioactive steroids were injected intravenously in 20 ml of saline over a period of 1 minute and blood and tissue samples were taken at 15, 30, 45, 60, 90, and 120 minutes after the injection. Pentobarbital sodium (60 mg/kg of body weight) administered intravenously was used for general anesthesia. For tissue deposition each of four dogs was injected with a mixture of ³H-labeled E_3 (50 μCi) and ¹⁴C-labeled T (10 μCi). The results were compared with those obtained in groups of control dogs.

The radioactivity in the tested tissues (expressed as dpm per gram of tissue) was determined with a tissue oxidizer (Kirdani *et al.*, 1972) capable of separating both ³H and ¹⁴C in relatively small samples of tissues (ca. 100 mg) or blood. The E_3-6,7-³H had a specific activity of 50 mCi/μmole; and the T-4-¹⁴C, 50 μCi/μmole.

C. Effects of Drugs on the Deposition of Labeled Estriol (E_3), Testosterone (T), and Dihydrotestosterone (DHT)

Table VI shows the doses and routes of administration of the various drugs given to dogs. Table VII and Fig. 16 present the results of the deposition of intravenously injected pairs of steroids. Based on our past experience, we interpret the results to be significant if there is a deviation of 40–60% from the control values. The data indicate that procarbazine

TABLE VI

Chemotherapeutic Agents Tested and Dose Administered to Dogs[a]

Drug	Dose (mg/kg/day)	Route of administration[b]
5-Fluorodeoxyuridine	15	Iv
Cyclophosphamide	20	Im
Vincristine	50[c]	Iv
Procarbazine	5	Iv
Hexamethylmelamine	50	Oral
CCNU	50	Oral
Isophosphamide	50	Iv
Bleomycin	1.5	Iv
NSC-45388	35	Iv
Streptozotocin	3	Iv
Adriamycin	2.5	Iv
Diglycolaldehyde	20	Iv

[a] Drugs given for 4.5 days; last administration occurred on day of labeled estriol and testosterone injection.

[b] Im, intramuscular; Iv, intravenously.

[c] Micrograms per kilogram per day.

TABLE VII

Deposition of Radioactivity in Dog Tissues after the Intravenous Injection of E_3-^{3}H and T-^{14}C (^{3}H/^{14}C = 5/1)[a]

	Deposition of radioactivity (dpm/gm)					
	Prostate		Pancreas		Testes	
Drug	E_3	T	E_3	T	E_3	T
Control	10,000	1700	20,000	1200	2900	720
5-Fluorodeoxyuridine	15,300	3900	23,800	1800	2700	1200
Cyclophosphamide	16,200	2100	26,800	1700	4700	1400
Vincristine	11,600	2000	26,100	1400	3000	1200
Procarbazine	5,400	950	22,800	1000	1800	500
Hexamethylmelamine	19,000	2000	23,900	1100	2600	700
CCNU	15,500	2400	24,000	1300	3200	900
Isophosphamide	14,000	1100	36,400	900	1800	600
Bleomycin	14,100	1800	33,600	1400	2900	800
NSC-45388	8,600	1400	22,600	900	1800	800
Streptozotocin	3,250	530	17,300	900	1200	430
Adriamycin	17,300	2800	33,700	2700	6700	1800
Diglycolaldehyde	10,700	1750	14,250	1500	2600	600

[a] E_3, estriol; T, testosterone.

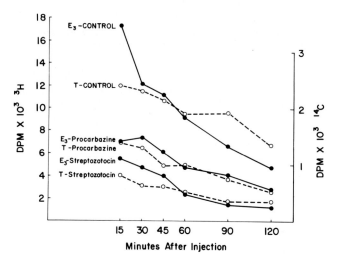

Fɪɢ. 16. Deposition of radioactivity in the dog prostate following the intravenous injection of ³H-labeled estriol (E₃) (50 μCi) and ¹⁴C-labeled testosterone (T) (10 μCi). Both streptozotocin and procarbazine caused markedly decreased deposition of radioactivity in the gland (Sandberg *et al.*, 1975). —³H;---, ¹⁴C.

and streptozotocin definitely interfere with the deposition of both E₃ and T. Hexamethylmelamine appears to cause a definite increase in E₃ deposition. The results in the testes and pancreas are shown for a comparison, since deposition of E₃ in the latter organ has been shown to be very extensive (Sandberg and Rosenthal, 1974; Kirdani *et al.*, 1972) and changes of deposition in the testes could reflect testicular changes that may affect prostatic parameters. None of the drugs inhibited the deposition of either E₃ or T in the pancreas; however, isophosphamide and bleomycin actually caused an increased E₃ concentration. Streptozotocin led to a definitely decreased deposition of E₃ and T in the testes, whereas cyclophosphamide caused an increase in T deposition. Since these studies were performed in intact dogs, it is difficult to ascertain whether some of the effects observed on the deposition of E₃ and T in the testes and prostate may not have been obtained through and partially contributed by the effects of the drugs on the hypothalamic–pituitary axis.

D. Effects of Estracyt and Flutamide on Steroid Deposition
in Dog Prostate

The effects of Estracyt (Kirdani *et al.*, 1974) and Flutamide (Varkarakis *et al.*, 1975b) on the deposition of labeled androgens and estrogens in the dog prostate were investigated. These agents probably produce antiprostatic effects through different mechanisms. Estracyt probably produces its effects by localization within the gland followed by hydrolysis of the molecule leading to freed E_2 and mustard, although in some species this hydrolysis may occur systemically, and, hence, the effects of the E_2 may be paramount. In the case of Flutamide, it probably produces its antiprostatic effects primarily by interfering with the association of T with prostatic intracellular receptor proteins, although there is some indication that the active form of Flutamide may be an *in vivo* metabolite of the drug (Liao *et al.*, 1974; Mainwaring *et al.*, 1974b; Varkarakis *et al.*, 1975b).

Estracyt showed a definite effect on the deposition of E_3 in the prostate (Fig. 17), i.e., a greatly decreased incorporation of the label by the gland. This was not true for T, in which case no significant changes in the deposition of the labeled steroid were observed. In the case of DHT, an actual increase in the deposition was observed. The results may be interpreted in at least two ways: (1) Estracyt entered the prostatic cells, in which the estrogen interfered with the deposition of E_3 by competing for binding sites; or (2) the effects were mediated via the pituitary (decreased LH release). We favor the former explanation.

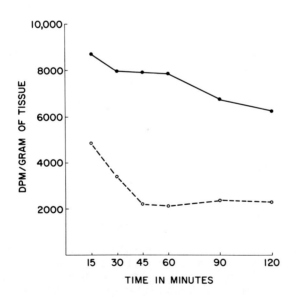

Fig. 17. Mean radioactivity levels in the canine prostate following treatment with Estracyt (○---○) (2.5 mg/kg/day iv for 2.5 days to 3 dogs). The pair of steroids estriol-^{14}C and dihydrotestosterone (DHT)-^{3}H was injected intravenously, 10 μCi and 50 μCi, respectively. The mean levels of untreated dogs (●——●) are shown for comparison. Estracyt caused a markedly decreased uptake of the estriol-^{14}C by the prostate. There was no decrease in the uptake of DHT-^{3}H (not shown in this figure) and, if anything, a somewhat increased concentration of radioactivity in the prostate (Kirdani *et al.*, 1974).

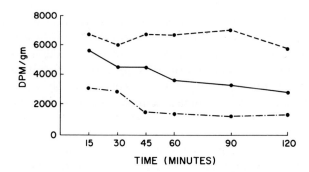

FIG. 18. Radioactivity in the prostate after 110×10^6 dpm of intravenously injected ³H-labeled dihydrotestosterone in dogs before (●---●, 2 dogs) and after the administration of either 5 mg/kg per day (●——●, 3 dogs) or 25 mg/kg per day (●—·—·●, 2 dogs) for 2 days of Flutamide (SCH 13521). The abscissa in this and in Fig. 19 indicates time after the injection of the radioactive steroid. Note the markedly decreased concentration of radioactivity in the prostate, particularly after the later dose of Flutamide (Varkarakis *et al.*, 1975b).

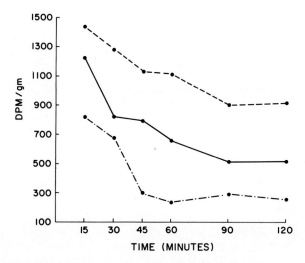

FIG. 19. Radioactivity in the prostate after 22×10^6 dpm of intravenously injected ¹⁴C-labeled testosterone (●---●, 2 dogs) and after the administration 5 mg/kg per day (●—●, 3 dogs) or 25 mg/kg per day (●—·—·●, 2 dogs) of Flutamide (SCH 13521). See legend to Fig. 18 for details (Varkarakis *et al.*, 1975b).

The effects of Flutamide on the deposition of labeled androgens and estrogens were of a different nature. There was definite inhibition of such deposition in the dog prostate of labeled T and DHT (Figs. 18 and 19), which appeared to be dose related. The interference with the deposition of E_2 or E_3 was less marked, though possibly significant.

V. COMMENTS

In expressing the effects of the various drugs on prostatic 5α-RA and arginase activity in terms of competitive, noncompetitive, and uncompetitive inhibition or activation, we have used these terms in an empirical sense. Hence, the terms and results are not to be construed as reflecting values, which in strict biochemical terms (Dawes, 1967) would have to be obtained *in vitro* with a partially or wholly purified enzyme system, and in which the effects of the various agents would be tested on the enzyme activity under appropriate conditions. Our aim in the present study was to establish *in vivo* effects of the drugs, and the terms used by us for inhibition or activation of the enzymes merely afford us an opportunity to classify the various drugs empirically into various categories, thus allowing us a more facile way of looking at the results. However, it should be pointed out, at the same time, that these drugs would probably not be effective in an *in vitro* system, as has been shown in some preliminary results by us (R. Y. Kirdani and A. A. Sandberg, unpublished data, 1975), since apparently their effects on the enzymes in the prostate require a period of time for expression. In addition, some of the drugs may possibly be "activated" in the body, e.g., through the formation of effective metabolites, as has been observed in the case of Flutamide. Furthermore, were we to isolate the enzymes for determining their quantitative kinetics *in vitro* under more acceptable conditions, we would be faced with the problem not only of loss of enzyme occurring under various conditions of isolation, but also with the problem of the distribution of the enzymes, particularly 5α-RA. It is known that most of the enzyme is associated with the nuclear membrane, but a significant part of it is also associated with the microsomes. Since an increased activity of the enzyme can be induced by various agents (e.g., T or DHT) in which only part of the intracellular enzyme (for example, microsomal in the case of T) may be influenced, it would be difficult to establish the exact location of the effects of the various chemotherapeutic agents in terms of the cellular distribution of the enzyme. Thus, we think that the presentation of the results in the present paper, even though based on several empirical assumptions, does afford a rather practical and useful approach to classifying various drugs possibly effective in cancer of the prostate.

A pessimistic evaluation of the results presented would point to the possibility that the various parameters measured in the studies presented may have little relevance or application to cancer of the prostate. This is based on the observation that not all human cancers have significant 5α-RA or arginase activity and, furthermore, that the levels of these enzymes may not have any relation to the development or biology of prostatic cancer. Nevertheless, a substantial number of prostatic cancers do have 5α-RA and arginase activity and receptor proteins for steroids, and it is inconceivable that these are not involved in the metabolic integrity of the cancer. Thus, we think that the agents that affect 5α-RA and arginase activities and those that interfere with the association or action of steroids with intracellular receptor proteins should have a definite effect in some cancers of the prostate. It is doubtful whether one model system, even one in an appropriate animal tumor, could serve as a testing system for drugs effective in every variety of prostatic cancer known to exist in the human (Györkey, 1973). Hence, various model systems for testing drugs effective in slow growing cancer of the prostate, as well as in those which have a rather rapid course or are hormonally dependent or independent, will have to be developed in the future in order to increase our confidence in selecting drugs effective in the various forms of prostatic cancer.

As stated above, even though the prostatic parameters measured, i.e., prostatic 5α-RA and arginase activity in dogs and rats and the deposition of E_3 and T in the dog, may not have any direct bearing on the treatment of prostatic cancer, particularly if the cancer does not contain substantial concentrations of the enzymes or receptor proteins for steroid hormones, we feel that the approaches we have utilized are worthy of application to therapy of cancer of the prostate. It is possible that the latter may have features that are comparable to some of those of cancer of the breast, e.g., the presence of receptor proteins for estrogens, which may serve as a reliable index for varying the endocrine *milieu* in patients with the disease. Hence, it is possible that those drugs which affect the deposition of E_3 and T, possibly through direct effects on the receptor protein, may be useful in cancer of the prostate, through their effects on hormonal conditions in the gland.

It is possible that some or all of the effects of some of the drugs administered may be mediated through the pituitary system and/or the testicular function. Thus, decreased T secretion by the testes, as a result of a drug's effect on LH release or synthesis, may be reflected in decreased 5α-RA and arginase activities, as observed with the administration of bleomycin.

The demonstration of certain unusual effects of the drugs on 5α-RA and arginase is of interest and deserves comment. The enhancement of 5α-RA by some agents has been reported by us previously (Saroff *et al.*, 1975), in which the results were based on a simple comparison of the percentage of conversion of T to DHT in prostatic tissue of normal rats vs that of animals which had received various drugs. In the present study, at least one-half of the drugs used caused activation of 5α-RA, as determined from the Lineweaver–Burk plots. In the case of two of the drugs (hydroxyurea, thiotepa) the effect actually led to some increase in prostatic weight. Even though the mechanism for this activation is not known, it is probable that these agents interfere with the synthesis or action of a substance(s) which inhibit 5α-RA in the prostate of the rat. Thus, it is conceivable that these drugs would lead to an increased 5α-RA and possibly aggravate (at least temporarily) some of the features of cancer of the prostate, particularly if these were T sensitive.

The most intense inhibition of 5α-RA in both rat prostates was produced by isophosphamide, with bleomycin and procarbazine inducing inhibition only in the dorsolateral gland. Adriamycin produced intense arginase inhibition in the latter prostate and 5-FU and NSC-45388 in the ventral gland.

The demonstration of competitive inhibition or arginase by several of these drugs is of interest, indicating an effect on the combination of the enzyme with its substrate. Such competitive inhibition was not observed with 5α-RA; this is not surprising in view of the difference in the tertiary structures of the drugs administered as compared to those of the steroidal hormones.

Except for bleomycin and isophosphamide, those drugs which caused the most intense decreases in 5α-RA and arginase activity did not lead to the most prominent decreases in either body or prostatic weight. Furthermore, except for bleomycin and procarbazine, those drugs which caused a significant reduction in arginase activity did not necessarily cause a decrease in 5α-RA.

The parameters in this study were measured after a rather short period of drug administration (4.5–14 days), and it is possible that even more profound effects might be seen with some of the chemotherapeutic agents, which were ineffective during short-term administration, if they were to be given for longer time periods (weeks or months). Of course, the untoward effects that might result from prolonged drug administration may preclude such a study or affect their clinical efficacy, but such an approach may be necessary in order to ascertain more specifically the effects of the various drugs on the rat prostate.

VI. CONCLUDING REMARKS

There is little doubt that in the future more appropriate and suitable model systems for testing drugs against cancer of the prostate will be developed, both *in vivo* and *in vitro*. These may involve prostatic cancer models in animals and the expansion of approaches similar to those pre-

A. A. SANDBERG

sented in this paper and by others. For example, at present a program based on the distribution of labeled zinc among the various prostatic proteins and the effects of hormones and chemotherapeutic agents on the distribution of such zinc are being investigated in our laboratory. Of great future promise is the development of methodologies in which prostatic cancer cells of varying origin can be maintained and grown in culture under conditions in which the cells will maintain their integrity and characteristics (Baulieu et al., 1969; Lasnitzki, 1970; Santti and Johansson, 1973; Lasnitzki et al., 1974). The effects of various drugs on such cells would prove to be an important advance in our armamentarium for developing drugs effective against cancer of the prostate. Such an in vitro system would afford considerable flexibility and sensitivity and be technically superior to in vivo model systems. However, it must be stressed that the maintenance of the biology and biochemistry of these cells in vitro is paramount, since if any of these characteristics are lost by the cells during their in vitro life, the effects of various drugs on these cells may be misleading and inconclusive. Thus, it behooves workers in this area to develop in vitro conditions that would maintain prostatic cancer cells as close as possible to their in vivo characteristics (Robel et al., 1971; McMahon et al., 1972; Johansson and Niemi, 1975), e.g., if 5α-RA is present in these cells, this enzyme must be maintained by the cells in vitro; the same applies to arginase and to the receptor proteins for various steroids in the cells.

An area requiring further exploration is the development of conjugate agents, similar to Estracyt, in which the unique properties of each constituent add an effective parameter to the other constituent of the molecule. In case of Estracyt, it is the property of E_2 for localization in certain cells (probably containing receptor proteins for E_2) that affords the mustard moiety an opportunity to be carried into such cells prior to systemic hydrolysis (Kirdani et al., 1974; Sandberg et al., 1975). By combining the most effective antimetabolite or any other chemotherapeutic agent with the proper steroid (or other substances for which certain cells have a high affinity) our armamentarium for treating cancer of the prostate, and those of other organs, will be immeasurably enhanced.

ACKNOWLEDGMENTS

The studies reported in this paper have been supported in part by grant CA-15436 from the National Cancer Institute. Much of the work reported in this paper has been done in collaboration with Drs. R. Y. Kirdani, J. Müntzing (now at AB Leo, Helsingborg, Sweden), G. P. Murphy, J. Saroff, M. J. Varkarakis (now at Athens, Greece), and H. Yamanaka (now at Gunma University School of Medicine, Maebashi, Japan). Miss Sue Beechler gave valuable clerical help.

REFERENCES

Armstrong, E. G., and Bashirelahi, N. (1974). *Biochem. Biophys. Res. Commun.* **61**, 578.

Baulieu, E.-E. (1973). *Proc. Int. Congr. Endocrinol., 4th, 1972* Int. Congr. Ser. No. 256, pp. 30–62.

Baulieu, E.-E., Lasnitzki, I., and Robel, P. (1969). *Nature (London)* **219**, 1155.

Baulieu, E.-E., Jung, I., Blondeau, J. P., and Robel, P. (1971). *Advan. Biosci.* **7**, 179–191.

Belham, J. E., and Neal, G. E. (1971). *Biochem. J.* **125**, 81.

Bonne, C., and Raynaud, J. P. (1973). *Biochimie* **55**, 227.

Boyns, A. R., Cole, E. N., Phillips, M. E. A., Hillier, S. G., Cameron, E. H. D., Griffiths, K., Shahmanesh, M., Feneley, R. C. L., and Hartog, M. (1974). *Eur. J. Cancer* **10**, 445.

Bruchovsky, N., and Wilson, J. D. (1968a). *J. Biol. Chem.* **243**, 2012.

Bruchovsky, N., and Wilson, J. D. (1968b). *J. Biol. Chem.* **243**, 5953.

Danutra, V., Harper, M. E., and Griffiths, K. (1973). *J. Endocrinol.* **59**, 539.

Davies, P., and Griffiths, K. (1974). *J. Endocrinol.* **62**, 385.

Dawes, E. A. (1967). "Quantitative Problems in Biochemistry," 4th ed. Williams & Wilkins, Baltimore, Maryland.

Dunning, W. F. (1963). *Nat. Cancer Inst., Mongr.* **12**, 351.

Dunning, W. F., Curtis, M. R., and Segaloff, A. (1946). *Cancer Res.* **6**, 256.

Fang, S., and Liao, S. (1969). *Mol. Pharmacol.* **5**, 420.

Fang, S., and Liao, S. (1971). *J. Biol. Chem.* **246**, 16.

Farnsworth, W. E. (1969). *Invest. Urol.* **6**, 423.

Frederiksen, D. W., and Wilson, J. D. (1971). *J. Biol. Chem.* **246**, 2584.

Ghanadian, R., and Fotherby, K. (1972). *Steroids Lipids Res.* **3**, 363.

Girogi, E. P., Grant, J. K., Stewart, J. C., and Reid, J. (1972a). *J. Endocrinol.* **55**, 421.

Giorgi, E. P., Stewart, J. C., Grant, J. K., and Shirley, I. M. (1972b). *Biochem. J.* **126**, 107.

Giorgi, E. P., Moses, T. F., Grant, J. K., Scott, R., and Sinclair, J. (1974). *Mol. Cell. Endocrinol.* **1**, 271.

Gloyna, R. E., Siiteri, P. K., and Wilson, J. D. (1970). *J. Clin. Invest.* **49**, 1746.

Griffiths, K., Harper, M. E., Groom, M. A., Pike, A. W., Fahmy, A. R., and Pierrepoint, C. G. (1970). *In* "Some Aspects of the Aetiology and Biochemistry of Prostatic Cancer" (K. Griffiths and C. G. Pierrepoint, eds.), pp. 88–96. Alpha Omega Alpha Publ., Cardiff, Wales.

Groom, B., Harper, M. E., Fahmy, A. R., Pierrepoint, C. G., and Griffiths, K. (1971). *Biochem. J.* **122**, 125.

Gustafsson, J.-Å., and Pousette, Å. (1974). *Biochemistry* **13**, 875.

Györkey, F. (1973). *Methods Cancer Res.* **10**, 279–368.

Haltmeyer, G. C., and Eik-Nes, K. B. (1972). *Acta Endocrinol. (Copenhagen)* **69**, 394.

Hansson, V., Tveter, K. J., Unhjem, O., and Djöseland, O. (1972). *J. Steroid Biochem.* **3**, 427.

Harding, B. W., and Samuels, L. T. (1962). *Endocrinology* **70**, 109.

Harik, S. I., Hollenberg, M. D., and Snyder, S. H. (1974). *Nature (London)* **249**, 250.

Higuchi, M., Uemura, K., Etō, K., Gōhara, S., and Hirata, S. (1972). *Kurume Med. J.* **19,** 205.

Horning, E. S. (1946). *Lancet* **2,** 829.

Huggins, C., and Hodges, C. F. (1941). *Cancer Res.* **1,** 293.

Isotalo, A., and Santti, R. S. (1975). *Acta Endocrinol. (Copenhagen)* **78,** 401.

Jenkins, J. S., and McCafferey, V. M. (1974). *J. Endocrinol.* **63,** 517.

Jensen, E. V., and de Sombre, E. R. (1972). *Annu. Rev. Biochem.* **41,** 203.

Jensen, E. V., and de Sombre, E. R. (1973). *Science* **182,** 126.

Jensen, E. V., Block, G. E., Smith, S., Kyser, K., and de Sombre, E. R. (1971). *Nat. Cancer Inst., Monogr.* **34,** 55.

Johansson, R., and Niemi, M. (1975). *Acta Endocrinol. (Copenhagen)* **78,** 766.

Jungblut, P. W., Hughes, S. F., Gorlich, L., Gowers, U., and Wagner, R. K. (1971). *Hoppe-Seyler's Z. Physiol. Chem.* **352,** 1603.

Karr, J. P., Kirdani, R. Y., Murphy, G. P., and Sandberg, A. A. (1974). *Life Sci* **15,** 501.

Kirdani, R. Y., Müntzing, J., Varkarakis, M. J., Murphy, G. P., and Sandberg, A. A. (1974). *Cancer Res.* **34,** 1031.

Kirdani, R. Y., Varkarakis, M. J., Murphy, G. P., and Sandberg, A. A. (1972). *Endocrinology* **90,** 1245.

Kirdani, R. Y., Sandberg, A. A., and Murphy, G. P. (1973). *Surgery* **74,** 84.

Kowarski, A., Shalf, J., and Migeon, C. J. (1969). *J. Biol. Chem.* **244,** 5269.

Lasnitzki, I. (1970). *In* "Some Aspects of the Aetiology and Biochemistry of Prostatic Cancer" (K. Griffiths and C. G. Pierrepoint, eds.), pp. 68–73. Alpha Omega Alpha Publ., Cardiff, Wales.

Lasnitzki, I., Franklin, H. R., and Wilson, J. D. (1974). *J. Endocrinol.* **60,** 81.

Lee, D. K. H., Young, J. C., Tamura, Y., Patterson, D. C., Bird, C. E., and Clark, A. F. (1973). *Can. J. Biochem.* **51,** 735.

Lee, D. K. H., Bird, C. E., and Clark, A. F. (1974). *J. Steroid Biochem.* **5,** 609.

Liao, S., Howell, D. K., and Chang, T.-E. (1974). *Endocrinology* **94,** 1205.

McCann, S., Gorlich, L., Janssen, U., and Jungblat, D. W. (1971). *Proc. Int. Congr. Horm. Steroids, 3rd, 1970* Int. Congr. Ser. No. 210, p. 150.

McMahon, M. J., Butler, A. V. J., and Thomas, G. H. (1972). *Brit. J. Cancer* **26,** 388.

Mainwaring, W. I. P., and Milroy, E. J. G. (1973). *J. Endocrinol.* **57,** 371.

Mainwaring, W. I. P., Mangan, F. R., Irving, R. A., and Jones, D. A. (1974a). *Biochem. J.* **144,** 413.

Mainwaring, W. I. P., Mangan, F. R., Feherty, P. A., and Freifeld, M. (1974b). *Mol. Cell. Endocrinol.* **1,** 113.

Mangan, F. R., Neal, G. E., and Williams, D. C. (1967). *Biochem. J.* **104,** 1075.

Mawhinney, M. G., Schwartz, F. L., Thomas, J. A., and Lloyd, J. W., III. (1974). *Invest. Urol.* **12,** 17.

Mirand, E. A., and Staubitz, W. J. (1956). *Proc. Soc. Exp. Biol. Med.* **93,** 457.

Mittelman, A., Shukla, S. K., Welvaart, K., and Murphy, G. P. (1975). *Cancer Chemother. Rep., Part 1* **59,** 219.

Moore, R. A., and Melchionna, R. H. (1937). *Amer. J. Cancer* **30,** 731.

Moore, R. J., and Wilson, J. D. (1972). *J. Biol. Chem.* **247,** 958.

Moore, R. J., and Wilson, J. D. (1973). *Endocrinology* **93,** 581.

Müntzing, J., Varkarakis, M. J., Yamanaka, H., Murphy, G. P., and Sandberg, A. A. (1974). *Proc. Soc. Exp. Biol. Med.* **146,** 849.

Murphy, G. P. (1974). *Ca* **24,** 282.

Nozu, K., and Tamaoki, B.-I. (1974a). *Biochim. Biophys. Acta* **348**, 321.
Nozu, K., and Tamaoki, B.-I. (1974b). *Acta Endocrinol. (Copenhagen)* **76**, 608.
Ofner, P. (1969). *Vitam. Horm. (New York)* **26**, 237.
Pegg, A. E., Lockwood, D. H., and Williams-Ashman, H. G. (1970). *Biochem. J.* **117**, 17.
Prout, G. E., J. (1973). *In* "Cancer Medicine" (J. F. Holland and E. Frei, eds.), pp. 1680–1694. Lea & Febiger, Philadelphia, Pennsylvania.
Rennie, P., and Bruchovsky, N. (1972). *J. Biol. Chem.* **247**, 1546.
Robel, P., Lasnitzki, I., and Baulieu, E.-E. (1971). *Biochimie* **53**, 81.
Roy, A. B. (1971). *Biochimie* **53**, 1031.
Sandberg, A. A., and Rosenthal, H. E. (1974). *J. Steroid Biochem.* **5**, 969.
Sandberg, A. A., Kirdani, R. Y. Yamanaka, H., Varkarakis, M. J., and Murphy, G. P. (1975). *Cancer Chemother. Rep., Part 1* **59**, 175.
Santii, R. S., and Johansson, R. (1973). *Exp. Cell Res.* **77**, 111.
Saroff, J., Yamanaka, H., Kirdani, R. Y., Sandberg, A. A., and Murphy, G. P. (1975). *In* "Normal and Abnormal Growth of the Prostate" (M. Goland, ed.), pp. 743–758. Thomas, Springfield, Illinois.
Schimke, R. T. (1964). *J. Biol. Chem.* **239**, 136.
Shearer, R. J., Hendry W. F., Sommerville, I. R., and Ferguson, J. D. (1973). *Brit. J. Urol.* **45**, 668.
Shimazaki, J., Furuya, N., Yamanaka, H., and Shida, K. (1969a). *Endocrinol. Jap.* **16**, 163.
Shimazaki, J., Matsushita, I., Furuya, N., Yamanaka, H., and Shida, K. (1969b). *Endocrinol. Jap.* **16**, 453.
Shimazaki, J., Ohki, Y., Matsuoka, M., Tanaka, M., and Shida, K. (1972a). *Endocrinol. Jap.* **19**, 69.
Shimazaki, J., Ohki, Y., Koya, A., and Shida, K. (1972b). *Endocrinol. Jap.* **19**, 585.
Shimazaki, J., Taguchi, I., Yamanaka, H., Mayuzumi, T., and Shida, K. (1973a). *Endocrinol. Jap.* **20**, 455.
Shimazaki, J., Ohki, Y., Kurihara, H., Furuya, N., and Shida, K. (1973b). *Endocrinol. Jap.* **20**, 489.
Siiteri, P. K., and Wilson, J. D. (1970). *J. Clin. Invest.* **49**, 1737.
Sinha, A. A., Blackard, C. E., Doe, R. P., and Seal, U. S. (1973). *Cancer* **31**, 682.
Sloan, W. R., Heston, W. D. W., and Coffey, D. S. (1975). *Cancer Chemother. Res., Part 1* **59**, 235.
Steins, P., Krieg, M., Hollmann, H. J., and Voigt, K. D. (1974). *Acta Endocrinol. (Copenhagen)* **75**, 773.
Tabor, H., and Tabor, C. W. (1972). *Advan. Enzymol.,* **36**, 203.
Varkarakis, M. J., Kirdani, R. Y., Murphy, G. P., and Sandberg, A. A. (1972). *J. Surg. Res.* **13**, 29.
Varkarakis, M. J., Kirdani, R. Y., Abramczyk, J., Murphy, G. P., and Sandberg, A. A. (1973). *Invest. Urol.* **11**, 106.
Varkarakis, M. J., Kirdani, R. Y., Murphy, G. P., and Sandberg, A. A. (1975a). *Proc. Soc. Exp. Biol. Med.* **148**, 904.
Varkarakis, M. J., Kirdani, R. Y., Yamanaka, H., Murphy, G. P., and Sandberg, A. A. (1975b). *Invest. Urol.* **12**, 275.
Voigt, W., and Dunning, W. F. (1974). *Cancer Res.* **34**, 1447.
Wilson, J. D. (1972). *N. Engl. J. Med.* **287**, 1284.
Yamanaka, H., Mayuzumi, T., Shimazaki, J., and Shida, K. (1971). *Endocrinol. Jap.* **18**, 487.

186 A. A. SANDBERG

Yamanaka, H., Mayuzumi, T., Matsuoka, M., Shimazaki, J., and Shida, K. (1972) *Gann* **63**, 693.

Yamanaka, H., Kirdani, R. Y., Saroff, J., Murphy, G. P., and Sandberg, A. A. (1975). *Amer. J. Physiol.* (in press).

DISCUSSION

K. Griffiths: Our approach was to find a compound which mimics the biological effects of diethylstilbestrol, but with less estrogenic effects. The estrogenic side effects of diethylstilbestrol—decreased libido, cardiovascular problems, breast development—are problems which the clinician must currently accept. A compound which we have synthesized, dihydrodibutylstilbestrol (DHBS), has many of the properties of diethylstilbestrol but is liss estrogenic (1/500×). DHBS decreases prostate weight in the rat and the weight of the seminal vesicles and decreases plasma testasterone, DHBS also displaces 5α-RHT from the 8 S-cytoplasmic receptor complex *in vitro*, with a 200-fold excess.

A. A. Sandberg: Even though the search for estrogenic compounds effective in cancer of the prostate, but without their untoward effects, is certainly a worthwhile undertaking, my personal opinion is that we should devote more effort toward finding agents that are potentially curative of the disease, rather than in the field of steroid hormones, which are only palliative for cancer of the prostate; of course, it is possible to utilize estrogens and other steroid hormones as "carriers" for chemotherapeutic drugs, e.g., as in the case of Estracyt, and we should probably take advantage of the properties of steroids and other compounds capable of uniquely entering a target cell for their possible ability to carry the antimetabolic agents into the cancer cells.

K.-D. Voigt: Do you think that 5α-DHT is the only active compound at the prostate level in dogs? Did you look into other androgen-dependent organs, like the levator ani muscle?

A. A. Sandberg: It is possible that other derivatives of testosterone, besides DHT, and other androgenic steroids affect prostatic physiology, but we only tested the 5α-reductase system. We did not look into other androgen-dependent organs or tissues.

C. G. Pierrepoint: I think that we have been persuaded that man and rat are not going to be suitable models for the study of prostatic hyperplasia in the dog. For those of us who are interested in the dog, we shall just have to work on it alone. With regard to Professor Griffiths' remarks on our dihydrodibutylstilbestrol, it is worth recording that this compound completely obliterated the binding of the active androgen in the dog, 5α-androstane-3α,17α-diol, to its cytoplasmic receptor at 50 times the concentration of the ligand. We have had little chance of testing this synthetic "estrogen" on dogs with prostatic hyperplasia, but one animal is worth recalling. A stud Dobermann pinscher was admitted with gross prostatic enlargement and urinary obstruction. Castration or stilbestrol therapy were obviously contraindicated if the animal was to continue as a fertile and potent stud dog. Dihydrodibutylstilbestrol was administered at the rate of 1 mg/day. The urinary trouble cleared up very quickly without loss of libido or fertility. Eventually (2-3 years later) the dog was destroyed because of gross enlargement of the prostate, but the quite lengthy respite was encouraging.

A. A. Sandberg: It is possible that some sort of modified estrogens (or other steroids) will be found of value in benign prostatic hypertrophy, but, again, I doubt that these substances per se will ultimately be curative of cancer of the prostate.

My opinion is that we must look to other areas of chemotherapy for agents potentially effective against cancer of the prostate.

E. E. Baulieu: If inhibition of 5α-reductase takes place, then testosterone will accumulate in the prostate. Have you evaluated the correlation between the effects of the chemotherapeutic agents and the effects of the inhibitor?

A. A. Sandberg: It is true that inhibition of the 5α-reductase system may lead to accumulation of testosterone in the prostatic gland, and this in itself may be deleterious in the case of cancer of the prostate. It is also possible that it may be beneficial in some cases of this disease. However, this is an area about which little is known or understood. I should point out that the so-called activation of 5α-reductase produced by a number of the drugs used by us may be indicative of their possible aggravating effect, if used in cancer of the prostate, at least in those cases in which DHT would tend to aggravate the disease. At the same time, however, it is also possible that the interference by the drugs with the inhibitor of 5α-reductase—particularly if it is indicative of interference with the synthesis and/or action of a protein—may in itself be of value as far as pointing to the possible efficacy of an antiprostatic cancer agent.

E. E. Baulieu: 5α-Reductase is a very nice indicator of androgen activity. Naturally, one should take into account the changes of the androgen status, as well as the direct effects on prostatic cells of all the chemotherapeutic agents which you introduced. Morever, I would like to know if you have any correlation between effects on growth of various compounds and on levels of 5α-reductase activity. This is because the formation of androstanolone may amplify testosterone action, which may eventually occur even without this metabolic step.

A. Mittelman: Dr. Sandberg has offered a rational approach to the beginning of chemotherapy of carcinoma of the prostate. The 5α-reductase and arginase systems offer the clinician a range of compounds for use in various clinical settings. In addition, we can evaluate the validity of Dr. Sandberg's and Dr. Coffey's systems. The dialogue between biochemists and clinicians, we hope, will lead to a rational program of chemotherapy of carcinoma of the prostate.

F. Neumann: Inhibition of 5α-reductase, does not say very much. Progesterone is a very potent inhibitor of 5α-reductase, but *in vivo* progesterone is almost inactive.

Another (synthetic) progestogen, 19-norhydroxyprogesterone caproate is also a very potent inhibitor of 5α-reductase. In the castrated testesterone-substituted rat, this compound has no effect on the prostate at all, his parameter (5α-reduction) is in my mind of very little value.

A. A. Sandberg: First we obviously did not rely solely on the 5α-reductase system (and its inhibitor) as the only index of possible efficacy of a drug in cancer of the prostate. This is the reason why we also employed the prostatic arginase system and steroid deposition in the dog prostate as other means of evaluating drugs. Second, it is possible that the 5α-reductase inhibitors you mentioned, though they are effective *in vitro,* may not enter the prostatic cell *in vivo,* and, thus, not produce the inhibition observed *in vitro.* I would like to hear what Dr. Eik-Nes has to say on this.

K. B. Eik-Nes: Nature has provided us with a model demonstrating the fact that an inhibitor of 5α-reductase must be in the tissue where you look for inhibition. The rat testis produces T via progesterone and produces and secretes less DHT than the dog producing T by a Δ^5-pathway not involving progesterone.

Moreover, a small point to Dr. Neumann: progesterone appears in the testis to inhibit 5α-reductase, some of the synthetic progestins seem to influence the 3-hydroxysteroid dehydrogenases in the testis of the rat. Thus, when speaking about inhibitors for DHT formation from T, one must also investigate whether the "inhibitor" influences further metabolism of DHT to the diols.

M. B. Lipsett: A number of therapeutic agents, having widely different types of action, activate 5α-reductase. You postulated that this was due to interference with synthesis of an inhibitor of 5α-reductase. However, among your agents was CCNU, and these hydroxyurea derivatives have no effect on nonmitosing cells. This seems to be a point against your hypothesis.

A. A. Sandberg: If CCNU does, indeed, produce its antimetabolic effects on mitotic cells, it may have produced its results in the rat (ventral) prostate possibly through another fortuitous mechanism. Maybe Dr. Coffey can tell us more about this compound or how it affects his DNA system?

D. S. Coffey: Our laboratory has observed that many of the nonhormonal cytotoxic drugs that block DNA synthesis will not decrease the size of the prostate when administered to normal intact rats; however, they are effective in blocking the restoration of the prostate by androgen administered to castrated rats. In the latter case, DNA synthesis is required for restoration and can be blocked by certain specific cancer therapeutic agents.

I. Lasnitzki: Did you mention a further conversion of DHT to 5α-androstanediol after long treatment?

A. A. Sandberg: We measured the total reduction of testosterone to its 5α-components, although we did not specially quantitate the 5α-androstanediol derived from testosterone.

H. J. Tagnon: I agree with Dr. Sandberg that we will have to use cytotoxic chemotherapy in addition to hormone therapy if we hope to make progress. We now have adequate hormone therapy in the form of estrogens and possibly Estracyt, and there is no great advantage to be expected from   search for new hormone agents. However, we are dealing with a group of patients who are old and, at the end of their course, have extensive bone invasion which precludes aggressive chemotherapy, and so does obstructive disease with the risk of infection. Therefore, I think the time has come to use chemotherapy along with hormone therapy and to use both at the beginning of the course, before extensive bone disease is present and obstruction is a problem. This, I think, is the direction for future pharmacological and clinical studies.

Round Table Discussion on the Evaluation of Drugs and Hormones Effective against Prostatic Disease

(*Rapporteur:* H. G. WILLIAMS-ASHMAN)

Many of the presentations during the first day of the symposium touched on laboratory test systems that might be used for evaluation of substances of potential value in the treatment of human prostatic proliferative disorders. The pertinent experiments related to various levels of biological organization, ranging from observations on normal or neoplastic prostate tissues growing in living animals or in organ cultures *in vitro*, to measurements on isolated enzyme systems. The two prostatic diseases that unfortunately plague the aging human male only too frequently—benign prostatic hyperplasia (BPH) and carcinoma of the prostate—exhibit species-specific attributes that render equivocal all available animal or biochemical model systems for the screening of new drugs, as was especially emphasized by Friedmund Neumann in his scholarly review. But we live in an imperfect world, and it would be foolish to dismiss some of the currently employed animal experimental approaches simply on the grounds that they do not reflect exactly all specialized features of human BPH or prostate cancer.

H. G. Williams-Ashman opened the general discussion by pointing out that most experimental work has been aimed at development of drugs active against already established BPH or prostate cancer. He mentioned the old cliché of medical science that an ounce of prevention is worth a ton of cure. The etiology of benign hyperplasia or carcinoma of the human prostate remains a big mystery. There is little or no evidence that abnormalities in the production, disposition, or metabolism of androgens or estrogens are true causative factors in these diseases, even though both types of neoplasm are sometimes androgen-responsive, and despite the fact that eunuchs seldom if ever develop BPH or prostate cancer. Again, there are, at present, no compelling reasons to believe that chemicals or radiation from the environment, or genetic, nutritional, and oncogenic viral factors, are paramount in the etiology of these human prostatic diseases. However, there is no question that all of these eventualities merit much further investigation in depth. Age is centrally related to the incidence of human prostate neoplasms but the mechanistic basis of this correlation is unclear. At all events, a plea was made for more intensive work on the controlled induction in experimental animals of prostate neoplasms that may resemble those in man, since this might provide test systems for prophylactic medicines that hopefully would hinder the appearance of prostate tumors.

Observations on the growth of the prostate and other male genital glands in living adult castrated rodents have uncovered, over the last decade, a number of potent antiandrogenic substances that are essentially devoid of estrogenic, antiestrogenic, and antigonadotropic activities, and which seem to act by competing with active androgens at the level of these target organs. Until recently, all antiandrogens of this type uncovered by such *in vivo* screens have been steroidal in nature. Rudolph Neri overviewed his discovery, with the aid of such tests, of a very active antiandrogen that is not a steroid. This is the substance Flutamide (Sch 13521, or α,α,α-trifluoro-2-methyl-4'-nitro-*m*-propionotoluidide). The inhibition of testosterone-induced prostate growth by Flutamide *in vivo* is evident from measurements of either the weight of the gland, or of rates of DNA synthesis by prostate according to the method of Sufrin and Coffey; either test system revealed that Flutamide is roughly equipotent with the steroid cyproterone acetate. Experiments involving administration of Flutamide *in vivo* indicated that, in analogy with the actions of cyproterone acetate, the nonsteroidal drug inhibits the uptake and nuclear retention of labeled testosterone or dihydrotestosterone (DHT) by the prostate of castrated rats. Flutamide *in vivo* also depressed the formation of a nuclear DHT–androgen receptor complex. However, in contrast to cyproterone acetate, which directly depresses the interaction of DHT with prostate androgen receptors *in vitro*, the direct effects of Flutamide in the test tube were not as pronounced as those *in vivo*, suggesting that Flutamide might act, at least in part, via an active metabolite. Administration of isotopically labeled Flutamide to man and several species of laboratory animals indeed revealed that the drug is metabolized to a fairly large number of derivatives, one of the most prominent being Sch 16423 (α,α,α-trifluoro-2-methyl-4'-nitro-*m*-lactotoluidide) or hydroxylated Flutamide. This is the only metabolite of Flutamide that exhibits powerful antiandrogenic activity *in vivo*. Moreover, the hydroxylated Flutamide exhibits a strong ability to compete *in vitro* with DHT in the formation of prostate androgen–receptor complexes.

Rudolph Neri also showed that prostate size and epithelial cell heights were markedly depressed by Flutamide after its administration to dogs with benign prostatic hyperplasia, and that these effects were reversible when treatment with the drug was stopped. Jonas Müntzing has made similar observations on the baboon prostate. Very recent preliminary clinical reports by Stoliar and Albert, and by Prout and Irwin, have indicated beneficial effects of Flutamide in some patients with prostate cancer with little evidence of toxicity. But it is too early to arrive at any unequivocal evaluation of the value of Flutamide in the treatment of human prostate disease.

Ian Mainwaring stated that he has also obtained evidence that the active form of Flutamide may be the aforementioned hydroxylated metabolite, this compound being more active than the parent drug in directly suppressing nuclear DHT–receptor complex formation by prosstate preparations *in vitro*.

The need for greater study of biochemical correlates of the extensive DNA synthesis and cell division that constitutes a relatively late yet transient phase of androgen-stimulated prostate growth was emphasized in some of the lectures. From a descriptive, yet alone a mechanistic standpoint, much less is known about the biochemistry of the proliferation of various cell types in the prostate in comparison with the functional differentiation and hypertrophy of epithelial cells. Furthermore, the dynamics of the postcastrate involution of the adult prostate are poorly understood.

Nicholas Bruchovsky mentioned some of his latest findings on estradiol-induced regression of rat ventral prostate. It is well known that estrogens effectively diminish testosterone output by the testis at the level of inhibition of gonadotropin secretion and at the level of the Leydig cell itself, but there are also hints in some species that estrogens may additionally interfere with the actions of androgens within prostate cells. Bruchovsky found that estradiol can be transported into prostate cell nuclei if sufficiently high cytoplasmic concentrations of the estrogen are attained. Under these conditions, estradiol appears to inhibit the nuclear sequestration of androgens. Intracellular transport of estradiol is accompanied by appearance of a receptor within the nucleus but its affinity for estradiol is low. Thus, according to Bruchovsky, estradiol might exert some of its effects on the prostate by interfering with androgen retention in the cell nuclei, or conceivably by producing an unstable receptor. Here it must be remembered that there are reports in the literature that estrogens can also directly inhibit the prostatic steroid 5α-reductase that converts testosterone to DHT.

Organ culture techniques, despite their obvious pitfalls, have many potential advantages for the study of human as well as animal prostate tissues, not only with regard to morphological and biochemical analyses, but also as tools for testing the direct actions of drugs and hormones. This was considered by Ilse Lasnitzki, who has recently correlated effects of testosterone, androgen metabolites, and estradiol-17β on epithelial morphology of BPH in organ culture with that on RNA synthesis. In organ cultures of BPH the epithelium grew well in the absence or in the presence of the steroids, but in control medium the cells often underwent squamous metaplasia while estradiol caused some cellular breakdown. Testosterone and DHT preserved the secretory character of the epithelium; in addition, DHT stimulated epithelial proliferation considerably. These changes were reflected in those of RNA synthesis determined by the incorporation of ^{3}H-labeled uridine in radioautographs of control and steroid-treated explants of BPH. Testosterone and DHT increased the number of labeled cells as well as the grain counts per cell whereas estradiol reduced them.

The experiments were extended to prostatic carcinomas in organ culture. In both moderately differentiated and anaplastic tumors, the percentage of labeled cells was similar to that found in the BPH, but the grain number per cell was considerably lower. Testosterone increased the number of grains, but estradiol did not reduce them below the control value. These interesting preliminary findings may have important clinical applications. Paul Robel also mentioned that, in his laboratory, new techniques of prostate perfusion of organ cultures of prostate are being studied in analogous situations of clinical relevance.

Androgen Metabolism by the Perfused Prostate

K. B. EIK-NES

Department of Biophysics, N.T.H., University of Trondheim, Trondheim, Norway

I. INTRODUCTION

Some time ago experiments *in vivo* demonstrated that the prostate will concentrate steroid androgen against a blood plasma gradient (Pearlman and Pearlman, 1961; Harding and Samuels, 1962). Moreover, when the prostate is incubated with androgens *in vitro*, androgen uptake (Hansson, 1971) and androgen metabolism (Farnsworth and Brown, 1963a) can be recorded. No one, however, has reported that the prostate will convert acetate or cholesterol to steroid hormones; thus it is difficult to determine a specific effect of the prostate on the overall steroid environment *in vivo* in contrast to glands producing specific steroids like the adrenal, the testis and the ovary. Incubation studies with prostatic tissue *in vitro* serve the purpose of showing what the gland *can* do, but not what it is doing under physiological conditions.

Much work will be reviewed during this symposium dealing with what the prostate *can* do. Now then, let us look at the other end of the scale. The prostate is fed steroids via its arterial blood, and many of these steroids may alter prostatic function (Table I). In so doing they may be retained by the gland, metabolized in the gland, and the products finally secreted by the gland. In order to investigate problems of this nature, we have to resort to experiments *in vivo*. Admittedly, experiments *in vitro* have distinct advantages: they can be performed under controlled conditions with respect to temperature, pH, ionic strength, cofactor concentration, and oxygen consumption. Moreover, the technique of high speed centrifugation permits experiments on intracellular localization of enzymic activities and detailed investigations of mechanisms

TABLE I

VENTRAL PROSTATE WEIGHT IN STEROID-TREATED
CASTRATED, MATURE RATS[a]

Treatment	Ventral prostate weight (mg/100 gm body weight)[b]
Sesame oil	16.5 ± 6.4
4-Androsten-17β-ol-3-one (T)	50.4 ± 2.8
4-Androsten-17α-ol-3-one	22.3 ± 3.6
4-Androstene-7α,17β-diol-3-one	18.2 ± 2.6
5α-Androstane	32.7 ± 7.2
5α-Androstan-3α-ol	20.9 ± 5.2
5α-Androstan-17β-ol	36.1 ± 9.6
5α-Androstan-17β-ol-3-one (DHT)	67.5 ± 1.8
5α-Androstane-3α,17β-diol(3α-diol)	66.4 ± 10.2
5α-Androstan-3α-ol,17-one	43.4 ± 2.5
5α-Androstan-3β-ol	21.9 ± 1.5
5α-Androstane-3β,17β-diol(3β-diol)	20.1 ± 3.3
5β-Androstane	16.2 ± 0.6
5β-Androstan-3α-ol	21.8 ± 4.4
5β-Androstan-3α-ol,17-one	20.2 ± 4.6
5β-Androstane-3α,17β-diol	22.1 ± 10.4

[a] Rats were treated subcutaneously daily with 100 μg of steroids per 100 gm body weight for 7 days. Treatment was started on the day of gonadectomy, and the steroids were administered in sesame oil solution. Three or more rats were used in each group. The data are from work by H. L. Verjans and K. B. Eik-Nes (unpublished, 1975).
[b] Mean ±SD.

underlying discrete reaction steps, in this case androgen metabolism in the prostate (Harding and Samuels, 1962). Finally, combining the technique of high speed centrifugation with high resolution microscopy, the structural nature of cell organelles or cell fragments, of interest for our incubation studies, can be evaluated critically (Leav et al., 1974). Data from such work assume less significance, however, when one notes that the technique of high speed centrifugation can result in tissue artifacts.

In experiments in vivo, blood is permitted to enter the organ via the arteries. With respect to steroid secretion and metabolism, control of blood flow through an organ is of paramount importance (Eik-Nes, 1970). Substances changing the metabolic activities of the organ can be delivered to the organ at a constant rate via the arterial blood. Such substances, as well as metabolic products of the organ, are removed via the venous drainage in a continuous fashion and not permitted to accumulate in the cells, as is often the case in experiments in vitro. Published information on end-product inhibition of enzymic activity has considerable bearing on this point (Monod *et al.*, 1963). The cofactors used by an organ *in vivo* are the physiological ones present in the proper cell compartments (Eik-Nes and Hall, 1965). Cofactor addition in studies *in vivo* is, however, a difficult task since most cofactors needed for steroid biotransformation show low permeability when infused via the artery of an organ (Eik-Nes, 1971). Finally, experiments *in vivo* allow investigation of the influence of the nervous and lymphatic systems of an organ. Since products of nerve action appear to direct blood flow in steroid-producing organs (Setchell *et al.*, 1966) and since such organs secrete steroids via the lymph (Lindner, 1963; Haltmeyer and Eik-Nes, 1974), these systems should not be overlooked or ignored when dealing with steroid-producing cells.

II. The Perfused Prostate

Owing to the difficult and rather complex anatomical localization of the prostate, all published prostate preparations *in vivo* require some surgical skill. Also, the needed surgical manipulations, use of anesthetics and anticoagulants, introduce artifacts (Eik-Nes, 1971). These artifacts should be carefully considered when deciding between prostatic experiments *in vivo* and *in vitro*. Already in 1950 Hudson *et al.* published a prostate preparation for perfusion studies. This preparation made use of the anesthetized dog, proper isolation of the prostatic blood vessels, and cannulation of the abdominal aorta and vena cava after the prostate had been severed from its connection with the urinary bladder and the prostatic urethra. This preparation as well as the prostatic perfusion preparation of Behnam and Hodges (1960) have been employed for investigating acid phosphatase activity (Hudson and Butler, 1950) and phosphorus metabolism (Behnam and Ocher, 1960) in the prostate. For purpose of looking at androgen metabolism by the prostate *in vivo*, the preparations described in Section II,A–D are available.

A. Preparation of Farnsworth *et al.* (1963)

Rats are anesthetized with Nembutal, and the arterial supply of all pelvic structures, except the prostate, are ligated through a midline incision. After the administration of heparin to the animal, the prostate is perfused via the abdominal aorta and vena cava with heterogenous rat blood containing radioactive testosterone. The blood used for perfusion is warmed to 37°C and oxygenated. Infusion pressure is monitored and by adjusting the speed of the infusion pump, a pressure between 90 and

120 mm Hg can be maintained. The preparation requires 2–3 hours and prostates can be perfused for 2–2.5 hours. Prostatic utilization of perfused testosterone depends on the completeness of arterial ligation of the pelvic organs. The preparation as such appears best suited for checking data on prostate metabolism of androgens *in vivo* versus such data *in vitro*. By criteria of paper chromatography the rat prostate will form radioactive metabolites from infused radioactive testosterone. As indicated by the authors: "On chromatographic analysis of the perfusate and the perfused gland, the distribution of products was essentially identical in blood and gland (except for unmetabolized testosterone in the blood) and also identical to the products obtained *in vitro*" (Farnsworth and Brown, 1963b).

With this system of perfusion, a considerable portion of the infused radioactivity will pass through the liver, and, in order to correct for this fact, incubation with minced liver tissue and radioactive testosterone is done. The testosterone metabolites from this incubation are subsequently incubated with minced prostatic tissue (Farnsworth and Brown, 1963b). This preparation is rather cumbersome, and one may wonder about the effect on prostatic metabolism of steroids of having all pelvic organs in the animal devoid of arterial blood. Will such organs produce toxins that can reach the prostate? It may, however, be useful to recall at this point that the preparation of Farnsworth and Brown is the first one for investigation of prostate metabolism of steroids *in vivo*. Since the rat is a well-explored laboratory animal, and since the major part of knowledge on prostate metabolism of steroids *in vitro* comes from work with the rat prostate, further refinements of the preparation of Farnsworth and Brown should be encouraged.

B. Preparation of Morfin *et al.* (1970a)

This preparation employs dogs anesthetized with intravenous sodium pentobarbital. Through a midline incision and retraction of the viscera, the prostate is reached. The umbilical and iliolumbar arteries are ligated, and via a catheter placed in the median sacral artery radioactive steroids can be added to the arterial blood irrigating the prostate and the urinary bladder. The arterial preparation, however, leaves structures supplied with arterial blood via the gluteal and the pudendal arteries as part of the infusion system. Shortly after stopping the infusion, the prostate is removed from the animal. Radioactive steroids in the infused tissues (prostate, urinary bladder) are determined and the prostate concentration of such compounds used as an index of organ metabolism *in vivo*. Control blood is obtained from the vena cava. The preparation is best for short term infusion studies. It offers no control of blood flow through the prostate and the infused radioactive steroids can be metabolized by organs outside the prostate.

In an extension of this method, Morfin *et al.* (1970b) have published a procedure for investigating steroid metabolism in the human prostate *in vivo*. This preparation, performed in association with retropubic prostatectomy, involves isolation of the hypogastric arteries distal to bifurcation from the external iliac arteries. The isolated hypogastric arteries are then used for infusion of radioactive steroids over 10 minutes, but as stated by the authors (Morfin *et al.*, 1970b), "A substantial portion of radiosteroids entered the gluteal arteries." This preparation suffers the same drawbacks as the one in the dog and can be employed only for rapid infusion. Within 8 minutes after the termination of steroid infusion the prostate can be removed. Side effects due to this preparation have not been observed. This approach to the prostate *in vivo* should aid knowledge of hormone metabolism in the diseased gland (Becker *et al.*, 1972).

C. Preparation of Haltmeyer and Eik-Nes (1972)

These investigators also make use of the sodium pentobarbital anesthetized dog. Through a midline incision from os pubis to umbilicus and retraction of visceral organs, the prostate is reached and freed of fat and connective tissue. The exposed prostatic arteries are dissected caudally from the urogenital arteries followed by ligation of the *rami urethrales*. The main prostatic veins are isolated and dissected and the prostate is freed from the ventral surface of the rectum. Arteries and veins in this region are severed between double ligatures. The prostatic ducts are now cannulated and the connection between the prostate and the urinary bladder is severed between double ligatures. Prior to this step the ureters are cannulated and the urine permitted to flow freely outside the animal. The connection between the prostate and the caudal part of urethra is then severed between double ligatures and the prostate removed from the dog. Cannulas are now placed in the prepared prostatic arteries and the gland is placed in a metabolic chamber maintained at 37.5°C (Eik-Nes, 1971). Arterial blood is obtained from a cannula in the femoral artery of the dog and oxygenated (Eik-Nes, 1971). The blood is warmed to 37.5°C and infused through the cannulas in the prostatic arteries at a constant rate. In prostates weighing between 30 and 90 gm, 7.8 ml of arterial blood are infused per minute. When working with normal-sized dog prostates (10–20 gm) it is advisable to reduce this flow. During an experiment the dog must be infused with 0.9% sodium chloride solution or, better, with a mixture of heterogenous dog blood and sodium chloride solution via a leg vein at the same rate as that of blood infusion via the prostatic arteries. In order to prevent clotting of blood the dog must be heparinized. Thus, extreme caution has to be exercised during preparation in severing all arteries and veins between double ligatures, and the preparation is time consuming (2–4 hours). The preparation suffers all the drawbacks associated with infusion of blood via arteries (Eik-Nes, 1971). Preliminary data indicate that dog prostates perfused with buffer via the arteries can metabolize and secrete infused steroids in effluent buffer. As for the perfused dog testis (Eik-Nes, 1971) the steroid metabolic activity is lower in prostates infused with buffer than in prostates infused with the animal's own arterial blood.

In spite of many shortcomings, this preparation offers control of blood flow through the prostate and exposure of exogenous material administered via the arteries to the prostate only. Prostatic venous blood can be examined for metabolic products, and perfusion experiments lasting for up to 150 minutes can be conducted without histological evidence of damage to the infused tissue. Via the cannulas in the prostatic ducts, the prostatic secretion can be obtained during perfusion. Agents stimulating this secretion (Smith, 1967), however, have not been tested in this preparation. The gland is without arterial blood during cannulation of the prostatic arteries and transfer of the gland from the dog to the metabolic chamber (10–15 minutes). Further, the prostate is without nerve connections during the perfusion and lacks anatomical connection with the urinary bladder and the caudal part of urethra. Whether these connections are needed for proper androgen function in the prostate is unknown.

D. PREPARATION OF RESNICK et al. (1974)

The vascular bed of the prostate is carefully prepared in anesthetized, castrated dogs. The gland is removed from the animal with intact vascular pedicles (distal aorta) and placed in an organ chamber maintained at 40°C. The prostate is then perfused, using a peristaltic perfusion pump, with a fluorocarbon-pluronic-electrolyte emulsion containing radioactive testosterone. Perfusion lasting for 4–6 hours can be done, and biopsy samples are obtained from the gland during perfusion. These samples are analyzed by the technique of radioautography. Infused radioactivity appears, however, to disappear from the prostatic tissue even when prolactin is added to the perfusate. The advantages of this preparation are that long-time perfusion studies can be conducted and that a controlled perfusion medium is used.

Preparations C and D employ the isolated prostate and are thus perfusion systems *in vitro*. During the last years it has been observed that the epididymis may in part direct androgen-dependent functions in the prostate (Pierrepoint *et al.*, 1974). This unilateral epididymal control mechanism of androgen function in the dorsolateral and ventral lobes of the prostate, seems to operate via an intact ductus deferens (Pierrepoint *et al.*, 1975a). Pierrepoint and associates (1975a,b) have also recorded high concentrations of androgens in the vein of the ductus deferens. Moreover, evidence has been obtained on transport of fluorescent material into the blood vessels of the prostate directly from the deferential vein in rats (Lewis and Moffat, 1975). This unilateral prostatic control system, depending apparently on a viable cauda epididymis, vas deferens, and deferential vein (Pierrepoint *et al.*, 1975a,b) is absent in animal preparations C and D. In spite of the fact that these preparations may fulfill many of the criteria for an adequate perfusion preparation, they do not incorporate this possible important gonadal control mechanism for prostatic function.

In prostate preparations B–D the dog is the preferred animal. The fact that dogs, like men, are unique among the species hitherto investigated in susceptibility to benign prostatic hyperplasia (Schlotthauer, 1937) and prostatic adenocarcinoma (Leav and Ling, 1968) makes these preparations rather useful when investigating steroid mechanisms responsible for these clinical conditions. The underlying reasons for such pathology, however, may not necessarily be identical in men and dogs. Predisposition to specific diseases in two species may or may not be casually related. Factors like ecology, environment, habitats, nutrition, previous diseases, biochemical and/or anatomical differences and similarities must be considered and evaluated. Moreover, Evans and Pierrepoint (1975) have found that the dog prostate contains a specific cytosol receptor for 5α-androstane-$3\alpha,17\alpha$-diol. This steroid may be the active androgen in the canine prostate (Harper *et al.*, 1970). Finally, a sex-binding β-globulin seems to be absent from dog blood plasma (Murphy, 1969). Thus, when working with preparations B, C or D, one should restrict conclusions from the data obtained to the dog only.

III. Androgen Metabolism in the Perfused Prostate

The perfused dog prostate will secrete 5α-dihydrotestosterone (DHT) into prostatic venous blood (Table II), as is also the case with the perfused testis (Folman *et al.*, 1972) and the perfused epididymis (Sowell and Eik-Nes, 1972). The perfused prostate will concentrate androgens

TABLE II

CHANGES IN BLOOD PLASMA CONCENTRATIONS OF 5α-DIHYDROTESTOSTERONE
ACROSS THE PERFUSED DOG PROSTATE[a]

| Dog index | 5α-Dihydrotestosterone (pg/ml blood plasma) | | |
	Effluent plasma	Affluent plasma	Changes across organ
A	480	404	+ 76
B	460	445	+ 15
C	300	308	− 8
D	110	140	− 30
E	530	510	+ 20
F	370	320	+ 50
G	690	610	+ 80
H	170	180	− 10
I	3020	1290	+1730
J	290	160	+ 130
K	192	78	+ 114
L	1330	120	+1210
M	707	541	+ 166

[a] The steroid androgen was measured in effluent and affluent blood plasma. Data are *in part* from an investigation by Haltmeyer and Eik-Nes (1972).

in the tissue (Morfin *et al.*, 1970a; Haltmeyer and Eik-Nes, 1972), and when radioactive testosterone (T) is perfused via the prostatic arteries, rapid metabolism of T to DHT and other radioactive metabolites can be observed (Morfin *et al.*, 1970a; Haltmeyer and Eik-Nes, 1972).

Secretion of DHT by the perfused dog prostate (Table II) was an unexpected finding, but superfused human prostatic tissue will form DHT and add it to the perfusate (Giorgi *et al.*, 1973). Also, lack of retention of infused radioactive testosterone in prostate preparation D has been published (Resnick *et al.*, 1974). It is well established that the rat prostate contains DHT-binding principles (Unhjem *et al.*, 1969; Mainwaring, 1969; Baulieu and Jung, 1970). If such binders exist in the dog prostate (Evans and Pierrepoint, 1975) and are saturated under the experimental conditions of animal preparation C, excess DHT is free to leave the prostatic cells via the venous drainage of the gland. Prostatic secretion of DHT could in addition reflect an orderly exchange of DHT between the nucleus and the cytoplasm of the prostatic cell. Unbound DHT in the cytoplasm would be a more likely candidate for penetration of the cell membrane than DHT associated with a cytosol binding principle. However, note should be taken of the fact that mechanisms of steroid secretion are largely unknown. In this respect, secretion of a steroid by a cell containing a specific receptor *for that steroid* merits special attention. The prevailing androgen in systemic, venous blood of mature, male animals is T; in the dog the ratio of circulating T/DHT varies between 8 and 45 (Folman et al., 1972). DHT is more potent than T in depressing circulating FSH and LH in castrated, mature male rats (Verjans et al., 1974). If secretion of DHT in animal preparation C is not an artifact produced by the preparation itself and if the dog prostate contains receptors for DHT, then the question must be asked whether secretion of DHT by the prostate reflects leakage of excess hormone from the gland or is serving some other physiological purpose. Moreover, the fact that androgens will leave the perfused prostate in preparations C and D could indicate that the androgen receptors of the gland are either destroyed or inactivated during preparation for perfusion or also by the techniques for perfusion employed in these preparations.

When radioactive T is perfused at a constant rate via the prostatic arteries in animal preparation C, the true specific radioactivity of T in venous blood is much higher than that of T in the prostatic tissue after the preparation has achieved metabolic equilibrium (Haltmeyer and Eik-Nes, 1972). Such data could indicate that the perfused prostate may have storage pools and secretory pools for T of different sizes. In these experiments the true specific radioactivities of secreted and stored DHT are more similar, pointing to the possibility that metabolism of T to DHT occurs in a specific prostatic compartment (Bruchovsky and Wilson, 1968) and that the release of DHT from this compartment is subject to other regulatory mechanisms than that of release of T. Moreover, whether prostatic secretion of DHT is sufficient to affect pituitary secretion of peptide hormones is currently unknown. Published data could support the view that some of these peptide hormones have effects on prostatic growth processes independent of the gonadal androgens (Lawrence and Landau, 1965; Riddle, 1963; Ishibe et al., 1968). Infusion of prolactin via the prostatic arteries in animal preparation C for 90 minutes did not alter T metabolism to DHT in a significant way (Haltmeyer and Eik-Nes, 1972). In prostate preparation D, perfusion with prolactin is associated with augmented cellular uptake of perfused testosterone (Resnick et al., 1974). Conflicting data exist, however, on the ability of prolactin to promote androgen uptake by the prostate (Boyns and Griffiths, 1972, see Lasnitzki, p. 200; Boyns and Griffiths, 1972, see Farnsworth, p. 217). Thus, available evidence at this juncture will not permit the conclusion that prostatic secretion of DHT serves a physiological purpose with respect to extragonadal control of prostatic function. The weight of experimental information favors overwhelmingly the view that the prostate "leaks" androgenic hormones into its venous blood.

Following infusion of radioactive T in animal preparation B, the androgenic hormone 5α-androstane-$3\alpha,17\beta$-diol (3α-diol) can be isolated from the prostate (Morfin *et al.*, 1970b). This steroid will promote growth of the prostate (Table I) and is a potent inhibitor of pituitary secretion of LH and FSH in castrated male rats (H. L. Verjans and K. B. Eik-Nes, unpublished, 1975). 5α-Androstane-$3\beta,17\beta$-diol (3β-diol) has little effect on these biological parameters. Whether 3α-diol is an important androgen can be questioned because of the ability of organs to convert 3α-diol to DHT. Such bioconversion takes place in the prostate *in vitro* (Robel *et al.*, 1971; Ofner and Vena, 1974). Experiments with proper inhibitors for this dehydrogenation reaction are called for in order to solve the problem of whether 3α-diol is an androgen per se in systems *in vivo*. The infused canine prostate will produce more 3β-diol than 3α-diol from radioactive T in animal preparation B (Morfin *et al.*, 1970b). The 3β-diol is active in maintaining epithelial height and secretory alveoli in prostate cells grown in tissue culture (Baulieu *et al.*, 1968). The mode of action of 3β-diol on these processes is currently not understood. No radioactive 3β-diol can be found in prostatic secrete of glands infused with radioactive T in animal preparation C (Haltmeyer and Eik-Nes, 1972).

Experiments *in vitro* with prostatic tissue have demonstrated that 3α-diol is a much better substrate for conversion to DHT than is 3β-diol (Robel *et al.*, 1971; Ofner and Vena, 1974). Ofner and Vena (1974) have reported that 3β-diol is the preferred substrate for hydroxylation reactions at C-6 and C-7 by the prostate *in vitro*. Whether these prostatic enzymes also operate *in vivo* awaits further work. 7-Hydroxylated androgens or androgen metabolites could be of importance for steroid metabolism in the prostate, since published information points to the fact that such metabolites can influence steroid metabolic enzymes in the testis (Inano *et al.*, 1973).

Prostates *in vivo* (Morfin *et al.*, 1970a,b) will convert T to Δ^4-androstenedione. This steroid androgen will be futher metabolized to 5α-androstanedione *in vivo* (Morfin *et al.*, 1970a,b), though 5α-androstanedione could also be formed from DHT. When dog prostates are infused with radioactive T in animal preparation C, the true specific radioactivity of secreted and tissue-stored DHT is much lower than that of secreted and tissue-stored T (Haltmeyer and Eik-Nes, 1972). If all of the DHT in these experiments was formed from T, one would expect that the true specific radioactivities would be more similar. Dogs subjected to animal preparation C are "stressed," and the "stressed" adrenal gland secretes substantial amounts of Δ^4-androstenedione (Wassermann and Eik-Nes, 1969). Adrenal secretion of Δ^4-androstenedione would in animal preparation C be delivered to the prostate via the infused blood, and in light of our data it is possible that metabolism of Δ^4-androstenedione $\rightarrow 5\alpha$-

androstanedione → DHT is of significance under the prevailing conditions of animal preparation C. Whatsoever the answer to this problem may be, compared to 5α-reductive metabolism of T, the activity of the oxidative pathway for initial T metabolism by the prostate *in vivo* is small. T metabolism to isoandrosterone will take place in the prostate *in vivo* (Morfin *et al.*, 1970b) ; either 5α-androstanedione or 3β-diol could be used as substrate for this conversion. Finally, the infused human and canine prostate can produce androsterone (Morfin *et al.*, 1970b).

Detailed investigations of preferred substrates for the above dehydrogenation reactions in the prostate have not been conducted *in vivo*. One should recognize that the hydroxysteroid dehydrogenases are reversible enzymes. A ratio of 17β-ol metabolites:17-one metabolites of 2.95 is obtained in work with animal preparation B using radioactive T as substrate (Morfin *et al.*, 1970b). When radioactive Δ⁴-androstenedione was infused in this preparation, a ratio of 17β-diol metabolites:17-one metabolites of 0.11 was found. These ratios of isotopic metabolites must, however, be considered in light of the fact that nonisotopic steroids were not measured in the prostatic tissue. Since the enzymes involved cannot distinguish between isotopic and nonisotopic steroids, the ratio between 17β-ol:17-one metabolites would be of physiological significance only if the substrate pool of all enzymes were similar.

At each prostate meeting this reviewer has attended, someone always brings up the problem of zinc and prostatic function. A zinc-binding protein from the cytosol fraction of the human prostate has been isolated (Reed and Stitch, 1973) which is rich in histidine (Heathcote and Washington, 1973). Since unknown radiometabolites are found in prostates infused with radioactive T (Morfin *et al.*, 1970b; Haltmeyer and Eik-Nes, 1972) and since steroids can be associated with zinc (Itabashi, 1960), we have investigated whether such association can occur with T or DHT. Using mass spectrometric and potentiometric titration techniques it was not possible to identify any complexes of these androgens with zinc (B. Mestvedt and K. B. Eik-Nes, unpublished, 1975) ; hence the unknown compounds from perfused prostates do not represent complexes between zinc and T or DHT. The androgen-dependent zinc uptake of the prostate *in vivo* (Prout *et al.*, 1959) is a problem warranting serious consideration.

In conclusion it can be stated that the perfused prostate preparations have promoted appreciable progress in understanding the biotransformations gonadal androgens are undergoing in this gland. Alternative models other than prostatic systems *in vitro* are needed in order to understand how the prostate handles important biomessengers for growth and function. The prostatic preparations discussed are far from perfect, and the true answers to prostatic metabolism of androgens must come from further experiments both *in vitro* and *in vivo*. With such answers we should be able to reexamine causes, relationships, and phenomena regarding our common problem: prostate and androgens.

ACKNOWLEDGMENTS

The work reviewed from the author's own laboratory was supported in part by research contract No-1-HD-42812 from National Institutes of Health, Bethesda, Maryland. I am greatly indebted to Dr. Leo T. Samuels, Department of Biological Chemistry, University of Utah, Salt Lake City, Utah, for his kind help during many years.

REFERENCES

Baulieu, E.-E., and Jung, I. (1970). *Biochem. Biophys. Res. Commun.* 38, 599.
Baulieu, E.-E., Lasnitzki, I., and Robel, P. (1968). *Nature (London)* 219, 1155.
Becker, H., Kaufmann, J., Klosterhalfern, H., and Voigt, K. D. (1972). *Acta Endocrinol. (Copenhagen)* 71, 589.
Behnam, A. M., and Hodges, C. V. (1960). *Surg. Forum* 11, 480.
Behnam, A. M., and Ocher, J. M. (1960). *J. Urol.* 84, 753.
Bruchovsky, N., and Wilson, J. D. (1968). *J. Biol. Chem.* 243, 2012.
Eik-Nes, K. B. (1970). *Amer. J. Physiol.* 217, 1764.
Eik-Nes, K. B. (1971). *Recent Progr. Horm. Res.* 27, 517.
Eik-Nes, K. B., and Hall, P. F. (1965). *Vitam. Horm. (New York)* 23, 153.
Evans, C. R., and Pierrepoint, C. G. (1975). *J. Endocrinol.* 64, 539.
Farnsworth, W. E. (1972). *In* "Prolactin and Carcinogenesis" (A. R. Boyns and K. Griffiths, eds.), p. 217. Alpha Omega Alpha Publ., Cardiff, Wales.
Farnsworth, W. E., and Brown, J. R. (1963a). *J. Amer. Med. Ass.* 183, 436.
Farnsworth, W. E., and Brown, J. R. (1963b). *Nat. Cancer Inst., Monogr.* 12, 323.
Farnsworth, W. E., Brown, J. R., and Lawrence, M. H. (1963). *Endocrinology* 73, 489.
Folman, Y., Haltmeyer, G. C., and Eik-Nes, K. B. (1972). *Amer. J. Physiol.* 222, 653.
Giorgi, E. P., Shirley, I. M., Grant, J. K., and Stewart, J. C. (1973). *Biochem. J.* 133, 465.
Haltmeyer, G. C., and Eik-Nes, K. B. (1972). *Acta Endocrinol. (Copenhagen)* 69, 394.
Haltmeyer, G. C., and Eik-Nes, K. B. (1974). *J. Reprod. Fert.* 36, 41.
Hansson, V. (1971). *Acta Endocrinol. (Copenhagen)* 68, 89.
Harding, B. W., and Samuels, L. T. (1962). *Endocrinology* 70, 109.
Harper, M. E., Pierrepoint, C. G., Fahmy, A. R., and Griffiths, K. (1970). *Biochem. J.* 119, 785.
Heathcote, J., and Washington, R. J. (1973). *J. Endocrinol.* 58, 421.
Hudson, P. B., and Butler, W. W. S. (1950). *J. Urol.* 63, 323.
Hudson, P. B., Butler, W. W. S., Brendler, H., and Scott, W. W. (1950). *J. Urol.* 63, 319.
Inano, H., Suzuki, K., Wakabayashi, K., and Tamaoki, B. I. (1973). *Endocrinology* 92, 22.
Ishibe, T., Fukushige, M., Takenaka, I., Misoguchi, M., and Kazuta, M. (1968). *Endocrinol. Jap.* 15, 181.

Itabashi, H. (1960). *Endocrinol. Jap.* **7**, 284.
Lasnitzki, I. (1972). *In* "Prolactin and Carcinogenesis" (A. R. Boyns and K. Griffiths, eds.), p. 200. Alpha Omega Alpha Publ., Cardiff, Wales.
Lawrence, A. M., and Landau, R. L. (1965). *Endocrinology* **77**, 1119.
Leav, I., and Ling, G. V. (1968). *Cancer* **22**, 1329.
Leav, I., Cavazos, L. F., and Ofner, P. (1974). *J. Nat. Cancer Inst.* **52**, 789.
Lewis, M. H., and Moffat, D. B. (1975). *J. Reprod. Fert.* **43**, (in press).
Lindner, H. R. (1963). *J. Endocrinol.* **25**, 483.
Mainwaring, W. I. P. (1969). *J. Endocrinol.* **45**, 531.
Monod, J., Changeux, J., and Jacob, F. (1963). *J. Mol. Biol.* **6**, 1095.
Morfin, R. E., Aliapoulios, M. A., Chamberlain, J., and Ofner, P. (1970a). *Endocrinology* **87**, 394.
Morfin, R. E., Aliapoulios, M. A., Bennett, A. H. Harrison, J. H., and Ofner, P. (1970b). *Excerpta Med. Found. Int. Congr. Ser.* **12**, 337.
Murphy, B. E. P. (1969). *Can. J. Biochem.* **46**, 299.
Ofner, P., and Vena, R. L. (1974). *Steroids* **24**, 261.
Pearlman, W. H., and Pearlman, M. R. J. (1961). *J. Biol. Chem.* **236**, 1321.
Pierrepoint, C. G., Davies, P., and Wilson, D. W. (1974). *J. Reprod. Fert.* **41**, 413.
Pierrepoint, C. G., Davies, P., Millington, D., and John, B. (1975a). *J. Reprod. Fert.* **43**, (in press).
Pierrepoint, C. G., Davies, P., Lewis, M. H., and Moffat, D. B. (1975b). *J. Reprod. Fert* (in press).
Prout, G. R., Sierp, M., and Whitmore, W. F. (1959). *J. Amer. Med. Ass.* **169**, 1703.
Reed, M. J., and Stitch, S. R. (1973). *J. Endocrinol.* **58**, 405.
Resnick, M. I., Walvoord, D. J., and Grayhack, J. T. (1974). *Surg. Forum* **25**, 70.
Riddle, O. (1963). *J. Nat. Cancer Inst.* **31**, 1039.
Robel, P., Lasnitzki, I., and Baulieu, E. E. (1971). *Biochimie* **53**, 81.
Schlotthauer, C. F. (1937). *J. Amer. Vet. Med. Ass.* **90**, 176.
Setchell, B. P., Waites, G. M. H., and Thorburn, G. D. (1966). *Circ. Res.* **18**, 755.
Smith, E. R. (1967). *J. Pharmacol. Exp. Ther.* **156**, 227.
Sowell, J. G., and Eik-Nes, K. B. (1972). *Proc. Soc. Exp. Biol. Med.* **141**, 827.
Unhjem, O., Tveter, K. J., and Aakvaag, A. (1969). *Acta Endocrinol. (Copenhagen)* **62**, 153.
Verjans, H. L., de Jong, F. H., Cooke, B. A., van der Molen, H. J., and Eik-Nes, K. B. (1974). *Acta Endocrinol. (Copenhagen)* **77**, 643.
Wassermann, G., and Eik-Nes, K. B. (1969). *Acta Endocrinol. (Copenhagen)* **61**, 33.

DISCUSSION

E. Diczfalusy: In order to add to the seeming confusion concerning the origin of 5α-dihydrotestosterone (DHT), I would like to call your attention to a dramatic decrease in the concentration of this steroid in seminal plasma following vasectomy (K. Purvis, S. K. Saksena, and E. Diczfalusy, *Clin. Endocrinol.* submitted for publication). This change is not accompanied by alterations in testosterone or androstenedione levels. What is hard to understand is why it takes as long as 6 months to arrive at these very low levels.

K. B. Eik-Nes: The contribution of DHT from the male sex organs to peripheral blood is rather small, and the purpose of this contribution is currently difficult to understand from a physiological standpoint. However, the long time needed for DHT to reach these low levels in your experiment may best be explained by organ secretion or lymph contribution of DHT to the seminal plasma independent of major organs of DHT production. How, I do not know.

C. G. Pierrepoint: An androgenic function for the epididymis seems to be highly probable. The work that Dr. Peter Davies and I have been involved in has certainly suggested that the androgen-maintained epididymis will synthesize androgens and that it plays a part in the local cortisol system of the prostate and seminal vesicles that we have reported. The epididymis, in the absence of the testes, will maintain the functional activity of these target organs at a higher level than is achieved in their absence. This gives evidence to the now discontinued practice of "cutting a horse proud" which was believed to retain one of the desirable qualities of the stallion in the gelding. Orchieectomy would seem to be less emasculinizing than orchi-epididymidectomy, which is again supported by the work of Gerald Lincoln on antler growth in red deer. Our evidence for a direct and unilateral cortisol system for the prostate via the vas deferens and the deferential vein is being supported by work now being reported in man and the examination of various parameters in seminal plasma following vasectomy. It is possible that your findings, Dr. Diczfalusy, of reduced DHT in seminal plasma after vasectomy is another reflection of the results of removing this direct pathway.

K.-D. Voigt: Did you find 17α-diols in prostates of other species also? Do you have any data on 17α-diol binding to dog plasma?

C. G. Pierrepoint: Yes, we have shown the formation of 5α-androstane-3α,17α-diol in the rat prostate as well as the 3β,17α. Dog plasma proteins do bind the α-diol as well as testosterone and 5α-dihydrotestosterone.

M. B. Lipsett: Two comments: First, in three large series examined one year after vasectomy, there were no changes in testosterone, estrogen, or gonadotropins in plasma.

Second, with respect to epididymal function in the absence of the testis, there is no evidence in men with nonfunctional Leydig cells that adrenal cortical secretions can substitute, in any appreciable degree, for the deficient Leydig cell secretion.

K. B. Eik-Nes: The epididymis has difficulties in forming steroids from cholesterol or acetate in most experiments *in vitro*. Thus, in the species of male animals where androgen function can be measured following castration, leaving the epididymis intact, this latter organ will probably form most of the androgens from adrenal steroids. As published by my laboratory, when we drain the adrenal venous blood of dogs into the spermatic artery, secretion of T will increase most significantly in spermatic venous blood. Therefore, in some animals the utilization of adrenal steroids for production of androgens by male sex organs should not be ignored nor overlooked.

M. Ritzen: The question of local androgen transport in the male duct system was brought up. The testicular androgen-binding protein (ABP) is secreted into and, in the rat, to some extent *through* the epididymis into the vas deferens. In other species, the situation is different. The rabbit ABP does *not* get through the epididymal duct, and consequently could not participate in androgen transport to the prostate or seminal vesicle.

K. B. Eik-Nes: We have no data on the role played by ABP in the dog. The epididymis of the dog will retain more DHT-^{3}H per gram of tissue when T-^{3}H is infused via the epididymal artery than the testis when that organ is also infused with T-^{3}H via the spermatic artery.

Under these experimental conditions, the testis secretes more DHT-^{3}H than the epididymis. Since the epididymis contains more androgen-binding principle per gram than the testis, there appears to be a relationship between secretion and binding of a steroid by organs infused via the arteries with precursors for that steroid.

E. E. Baulieu: What could be the physiological significance of other steroids than testosterone for DHT formation? Would you find the same for the androstanediols?

K. B. Eik-Nes: The facts are that the infused dog prostate secretes DHT, and these dogs are "stressed" and have adrenals secreting relatively large amounts of Δ^4-androstenedione. It may be that prostatic secretion of DHT in our preparation is an artifact due to the "stressed" adrenal secretion of Δ^4-androstenedione, and thus our preparation is not an adequate armamentarium for understanding prostatic function *in vivo*. Our knowledge depends on our technology, and I should like to bring this point of adrenal Δ^4-androstenedione to the attention of people who would like to use our preparation infusing the animal's own arterial blood via the prostatic arteries. As discussed in my lecture, 5α-androstane-3α,17α-diol may be the *active androgen* in the dog prostate, not DHT; thus DHT is secreted by the gland.

C. G. Pierrepoint: The information has been available in the literature for quite a few years that 5α-androstane-3α,17α-diol (the α-diol) was probably the active androgen in the dog prostate. It had been shown that it stimulated DNA and RNA polymerases in this gland and that it was located mainly in the nuclei. This evidence has been considerably strengthened by the work of Dr. C. R. Evans in my laboratory, who has demonstrated a 4–5 S cytoplasmic receptor for the α-diol which appears to be specific and is well competed for by testosterone, 5α-dihydrotestosterone, epitestosterone, androsterone, 5α-androstane-3α,17β-diol (slightly), or 5α-androstane-3β,17β-diol. Transfer to the nucleus has been demonstrated with consequent binding to a nuclear protein. Prostatic cytosol preincubated with the α-diol stimulates RNA polymerase in the nuclei from castrated dog prostates, whereas a reduction in activity apparently occurred when the experiment was repeated with DHT. Further evidence for the androgenicity of this steroid has been the demonstration of a cytoplasmic receptor for it alone in an anal adenoma from a dog, a known androgen-dependent tumor.

K. B. Eik-Nes: The dog prostate produces DHT, and, as indicated, the reason why the perfused dog prostate secretes DHT in effluent blood may be that DHT is not *the androgen* in this gland. It would be of interest to know whether other androgen-sensitive organs in the dog also have specific receptors for 5α-androstane-3α,17α-diol rather than for DHT. As you may recall, we have reported the secretion of DHT by the dog testis and epididymis.

Production of Testosterone by Prostate and Other Peripheral Tissues in Man

MORTIMER B. LIPSETT

The Cancer Center, Inc., Case Western Reserve University School of Medicine, Cleveland, Ohio

I. Introduction

The major circulating androgens in adult men are testosterone,* dihydrotestosterone, androstanediol, and androstenediol. The concentrations are such that the net androgenicity of plasma steroids in men is chiefly a function of plasma testosterone concentration. Only when plasma testosterone concentration reaches the hypogonadal range could the other steroids exert significant androgenic effects. Since all androgens are both secreted and derived from the peripheral metabolism of other steroids, one must consider the origins of the androgens and proandrogens as well as their secretion and production rates. The basic methods for these analyses were outlined by Tait in his first papers (Tait, 1963; Tait and Burstein, 1964) and have recently been elegantly formulated (Gurpide, 1975).

* The chemical names for the steroids are as follows: testosterone, 17β-hydroxyandrost-4-en-3-one; dihydrotestosterone, 17β-hydroxyandrostan-3-one; androstanediol, 3α,17β-dihydroxyandrostanediol; androstenediol, 3β,17β-dihydroxyandrost-5-en-17-one; androstenedione, androst-4-ene-3,17-dione.

II. METHODOLOGY

A. INTRODUCTION

Secretion rate is defined as the rate of entry of a steroid into the blood from an endocrine gland. Secretion can be proved by the demonstration of a gradient between the concentration of a steroid in the glandular venous effluent and the peripheral venous blood. The *production rate* is the irreversible rate of entry of the steroid into the blood from all sources. For example, androstenediol is both secreted by the adrenal cortex and derived from the metabolism of dehydroepiandrosterone in peripheral tissues. The net of the rates of entry into the blood compartment from both sources is the production rate.

Horton and Tait (1966) initially utilized a model for androgen metabolism consisting of two anatomical and two chemical compartments. Although this is the simplest model that can describe the secretion and production rates, and interconversions of testosterone and androstenedione, it is readily apparent that when other precursors of plasma testosterone, such as dehydroepiandrosterone are included, the model will become increasingly complex. The interconversions of two steroids in the same and between anatomical compartments are given by ρ values. Although the tissue compartment of this and other systems has not been fully characterized, the blood production rates and the overall interconversions (ρ values) can be determined from the specific activity of androgens in the blood compartment following introduction of the appropriate radioactive steroids.

B. METABOLIC CLEARANCE RATES

The production of steroids in the blood compartment can be estimated as the product of the *metabolic clearance rate* (MCR) and the plasma steroid concentration. The MCR is defined as the volume of blood or plasma irreversibly cleared of steroid per unit time. The relationship of the MCR to the production rate and plasma concentration of steroid can be visualized by considering the blood flow through a hypothetical organ that removes steroid irreversibly from blood (Tait, 1963). Thus if the concentration of steroid in blood entering the organ is S, then, by definition, in the effluent blood it is zero. The MCR of S (MCR^S) is then equal to the blood flow through the organ. From application of the Fick principle, the product of the MCR (liters per day) $\times$ S (μg per liter) gives the mass of S removed from the blood in micrograms per 24 hours. Under steady state conditions this will also equal the rate of irreversible entry of steroid into the blood, or the production rate. The MCR is thus determined by infusing radioactive S^* at rate RS^* until the plasma level is constant at S^*. Then $MCR^S = RS^*/[S^*]$.

Experimentally, ρ^* values (transfer factors) are determined by infusing two steroids with different labels and measuring the ratio of isotopes in the product. For example, if ^{14}C-labeled testosterone and ^3H-labeled androstenedione are infused into the blood, then

$$\rho_{BB}^{AT} = (^3H/^{14}C \text{ in plasma testosterone})/(^3H/^{14}C \text{ of infused isotopes})$$

From this general expression, Tait and Horton (1964) showed that:

$$\rho_{BB}^{AT} = (MCR^T/MCR^A)(X^T/X^A)$$

where MCR^T and MCR^A equal the MCRs of testosterone and androstenedione and X^T/X^A equals the isotope ratio of testosterone to androtenedione following infusion of isotope X in androstenedione. A detailed discussion of these formulations has been presented (Tait and Burstein, 1964). The MCR should be expressed as a function of surface area (Bardin and Lipsett, 1967) to facilitate comparisons.

These techniques have been used to determine the production rates of testosterone, androstenedione, dihydrotestosterone, dehydroepiandrosterone, androstenediol, and androstanediol, and the contributions of precursors to their production rates. It should be noted that the determination of MCR takes about 2 hours with the subjects in the supine position, but the calculated production rates are expressed for a 24-hour period.

1. Uncertainties of MCR Estimates

As will be discussed below, the metabolic clearance may vary with position and possibly with exercise. In addition, there is a diurnal variation of plasma steroid levels as shown for dehydroepiandrosterone, for example (Nieschlag et al., 1973), as well as short-term fluctuations in its concentration (Rosenfield et al., 1975).

Therefore, even though the steady-state assumptions for the metabolic clearance model hold for a short time with the subjects in basal state, they will not be accurate for a 24-hour period with normal activity. The

---

$^*\rho$ is defined as the fraction of one compartment, pool, or production rate that is converted to another compartment, pool, or production rate (Gurpide, 1975). When written according to Tait and Horton (1964) the superscripts represent the steroids or chemical compartments involved, e.g., TA = testosterone to androstenedione; and the subscripts, the anatomical compartments involved, e.g., BB = blood to blood. With the use of both superscripts, the entire process is described. For example, ρ_{BB}^{AT} = fraction of androstenedione converted to testosterone in the blood compartment. The ρ values are those obtained in vivo irrespective of the number of paths and compartments.

urinary isotope dilution technique for estimating the production rate of a steroid obviates corrections for hourly variation of the plasma levels and MCRs, but, as has been shown, this method is not generally applicable to the androgens (Koreman and Lipsett, 1964; Tait and Horton, 1964). The use of mean plasma level in the calculation of the production rate can correct for the variations of plasma steroid levels. Estimation of the metabolic clearance in supine and erect positions and during light work gives the range over which the MCR could vary. From these estimates, a mean production rate can be calculated. Although this approach would yield a valid estimate of the 24-hour production rate, it is cumbersome for the comparison of production rates among individual subjects with disorders of androgen metabolism. This problem may be resolved by studying all subjects in the basal state at the same time of day and calculating the production rate from a plasma sample obtained just prior to the metabolic clearance determination. This gives a production rate per 2 hours, a time during which the requirements for the steady state may be fulfilled. Even though the calculated values are expressed on a 24-hour basis, the assumptions implicit in this expression should be recognized. Given these problems, production rates and interconversion rate contain appreciable statistical uncertainty.

2. Value of MCR

The relationship between the plasma concentration and the production rate of a steroid has been used for many years as an indication of rate of metabolism. One of the most useful ways of describing this relationship is the MCR since, as noted above, PR=MCR × (S). The MCR remains valid regardless of the routes of removal of the steroid, or of the model needed to describe its metabolism (Tait, 1963). It is this feature and the relative simplicity of the calculations that has led to wide acceptance of the MCR for comparisons of *in vivo* steroid metabolism.

C. Hepatic Blood Flow

Because the liver is the important site of metabolism of steroids, the rate of removal from the blood will depend on hepatic blood flow. For example, the MCR of androstenedione is about 2200 liters per 24 hours and the hepatic extraction is 82% (Rivarola *et al.*, 1967). With both a high clearance and hepatic extraction, one would expect that the clearance of androstenedione would vary directly with hepatic blood flow. In this respect, androstenedione is similar to aldosterone, which also has a high clearance and extraction. By contrast, testosterone has a lower MCR

(Bardin and Lipsett, 1967) and a lower hepatic extraction (44%) (Rivarola et al., 1967). Since hepatic blood flow is lower while the subject is standing (Culbertson et al., 1951), the MCR_T of normal men was measured in the supine and erect positions to determine whether changes in hepatic blood flow significantly altered clearance. There was a 21–32% decrease in the MCR_T when the men changed from supine to erect. Southren et al. (1968) and Flood et al. (1973) found similar decreases of MCR_T and the MCR for androstenedione. These observations suggest that under the conditions of study the assumption of the erect position may variably lower hepatic blood flow and clearance rates. Therefore the effect of postural changes on the metabolic clearance rates of two steroids is difficult to compare unless the two steroids are studied simultaneously.

D. Tissue Extraction

Although the liver is the major organ for the extraction and metabolism of most steroids, there is direct as well as inferential evidence for extrahepatic metabolism of the androgens (see below). The MCR of androstenedione is greater than hepatic plasma flow, which indicates that some androstenedione is metabolized outside the liver. In addition, Horton and Tait (1966) compared the conversion of orally and intravenously administered labeled androstenedione to testosterone and concluded that the primary site of conversion of blood androstenedione to blood testosterone is extrasplanchnic tissue. Since 17β-hydroxylase is widely dispersed, and since in many organs oxidation of the 17-hydroxyl group is favored over reduction of the 17-ketone, extrahepatic metabolism of testosterone is a reasonable possibility. Evidence for this has been obtained by Mauvais-Jarvis and his co-workers (1970), who compared the metabolism of testosterone given by inunction with its metabolism after intravenous injection. Because the factors that influence both hepatic and extrahepatic extraction have not been studied independently, they must be discussed together, and it is recognized that a change in hepatic extraction might not necessarily be associated with a similar change in extrahepatic extraction. "Tissue extraction" is understood to be the sum of hepatic and extrahepatic extractions for a given steroid.

Tissue extraction is determined both by the rate of steroid transport from plasma and by the rate of enzymic metabolism in the cells. The transport of steroids from plasma is in turn influenced by steroid binding to plasma proteins. In a given situation it may be difficult to ascertain whether plasma protein binding or intracellular metabolism is rate limiting in overall tissue extraction, especially since these two processes can rarely be studied simultaneously. For example, the decreased MCR of testosterone during estrogen administration may be due, in part, to the increased testosterone-binding capacity of the plasma protein, which is increased 4-fold by estrogen (Pearlman and Crepy, 1967). It is well known, however, that estrogens suppress many enzyme systems, and some or all of the effect of estrogen on the testosterone clearance could be due to decreased celllular metabolism (Kumagai et al., 1959; Yates and Urquhart, 1962). Another example is the finding that hirsute women and men have higher testosterone MCRs than normal women (Bardin and Lipsett, 1967), and an increase in the MCR of testosterone has also been observed following exogenous androgen administration (Southren et al., 1968; Vermeulen et al., 1969). In this instance, the change in clearance could result from decreased plasma protein binding, increased saturation, or increased cellular metabolism, and Vermeulen et al. 1969) offered evidence that this last mechanism was also operative. Pearlman and Crepy (1967) first demonstrated that the testosterone-binding activity of plasma from men was lower than that of women, and Dray et al. (1968) noted similarly low binding activities in hirsute as opposed to normal women. These observations suggested that decreased testosterone binding could account for the increased testosterone MCR. The decreased testosterone MCR in hyperthyroidism is associate with increased testosterone binding to plasma protein (Dray et al., 1967; Crepy et al., 1967).

E. TESTOSTERONE-ESTRADIOL BINDING GLOBULIN (TEBG)

Testosterone binding to plasma proteins has been recognized for many years (Antoniades et al., 1960). Mercier and Baulieu (1968) using DEAE-cellulose column chromatography identified testosterone binding to albumin and β-globulin fractions.

Other investigators have subsequently confirmed the existence of this β-globulin fraction by column chromatography (Gueriguian and Pearlman, 1968) and electrophoresis (Steeno et al., 1968). On polyacrylamide gel electrophoresis, a protein that binds testosterone migrates with transferrin and is widely separated from cortisol-binding globulin, CBG (Corvol et al., 1971).

TEBG is inactivated at 60°C and in buffers below pH 5 (Pearlman and Crepy, 1967; Kato and Horton, 1968). From the studies of Vermeulen and Verdonck (1968), Kato and Horton (1968), and Steeno et al. (1968), it is apparent that TEBG has a high degree of stereospecificity for certain functional groups on the steroid nucleus. An unhindered 17β-hydroxyl group is essential for binding, and an oxygen at the 3 position is also important. Other polar groups, such as double bonds at the Δ^1,

Δ^4, Δ^5 position or 11- or 21-hydroxyl groups, tend to interfere with binding. It is important to note that other androgens, dihydrotestosterone (Kato and Horton, 1968), androstanediol (Clark and Bird, 1973), and androstenediol (Murphy, 1970) are bound to TEBG.

Testosterone is also known to bind to other proteins in plasma but with less affinity than to TEBG. The association constant with albumin is about 3×10^9 liters/mole (Pearlman and Crepy, 1967; Vermeulen and Verdonck, 1968). From these constants it is estimated that at physiological levels of testosterone and at normal plasma protein concentrations of cortisol less than 5% of testosterone is bound to CBG. However, at higher testosterone concentrations or at lower plasma cortisol levels a significant fraction of testosterone may be bound to CBG.

If the binding of testosterone to TEBG is analogous to cortisol binding to CBG, then one would expect that nonprotein-bound testosterone would be the biologically active portion of the total plasma testosterone and that the capacity of the binding protein might influence the level of the free steroid as well as its overall metabolism. There is evidence for this in the studies relating free testosterone or similar indexes to virilization (Rosenfield, 1973). Although steroids are bound to albumin, the affinity is low, tissue extraction is high, and this binding therefore may be neglected for physiological considerations.

III. Origin of Androgens

A. Testosterone

In normal men, over 95% of the testosterone production rate of 7 mg. daily is a result of Leydig cell secretion. Testosterone precursors thus contribute little to the production rate. In orchiectomized men, however, the situation is quite different. The adrenal cortex secretes only small amounts of testosterone (Baird *et al.*, 1969), so that most of the testosterone in blood is produced by peripheral metabolism of steroids secreted by the adrenal cortex. Although pertinent studies have not been made in orchiectomized men, data obtained from normal women can be used to give reasonable estimates (see Table I). There may be some overestimations of production rates of several steroids due to ovarian contributions; this is particularly pertinent when considering androstenedione, since the ovary secretes about 20% of the production rate.

The production rate of androstenedione is about 3 mg daily (Bardin and Lipsett, 1967), and of this about 2 mg is secreted by the adrenal cortex. Since the transfer factor, ρ_{BB}^{AT} is about 5%, about 100 μg of testosterone

TABLE I

PARAMETERS OF ANDROGEN METABOLISM IN WOMEN[a]

Steroid	MCR (liters/ day)	Plasma conc. (ng/ 100 ml)	PR (μg/day)	Transfer factor, ρ[b]	Percent of PR from precursor[b]
T	700	43	300	Δ-T 0.06	Δ, 60
				DHA-T 0.007	DHA, 17
DHT	400	20	80	T-DHT 0.02	T, 8
				Δ-DHT 0.003	Δ, 30
Δ	1600	120	3000	DHA-Δ 0.06	DHA, 14
DHA	1600	450	7200	—	—
Δ^5-diol	600	90	540	DHA-Δ^5 0.03	DHA, 40
A-diol	1300	2	26	DHT-A 0.22	DHT, 60
				Δ-A	

[a] T = testosterone, DHT = dihydrotestosterone, Δ = androstenedione, DHA = dehydroepiandrosterone, Δ^5-diol = Δ^5-androstenediol, A-diol = androstanediol; PR = Blood production rate; MCR = metabolic clearance rate.

[b] Only quantitatively important precursors are listed. The precursor is listed first, followed by the product.

would be produced daily. This is the major source of testosterone in women and, by inference, in orchiectomized men.

Dehydroepiandrosterone is metabolized to testosterone via androstenedione. The transfer factor, ρ_{BB}^{DT}, is 0.007. Thus, given the dehydroepiandrosterone production rate of 7 mg daily, 50 μg of testosterone is produced. This is about 17% of the testosterone production rate in normal women (Table I) and a larger fraction in orchiectomized men.

Estimates for androstenediol contributions in women are not as firm. The transfer factor for the group reaction (Δ^5-3β-hydroxysteroid to Δ^4-3-ketosteroid) is 6% (Horton and Tait, 1967) based on their studies of dehydroepiandrosterone. Thus, another 60 μg of testosterone could be produced by transformation of androstenediol. From these estimates, the orchiectomized man should have a testosterone blood production rate of about 200 μg daily, about two-thirds of the production rate in normal women with ovarian function.

B. DIHYDROTESTOSTERONE

The production rate of this putative intracellular androgen is about 400 μg daily (Saez et al., 1972). About 50% is derived from plasma testosterone and an additional 25% from androstenedione (Mahoudeau et *al.*, 1971). The testis also secretes some dihydrotestosterone. In agonadal men, dihydrotestosterone production rates should be about two-thirds those of normal women (Table I), or between 50 and 60 μg daily. The role of other precursors, such as the Δ^5-3β-hydroxysteroids, can be ignored since dihydrotestosterone is produced via testosterone in peripheral tissues (Saez *et al.*, 1972).

The metabolism of testosterone to dihydrotestosterone within the prostate is now well appreciated. Mahoudeau *et al.* (1974) catheterized a prostatic vein in nine men with benign prostatic hypertrophy. Although they demonstrated secretion of dihydrostestosterone, the gradient between prostatic vein and peripheral vein was so low that, even making an overestimate for blood flow, one would not estimate a significant prostatic secretion rate for dihydrostestosterone. However, it should be recognized that sampling prostatic venous blood is difficult and that there may have been dilution with peripheral blood, thereby reducing the apparent gradient. Barberia *et al.* (1975) have reported that the ratio of dihydrotestosterone to testosterone was increased in elderly men with benign prostatic hypertrophy although their testosterone concentrations were decreased. Prostatectomy reduced dihydrotestosterone concentrations to normal, implying that the prostate produced 50% of the blood dihydrotestosterone. These sets of opposing data will have to be reconciled by further study.

C. Dehydroepiandrosterone

This steroid is secreted primarily by the adrenal cortex, both free and as the sulfate (Nieschlag *et al.*, 1973), and small amounts are secreted by the ovary (Kirschner *et al.*, 1973) and by the testis (Nieschlag *et al.*, 1973). The only possible precursor of dehydroepiandrosterone is 17-hydroxypregnenolone; the transfer factor is so low (Strott *et al.*, 1970) that it can be ignored.

D. Androstenediol

Plasma concentrations of this steroid are twice as high in men as in women (Loriaux and Lipsett, 1973), and it has been shown that this steroid is secreted by the testis (Laatikainen *et al.*, 1971) and the ovary (Kirschner *et al.*, 1973), but not by the adrenal cortex (Kirschner *et al.*, 1973). Thus in an orchiectomized man one would predict that the origin of androstenediol was almost entirely from the peripheral metabolism of dehydroepiandrosterone.

E. Androstanediol

It has been shown that androstanediol originates from plasma testosterone and from androstenedione (Mahoudeau *et al.*, 1971). In women the production rate is low (Kinouchi and Horton, 1974) (Table I). As described elsewhere in this volume, the androstanediols may have important intracellular functions. It seems unlikely that the peripheral production of the 3α-androstanediol and the 3β-androstanediol (Mahoudeau *et al.*, 1971) are important for these functions. The kinetics of metabolism are of interest, since there is considerable binding to albumin (Bird *et al.*, 1974).

IV. Androgenicity

The reasons for discussing these steroids and their transformation in some detail is to attempt to estimate total androgenic effects on tissue. The word androgen is an operational definition for a steroid that exhibits certain characteristics, e.g., stimulates growth of prostate and seminal vesicle and has a high affinity for the cytosol receptor in these tissues. The steroids discussed above demonstrate biological androgenicity in the rodent bioassay systems but may have low binding affinity for cytosol receptor. This apparent discrepancy is due to peripheral transformations of the steroid as well as the quantitatively modified transformations occurring in target tissue, e.g., dehydroepiandrosterone to dihydrotestoster-

TABLE II

APPARENT CONTRIBUTIONS OF 17-HYDROXYSTEROIDS TO
PLASMA ANDROGENICITY IN WOMEN[a]

Steroid[b]	(1) Plasma conc. (ng/100 ml)	(2) Androgenic potency[c]	(3) Percent free in plasma	Index ($1 \times 2 \times 3$)	Percent contribution to androgenicity
T	40	1.0	1.3	52	37
DHT	20	1.3	1.2	31	22
Δ⁵-Diol	90	0.3	2.1	56	40
A-diol	2	0.5	1.3	1.3	1

[a] Table modified from Rosenfield (1973).

[b] T = testosterone; DHT = dihydrotestosterone; Δ^5-diol = Δ^5-androstenediol; A-diol = androstenediol.

[c] Bioassay data from rodents, expressed relative to testosterone (Dorfman and Shipley, 1956).

one in the prostate. But there are discrepancies between androgenicity as defined by the rat bioassay and the calculated androgenicity of a steroid based on its conversion to testosterone or dehydrotestosterone. This is due in part to the fact that the rat has no TEBG. The presence of this protein in human plasma means that calculation of androgenicity must take into account the distribution of the steroid between binding protein and solution.

Rosenfield (1973) attempted to do this using estimates of free (non-protein-bound) steroid in plasma. In Table II, it is apparent that androstenediol makes a considerable contribution to the androgenicity of plasma steroids. The most potent androgen, dihydrotestosterone, has a lesser contribution owing to its high affinity for TEBG. Unfortunately, the interconversions known to occur within target tissues are not perceptibly reflected in these estimates.

REFERENCES

Antoniades, N. H., Daughaday, W. H., and Slaunwhite, W. R. (1960). *In* "Hormones in Human Plasma" (H. N. Antoniades, ed.), p. 455. Little, Brown, Boston, Massachusetts.

Baird, D. T., Uno, A., and Melby, J. C. (1969). *J. Endocrinol.* **45,** 135.

Barberia, J., Hsieh, P., Cosgrove, M. T., and Horton, R. (1975). *Clin. Res.* **23,** 233A.

Bardin, C. W., and Lipsett, M. B. (1967). *J. Clin. Invest.* **46,** 891.

Bird, C. E., Choong, A., Knight, L. and Clark, A. F. (1974). *J. Clin. Endocrinol. Metab.* **38,** 372.

Clark, A. F., and Bird, C. (1973). *J. Endocrinol.* **57,** 298.

Corvol, P. L., Chrambach, A., Rodbard, D., and Bardin, C. W. (1971). *J. Biol. Chem.* **246,** 3435.

Crepy, O., Dray, F., and Sebaoun, J. (1967). *C. R. Acad. Sci., Ser. D* **264,** 2651.

Culbertson, J. W., Wilkins, R. N., Ingelfinger, F. J., and Bradley, S. E. (1951). *J. Clin. Invest.* **30,** 305.

Dorfman, R. I., and Shipley, R. A., eds. (1956). "Androgens." Wiley, New York.

Dray, F., Sebaoun, J., Mowszowicz, I., Delzant, G., Desgrez, P., and Dreyfus, G. (1967). *C. R. Acad. Sci., Ser. D* **264,** 2578.

Flood, C., Hunter, S. A., Lloyd, C. A., and Longcope, C. (1973). *J. Clin. Endocrinol. Metab.* **36,** 1180.

Gueriguian, J. L., and Pearlman, W. (1968). *J. Biol. Chem.* **243,** 5226.

Gurpide, E. (1975). —Tracer Methods in Hormone Research." Springer-Verlag, Berlin and New York.

Horton, R., and Tait, J. F. (1966). *J. Clin. Invest.* **4,** 301.

Horton, R., and Tait, J. F. (1967). *J. Clin. Endocrinol. Metab.* **27,** 79.

Kato, T., and Horton, R. (1968). *J. Clin. Endocrinol. Metab.* **8,** 1160.

Kinouchi, T., and Horton, R. (1974). *J. Clin. Invest.* **54,** 646.

Kirschner, M. A., Sinhamahapatra, S., Zucker, I. F., Loriaux, L., and Nieschlag, E. (1973). *J. Clin. Endocrinol. Metab.* **37,** 183.

Korenman, S. G., and Lipsett, M. B. (1964). *J. Clin. Invest.* **43,** 2125.

Kumagai, A., Otomo, M., Yano, S., Takeuchi, N., Nishino, K., Ueda H., Ko, S. and Kitamura, M. (1959). *Endocrinol. Jap.* **6,** 86.

Laatikainen, T., Laitinen, E. A., and Vihko, R. (1971). *J. Clin. Endocrinol. Metab.* **32,** 59.

Loriaux, D. L., and Lipsett, M. B. (1973). *Steroids* **19,** 681.

Mahoudeau, J. A., Bardin, C. W., and Lipsett, M. B. (1971). *J. Clin. Invest.* **50,** 1338.

Mahoudeau, J. A., Delassalle, A., and Bricaire, H. (1974). *Acta Endocrinol. (Copenhagen)* **77,** 401.

Mauvais-Jarvis, P., Bercovici, J. P., Crepy, O., and Gauthier, F. (1970). *J. Clin. Invest.* **49,** 31.

Mercier, C., and Baulieu, E. E. (1968). *Ann. Endocrinol.* **29,** 159.

Murphy, E. E. P. (1970). *Steroids* **16,** 791.

Nieschlag, E., Loriaux, D. L., Ruder, H. J. Zucker, I. R., Kirschner, M. A., and Lipsett, M. B. (1973). *J. Endocrinol.* **57,** 123.

Pearlman, W. H., and Crepy, O. (1967). *J. Biol. Chem.* **242,** 182.

Rivarola, A. M., Singleton, R. T., and Migeon, C. J. (1967). *J. Clin. Invest.* **46,** 2095.

Rosenfield, R. L. (1973). *J. Reprod. Med.* **11.**

Rosenfield, R. S., Rosenberg, R. J., Fukushima, D. K., and Hellman, L. (1975). *J. Clin. Endocrinol. Metab.* **40,** 850.

Saez, J. M., Forest, M. G., Morera, A. M., and Bertrand, J. (1972). *J. Clin. Invest.* **51,** 1226.

Steeno, O., Heyns, W., VanBaelen, H., and DeMoor, P. (1968). *Ann. Endocrinol.* **29,** 141.

Strott, C. A., Bermudez, J. A., and Lipsett, M. B. (1970). *J. Clin. Invest.* **49,** 1999.

Southren, A. L., Gordon, G. G., and Tochimoto, S. (1968). *J. Clin. Endocrinol. Metab.* **28,** 1105.

Tait, J. F. (1963). *J. Clin. Endocrinol. Metab.* **23,** 1285.

Tait, J. F., and Burstein, S. (1964). *In* "The Hormones" (G. Pincus, K. V. Thimann, and E. B. Astwood, eds.), Vol. 5. Academic Press, New York.

Tait, J. F., and Horton, R. (1964). *Steroids* **4,** 365.

Vermeulen, A., and Verdonck, L. (1968). *Steroids* **11,** 609.

Vermeulen, A., Verdonck, L., Vander Straeten, M., and Orie, N. (1969). *J. Clin. Endocrinol. Metab.* **29,** 1470.

Yates, F. E., and Urquhart, J. (1962). *Physiol. Rev.* **42,** 359.

DISCUSSION

P. Robel: Horton reported at a meeting in Bethesda that in patients undergoing prostatectomy for benign prostatic hyperplasia circulating DHT is significantly reduced. Therefore, it seems that, at least in these patients, the prostate may contribute significantly to circulating DHT.

M. B. Lipsett: These data need confirmation, particularly in view of the report of Mahoudeau *et al.* [J. A. Mahoudeau, A. Delassalle, and H. Bricaire, *Acta Endocrinol.* **77,** 401 (1974)] and some data of Voigt. For the plasma DHT to decrease 50% after prostatectomy would mean a large production of DHT with a high gradient between prostatic and spermatic veins.

M. Ritzén: I would like to stress the point that Dr. Lipsett made concerning the methodology of measuring steroid binding to plasma proteins. If examined by steady-state polyacrylamide gel electrophoresis, albumin is revealed as the major testosterone binding protein in the male, owing to the high concentration of albumin that compensates for the low binding affinity [M. Ritzén *et al., J. Biol. Chem.* **249**, 6597 (1974)].

M. B. Lipsett: I would agree. It is of interest that if the binding affinity is greater than that of testosterone, the MCR is higher. The MCR depends, of course, on concentrations of ligands in the blood as well.

H. G. Williams-Ashman: In adult men with indications of normal gonadal and liver functions, to what extent are production rates and metabolic clearance rates of androgens influenced by drugs, especially drugs that can be obtained without prescription and that are ingested by large sections of the population?

M. B. Lipsett: This has not been systemically examined. In man, in contrast to the rat, inducers of hepatic mixed-function oxidases have only small effects on the rate of metabolism. Rather, the routes of metabolism are altered by differing hydroxylation patterns.

E. Diczfalusy: In castrated rats, 5α-androstane-3α, 17β-diol is a very powerful inhibitor of LH secretion. Are you aware of any data on a similar effect in clinical experiments?

M. B. Lipsett: I have not seen any reports of the infusion of this steroid in man.

K. B. Eik-Nes: The flow of blood in dog prostates weighing between 20 and 30 gm is about 8 ml per minute. Thus, this is a small portion of the total minute-volume of the heart.

As to the problem of prostates afflicted with BHP, we have not been able to show that secretion of DHT by dog prostates weighing more than 30 gm is consistently higher than that by prostates of normal, non-BHP size (less than 20 gm).

M. B. Lipsett: The blood flow data mean that there should be a large gradient for DHT between prostatic and peripheral veins in order for there to be an important contribution of the prostate to circulating DHT. In Mahoudeau's study this was not demonstrated.

Steroid Hormone Receptors: A Survey

W. I. P. MAINWARING

Androgen Physiology Department, Imperial Cancer Research Fund,
Lincoln's Inn Fields, London, England

I. INTRODUCTION

Recent years have witnessed a dramatic extension in our knowledge of the binding and mechanism of action of steroid hormones. Progress in this discipline of endocrinology was founded on the now classical study of Jensen and Jacobsen (1962) in which the interaction of a tritiated steroid hormone with its target organ was investigated for the first time. The value of their contribution may be likened to the dramatic effect of adding a judiciously selected seeding crystal to a quiescent and saturated salt solution.

The elucidation of the discrete stages of the hormonal responses has proceeded rapidly; for a detailed survey of the earlier literature, the recent summary presented by King and Mainwaring (1974) should be consulted. The generation of this widespread interest may be attributed to many factors. First, the ubiquitous description of high-affinity binding mechanisms for all major classes of steroid hormones, the so-called steroid receptor systems, provoked a novel and exciting insight into the regulation of important biological processes where only relatively small numbers of hormone molecules were involved. Second, by an element of

223

serendipity, developments in the field of hormone action followed in the wake of the impressive advances being made in the underlying processes of macromolecular syntheses, notably in bacteria and cultured mammalian cells; thus, findings in hormone-response systems could be rapidly exploited by new technological procedures, particularly with respect to nucleic acid metabolism. Third, the work on steroid receptor systems offered new hope in the diagnosis and chemotherapy of clinical disorders with a hormonal etiology.

At the risk of bing stigmatized as a prophet of doom, it could be that the halcyon days of hormone action are temporarily drawing to a close. Investigators in this area of contemporary research are now confronted with daunting problems whose final solution will prove to be a test of enterprise and determination. The present survey is an attempt to define the areas of particular importance in future work. As a more hopeful leitmotif, the following quotation seems appropriate:

> Whatever you can do,
> Or dream you can,
> Begin it.
> Boldness has genius,
> Power and
> Magic in it.
>
> (W. H. Murray, 1921)

A. DEFINITIONS

As in all scientific subjects, a working parlance has evolved in work relating to hormone action. Subject to definition, the following terms are acceptable. *Receptor:* an intracellular component, almost certainly proteinaceous, responsible for the specific and high-affinity binding of a selected steroid hormone and playing an integral part in its mechanism of action. *Acceptor:* a nuclear component, responsible for the high affinity but finite retention of steroid-hormone receptor complexes in chromatin. *Induction:* the sequence of processes through which the synthesis *de novo* of a macromolecule is accelerated by a steroid hormone. Deinduction describes the reverse. *Target cell:* cell known by classical bioassay procedures to be under the regulation of a given type of steroid hormone.

B. GENERAL MODEL FOR THE MECHANISM OF ACTION OF STEROID HORMONES

Based on a consensus of current opinion, a schematic model of hormone action may be proposed, as in Fig. 1.

The interaction and retention of a steroid hormone with its target cells

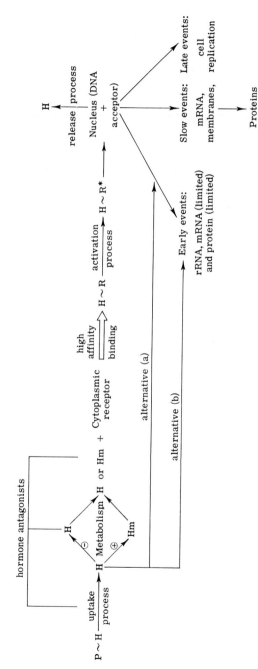

FIG. 1. A simplified mechanism of action of asteroid hormones. This model places particular importance on the nuclear binding of steroids, resulting in the enhancement of processes mandatorily involving DNA as template. This is clearly an oversimplification, and alternative (a) suggests that nuclear processes may be stimulated by hormones without the involvement of a cytoplasmic receptor system whereas alternative (b) imputes direct hormonal stimulation of metabolic processes without involvement of the receptor system at all. Abbreviations: P, steroid-binding protein in plasma; H, steroid hormone; Hm, hormone metabolite; ⊖ and ⊕, indicate absence or requirement of intracellular metabolism of the hormone; R, receptor protein; R*, activated configuration of receptor.

is not a random process but is mediated by an integrated sequence of molecular events. (1) Secreted hormones are transported in the plasma as relatively stable complexes, resulting from their association with plasma proteins. (2) Steroid hormones enter all cells to some extent by a process that is currently ill-defined. (3) Within the target cell, the hormone may or may not be subjected to extensive metabolism. (4) The parent hormone or a selected metabolite is specifically bound with a high affinity to a cytoplasmic receptor protein, forming a hormone-receptor complex. (5) By subtle alterations in tertiary or quaternary structure, a change in the configuration of the receptor complex occurs, resulting in an activated complex with a higher propensity for the nuclear acceptor sites. (6) The activated complex is retained for a significant but finite period of time at precisely defined sites within cromatin. (7) The receptor complex triggers an enhancement of genetic transcription and thereby initiates a spectrum of processes responsible for the manifestation of the hormonal responses; these responses proceed at markedly different rates. (8) The hormone leaves chromatin and ultimately, the cell, by processes yet unknown. To comply with the fundamental tenets of endocrinology, the entire system must be reversible; as a corollary, despite the high affinity of steroid–receptor and receptor complex–acceptor interaction, these are not permanent and thus do not involve covalent linkage.

In a review of this type, it is not possible to broach all aspects of the binding of steroid hormones in depth, and excellent reviews of certain facets of the overall binding process may be found elsewhere. The binding of steroids in plasma is presented in the authoritative treatise by Westphal (1971), and only two features of the sex steroid-binding β-globulin (SBG) and corticosteroid-binding α_2-globulin (CBG) warrant further comment. First, since they bind steroid hormones with a high affinity, they provide admirable controls for investigations on the regulation of metabolic processes by steroid hormones. Unlike receptor proteins, the plasma proteins cannot promote the attachment of steroid hormones to chromatin (Steggles *et al.*, 1971; Mainwaring and Peterken, 1971), DNA (Mainwaring and Irving, 1973), or nuclear acceptor (Mainwaring and Symes, 1975). Second, CBG may be purified in quantity in a form approaching homogeneity (Muldoon and Westphal, 1967; Chader and Westphal, 1968) and will probably prove to be the first high-affinity binding protein to be subjected to sequence analysis and studies on the nature and geometry of its single binding site. The chances of success have been expedited by the facile purification of CBG by affinity chromatography (Trapp *et al.*, 1971).

For a survey of steroid metabolism, the reference works by Dorfman and Ungar (1965) and Ofner (1968) are recommended. The background

TABLE I

THE ACTIVATION OF CYTOPLASMIC HORMONE–RECEPTOR COMPLEXES

Class of hormones	Experimental system	References
Estrogens	Rat uterus	Brecher et al. (1970); Jensen et al. (1971)
	Calf uterus	Puca et al. (1972)
Androgens	Rat prostate	Mainwaring and Irving (1973)
Mineralocorticoids	Rat kidney	Marver et al. (1972)
Glucocorticoids	Hepatoma (HTC) cells	Higgins et al. (1973)
	Rat liver	Kalimi et al. (1975)

history of the mechanism of action of steroid hormones may be found in Liao and Fang (1969), Baulieu et al. (1971a), and King and Mainwaring (1974).

The so-called "activation" of hormone–receptor complexes seems to be a general feature of the hormone-binding mechanism in a diversity of experimental systems. This phenomenon, usually resulting in other changes in the physicochemical properties of the complex apart from its affinity for chromatin acceptor sites, may be simulated in cell-free systems by careful manipulation of temperature or ionic strength; examples in the current literature are presented in Table I. The report by Kalimi et al. (1975) is particularly noteworthy for two reasons: first, activation can be promoted at low temperature by Ca^{2+} ions; and, second, activation does not result in a decrease in the sedimentation coefficient of the complex, as widely reported in all other systems. Puca et al. (1972) have identified a receptor-transforming factor in calf uterus, and it will be of great interest if similar activities can be found in other hormone-responsive cells.

C. LIMITATIONS OF THE SIMPLISTIC MODEL

The foundations of the receptor hypothesis currently rest on impressive, but nevertheless circumstantial, evidence. Rigorous proof of the importance of receptor complexes is in abeyance until they may be purified to a state approaching homogeneity, but several independent lines of enquiry have promulgated the putative importance of the receptor systems. First, antagonists for many classes of steroid hormones are now available which counter the formation of the receptor complex and negate virtually all manifestations of the hormonal response. For example, the synthetic spirolactone, SC 14266, is a competitor for the high-affinity binding sites for aldosterone in rat kidney (Swaneck *et al.*, 1970) at concentrations known to suppress the natriuretic effects of mineralocorticoids (Kagawa *et al.*, 1964). Similarly, the antiandrogen cyproterone acetate curtails the formation of androgen receptor complexes (Fang and Liao, 1969) and ablates most parameters of androgen induction in rat prostate, including the synthesis of polyamines and ribosomes (Mangan *et al.*, 1973), messenger RNA (Mainwaring *et al.*, 1974b), and DNA (Rennie *et al.*, 1975). Second, striking differences may be cited in the receptor contents of experimental tumors which may exist in glucocorticoid-sensitive and -insensitive sublines. The hormone-sensitive cells contain glucocorticoid receptors whereas the hormone-insensitive cells do not; this distinction persists in L929 fibroblasts (Hackney *et al.*, 1970), P1798 lymphosarcomas (Kirkpatrick *et al.*, 1971), and lymphomas (Roseanau *et al.*, 1972). Third, credence in the receptor systems may be drawn from the striking correlation between the binding of steroids to the high-affinity receptor systems and their known biological activities. Many such examples may be quoted, but the work of Munck and Wira (1971) on the binding of glucocorticoids relative to the hormone-induced suppression of glucose uptake in lymphocytes has been selected (Table II).

TABLE II

COMPARISON OF THE RELATIVE BINDING OF STEROIDS IN LYMPHOCYTES
WITH THEIR EFFECTS ON GLUCOSE UPTAKE[a,b]

Steroid	Specific binding	Metabolic activity
Cortisol (arbitrary standard)	1.0	1.0
Dexamethasone	4.8	10
9α-Fluoroprednisolone	3.6	18
Prednisolone	1.3	1.2
Corticosterone	0.5	0.4
11-Deoxycorticosterone	0.5	
Progesterone	0.4	
11-Deoxy-17α-hydroxycorticosterone	0.3	
17α-Hydroxyprogesterone	0.1	< 0.02
Testosterone		
Cortisone	< 0.05	
Epicortisol		
Tetrahydrocortisol		

[a] The relative binding of steroids was determined by their ability to displace the binding of steroids was determined by their ability to displace the binding of 7.5 nM [1]H-labeled cortisol. With respect to metabolic activities, potent glucocorticoids suppress the uptake of glucose in these cells. The data are expressed relative to the activity of cortisol.

[b] From Munck and Wira (1971).

The criticisms that may be leveled at the simplistic model will now be discussed.

1. Redundant binding. There are anomalous but interesting instances where high-affinity binding of steroids occurs without a resultant hormonal response. These include the nuclear binding of the biologically inactive 11-deoxy-17α-hydroxycorticosterone in lymphocytes (Munck and Brinck-Johnson, 1968) and HeLa cells (Melnykovych and Bishop, 1968); the lack of response to estrogen binding in animals demonstrating obligatory delayed implantation (O'Farrell and Daniel, 1971); and the constancy of the receptor content of the transitorily sensitive lymphoma subline, S1AT.8, irrespective of its sensitivity to glucocorticoids (Baxter et al., 1971). In all cases, binding is not equatable with a hormonal response.

2. Obligatory presence of cytoplasmic receptors. Hormonal responses can be evoked in certain cells where nuclear binding seemingly proceeds in the absence of cytoplasmic receptors, for example, chick liver (Mester and Baulieu, 1972) and bone marrow (Minguell and Vallandares, 1974).

3. Receptor-independent processes. Certain hormone-sensitive processes can proceed without the mandatory involvement of receptors or, indeed, dramatic changes in RNA synthesis; cases in point include the imbibition of water by estrogens and the induction of liver tyrosine aminotransferase (Levitan and Webb, 1969, 1970). In contrast to polypeptide hormones (see review by Robison and Sutherland, 1972), a convincing case cannot be made for the comprehensive involvement of the classical second messenger, adenosine 3':5'-cyclic monophosphate (cAMP) in cellular responses to steroid hormones. Exceptions include the induction of glycolytic enzymes by androgens (Singhal et al., 1971; Mangan et al., 1973); these changes may be promoted by the administration of either testosterone or cAMP, in vivo, but they are not prevented by the antiandrogen cyproterone acetate (Mangan et al., 1973).

4. Synergism between hormones. Examples are known where the presence of a hormone (sometimes a polypeptide hormone) may enhance the activity of another (Grayhack and Lebovitz, 1967; Rochefort et al., 1972). Such observations are difficult to reconcile with the simple model.

5. Developmental changes. Certain steroid-mediated phenomena are intimately associated with developmental processes, the onset of erythropoiesis by 5β-reduced steroids in cultured blastoderm being a suitable example (Levere et al., 1967). The cells suddenly become refractory to steroids, but the molecular basis for the suppression of the response cannot be predicted simply by inspection of the model.

6. Requirement for transcription changes. 5α-Androstane-3β,17β-diol can induce β-glucuronidase in mouse liver, but the process is not sensitive

to antiandrogens (Ohno and Lyon, 1971), as indeed is the nuclear binding process (Fang and Liao, 1969). This androgen does not enter the nucleus in the mouse (Bullock et al., 1971) or rat (Baulieu et al., 1971b), and hence this androgenic induction depends exclusively on cytoplasmic or translational mechanisms alone.

7. Aberrant binding. The Tfm mouse provides a stable mutation (male genotype; female phenotype) in which the male urogenital system fails to develop, despite the presence of the X chromosome. The 7 S androgen receptor, present in normal male and female mice, is totally absent in kidney of the Tfm mutant (Bullock and Bardin, 1972), yet prominent binding to an atypical 3 S species of protein was reported in the submandibular gland (Wilson and Goldstein, 1972). Such acute differences extend beyond methodological differences and are incompatible with the simple model of hormone uptake and retention given in Fig. 1.

8. Differential steroid responses. In essence, steroids may act in two fundamental ways; operating switch mechanisms, effecting qualitative changes, or by amplification mechanisms, promoting quantitative changes. Switch mechanisms are well illustrated by the induction of avidin synthesis in chick oviduct (O'Malley et al., 1969) and an amplification process by the induction of aldolase synthesis in rat prostate (Mainwaring et al., 1974c). The subtle difference in mechanism, centered on the high-affinity binding of steroids, is not self-evident in the simple model.

9. Acute tissue specificity of hormonal responses. This is the principal stricture to the model in Fig. 1, for steroids can have diametrically opposed effects on different organs and cell types within the same animal. Dramatic examples include the anabolic action of glucocorticoids on liver, inducing many enzymes (Knox and Auerbach, 1955), contrasted with their catabolic or lytic effects on lymphocytes (Dougherty, 1952). Among androgen-sensitive organs in the mouse, alcohol dehydrogenase is inducible only in the kidney (Ohno et al., 1970). These differences in hormonal response provoke serious and penetrating criticisms of the simple model of hormone action.

II. Entry and Release of Steroid Hormones

As recently as 1971, Baulieu and his collaborators could justifiably state that little evidence supported the presence of a facilitated entry mechanism for steroids into mammalian cells (Baulieu et al., 1971a). In general terms, there does not appear to be a permeability barrier to steroid entry at 37°C (see many citations in King and Mainwaring, 1974).

However, certain observations suggest that an entry mechanism may exist, as was proposed many years ago (Greer, 1959; Bellamy et al., 1962). Estrogen uptake is severely impaired at 0°C and may represent its distribution in the intercellular spaces (Williams and Gorski, 1971). Other studies invoke a specific membrane protein in estrogen entry (Milgrom et al., 1972) of the class of membrane proteins described by Riggs and Pan (1972).

Far more convincing evidence for an entry mechanism is available from the elegant work conducted by Giorgi and her colleagues (Giorgi et al., 1971, 1973, 1974) on the dynamics of androgen–tissue relationships in normal canine and hypertrophied human prostate gland maintained under conditions of superfusion, in vitro. These innovative studies unequivocally support the existence of a surface carrier mechanism in the hypertrophied human prostate. Even if it transpires that this mechanism is significant only in hypertrophied rather than normal tissue, it opens up an exciting avenue for prostate chemotherapy, directed against androgen entry rather than androgen binding within the cell. Potential candidates for such studies include cyproterone rather than cyproterone acetate (Giorgi et al., 1973) and the 19-norprogesterone derivative, gestonorone caproate (Orestano et al., 1975). It is important to stress that the identification of a temperature-dependent entry process for glucocorticoids, such as triamcinolone acetonide, has recently been reported by Harrison et al. (1975) in cultures of a pituitary adenocarcinoma.

Our knowledge of the release of steroid hormones is even more fragmentary, largely because it is difficult to devise experimental systems in which the release mechanism can be simulated with a degree of fidelity. Clues purporting to an exit mechanism for glucocorticoids in fibroblasts have been presented by Gross et al. (1968, 1970), and certain evidence for a displacement mechanism for testosterone may be found in the study by Kirdani et al. (1972). One possible means for promoting the release of a hormone from nuclear chormatin would be its metabolism to a form of lower affinity for the receptor and acceptor sites. This now seems unlikely in view of the careful study conducted by Munck and Brinck-Johnson (1974) in lymphocytes; cortisol is extremely prone to metabolism yet no indication of metabolic conversion was detectable during its release from the specific nuclear sites.

III. Steroid Antagonists

These compounds are of interest as potential chemotherapeutic agents and also because they are invaluable tools for basic research on model

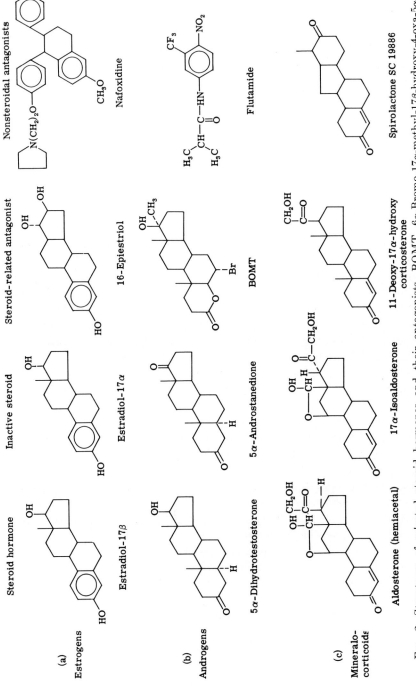

FIG. 2. Structures of selected steroid hormones and their antagonists. BOMT, 6α-Bromo-17α-methyl-17β-hydroxy-4-oxa-5α-androstane-3-one.

binding systems. A structural survey of antagonists for three major classes of steroid hormones is presented in Fig. 2. Clinically useful antagonists must satisfy three essential criteria; high potency at low concentrations, negligible intrinsic hormonal activity, and low toxicity. On such grounds, nonsteroidal antagonists are of particular interest. The development of Flutamide (Neri and Monahan, 1972) is likely to be advantageous in the treatment of many disorders, including prostatic carcinoma, since it is the most potent antiandrogen available and competes for the binding sites in the androgen-receptor system (Neri et al., 1974; Liao et al., 1974; Mainwaring et al., 1974a). In the main, steroid antagonists need to be present in considerable excess in order to suppress hormone binding, but the remarkable competition displayed by spirolactone SC 26304 for mineralocorticoid-specific binding sites (Marver et al., 1974) demonstrates the potential efficiency of steroid antagonists. The provision of potent antagonists for all principal classes of steroid hormones now seems a distinct possibility.

Implicit in the receptor hypothesis is a close geometric fit between the receptor site and its appropriate ligand. Detailed physical comparison of the compounds given in Fig. 2 may provide invaluable clues to the three-dimensional structure of steroid binding sites. Such reports are few, but the fact that a plausible explanation of the biological activity of the potent but nonsteroidal estrogen diethylstilbestrol was gained only after exacting X-ray crystallographic analysis (Hospital et al., 1972) should inspire more work in this area.

Somewhat surprisingly, the reversibility of the suppression achieved by nonsteroidal antagonists has not been extensively documented. For certain specific purposes, it should be possible to synthesise derivatives of antagonists suitable for the affinity labeling of the steroid-binding sites in many proteins. Covalent attachment of these compounds could be advantageous in the purification of binding proteins, including receptors, because the antagonists are singularly less sensitive to steroid-catabolizing systems. Suitable derivatives for affinity labeling could include bromo- (Arias et al., 1973) and iodo- (Ganguly and Warren, 1971) substituted forms.

IV. STEROID METABOLISM

Only in the mechanism of action of androgens can a convincing case be made for the mandatory involvement of steroid metabolism (King and Mainwaring, 1974). This provides a novel dimension to androgen action in that androgen binding is limited not only by the presence or the absence of receptor systems, but also on the metabolic potential of the cells in question. In most male accessory sexual glands, the critical enzyme, 5α-reductase, is conspicuously active and the supply of important 5α-reduced steroids, especially 5α-dihydrotestosterone, exceeds biological demands. This is not the case in all androgen-sensitive organs, including adult bull and rabbit prostate (Wilson and Gloyna, 1970), skeletal muscle (Wilson and Gloyna, 1970; Mainwaring and Mangan, 1973), or adult rat testis (Folman et al., 1973). In striking contrast, appreciable 5α-reductase activity is present in the prostate glands (Wilson and Gloyna, 1970) and testis (Inano and Tamaoki, 1966; Shikita and Hall, 1967) of immature animals. Since adult testes (Mainwaring and Mangan, 1973; Hansson et al., 1974a,b) contain high-affinity androgen receptors, these collective findings have developmental significance. First, androgen receptors may be nonfunctional in certain adult organs with respect to 5α-reduced metabolites. Second, the formation and binding of 5α-dihydrotestosterone may be important only during periods of maximum growth, as during the acquisition of sexual maturity. A corollary to this premise is that 5α-dihydrotestosterone is the principal mitogenic androgen, as indeed seems to be the case (Baulieu et al., 1968; Roy et al., 1972). Third, the growth of androgen-sensitive cells may be modulated by the nuclear retention of either testosterone or 5α-dihydrotestosterone; Rennie and Bruchovsky (1972) have reported the binding of testosterone in prostate nuclei, for example. Developmental changes in androgen metabolism provide different modes of androgenic stimulation depending on the demands for growth, regeneration, or secretion. Such a subtle mechanism appears to be unique to the androgens.

Androgen metabolism is negligible in muscle, and currently available evidence suggests that testosterone itself provides the androgenic stimulus (Jung and Baulieu, 1972; Kreig et al., 1974).

Overwhelming interest in 5α-reduced steroids has tended to obscure the specific induction of heme synthesis in many erythropoietic systems by 5β-reduced steroids (Levere et al., 1967; Granick and Kappas, 1967). The biological activities of the stereoisomers of dihydrotestosterone provide an impressive illustration of the importance of steroid structure in hormonal responses, attributable to the planar (5α-) or extremely angular (5β-) orientation of the A and B rings of the steroid skeleton. The 5β-isomer cannot compete for the 5α-specific binding sites in prostate (Mainwaring and Mangan, 1973) whereas the 5α-isomer is totally inactive in the induction of heme (Granick and Kappas, 1967). The absolute sterospecificity of responses in erythropoietic cells, both in terms of heme induction and steroid binding, has been demonstrated by recent work in this laboratory (Table III).

TABLE III

RELATIVE BINDING OF ^{3}H-LABELED STEROIDS IN CYTOPLASMIC EXTRACTS OF CHICK BLASTODERM AND THEIR ABILITY TO INDUCE HEMOGLOBIN[a]

Steroid	Induction of hemoglobin (μg/20 μg of DNA)	Binding (cpm ^{3}H-labeled steroid/500 mg wet wt. of matrix)
None	10.5	—
5β-Dihydrotestosterone	37.3	760
Etiocholanolone	38.5	ND
5α-Dihydrotestosterone	11.5	280
Cortisol	15.4	220
Estradiol-17β	7.1	190
Progesterone	23.0	ND[b]
Testosterone	ND[b]	180

[a] Chick blastoderms, dissected from fertilized eggs after 24 hours of incubation, were maintained in organ culture. For induction experiments, nonradioactive steroids were added to 30 nM concentration (six blastoderms per group), and hemoglobin was determined 48 hours later. In binding experiments, cytoplasmic extracts were prepared and incubated with ^{3}H-labeled steroids (10,000 cpm/0.25 ml) for 2 hours at 0°C; specific binding was estimated by DNA-Sepharose chromatography (500 mg wet weight per column; 150 μg of immobilized DNA). The data are taken from Irving et al. (1975).

[b] ND indicates not determined.

V. PURIFICATION OF STEROID-RECEPTOR COMPLEXES

Indubitably, this now assumes the most urgent priority in the further elucidation of the mechanism of action of steroid hormones. Horrendous problems have to be faced, and these are compounded of the small amounts of the receptor proteins and their notorious lability. In addition, an important stricture to future progress remains the paucity of reliable means for assaying receptors save for their binding of steroid hormones per se.

A. CONVENTIONAL APPROACHES

Creditable attempts have been made at receptor purification employing conventional means of protein fractionation (de Sombre et al., 1969; Puca et al., 1971), and the properties of cytoplasmic receptor complexes were satisfactorily maintained throughout these partial purification procedures. It now seems clear, however, that such standard procedures were extended beyond their real limits of resolution in the course of these studies.

B. AFFINITY CHROMATOGRAPHY

Purification of receptor complexes is perhaps only feasible by rigorous exploitation of their extreme biological specificity as compared to their limited chemical specificity. A parallel may be adroitly drawn with the resounding success of radioimmune assays over classical procedures in the quantitative determination of steroid hormones. Affinity chromatography, centered on the immobilization of intracellular components involved in the expression of the biological specificity of steroid-binding mechanisms, offers the only practical solution to this daunting analytical problem. Rapid and considerable purification of receptor complexes may be achieved by DNA-cellulose chromatography (Mainwaring and Mangan, 1971; Mainwaring and Irving, 1973). Despite justifiable criticisms of this approach with respect to the type of receptor complexes retained (Yamamoto, 1974) and the lack of apparent saturability (Andre and Rochefort, 1975), the method has the advantage that steroids bound to all plasma proteins, including SBG, are not retained. The extreme flexibility of the immobilization of proteins to CNBr-activated Sepharose (Cuatrecasas, 1970) offers the most hopeful line of approach in the immediate future. Depending on the nature of the matrix, either steroid-saturated or steroid-free receptor preparations may be purified in three different ways.

1. *Immobilization of antibodies.* An ideal solution to receptor purification is to link antibodies raised against partially purified receptor complexes to an insoluble matrix. Success depends on the availability of suitably enriched receptor preparations for raising the antibodies, and this seems to be beyond present capabilities. The use of antibodies raised against steroid hormones alone does not offer much hope of success because the recent studies by Castañeda and Liao (1975) suggest a unique environment for steroid-binding sites in receptor proteins. The envelopment of these high-affinity sites within the protein suggests that they may not be accessible through steric factors to immobilized steroid antibodies. Nevertheless, the conspicuous success of Cittanova *et al.* (1974) in purifying the estrogen-binding rat α-fetoprotein by such means augurs auspiciously for future work.

2. *Immobilization of appropriate ligand.* This method has extreme promise because serum albumin or other "spacer" may be first linked to the matrix and then coupled with steroid hemisuccinates or other suitable derivatives by use of water-soluble agents such as 1-ethyl-3-(3-dimethylaminopropyl) carbodiimide. Impressive advances have been

made using such procedures in the purification of estrogen (Sica *et al.*, 1973) and progesterone (Smith *et al.*, 1975) receptor complexes. In this procedure, elution of the adsorbed receptor protein is achieved by the appropriate steroid hormone, usually in the tritiated form of high specific radioactivity. Subsequent analysis requires the separation of receptor-bound radioactivity from the free ^{3}H-labeled steroid.

3. Immobilization of acceptor molecules. This procedure has not been used thus far, but it would seem to have a promising future in receptor purification, particularly in conjunction with method (2), described above.

By judicious combination of these affinity-chromatography procedures, the extensive purification of receptor complexes may be a practical reality. Extensive purification is essential for further progress in the elucidation of the structure of steroid-binding sites and in studies on the possible regulation of transcriptional events by steroid-receptor complexes. To date, studies on the latter have been conducted with impure receptor preparations (Mohla *et al.*, 1972; Davies and Griffiths, 1973; Mainwaring and Jones, 1975) and the results are open to certain criticism.

VI. Specificity of Hormonal Responses

The remarkable specificity of hormonal responses exists at two levels; *overt* specificity of the circulating hormones for their target cells and *subtle* specificity among a group of responsive cell types to a given hormonal stimulus.

A. Specificity in Cytoplasmic Receptors

An important measure of specificity is imparted by the remarkable ligand preference of a given receptor system, say for glucocorticoids, but not other classes of steroid hormones. This general premise has been extensively discussed elsewhere (King and Mainwaring, 1974), and overt specificity may be largely attributed to the specificity of cytoplasmic binding.

The question, then, is whether the specificity of cytoplasmic receptors in terms of ligand specificity and tissue distribution is sufficient to explain the subtle differences in cellular responses. In general terms, the physico-chemical properties of the cytoplasmic receptor complexes are remarkably similar (Table IV), at least using present methods of analysis. This suggests that differences in the structure of individual receptor complexes

TABLE IV

SIMILARITIES IN THE PHYSICOCHEMICAL PROPERTIES OF CYTOPLASMIC RECEPTOR–STEROID COMPLEXES[a]

Steroid	Tissue	s_{20w}	f/f_0	pI	MW	Effect of KCl	Reference
1. Estradiol-17β	Calf uterus	8.0	ND[b]	5.8	ND	+	de Sombre et al. (1969)
	Rat uterus	8.6	1.65	6.2	236,000	+	Puca et al. (1971)
	Rat uterus	8.0	1.69	5.8	220,000	ND	Mainwaring and Irving (1973)
2. Dexamethasone	HTC[c] cells	6–8	ND	ND	ND	+	Baxter and Tomkins (1971)
	Liver	7.0	ND	ND (unstable)	200,000	+	Koblinsky et al. (1972)
3. Progesterone	Guinea pig uterus	7.0	1.51	5.8; 4.5 (trace)	210,000	ND	Mainwaring and Irving (1973)
	Chick oviduct	8.0; 5.0	ND	4.0; 4.5	100,000; 357,000	+	Sherman et al. (1970)
4. 5α-Dihydrotestosterone	Male accessory sexual glands	8.0	1.96	5.8	290,000	+	Mainwaring and Irving (1973)
5. Aldosterone	Rat kidney	8.5	ND	ND	ND	=	Marver et al. (1972)

[a] In all cases, cytoplasmic extracts (105,000 g supernatant) were isolated in the cold (0–4°C). In KCl effects, + indicates that the s_{20w} is reduced in gradients run at high ionic strength.
[b] ND indicates not determined.
[c] HTC, hepatoma tissue culture cells.

are probably not a tenable explanation of discrete variations in hormonal responses. In the absence of more direct means, ligand specificity remains the only probe for tissue-specific differences in the structure of cytoplasmic receptors. Inspection of the current literature reveals few examples in support of such a viewpoint. Among glucocorticoid-sensitive cells, testosterone can suppress receptor binding and the induction of tyrosine aminotransferase (Samuels and Tomkins, 1970), yet it is a completely inactive steroid by both binding and metabolic criteria in lymphocytes (Munck and Brinck-Johnson, 1968). In androgen-receptor systems, cyproterone acetate is an almost universal antiandrogen; the unique exception is the androgen-receptor system, essentially specific for testosterone, in rat uterus (Giannopoulos, 1973).

B. SPECIFICITY IN NUCLEAR ACCEPTORS

Despite certain evidence to the contrary (Chamness *et al.*, 1973), the acceptor sites in chromatin are tissue specific (see extensive review in King and Mainwaring, 1974). This concept was largely formulated on the results of reconstituted, cell-free systems which demonstrated that nucelar components tended to recognize and bind more extensively receptor complexes from homologous (same tissue) rather than heterologous sources.

Puca *et al.* (1974) revolutionized studies of receptor complex–acceptor interactions by the application of the principles of affinity chromatography. In their innovative procedure, they covalently attached nuclear proteins to Sepharose 4B and demonstrated further that the proven specificity of the binding of ^{3}H-labeled estradiol-17β could be simulated entirely using the immobilized acceptor and estradiol-receptor complexes. The striking advantages of affinity chromatography ensure the widespread adoption of this novel technique. In particular, large batches of stable matrix can be easily prepared, thereby ensuring experimental consistency. Large numbers of columns may be run concomitantly, and this is a great practical advantage over previous procedures in which chromatin or nuclei served as the source of acceptor sites. Furthermore, the columns may be readily yet extensively washed to remove traces of unbound ^{3}H-labeled steroid, thus providing accurate and reproducible assessment of receptor–acceptor interactions.

Recent studies in this laboratory (Mainwaring and Symes, 1975) have confirmed and extended the observations made by Puca *et al.* (1974). Using male accessory sexual glands as our model system, we extensively investigated the interaction of immobilized acceptor sites with cytoplasmic receptor complexes labeled with [^{3}H]5α-dihydrotestosterone. Our findings may be summarized as follows:

1. The acceptor sites are limited in number, saturable, and of high affinity (K_d 3 × 10^{-9} M).

2. Acceptor–receptor complex interactions are abolished at concentrations of KCl known to dissociate such processes in whole nuclei.

3. The process is stringently dependent on the presence of the cytoplasmic receptor protein, and its function cannot be mimicked by SBG.

4. Acute steroid specificity is evident in that 5α-dihydrotestosterone cannot be replaced by 5β-dihydrotestosterone, androsterone, dexamethasone, or estradiol-17β. Conversely, binding of [³H]5α-dihydrotestosterone may be negated by a 100-fold excess of its nonradioactive counterpart and by the antiandrogen cyproterone acetate; 5β-dihydrotestosterone was inactive in competition studies.

5. The 5α-dihydrotestosterone-receptor complex must be presented intact for binding to the acceptor site. When the cytoplasmic extract and ³H-labeled steroid are not applied to the matrix concomitantly, no binding occurs. Prior treatment of the steroid-receptor complex with N-ethylmaleimide or N-bromosuccinimide, known to destroy the receptor complex, predictably prevent interaction with the acceptor.

6. By performing crossover experiments with acceptor and receptor preparations from a variety of accessory sexual glands, including seminal vesicle, prostate, epididymis, and preputial gland, evidence for the tissue-specific nature of receptor–acceptor interactions was obtained. Prostate androgen receptor, for example, was more efficiently retained by insoluble matrices containing prostate nuclear components than similar preparations from other tissues.

7. The content of androgen acceptor sites was significantly higher in nuclear extracts from androgen-dependent tissues (prostate) than androgen-independent tissues (spleen, kidney, liver, lung, and pancreas).

These studies provide evidence that a second level of specificity in hormonal responses, even among tissues responsive to the same hormone, may exist in the nature of the nuclear acceptor sites. The further application of the procedure devised by Puca *et al.* (1974) is likely to provide a more penetrating insight into the molecular mechanisms responsible for the expression of different hormonal responses. Future prospects in this aspect of hormone action currently appear hopeful.

VII. Conclusions

Purification of the steroid-receptor complexes is of pressing urgency for the solution of many outstanding problems pertaining to the mechanism of action of steroid hormones. Purified receptor preparations are particularly required for studies on the hormonal regulation of metabolic processes and for investigations on the high-affinity steroid-binding sites. Further effort is also required to provide a satisfactory explanation for the tissue specificity of hormonal responses. As a rider to this future investigation, the nature of the nuclear acceptor must be unequivocally defined.

ACKNOWLEDGMENT

The author is deeply indebted to Mrs. Margaret Barker for her patient and painstaking assistance in the preparation of the manuscript.

REFERENCES

Andre, J., and Rochefort, H. (1975). *FEBS (Fed. Eur. Biochem. Soc.) Lett.* **50**, 319.

Arias, F., Sweet, F., and Warren, J. C. (1973). *J. Biol. Chem.* **248**, 5641.

Baulieu, E.-E., Lasnitzki, I., and Robel, P. (1968). *Nature (London)* **219**, 1155.

Baulieu, E.-E., Alberga, A., Jung, I., Lebeau, M.-C., Mercier-Bodard, C., Milgrom, E., Raynaud, J.-P., Raynaud-Jammet, C., Rochefort, H., Truong, H., and Robel, P. (1971a). *Recent Progr. Horm. Res.* **27**, 351.

Baulieu, E.-E., Jung, I., Blondeau, J. P., and Robel, P. (1971b). *Advan. Biosci.* **7**, 179.

Baxter, J. D., and Tomkins, G. M. (1971). *Proc. Nat. Acad. Sci. U.S.* **68**, 932.

Baxter, J. D., Harris, A. W., Tomkins, G. M., and Cohn, N. (1971). *Science* **171**, 189.

Bellamy, D., Phillips, J. G., Jones, I. C., and Leonard, R. A. (1962). *Biochem. J.* **85**, 537.

Brecher, P. I., Numata, M., de Sombre, E. R., and Jensen, E. V. (1970). *Fed. Proc., Fed. Amer. Soc. Exp. Biol.* **29**, 249.

Bullock, L. P., and Bardin, C. W. (1972). *J. Clin. Endocrinol. Metab.* **35**, 935.

Bullock, L. P., Bardin, C. W., and Ohno, S. (1971). *Biochem. Biophys. Res. Commun.* **44**, 1531.

Castañeda, E., and Liao, S. (1975). *J. Biol. Chem.* **250**, 883.

Chader, G. J., and Westphal, U. (1968). *J. Biol. Chem.* **243**, 928.

Chamness, G. C., Jennings, A. W., and McGuire, W. L. (1973). *Nature (London)* **241**, 258.

Cittanova, N., Grigorova, A. M., Benassyag, C., Nunez, E., and Jayle, M. F. (1974). *FEBS (Fed. Eur. Biochem. Soc.) Lett.* **41**, 21.

Cuatrecasas, P. (1970). *J. Biol. Chem.* **245**, 3059.

Davies, P., and Griffiths, K. (1973). *Biochem. J.* **136**, 611.

de Sombre, E. R., Puca, G. A., and Jensen, E. V. (1969). *Proc. Nat. Acad. Sci. U.S.* **64**, 148.

Dorfman, R. I., and Ungar, F. (1965). "Metabolism of Steroid Hormones." Academic Press, New York.

Dougherty, T. F. (1952). *Physiol. Rev.* **32**, 379.

Fang, S., and Liao, S. (1969). *Mol. Pharmacol.* **5**, 428.

Folman, Y., Ahmad, N., Sowell, J. G., and Eik-Nes, K. B. (1973). *Endocrinology* **92**, 41.

Ganguly, M., and Warren, J. C. (1971). *J. Biol. Chem.* **246**, 3646.

Giannopoulos, G. (1973). *J. Biol. Chem.* **248**, 1004.

Giorgi, E. P., Stewart, J. C., Grant, J. K., and Scott, R. (1971). *Biochem. J.* **123**, 41.

Giorgi, E. P., Shirley, I. M., Grant, J. K., and Stewart, J. C. (1973). *Biochem. J.* **132**, 465.

Giorgi, E. P., Moses, T. F., Grant, J. K., Scott, R., and Sinclair, J. (1974). *Mol. Cell. Endocrinol.* **1**, 271.

Granick, S., and Kappas, A. (1967). *J. Biol. Chem.* **242**, 4587.

Grayhack, J. T., and Lebovitz, J. M. (1967). *Invest. Urol.* **5**, 87.

Greer, D. S. (1959). *Endocrinology* **64**, 898.

Gross, S. R., Arnonow, L., and Pratty, W. B. (1968). *Biochem. Biophys. Res. Commun.* **32**, 66.

Gross, S. R., Aronow, L., and Pratt, W. B. (1970). *J. Cell Biol.* **44**, 103.

Hackney, J. F., Gross, S. R., Aronow, L., and Pratt, W. B. (1970). *Mol. Pharmacol.* **6**, 500.

Hansson, V., McLean, W. S., Smith, A. A., Tindall, D. J., Weddington, S. C., Nayfeh, S. N., and French, F. S. (1974a). *Steroids* **23**, 823.

Hansson, V., Trygstad, O., French, F. S., McLean, W. S., Smith, A. A., Tindell, D. J., Weddington, S. J., Petrusz, P., Nayfeh, S. N., and Ritzén, E. M. (1974b). *Nature (London)* **250**, 387.

Harrison, R. W., Fairfield, S., and Orth, D. N. (1975). *Biochemistry* **14**, 1304.

Higgins, S. J., Rosseau, G. G., Baxter, J. D., and Tomkins, G. M. (1973). *J. Biol. Chem.* **248**, 5866.

Hospital, M., Busetta, B., Bucourt, R., Weintraub, H., and Baulieu, E.-E. (1972). *Mol. Pharmacol.* **8**, 438.

Inano, H., and Tamaoki, B.-I. (1966). *Endocrinology* **79**, 579.

Irving, R. A., Spooner, P. M., and Mainwaring, W. I. P. (1975). *Biochem. J.* (in press).

Jensen, E. V., and Jacobson, H. I. (1962). *Recent Progr. Horm. Res.* **18**, 387.

Jensen, E. V., Numata, M., Brecher, P. I., and de Sombre, E. R. (1971). *Biochem. Soc. Symp.* **32**, 133.

Jung, I., and Baulieu, E.-E. (1972). *Nature (London) New Biol.* **237**, 24.

Kagawa, C. M., Bouska, D. J., Anderson, M. L., and Krol, W. F. (1964). *Arch. Int. Pharmacodyn. Ther.* **149**, 8.

Kalimi, M., Colman, P., and Feigelson, P. (1975). *J. Biol. Chem.* **250**, 1080.

King, R. J. B., and Mainwaring, W. I. P. (1974). "Steroid-Cell Interactions." Butterworth, London.

Kirdani, R. Y., Varkarakis, M. J., Murphy, G. P., and Sandberg, A. A. (1972). *Endocrinology* **90**, 1245.

Kirkpatrick, A. F., Milholland, R. J., and Rosen, F. (1971). *Nature (London), New Biol.* **232**, 216.

Knox, W. E., and Auerbach, V. U. (1955). *J. Biol. Chem.* **214**, 307.

Koblinsky, M., Beato, M., Kalimi, M., and Feigelson, P. (1972). *J. Biol. Chem.* **247**, 7897.

Kreig, M., Szalay, R., and Voigt, K. D. (1974). *J. Steroid Biochem.* **5**, 453.

Levere, R. D., Kappas, A., and Granick, S. (1967). *Proc. Nat. Acad. Sci. U.S.* **58**, 985.

Levitan, I. B., and Webb, T. E. (1969). *Biochim. Biophys. Acta.* **182**, 491.

Levitan, I. B., and Webb, T. E. (1970). *Biochim. Biophys. Acta* **207**, 283.

Liao, S., and Fang, S. (1969). *Vitam. Horm. (New York)* **26**, 237.

Liao, S., Howell, D. K., and Chang, T.-M. (1974). *Endocrinology* **91**, 427.

Mainwaring, W. I. P., and Irving, R. A. (1973). *Biochem. J.* **134**, 113.

Mainwaring, W. I. P., and Jones, D. A. (1975). *J. Steroid Biochem.* **6**, 475.

Mainwaring, W. I. P., and Mangan, F. R. (1971). *Advan. Biosci.* **7**, 165.

Mainwaring, W. I. P., and Mangan, F. R. (1973). *J. Endocrinol.* **59**, 121.

Mainwaring, W. I. P., and Peterken, B. M. (1971). *Biochem. J.* **125**, 285.

Mainwaring, W. I. P., and Symes, E. K. (1975). *Biochem. J.* (in press).

Mainwaring, W. I. P., Mangan, F. R., Feherty, P. A., and Freifeld, M. (1974a). *Mol. Cell. Endocrinol.* **1**, 113.

Mainwaring, W. I. P., Wilce, P. A., and Smith, A. E. (1974b). *Biochem. J.* **137**, 513.

Mainwaring, W. I. P., Mangan, F. R., Irving, R. A., and Jones, D. A. (1974c). *Biochem. J.* **144**, 413.

Mangan, F. R., Pegg, A. E., and Mainwaring, W. I. P. (1973). *Biochem. J.* **134**, 129.

Marver, D., Goodman, D., and Edelman, I. S. (1972). *Kidney Int.* **1**, 210.

Marver, D., Stewart, J., Funder, J. W., Feldman, D., and Edelman, I. S. (1974). *Proc. Nat. Acad. Sci. U.S.* **71**, 1431.

Melnykovych, G., and Bishop, C. E. (1968). *Biochem. Biophys. Res. Commun.* **32**, 233.

Mester, J., and Baulieu, E.-E. (1972). *Biochim. Biophys. Acta* **261**, 236.

Milgrom, E., Atger, M., and Baulieu, E.-E. (1972). *C. R. Acad. Sci.* **274**, 2771.

Minguell, J., and Vallandares, L. (1974). *J. Steroid Biochem.* **5**, 649.

Mohla, S., de Sombre, E. R., and Jensen, E. V. (1972). *Biochem. Biophys. Res. Commun.* **46**, 661.

Muldoon, T. G., and Westphal, U. (1967). *J. Biol. Chem.* **242**, 5636.

Munck, A., and Brinck-Johnson, T. (1968). *J. Biol. Chem.* **243**, 5556.

Munck, A., and Brinck-Johnson, T. (1974). *J. Steroid Biochem.* **5**, 203.

Munck, A., and Wira, C. (1971). *Advan. Biosci.* **7**, 301.

Neri, R., and Monahan, M. (1972). *Invest. Urol.* **10**, 123.

Neri, R., Florance, K., Koziol, P., and van Cleave, S. (1974). *Endocrinology* **91**, 427.

O'Farrell, P. H., and Daniel, J. C. (1971). *Endocrinology* **88**, 1104.

Ofner, P. (1968). *Vitam. Horm. (New York)* **26**, 237.

Ohno, S., and Lyon, N. F. (1971). *Clin. Genet.* **1**, 121.

Ohno, S., Stenius, C., Christian, L., Harris, C., and Ivey, C. (1970). *Biochem. Genet.* **4**, 565.

O'Malley, B. W., McGuire, W. L., Kohler, P. O., and Korenman, S. G. (1969). *Recent Progr. Horm. Res.* **25**, 105.

Orestano, F., Altwein, J., Knapstein, P., Klose, K., and Bandhauer, K. (1975). *J. Steroid Biochem.* **6**, 898.

Puca, G. A., Nola, E., Sica, V., and Bresciani, F. (1971). *Biochemistry* **10**, 3769.

Puca, G. A., Nola, E., Sica, V., and Bresciani, F. (1972). *Biochemistry* **11**, 4157.

Puca, G. A., Sica, V., and Nola, E. (1974). *Proc. Nat. Acad. Sci. U.S.* **71**, 979.

Rennie, P. S., and Bruchovsky, N. (1972). *J. Biol. Chem.* **247**, 1546.

Rennie, P. S., Symes, E. K., and Mainwaring, W. I. P. (1975). *Biochem. J.* **132**, 1.

Riggs, T. R., and Pan, M. W. (1972). *Biochem. J.* **128**, 19.

Robison, G. A., and Sutherland, E. W. (1972). *Ann. N.Y. Acad. Sci.* **185**, 5.

Rochefort, H., Lignon, F., and Capany, F. (1972). *Biochem. Biophys. Res. Commun.* **47**, 662.

Rosenau, W., Baxter, J. D., Rousseau, G. G., and Tomkins, G. M. (1972). *Nature* (*London*), *New Biol.* **237**, 20.

Roy, A. K., Baulieu, E.-E., Feyel-Cabanes, T., Le Goascoyne, C., and Robel, P. (1972). *Endocrinology* **91**, 396.

Samuels, H. H., and Tomkins, G. M. (1970). *J. Mol. Biol.* **52**, 57.

Sherman, M. R., Corvol, P. L., and O'Malley, B. W. (1970). *J. Biol. Chem.* **245**, 6085.

Shikita, M., and Hall, P. F. (1967). *Biochim. Biophys. Acta* **136**, 484.

Sica, V., Parikh, I., Nola, E., Puca, G. A., and Cuatrecasas, P. (1973). *J. Biol. Chem.* **248**, 6543.

Singhal, R. L., Parulekar, M. R., Vijayvaragiya, R., and Robison, G. A. (1971). *Biochem. J.* **125**, 329.

Smith, R. G., Iramain, C. A., Buttram, V. C., and O'Malley, B. W. (1975). *Nature* (*London*), *New Biol.* **253**, 271.

Steggles, A. W., Spelsberg, T. C., Glasser, S. R., and O'Malley, B. W. (1971). *Proc. Nat. Acad. Sci. U.S.* **68**, 1479.

Swaneck, G. E., Chu, L. L. H., and Edelman, I. S. (1970). *J. Biol. Chem.* **245**, 5382.

Trapp, G. A., Seal, U. S., and Doe, R. P. (1971). *Steroids* **18**, 421.

Westphal, U. (1971). "Steroid-Protein Interactions." Springer-Verlag, Berlin.

Williams, D., and Gorski, J. (1971). *Biochem. Biophys. Res. Commun.* **45**, 258.

Wilson, J. D., and Gloyna, R. E. (1970). *Recent Progr. Horm. Res.* **26**, 309.

Wilson, J. D., and Goldstein, J. L. (1972). *J. Biol. Chem.* **247**, 7342.

Yamamoto, K. R. (1974). *J. Biol. Chem.* **249**, 7068.

DISCUSSION

P. Davies: Concerning the tissue specificity and species specificity of the acceptor proteins, we have shown that human hypertrophic prostatic cytosol or rat ventral prostatic cytosol labeled with [^{3}H]5α-DHT can transfer radioactivity in a protein-bound form into isolated nuclei from either tissue with equal facility. A peak of specifically bound steroid is observed in crossover experiments in each case, and effects on transcription can be observed. Would you comment on these findings?

In our studies on the stimulation of prostatic RNA polymerase by prostatic DHT-receptor complexes using modified templates, no stimulation was observed using calf thymus DNA, liver chromatin, or prostatic DNA. Stimulation was achieved using prostatic chromatin, intact, with histones removed, and with the rule of non-histones removed at this latter stage, only a minor portion of nonhistones, removable by phenol, remains. Since stimulation occurs under these conditions, it is probable that any acceptor protein is among this small proportion of tightly bound proteins.

I. Mainwaring: Your evidence accords with mine in that stimulation would not necessarily be predicted to occur with purified DNA or liver chromatin. Despite evidence that receptor complexes may bind to DNA, the specificity is not commensurate with that achieved with immobilized acceptor protein. In addition, purified DNA and liver chromatin are deplete in acceptor protein. With respect to your crossover experiments, one would predict some measure of acceptor activity in both sources of nuclei, human and rat; the critical question is the quantitation and specificity of the interaction, and this will only be evident in more detailed or specific analysis.

B. Uvnäs: Were all membrane receptors formed in the membrane itself or intracellularly?

I. Mainwaring: I cannot answer your question directly as no one has evidence on this point. To the best of my knowledge, membrane receptors of the type delineated for polypeptide hormones have not been established for steroid hormones. While a transport mechanism for steroid hormones may exist in cell membranes, this system would not qualify for description as a receptor system in my view.

E. E. Baulieu: We have been interested by a step of "entry" of steroids into target cells and mainly worked with estrogens and uterus [E. Milgrom, M. Atger, and E. E. Baulieu, *Biochim. Biophys. Acta* 320, 267 (1973)]. This work indicates that there is very likely a protein-mediated facilitated transport system "before" the receptor. It is interesting to see such a step confirmed in other systems, but one cannot say what is its molecular basis and its potential interest for the physiopathological behavior of hormone-responsive cells.

A. Mittelman: The cochromatography of the nonhistone protein with the histone fraction implies basicity for the acceptor protein. Have you examined this possibility in your studies? A protein with strongly basic amino acids, i.e., methylhistidine, actin, possibly?

I. Mainwaring: Preliminary data indicate that after isoelectric focusing of nuclear extracts the acceptor activity is associated with protein of isoelectric point within the range 8 to 9. This implies a somewhat basic protein, but the isoelectric point is not compatible with the acceptor being a classical histone; their isoelectric point range is 9.5 to 10.

E. E. Baulieu: I like the word "acceptor," but to me it means essentially an entity which "accepts." Indeed, your technology, after Puca, is directly related to binding of the receptor by something, apparently a protein, which is then well named "acceptor." However, the acceptor may not be the "executive" entity, and one should still make a distinction between an acceptor site, which means only binding, and an eventual point of action in terms of cellular response. In the future maybe one can demonstrate that the two sites are one and the same, but until then the distinction is logically safe. Moreover, the proteins among which you find an acceptor entity are extracted from nuclei with 2 M NaCl containing buffer. However, from our work [M. C. Lebeau, N. Massol, and E. E. Baulieu, *Eur. J. Biochem.* 36, 294 (1973)], now confirmed in a variety of systems, there is nuclear "residual" or "insoluble" receptor, which apparently is so tightly bound to some nuclear elements that those could also be named "acceptors," and naturally, you cannot study this sort of acceptor with your extraction.

S. Liao: I am happy to see that your results are in complete agreement with what Dr. Tymoczko found when he was in my laboratory. He found [*BBA, (Biochem. Biophys. Acta) Libr.* 252, 607 (1971)] that the acceptor protein in the nuclear acidic protein fraction can be fractionated by salt and ethanol and precipitated by acids.

I. Mainwaring: The measure of agreement on this point is, I agree, very heartening.

D. S. Coffey: Did all these measurements of acceptor profiles on your sucrose gradient represent the specific high-affinity, low-capacity component?

I. Mainwaring: Yes, the experiments were designed in such a manner in terms of input of receptor complex that the high-affinity, low-capacity acceptor sites would be occupied preferentially.

Androgen Binding and Metabolism in the Human Prostate

A. ATTRAMADAL, K. J. TVETER, S. C. WEDDINGTON,
O. DJÖSELAND, O. NAESS, V. HANSSON, AND O. TORGERSEN

*Laboratory of Histochemistry, Institute of Pathology,
Surgical Department A, and the Laboratory of Endocrinology,
Medical Department B, Rikshospitalet, Oslo, Norway*

I. Introduction

At a workshop on the biology of the prostate about a decade ago, Dr. Huggins (1963) characterized our knowledge of prostatic physiology as fragmentary and primitive. Although our understanding of the basic processes involved in the pathogenesis of prostatic disease still is insufficient, we now know significantly more about the interrelationship between the organ and the hormones regulating its growth, as evidenced by the numerous papers presented at this symposium.

The present paper summarizes our results on hormone binding and metabolism in the human prostate, with comparison of the findings in neoplastic and nonneoplastic tissue.

II. The Nonneoplastic Prostate

A. Androgen Uptake in Benign Nodular Prostatic Hyperplasia (BNPH)

Several years ago, we demonstrated that there was a principal difference between prostatic tissue and muscle with regard to their ability to

247

TABLE I

Uptake and Retention of Radioactivity in Slices from Benign Nodular Prostatic Hyperplasia and the Pyramidalis Muscle[a,b]

| Patient No. | No washing | | | Washing time | | | | | |
| | | | | 30 Minutes | | | 60 Minutes | | |
	Prostate	Muscle	Ratio	Prostate	Muscle	Ratio	Prostate	Muscle	Ratio
1	3565 ± 260	3855 ± 171	0.92	3090 ± 135	763 ± 56	4.1	2775 ± 123	287 ± 70	9.7
2	3984 ± 323	2995 ± 127	1.33	2008 ± 153	775 ± 20	2.6	2042 ± 128	450 ± 33	4.5
3	1720 ± 58	1588 ± 65	1.1	1157 ± 94	436 ± 92	2.7	1063 ± 36	316 ± 23	3.3
4	2238 ± 199	1588 ± 65	1.4	1534 ± 61	436 ± 92	3.52	1282 ± 95	316 ± 23	4.1

[a] From Hansson et al. (1971), with permission.
[b] Tissues were incubated for 2 hours in Eagle's medium at 37°C with [3H]testosterone (7.3×10^{-10} M) followed by washing in a hormone-free medium for different periods at 25°C. The results are given as dpm/mg ± SEM.

accumulate radioactive androgens by incubation *in vitro* (Hansson *et al.*, 1971). When slices from human benign nodular prostatic hyperplasia (BNPH) were incubated at 37°C with [³H]testosterone *in vitro*, there was a selective accumulation and retention of radioactivity in the prostatic slices in contrast to the significantly lower uptake by the pyramidalis muscle (Table I). After incubation for 2 hours, the mean ratio between the uptake of androgen in the prostate and in muscle was 1.2, and the difference in androgen uptake in these two tissues was significant only in two patients ($p < 0.05$). When the slices were washed in a hormone-free medium for 30 minutes, the ratio between androgen uptake in the prostate and in the muscle increased to 3.2. After washing for 60 minutes, the mean ratio increased to more than 5. These findings, therefore, indicated that human BNPH tissue is able to accumulate androgen in a way very similar to what has been shown for the rat prostate (Tveter and Attramadal, 1968; Hansson, 1971).

B. ANDROGEN BINDING IN HUMAN BNPH

Human hyperplastic prostatic tissue removed by retropubic prostatectomy, was placed in ice-cold saline and immediately brought to the laboratory. The tissues were minced and homogenized in 4 volumes of buffer (TEMG: 50 mM Tris-HCl, pH 7.4, containing 1 mM EDTA, 12 mM thioglycerol, and 10% glycerol), and a 105,000 g supernatant fraction was prepared. This supernatant fraction was equilibrated with 4 nM [³H]5α-dihydrotestosterone ([³H]5α-DHT; 150Ci/mmole) and placed at −70°C until examined.

C. POLYACRYLAMIDE GEL ELECTROPHORESIS

When aliquots of 105,000 g supernatants labeled with [³H]5α-DHT were analyzed by polyacrylamide gel electrophoreses (PAGE), we constantly found a large peak of bound radioactivity migrating at the same speed as serum testosterone-binding globulin (TBG). In several of the samples we also saw a slower migrating peak of bound radioactivity, as illustrated in Fig. 1. The second peak had the same mobility as the intracellular receptors of the rat prostate. The results obtained by using PAGE was indicative of at least two different binding proteins for androgens in the 105,000 g supernatant fractions. However, the results obtained using this method were not consistent. In our opinion, the soluble receptor protein in human BNPH very easily forms aggregates that will not penetrate into the gel. According to our experience, PAGE is not a suitable method for investigating the intracellular androgen receptors in human prostate gland.

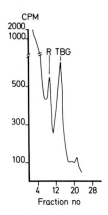

FIG. 1. Polyacrylamide gel electrophoresis (PAGE) of cytosol fraction from human benign nodular prostatic hyperplasia (BNPH). Slices of BNPH were incubated with 4 nM [^{3}H]5α-DHT in Eagle's tissue culture medium overnight at 0°C The tissue was then homogenized in 50 mM Tris-HCl, pH 7.4, containing 0.32 M sucrose and 3 mM MgCl$_2$. A cytosol fraction was prepared; 300 μl of the cytosol fraction, containing 3.5 mg of protein per milliliter was examined by PAGE. The gel contained 3.25% acrylamide and 0.5% agarose, and measured 70 × 8 mm. Tris-glycine, pH 8.6, was used as buffer. A current of 1.5 mamp per gel was applied at 125 V, and electrophoresis was performed at 0–2°C for 2.5 hours. Bromophenol blue served as marker. After electrophoresis, the gels were sliced into 2.2-mm segments, and the radioactivity was determined in each segment. TBG, testosterone-binding globulin; R, receptor.

D. Sucrose Gradient Analysis

By subjecting cytosol fractions labeled with [^{3}H]5α-DHT to sucrose density gradient centrifugation, radioactivity was found as heavy aggregates and as an 8 S and a 4 S peak. The size of the 8 S and the 4 S peaks varied from patient to patient, probably reflecting differences in the amounts of circulating endogenous androgens in different individuals. Typical sucrose gradient profiles are illustrated in Fig. 2. When a 200-fold excess of unlabeled 5α-DHT was added before the radioactive 5α-DHT, the aggregates in the lower parts of the gradients were completely inhibited, as was the 4 S peak. However, a small 8 S complex could still be observed. If the unlabeled hormone was added after the labeled steroid, the 4 S peak was still completely displaced, whereas very little effect was seen on the heavy aggregates in the bottom of the tubes and on the binding in the 8 S region. A 200-fold excess of cyproterone acetate added before the radioactive 5α-DHT reduced the binding in the lower part of the sucrose gradient, similarly to unlabeled 5α-DHT, whereas it had little effect on the binding in the 4 S region. Our findings appear to be different from those reported by Mainwaring and Milroy (1973). In their

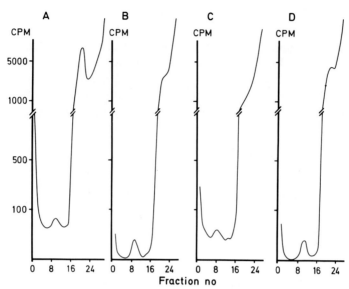

Fig. 2. Sucrose gradient analyses of cytosol fractions from human benign-nodular prostatic hyperplasia (BNPH). The tissue was homogenized at 0°C in TEMG buffer. A cytosol fraction was prepared and labeled with 4 mM [³H]5α-DHT at 0°C overnight. In one experiment a 200-fold excess of unlabeled 5α-DHT was added 20 minutes before the labeled compound. In another, the same amount of unlabeled 5α-DHT was added after the cytosol fraction had been equilibrated overnight with [³H]5α-DHT. In a third experiment a 200-fold excess of cyproterone acetate was added 20 minutes before the addition of [³H]5α-DHT. After the incubation the cytosol fractions were kept at −70°C until examined. Samples of 250 μl were layered on the top of 5 to 20% (w/v) sucrose gradients prepared in 10 mM Tris containing 1 mM EDTA, 12 mM monothioglycerol, and 10% glycerol. The protein content of the samples were 7.6 mg/ml. The gradients were centrifuged in a Beckman L2 65B ultracentrifuge at 50,000 rpm for 20 hours at 0–2°C, using an SW 56 rotor. Fractions of 10 drops were collected from the bottom of the tubes. IgG (7 S) and bovine serum albumin (BSA) (4.6 S) were used as markers. The radioactivity in each fraction was determined. (A) BNPH-cytosol fraction labeled with [³H]-5α-DHT. (B) Unlabeled 5α-DHT added to the cytosol fraction 20 minutes prior to labeling with [³H]5α-DHT. (C) Unlabeled 5α-DHT added after labeling with [³H]5α-DHT. (D) Effect of cyproterone acetate added to the cytosol fraction 20 minutes before labeling with [³H]5α-DHT.

experiments a 100-fold excess of nonradioactive 5α-DHT reduced the 8 S peak by 90%.

These studies indicated that there are specific androgen-binding proteins moving as heavy aggregates that can be blocked by unlabeled testosterone as well as by cyproterone acetate, while the 8 S component could hardly be displaced by unlabeled steroid. Thus, there are apparently differences in the binding properties of the androgen-binding components sedimenting fast in sucrose gradient compared to those sedimenting in the 4 S region. The latter could be displaced within 4 hours regardless of the unlabeled steroid being added before or after the radioactive 5α-DHT. The androgen binding aggregates at the bottom of the tubes as well as the 8 S peak were destroyed by heating at 50°C for 30 minutes, but were not destroyed by RNase or DNase. Protease completely destroyed the binding both in the 8 S and in the 4 S region.

E. SEPHADEX G-200 CHROMATOGRAPHY

When cytosol fractions from human BNPH were incubated directly with [³H]5α-DHT for 2 hours at 0°C, there was a heavy labeling of macromolecules when examined by Sephadex G-200 gel chromatography. As seen in Fig. 3, most of the radioactivity was eluted between IgG and albumin, and the distribution coefficient (K_{av}) was identical to that of human TBG. After incubating similar BNPH cytosol fractions with increasing amounts of [³H]5α-DHT (equilibrated at 0°C for 2 hours) and removing the free hormone by charcoal absorption or Sephadex G-25 gel filtration, the Scatchard plot showed a single high-affinity binding component with dissociation constant (K_d) of about 7–8 $\times$ 10⁻¹⁰ M, which was

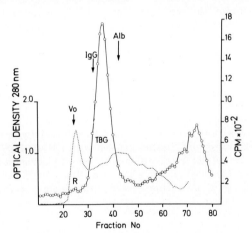

FIG. 3. Binding of [³H]5α-DHT in benign nodular prostatic hyperplasia (BNPH) cytosol. Gel filtration on Sephadex G-200 (2.5 x 37.2 cm) of a 4 ml of BNPH cytosol fraction labeled with 2 nM [³H]5α-DHT. Elution volumes of blue dextran (V_o), human γ-globulin (IgG), and albumin (Alb) are indicated by arrows. All the bound [³H]5α-DHT is eluted between IgG and albumin, very similar to human TBG. ····, OD 280 nm; O——O, cpm. From Hansson *et al.*, in "Normal and Abnormal Growth of the Prostate" (L. R. Axelrod, ed.) 1975. Courtesy of Charles C Thomas, Publisher, Springfield, Illinois.

identical to that obtained for human serum (Hansson *et al.*, 1973; Tveter *et al.*, 1975).

As illustrated in Fig. 3, we were not able to demonstrate intracellular androgen receptors different from TBG when cytosol fractions obtained from BNPH were incubated for 2 hours with [³H]5α-DHT at 0°C. However, when slices of BNPH were incubated with [³H]testosterone for 1–2 hours at 37°C and the supernatant fraction was examined by Sephadex G-200 gel filtration, the protein-bound radioactivity was eluted as two well separated peaks (Hansson *et al.*, 1973; Tveter *et al.*, 1975). One peak was eluted in the void volume, similarly to the intracellular receptors in the prostate and the epididymis of the rat. The other peak was eluted between human IgG and albumin similarly to TBG (Fig. 4). By thin-layer chromatography and recrystallizations to constant specific activity, it was found that about 90% of the protein-bound radioactivity in the excluded peak (receptor) was [³H]5α-DHT. The retained peak (TBG) contained about 68% 5α-DHT, while the peak of free radioactivity contained several different metabolites including 5α-DHT (48%) (Table II). When the cytosol fractions were heated at 50°C for 30 minutes, the excluded peak was completely destroyed, whereas the TBG peak was only slightly reduced in size. These experiments showed differences in heat stability as well as in steroid specificity of these two complexes, and strengthened the belief that the excluded peak represented the intracellular androgen receptor.

TABLE II

PERCENTAGE OF RADIOACTIVE COMPONENTS FROM BENIGN NODULAR PROSTATIC HYPERPLASIA (BNPH) TISSUE[a,b]

Component	Peak v (%)	Peak r (%)	Peak f (%)
Polar compounds	2.4	0.5	9.4
5α-Androstane-3α,17β-diol	1.5	3.5	12.3
Testosterone	5.4	26.9	1.9
5α-Androstan-17β-ol-3-one	87.2	68.1	48.3
4-Androstene-3,17-dione	—	—	2.1
5α-Androstane-3,17-dione	3.0	—	26.1

[a] From Hansson *et al.* (1975) Courtesy of Charles C Thomas, Publisher.

[b] Slices of BNPH were incubated for 60 minutes at 37°C in Eagle's tissue culture medium containing 2 nM [³H]-testosterone. The tissue was homogenized in 3 volumes 0.1 M Tris, and the cytosol fraction prepared was subjected to Sephadex G-200 gel filtration. The column was eluted with 0.1 M Tris-HCl buffer, and fractions of 40 drops (2.6 ml) were collected. The radioactivity was eluted in three different peaks: one peak eluted in the void volume (v), one was slightly retained (r), and the final peak represented free steroid (f) (cf. FIG. 4). The radioactive substances in the three different peaks were extracted and characterized by thin-layer chromatography and recrystallizations to constant specific activity.

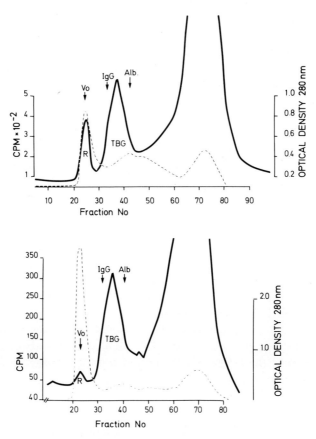

Fig. 4. Binding of androgens in benign nodular prostatic hyperplasia (BNPH) cytosol. Gel filtration of a BNPH cytosol fraction (6 ml) on a column of Sephadex G-200 (2.5 × 36.2 cm). Slices of BNPH were incubated for 60 minutes at 37°C in Eagle's tissue culture medium containing 2 nM [³H]testosterone (90 Ci/mmole). After homogenization in 3 volumes of 0.1 M Tris, the cytosol fraction was divided in two equal parts. One was subjected to Sephadex G-200 gel filtration without heating (upper panel) and the other was heated at 50°C for 30 minutes before the gel filtration. The column was eluted with 0.1 M Tris-HCl buffer, and fractions of 40 drops (mean volume 2.56 ml) were collected. Elution positions of blue dextran (Vₒ), IgG, and albumin (Alb) are given by arrows. As seen, heating destroyed the excluded peak (R) containing receptor proteins but had no effect on the retained peak of labeled steroid bound to TBG. ——, Cpm; ---, OD 28 nm. From Hansson *et al.*, in "Normal and Abnormal Growth of the Prostate" (L. R. Axelrod, ed.) 1975. Courtesy of Charles C Thomas, Publisher, Springfield, Illinois.

A very similar picture to that in Fig. 4 was found when prostate supernatant fractions from human BNPH were equilibrated with [³H]5α-DHT overnight at 0°C and stored at −70°C for several days before being examined by Sephadex G-200 gel filtration. Also by this technique we obtained two labeled androgen–protein complexes eluted from the G-200 column. One was excluded from the column and eluted in the void volume, whereas the other behaved like serum TBG (Fig. 5). It was shown that the excluded peak was heat sensitive, but nondisplaceable, whereas the second peak was less sensitive to heat but could easily be displaced by unlabeled 5α-DHT, when the latter was added after radioactive 5α-DHT.

When the void volume peak obtained by Sephadex G-200 gel filtration (containing androgen-receptor complexes), was pooled and aliquots were subjected to treatment with different enzymes, the complexes were completely destroyed by protease, but not affected by RNase or DNase (Fig. 6). Treatment with a sulfhydryl reagent, *p*-chloromercuriphenyl sulfonic acid (PCMPS), also abolished the binding. Similar results were obtained by Mainwaring and Milroy (1973).

As illustrated in Fig. 7, the androgen receptor complexes recovered from the void volume of Sephadex G-200 show a very slow rate of dissociation. To the sample containing labeled androgen-receptor complexes an excess

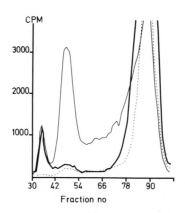

FIG. 5. Androgen binding in human benign nodular prostatic hyperplasia (BNPH) cytosol fraction. Cytosol fractions from two patients were pooled and subjected to Sephadex G-200 gel filtration. The cytosol fractions were prepared and labeled with [³H]5α-DHT as described in the legend to Fig. 1. After having been kept at −70°C, the cytosol fraction was precipitated with equal volumes of saturated (NH₄)₂SO₄, and centrifuged at 0–2°C for 30 minutes at 9000 rpm. The precipitate was dissolved, without washing, in 3 ml of 50 m*M* Tris containing 10% glycerol and 1 m*M* EDTA. Of this solution, 1 ml was put on a Sephadex G-200 column measuring 1.6 × 58 cm. The column was eluted with 10 m*M* Tris-HCL, pH 7.4, containing 0.02% NaN₃, at 0–2°C. Fractions of 2 ml were collected. The flow rate was 7 ml/hour. ——, Control; ▬▬, the effect of excess of unlabeled 5α-DHT (× 200) ; - - -, the effect of heating at 50°C for 30 minutes.

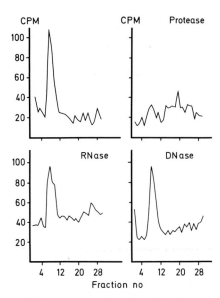

FIG. 6. Effect of enzymes on the binding of [³H]5α-DHT to receptors in benign nodular prostatic hyperplasia (BNPH) cytosol fraction. Aliquots (0.5 ml) of excluded androgen–protein complexes from Sephadex G-200 gel filtration (see Fig. 4) were treated with protease (100 μg/ml), RNase (20 μg/ml), and DNase (20 μg/ml) for 4 hours at 0°C, and binding was assayed by Sephadex G-25 gel filtration at 0°C. Flow: 30 ml/hour; column size 0.9 × 13 cm; buffer 10 mM Tris-HCl, pH 7.4, Protein in sample: 1.0 mg/ml. Fractions of 0.55 ml each were collected.

of unlabeled 5α-DHT was added, and binding was assayed by Sephadex G-25 gel filtration at different time intervals after the addition of the labeled steroid. Within a 48-hour period, there was only about 25% dissociation at 0°C. Hence the androgen-receptor complexes in BNPH are characterized by a slow rate of dissociation at 0°C similar to the intracellular androgen receptors in rats (Hansson et al., 1974a). This is very different from androgen bound to "carrier" proteins like androgen-binding protein (ABP) or TBG, which show a rapid rate of dissociation.

The androgen-receptor complexes eluted in the void volume of Sephadex G-200, were converted to a distinct 4 S peak in 0.4 M KCl.

Thus, the androgen receptors in the human BNPH appear to be very similar to those in the rat tissues. They exhibit slow electrophoretic mobility by gel electrophoresis, are very sensitive to heat, and are destroyed by proteolytic enzymes and PCMPS, but not by RNase or DNase. They also show a high degree of steroid specificity binding 5α-DHT very firmly. Finally, the rate of dissociation of the androgen-receptor complexes is very slow ($t_{1/2}$ at 0°C > 2 days) indicating that they might function as a complex that is not exchanged during the translocation into

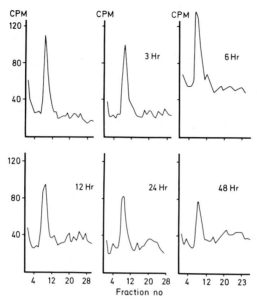

Fɪɢ. 7. Dissociation of [³H]DHT-receptor complexes in benign nodular prostatic hyperplasia (BNPH) cytosol fractions. Aliquots (0.5 ml) of excluded androgen-protein complexes from Sephadex G-200 gel filtration (see Fig. 4) were subjected to Sephadex G-25 gel filtration at various intervals after the addition of unlabeled steroid ($\times$1000). Details as in Fig. 4. As seen from the figure, there is less than 25% dissociation of androgen-receptor complexes after 48 hours.

the nucleus. This is strikingly different from androgen transport proteins like serum TBG or testicular ABP, which most probably do not enter the cells (Table III).

TABLE III

Rᴀᴛᴇ ᴏғ Dɪssᴏᴄɪᴀᴛɪᴏɴ ᴏғ 5α-DHT ғʀᴏᴍ Vᴀʀɪᴏᴜs Sᴛᴇʀᴏɪᴅ Pʀᴏᴛᴇɪɴ
Cᴏᴍᴘʟᴇxᴇs ᴀs Eᴠɪᴅᴇɴᴄᴇᴅ ʙʏ $t_{1/2}$ ᴀᴛ 0°C[a]

Complex	$t_{1/2}$OC	Reference
5α-DHT-receptor complexes in rat prostate	>2 Days	Hansson et al. (1974a)
5α-DHT-receptor complexes in human BNPH and prostatic cancer	>2 Days	Present study
Rat ABP	6 Minutes	Hansson et al. (1974a)
Rabbit ABP	~6 Minutes	Unpublished data
Rabbit TBG	~5.2 Minutes	Hansson et al. (1974b)
Human TBG	67 Minutes	Hansson et al. (1974b)

[a] DHT, dihydrotestosterone; BNPH, benign nodular prostatic hyperplasia; ABP, androgen-binding protein; TBG, testosterone-binding globulin.

III. The Neoplastic Prostate

In many patients operated upon for BNPH, the histological examination revealed areas of malignancy. Also in such cases high-affinity androgen-binding proteins were demonstrated in the cytosol fractions (Tveter et al., 1971). We have more recently examined 6 cases of advanced prostatic carcinoma, some with distant metastases, and have demonstrated specific androgen-binding proteins different from serum TBG.

A. Polyacrylamide Gel Electrophoresis

The prostatic tissue was homogenized in four volumes of TEMG buffer, equilibrated with 4 nM [³H]5α-DHT overnight, and stored at −70°C until examined. Just like the supernatant fractions from BNPH, we found a 5α-DHT–protein complex migrating with the same relative mobility as serum TBG. In some of the patients we also observed the more slowly moving component. One such case is illustrated in Fig. 8. This patient had advanced prostatic carcinoma and was operated upon because of obstruction of the rectum owing to local tumor infiltration in the pelvis. Metastatic tissue from the abdomen was homogenized, and the cytosol labeled with [³H]5α-DHT was subjected to PAGE. Two peaks of radioactivity were observed, one migrating as serum TBG whereas the other had a much slower electrophoretic mobility. Addition of a large excess of unlabeled 5α-DHT to one sample for 4 hours completely inhibited the binding to the TBG peak, whereas the more slowly moving complex was not affected. From a clinical point of view, it is interesting that the metastatic tissue thus seems to contain receptorlike proteins similar to those observed in cancer tissue removed from the prostate gland.

We have further characterized the androgen receptors in prostatic cancer by sucrose gradient centrifugation and gel filtration.

B. Sucrose Gradient Centrifugation

Sucrose gradient centrifugation consistently showed androgen-binding components sedimenting as heavy aggregates, as 8 S and 4 S complexes. The complexes sedimenting faster than 4 S were heat sensitive and displaced by unlabeled 5α-DHT as well as cyproterone acetate. Just as for the human BNPH, displacement of the 8 S peak was not complete. Almost identical sucrose gradient profiles were found in all six patients ex-

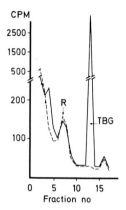

FIG. 8. Polyacrylamide gel electrophoresis (PAGE) of cytosol fraction from metastatic prostatic cancer tissue. The patient, treated with estrogen for several months, got bowel obstruction due to pelvic infiltration of prostatic carcinoma. During the operation (sigmoideostomia), metastatic nodules from the mesosigmoideum were removed. Histologically the nodules consisted of prostatic cancer tissue. The nodules were sliced and incubated in Eagle's tissue culture medium containing 5 nM [³H]testosterone overnight at 0°C. Then incubation was continued at 37°C for 1 hour. The slices were homogenized in 4 volumes of 0.32 M sucrose in 50 mM Tris containing 3 mM MgCL₂, pH 7.4. A cytosol fraction was prepared. Of this fraction, 500 μl containing 1 mg of protein per milliliter, was examined by PAGE. The gel contained 3.25% acrylamide and 0.5% agarose, and measured 8 mm × 70. Tris/glycine (1:10), pH 8.6 was used as buffer. A current of 4 mamp per gel was applied, and electrophoresis was performed at 0–2°C for 2¾ hour at 120 V. Bromophenol blue was used as marker. After electrophoresis, the gels were sliced into 2.2-mm segments, and radioactivity was determined in each segment. ——, Control; - - -, excess unlabeled 5α-dihydrotestosterone. R, receptor.

amined, although some variation in the size of the 8 S peak was observed (Fig. 9).

C. SEPHADEX G-200 GEL FILTRATION

After labeling of the supernatant fraction as described above, the cytosol was precipitated with ammonium sulfate at 0°C, and the resuspended precipitate was chromatographed on Sephadex G-200 columns. Pooled supernatant fractions from two patients showing high binding by sucrose gradient centrifugation were used. As illustrated in Fig. 10, two peaks of radioactivity occurred. The androgen-protein complex in the void volume was heat sensitive but nondisplaceable, whereas the retained androgen-protein complex, having a distribution coefficient (K_{av}) similar to TBG, was easily displaced. The rate of dissociation of [³H]5α-DHT bound by the receptor was measured by Sephadex G-25 gel filtration.

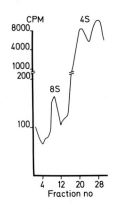

FIG. 9. Sucrose gradient analyses of a cytosol fraction obtained from prostatic cancer. The tissue was homogenized in TEMG buffer and incubated with 4 nM [^{3}H]5α-dihydrotestosterone at 0°C, overnight. Samples of 250 μl were layered on the top of 5–20% (w/v) sucrose gradients prepared in 10 mM Tris containing 1 mM EDTA, 12 mM monothioglycerol, and 10% glycerol. The protein content of the sample was 7.8 mg/ml. The gradients were centrifuged in a Beckman L2 65B ultracentrifuge at 50,000 rpm for 20 hours at 1°C, using an SW 56 rotor. Fractions of 10 drops were collected from the bottom of the tubes. IgG (7 S) and bovine serum albumin (4.6 S) were used as references. The radioactivity in each fraction was determined.

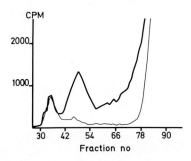

FIG. 10. Sephadex G-200 gel filtration of pooled cytosol fractions from two patients with prostatic cancer. The cytosol fraction from each patient was incubated with 4 nM [^{3}H]5α-dihydrotestosterone in TEMG buffer. The cytosol fractions, kept at −70°C, were pooled after thawing and precipitated with equal volumes of saturated (NH$_4$)$_2$SO$_4$. After centrifugation at 9000 rpm for 30 minutes at 0–2°C, the precipitate was dissolved in 3 ml of 50 mM Tris with 1 mM EDTA and 10% glycerol. One milliliter of the solvent was put on a Sephadex G-200 gel column measuring 1.6 × 58 cm. The column was eluted with 10 mM Tris-HCl, pH 7.4, containing 0.02% NaN$_3$. Fractions of 2 ml were collected. The flow rate was 7 ml/hour. The radioactivity in each fraction was determined. ——, control; ——, excess of unlabeled 5α-DHT (times 100) added 4 hours before gel filtration.

The fractions of the void volume obtained by the Sephadex G-200 gel filtration were pooled. The subsequent analysis by Sephadex G-25 gel filtration performed at 0°C at various intervals after the addition of a surplus of unlabeled steroid revealed a slow rate of dissociation ($t_{1/2}$ 0°C > 48 hours). Furthermore, treatment with enzymes (protease, RNase and DNase) and PCMPS showed the same effects as those observed in human prostatic hyperplasia. Likewise, this complex was converted to a 4 S peak in 0.4 M KCl. Thus, so far the results do not indicate any qualitative differences between androgen receptors in neoplastic and nonneoplastic tissue. Moreover, all the patients studied appear to have specific androgen-binding proteins with properties similar to "receptors" and different from TBG.

IV. Androgen Metabolism in Human Prostate

In order to study the androgen metabolism in the human accessory sex organs, various types of tissue were incubated with [³H]testosterone

TABLE IV

Formation of 5α-Androstane-3α,17β-diol (3α-diol), Dihydroxytestosterone (DHT) and Oxidative Metabolites (4-Androstene-3,17-dione, 5α-Androstane-3,17-dione) in the Ether Phase after Incubation of Prostatic Tissue from Hyperplasia and Cancer with Tritiated Testosterone (T)[a,b]

Tissue		Distribution of each metabolite as per cent of total ether extractable radioactivity			
		3α-Diol	T	DHT	Oxidative
BNPH[b]	(8)	6	39	44	9
Cancer	(3)	<1	81	16	3
Normal tissue					
Lateral prostate	(2)	<1	62	34	3
Dorsal prostate	(2)	<1	56	36	7
Seminal vesicle	(2)	ND	86	9	3

[a] Tissue was incubated under continuous shaking at 37°C in Eagle's basal medium to which [³H]testosterone and potassium penicillin had been added. After 2 hours the incubation was stopped by addition of acetone. The tissue was then homogenized, extracted with acetone, and partitioned between diethyl ether and water (Djøseland et al., 1974). Procedures for TCL, derivative formation, localization, and identification of the radioactive metabolites were performed as previously described (Djøseland et al., 1973). Normal prostate and seminal vesicle were used as controls. Number of patients indicated in parentheses.

[b] Benign nodular prostatic hyperplasia.

(Table IV). Normal prostatic tissue and seminal vesicles were obtained from patients having carcinoma of the urinary bladder, treated with radical cystectomy.

The metabolic conversion of [³H]testosterone in BNPH is very similar to that seen in the different lobes of the normal prostate. In both tissues there is a rather extensive conversion of testosterone to 5α-DHT. 5α-DHT formation in BNPH has been reported by Ofner et al. (1970), Pike et al. (1970), and Becker et al. (1972). The studies of Siiteri and Wilson (1970) indicate that 5α-DHT might play an etiological role in the development of BNPH. The seminal vesicles, on the other hand, have apparently a much lower transformation of testosterone into 5α-reduced metabolites. In this respect one might recall that while neoplasms of the seminal vesicle are medical rarities, they are very common in the human prostate. Table IV and Fig. 11 also show that the conversion of testosterone to 5α-DHT is significantly slower in prostatic cancer than in prostatic hyperplasia and in normal tissue. The reason for this difference is obscure, but transformation of the normal prostatic cells into the less differentiated cancer cell might be one possible explanation.

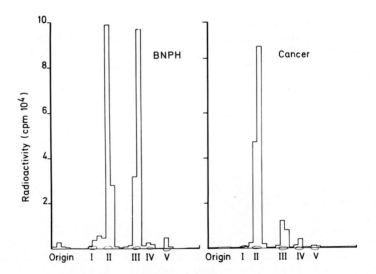

Fig. 11. Radiochromatogram obtained after incubation of prostatic tissue from benign nodular prostatic hyperplasia (BNPH) and cancer with tritiated testosterone. After incubation the radioactivity was partitioned between water and ether. The ether extract was subjected to thin-layer chromatography in system A (methylene chloride:diethyl ether 4:1, on silica gel). The radioactive peaks correspond to authentic 5α-androstane-3α,17β-diol (I), testosterone (II), 5α-dihydrotestosterone (III), 4-androstene-3,17-dione (IV), and 5α-androstane-3,17-dione (V).

V. Summary and Conclusions

Human prostatic tissue, both neoplastic and nonneoplastic, contains at least two soluble androgen-binding proteins. One has characteristics very similar to those of the intracellular receptors in accessory sex organs of the male rat, whereas the other has properties very similar to those of serum TBG. We have not been able to demonstrate differences in physicochemical properties between the receptors in neoplastic and non-neoplastic tissues. Human prostatic tissue contains enzymes capable of metabolizing testosterone to reductive and oxidative metabolites. The formation of 5α-DHT is apparently higher in hyperplastic tissue than in cancer. Further measurements of receptor concentrations and 5α-reductase activity in prostatic tissue might be useful in selecting patients for endocrine therapy.

ACKNOWLEDGMENTS

This work has been supported by The Norwegian Cancer Society (Landsforeningen mot Kreft), Norwegian Research Council for Science and the Humanities (NAVF), the Nordic Insulin Foundation, and Norwegian Society for Fighting Cancer.

REFERENCES

Becker, H., Kaufmann, J., Klosterhalfen, H., and Voigt, K. D. (1972). *Acta Endocrinol. (Copenhagen)* **71**, 589.

Djøseland, D., Hansson, V., and Haugen, H. N. (1973). *Steroids* **21**, 773.

Djøseland, D., Hansson, V., and Haugen, H. N. (1974). *Steroids* **23**, 397.

Hansson, V. (1971). *Acta Endocrinol. (Copenhagen)* **68**, 89.

Hansson, V., Tveter, K. J., Attramadal, A., and Torgersen, O. (1971). *Acta Endocrinol. (Copenhagen)* **68**, 79.

Hansson, V., Tveter, K. J., Unhjem, O., Djøseland, O., Attramadal, A., Reusch, E., and Torgersen, O. (1975). *In* "Normal and Abnormal Growth of the Prostate" (L. R. Axelrod, ed.), p. 676. Thomas, Springfield, Illinois.

Hansson, V., Trygstad, O., French, F. S., McLean, W. S., Smith, A. A., Tindell, D. J., Weddington, S. C., Petrusz, P., Nayfeh, S. N., and Ritzen, E. M. (1974a). *Nature (London)* **250**, 387.

Hansson, V., Ritzen, E. M., Weddington, S. C., McLean, W. S., Tindall, D. J., Nayfeh, S. N., and French, F. S. (1974b). *Endocrinology* **95**, 690.

Huggins, C. (1963). *Nat. Cancer Inst., Monogr.* **12**, XI.

Mainwaring, W. I. P., and Milroy, E. J. G. (1973). *J. Endocrinol.* **57**, 371.

Ofner, P., Morfin, R. F., Vena, R. L., and Aliapoulios, M. A. (1970). *In* "Some Aspects of the Aetiology and Biochemistry of Prostatic Cancer" (K. Griffiths and C. G. Pierrepoint, eds.), p. 55. Alpha Omega Alpha Publ., Cardiff, Wales.

Pike, A., Peeling, W. B., Harper, M. E., Pierrepoint, C. G., and Griffiths, K. (1970). *Biochem. J.* **120**, 443.

Siiteri, P. K., and Wilson, J. D. (1970). *J. Clin. Invest.* **49**, 1737.

Tveter, K. J., and Attramadal, A. (1968). *Acta Endocrinol. (Copenhagen)* **59**, 218.

Tveter, K. J., Uhjem, O., Attramadal, A., Aakvaag, A., and Hansson V. (1971). *Advan. Biosci.* **7**, 193.

Tveter, K. J., Hansson, V., and Unhjem, O. (1975). *In* "Molecular Mechanisms of Gonadal Hormone Action" (J. A. Thomas and R. L. Singhal, eds), Advan. Sex Horm. Res., Vol. I, p. 17. Univ. Park Press, Baltimore, Maryland.

DISCUSSION

P. Robel: Your data suggest that the cytosol receptor from BPH is largely occupied by endogenous androstanolone. Indeed, I have collected the 8 S peak of sucrose gradients and measured DHT, and shown that more than 90% of receptor sites are occupied by endogenous androgen. Have you performed competitive experiments to see whether you are dealing with an estradiol receptor or with the binding of estradiol to an androgen receptor?

K. J. Tveter: Unfortunately, we have not had the opportunity to do that yet. We will do this as soon as possible to get an idea of the specificity of the receptor.

H. J. de Voogt: How much tissue did you use for these experiments? For the examination of prostatic cancer it is very important to be able to do receptor analysis from as little tissue as possible (biopsy).

K. J. Tveter: Our techniques require several grams of tissue. If other techniques (e.g., that of Wagner), requiring only milligrams of tissue, prove to be reliable, it would be easier to do follow-up studies of patients given different kinds of antiandrogenic treatment.

H. J. Tagnon: Does the proteolytic activity present in the prostate and in the cytosol interfere with the receptor detection or measurement? Do you use inhibitors?

K. J. Tveter: We have not used PMSF or similar agents. Immediately after removal of the surgical specimen, it was put in ice-cold saline in the operating theatre and brought to the laboratory as soon as possible. Homogenization of the tissue was performed within a few minutes.

H. J. Tagnon: Hawkins in our laboratory has data indicating the presence of an estradiol receptor in prostate cytosol under conditions in which the presence of androgen receptors could not be demonstrated. The use of competitors confirmed this.

L. Andersson: Since a sample from the primary tumor in prostatic carcinoma may contain normal prostatic tissue as well, your finding of TBG in the metastasis, where only abnormal prostate cells occur, is of particular interest. Have you investigated whether such androgenic receptors are present even in anaplastic carcinoma? In this tumor form the cellular pattern deviates considerably from normal, and it is also believed that biochemical behavior would be abnormal.

K. J. Tveter: Until now we have investigated too few patients to make any correlation between the histological appearance and our biochemical findings. I think this is a very important problem from a clinical point of view. I would suggest that in order to do such comparative studies, several urological centers should cooperate, using the same experimental protocol. Within a relatively short period of time it might then be possible to see whether the more anaplastic forms of the tumor might contain fewer androgen-binding sites. Such studies might also indicate a possible correlation between the presence of receptors and the prognosis in each individual patient.

T. Nilsson: We have attempted to quantify the specific binding sites E_2 and DHT in human BPH and carcinoma for clinical use (as it has been used in breast cancer). These preliminary data indicate that there are patterns defining the tissue of BPH as well as the carcinomatous tissue.

Testosterone Receptors in the Prostate and Other Tissues

G. VERHOEVEN, W. HEYNS, AND P. DE MOOR

Laboratorium voor Experimentele Geneeskunde, Rega Instituut, Leuven, Belgium

I. GENERAL INTRODUCTION

Androgens have classically been defined as steroid hormones that are able to stimulate the development of male secondary sex characteristics. It was recognized very early, however, that nearly all tissues of the body are to a certain extent influenced by male sex hormones (Kochakian, 1946). The major androgen target tissues (prostate, seminal vesicles, epididymis) belong to the male genital tract, and their differentiation depends completely on androgen activity during critical periods of embryonic development. During recent years increased interest has been shown in androgen target organs outside the genital tract. In fact, in

265

disorders of sexual differentiation that are primarily characterized by androgen unresponsiveness—such as the testicular feminization syndrome—accessory sex glands do not develop, and the only tissues we can rely upon to identify the underlying molecular defect are those tissues that, although androgen responsive, do not depend upon androgens for their differentiation. Moreover, the role of androgens in these tissues is physiologically important (e.g., muscles, skin) and may become of major clinical concern in disorders such as hirsutism, acne, baldness, anemia, and osteoporosis.

A question that is clinically and therapeutically important is whether the enormous variety of androgen effects on tissues of the genital tract and on other tissues is mediated by the same cellular mechanisms. Evidence has been presented that the *relative* activity of different androgens in different target tissues varies widely (Liao and Fang, 1969) and that different androgenic compounds may even have *qualitatively* different effects on the same target tissue (Huggins, *et al.*, 1954; Robel *et al.*, 1971; Gonzales-Diddi *et al.*, 1972). Moreover, striking differences have been described in the metabolism and binding of androgens in different target organs. In the following sections we will discuss whether the cytoplasmic receptor proteins for androgens in different target tissues are identical. Metabolism will be covered insofar as it may influence receptor binding.

II. Testosterone and Its "Active Metabolites"

Testosterone, the major androgen secreted by the testis, is peripherally metabolized to at least three distinct classes of hormones with biological activity. 5α-Reduction leads to the formation of potent virilizing and anabolizing compounds, aromatization yields estrogens, and 5β-reduction results in the formation of steroids with hematopoietic activity (Kappas *et al.*, 1972). Both 5α-reduction (Gloyna and Wilson, 1969) and aromatization (Naftolin *et al.*, 1971; Schweikert *et al.*, 1975) take place in the target cells themselves. As a consequence, these reactions may be regarded as an integral part of the receptor mechanisms of the cell. Actual "receptor proteins" have not yet been described for 5β-reduced androgen derivatives, and the activity of aromatized testosterone metabolites is probably mediated by distinct estrogen receptor proteins. Accordingly, the following discussion will focus on receptor molecules for testosterone and its 5α-reduced transformation products.

The concept that steroid hormone activity is related to the modulation of the expression of the genome and the finding of Bruchovsky and Wilson (1968) and Anderson and Liao (1968) that after *in vivo* or *in vitro* administration of ^{3}H-labeled testosterone 80% or more of the radioactivity in rat prostate nuclei can be accounted for by DHT (dihydrotestosterone, 17β-hydroxy-5α-androstan-3-one) stimulated an enormous amount of investigation concerning the formation and activity of 5α-reduced testosterone derivatives in different target tissues (for review, see Verhoeven, 1974). DHT is considerably more active than testosterone in several bioassay systems (Dorfman and Shipley, 1956), its formation is most prominent in accessory sex glands (Gloyna and Wilson, 1969), and DHT accumulation has specifically been related to cell growth and proliferation (Gloyna and Wilson, 1969; Wilson and Walker, 1969; Robel et al., 1971; Lesser and Bruchovsky, 1971). The concept of "active 5α-reduced metabolites" has been extended to other testosterone metabolites by Robel et al. (1971) on the basis of the effects of these compounds on prostatic explants in tissue culture. The actual contribution of these other metabolites to the overall effect of androgens awaits elucidation. All these studies, however, raise two important questions. (1) Is testosterone itself active at the level of the target cells? (2) What is the biological significance of the secretion of testosterone as the major testicular androgen?

III. Evidence for a Biological Role for DHT and Testosterone

. Three different series of investigations have presented suggestive evidence that in some target tissues testosterone functions as the active mediator of androgen action, whereas other organs require the formation of DHT.

A. Cellular Uptake and Nuclear Retention of DHT and Testosterone

Although DHT is undoubtedly the major androgen observed in nuclei from male accessory organs of reproduction (Wilson and Gloyna, 1970), testosterone has been found to be the predominant androgen in nuclei from several target tissues outside the male genital tract. Nuclear retention of testosterone has been reported in mouse and rat kidney (Bullock et al., 1971; Ritzén et al., 1972), mouse submandibular gland (Goldstein and Wilson, 1972), immature rat uterus (Giannopoulos, 1973), rat anterior hypophysis (Jouan et al., 1973), rat testis (Hansson et al., 1974), rat bone marrow (Valladares and Minguell, 1975), erythropoietic mouse spleen (Hadjian et al., 1974), and Shionogii carcinoma (Bruchovsky,

1972). Cellular uptake of testosterone has also been demonstrated in levator ani and bulbocavernosus muscle (Jung and Baulieu, 1972; Krieg *et al.*, 1974b), mature rat uterus (Heyns, 1974), and rabbit Wolffian ducts (Wilson, 1973). It should be noted that the percentage of the cellular radioactivity concentrated in the nuclei of these tissues is low when compared with male accessory sex glands. Usually it does not exceed 5%. However, considerably lower nuclear uptake of testosterone is noted in several of these organs in animals with the testicular feminization syndrome (Bullock *et al.*, 1971; Ritzén *et al.*, 1972; Goldstein and Wilson, 1972). This supports the contention that the observed uptake is really related to androgen action. The smaller fraction of androgens in the nuclei of these tissues may reflect a lower concentration of cytoplasmic receptor proteins or nuclear acceptor sites, a smaller number of androgen-responsive cells, or the higher dissociation rate of testosterone-receptor complexes (see further).

B. The Intracellular Levels of Testosterone and DHT in Different Target Tissues

The specific uptake and retention of androgens in target tissues results in organ levels of male sex hormones that exceed the circulating levels. Although the data concerning the concentration of androgens in different target tissues are relatively scarce, it has clearly been established that the concentration of DHT in normal and hypertrophic dog prostate (Gloyna *et al.*, 1970), normal and hyperplastic human prostate (Siiteri and Wilson, 1970; Giorgi *et al.*, 1971), rat prostate (Robel *et al.*, 1973), and rat prostatic explants (Lasnitzki *et al.*, 1974) considerably exceeds the corresponding concentration of DHT in plasma or in the medium. In contrast, none of the mentioned tissues displays important intracellular/extracellular gradients for testosterone. Although the concentration of testosterone in blood is some 10 times higher than the concentration of DHT, this results in prostatic levels of DHT that equal or even considerably exceed the levels of blood testosterone. In several other tissues, however, such as levator ani muscle, hypothalamus, hypophysis, and kidney, the tissue concentration of testosterone exceeds the tissue concentration of DHT and the circulating level of testosterone (Robel *et al.*, 1973). These findings suggest a relatively more important contribution of testosterone in the overall effect of androgens in these tissues. The question whether these differences in the accumulation of testosterone or DHT reflect the presence of binding proteins with different ligand specificity or differences in target cell metabolism will be discussed further.

C. Embryological and Clinical Evidence for a Dissociation of Testosterone and DHT Effects

Several findings indicate that testosterone itself is responsible for the development of the internal organs of male reproduction, whereas DHT mediates the development of the external male genitalia. In fact, in the Wolffian ducts 5α-reductase activity is undetectably low at the time of sexual differentiation both in the rabbit (Wilson and Lasnitzki, 1971) and in man (Kelch et al., 1971; Siiteri and Wilson, 1974). Moreover, the Wolffian ducts concentrate testosterone (Wilson, 1973). These observations have received considerable support from the recent identification of a form of male pseudohermaphroditism characterized by the absence of 5α-reductase activity in male accessory sex tissues (Walsh et al., 1974; Imperato-McGinley et al., 1974). In this disease the external genitalia that depend on the formation of DHT fail to develop. The derivatives of the Wolffian ducts, however, undergo normal differentiation. At puberty the patients undergo partial masculinization, but DHT-dependent tissues such as the prostate remain hypotrophic.

IV. Methodological Problems in the Study of Androgen-Receptor Proteins in Different Target Tissues in Vitro

Our present knowledge on androgen-receptor proteins in different tissues relies almost completely on studies in unfractionated cytosol preparations. This kind of investigation is complicated by three factors: the extremely low concentrations of androgen-receptor sites (even in rat prostate the number of receptor sites is approximately 10 times lower than in target tissues for some steroid hormones), the previously mentioned differences in target cell metabolism, and the presence in the cytosol from several tissues of binding proteins other than the actual receptor proteins. The latter proteins include both nonspecific binding proteins, which are present in all tissues investigated, and specific binding proteins, such as androgen-binding protein (ABP) in epididymis (Hansson, 1972; Danzo et al., 1973), the 3 S binding protein in mouse submandibular gland (Wilson and Goldstein, 1972), and the "α-protein" in rat prostate (Fang and Liao, 1971); the relationship of the latter proteins to the actual androgen receptor is obscure and merits further investigation.

Until recently the only technique that more or less successfully distinguished between putative receptors and other ABPs was sucrose density gradient centrifugation. This technique is hardly suited for quantitative investigations, however, and minor differences in the preparation of the cytosol fractions have resulted in an enormous confusion concerning the actual sedimentation coefficient of androgen receptors. Both charcoal adsorption (Bullock and Bardin, 1974) and Sephadex chromatography (Giannopoulos, 1971) have successfully been applied in some target organs but are of limited use in tissues containing several ABPs. Recently several new techniques have been advanced. Agar gel electrophoresis (Krieg et al., 1974a), protamine sulfate precipitation (Blondeau and Corpechot, 1974), and androgen antibodies (Castañeda and Liao, 1975) have been used in studies concerning the rat prostate receptor. Verhoeven (1974) compared androgen receptors in different tissues, using an ammonium sulfate precipitation technique. The latter method relies on the well known fact that androgen-receptor proteins can be precipitated quite selectively at low concentrations of ammonium sulfate (Fang and Liao, 1971; Mainwaring and Peterken, 1971). In the following sections we shall discuss some results obtained with this technique in rat prostate and mouse kidney and parallel data for rat uterus obtained by a gel filtration technique.

V. Factors That Favor the Binding of Testosterone or DHT to Receptor Proteins in Vitro

It has been suggested that some target tissues contain receptor proteins that bind specifically DHT, whereas other tissues are endowed with "testosterone receptors." Fang and Liao (1971) reported a nearly absolute specificity of the rat prostate receptor (β-protein) for DHT. Several other authors, however, observed less striking differences in the relative binding of testosterone and DHT to prostatic receptors in vitro (Mainwaring, 1969; Jung and Baulieu, 1971; Sullivan and Strott, 1973; Krieg et al., 1974a; Verhoeven, 1974). Preferential binding of DHT in vitro was also observed in rat epididymis (Blaquier, 1971; Hansson et al., 1973), rat seminal vesicles (Stern and Eisenfeld, 1969), rat preputial gland (Bullock and Bardin, 1972), rat hypothalamus (Kato and Onouchi, 1973), hamster sebaceous gland (Adachi and Kano, 1972), and cock ear lobe (Dubé and Tremblay, 1974). On the contrary, receptor proteins that preferentially bind testosterone in vitro have been reported in rat uterus (Giannopoulos, 1971), levator ani muscle (Jung and Baulieu, 1972), mouse kidney (Bullock and Bardin, 1974), and rat bone marrow (Valladares and Minguell, 1975). Direct comparison of the binding of testosterone and DHT to binding proteins in tissues containing "DHT receptors" (prostate) and "testosterone receptors" (mouse kidney, rat uterus) revealed three important factors that favor the binding of either the former or the latter ligand *in vitro* (De Moor *et al.*, 1975).

1. The influence of the duration of the incubation and separation procedure on the binding of testosterone and DHT. Using fast procedures such as ammonium sulfate precipitation and gel filtration, we studied in detail the influence of time on the binding of testosterone and DHT. After 4 hours of incubation at 0°C, both ligands were bound to receptor proteins in mouse kidney, rat uterus, and rat prostate. Moreover, at this time point testosterone binding consistently exceeded DHT binding even in the prostate. After longer incubation periods, however, testosterone binding declined progressively while DHT binding remained unaltered for at least 24 hours (Table I). The decrease in testosterone binding can at least partly be accounted for by the considerably higher dissociation rate of the testosterone–receptor complex (Baulieu *et al.*, 1971; De Moor *et al.*, 1975) and by the instability of the free receptor molecule (Heyns, 1974). These findings explain why in methods such as density gradient centrifugation, where the separation of bound and free steroid takes 14–20 hours and where reassociation is limited, DHT binding is favored. Two other factors explain why testosterone binding prevails after short periods of incubation and rapid separation of bound and free steroids.

2. The influence of the extensive metabolism of DHT at 4°C. Bullock and Bardin (1974) stressed the fact that even at 4°C DHT is extensively metabolized by mouse kidney cytosol. These findings have been extended by us to several other tissues. After 4 hours of incubation of prostate, kidney, and uterus cytosol at 4°C only 56, 20, and 10%, respectively, of the incubated ^{3}H-labeled DHT remained unaltered. The major metab-

TABLE I

INFLUENCE OF THE INCUBATION TIME ON TESTOSTERONE AND
DIHYDROTESTOSTERONE (DHT) BINDING IN PROSTATE CYTOSOL[a]

		Incubation time	
Ligand	Temperature (°C)	4 Hours % Receptor bound	20 Hours % Receptor bound
DHT-^{3}H	0	17.2	17.1
	4	16.0	16.8
Testosterone-^{3}H	0	21.2	14.3
	4	18.5	13.1

[a] Percentage of the incubated testosterone-^{3}H or DHT-^{3}H associated with receptor proteins precipitable at 40% of saturation with ammonium sulfate after various periods of incubation at 0° or 4°C. Values represent the mean of duplicate determinations.

olite in all tissues investigated was 5α-androstane-3α,17β-diol. ³H-labeled testosterone, on the contrary, was not metabolized, and in the receptor-bound fraction (40% ammonium sulfate precipitate or void volume of the Sephadex column) only DHT or testosterone was identified. The metabolism of DHT to compounds that bind poorly to the receptor protein undoubtedly lowers the concentration of this ligand that is available for receptor binding and may simulate preferential binding of testosterone. It may be concluded that testosterone should be utilized for studies on receptor proteins in tissues where DHT is extensively metabolized.

3. The influence of the binding of testosterone and DHT to cytosol proteins other than the receptor proteins. Equilibrium dialysis experiments both for mouse kidney, rat uterus, and rat prostate cytosol showed that at ligand concentrations that clearly exceed the binding capacity of the receptor proteins—in other words, at concentrations where mainly high-capacity binding is measured—the bound:unbound ratios for DHT are 2 to 4 times higher than for testosterone. This preferential binding of DHT to nonreceptor proteins leads again to underestimation of the affinity of receptor proteins for DHT.

In conclusion, long-term methods such as gradient centrifugation may fail to show testosterone binding even if it was originally present. The binding of DHT, on the other hand, is underestimated to a variable degree in different tissues in short-term as well as in long-term experiments. The data presented show that both testosterone and DHT are bound to high-affinity, low-capacity binding sites in the three tissues investigated. However, they do not prove that the binding occurs to the same receptor protein.

VI. THE STRIKING SIMILARITY OF TESTOSTERONE AND DHT RECEPTOR PROTEINS IN DIFFERENT TISSUES

The androgen-receptor proteins in rat prostate, rat uterus, and mouse kidney displayed identical behavior on ammonium sulfate precipitation and density gradient centrifugation. In the three tissues receptors were precipitated at 30–40% of saturation. At higher salt concentrations only high-capacity binding was salted out. Only in prostate could the precipitation behavior of [³H]DHT and [³H]testosterone-receptor complexes be compared directly. In the other tissues the data for [³H]DHT varied markedly because of the extensive metabolism. In the prostate, however, the precipitation curves for both androgens were exactly parallel (Verhoeven, 1974). In the three tissues, receptor proteins migrated in the 8–10 S region of 5 to 20% sucrose gradients of low ionic strength. Although the binding was very low in kidney and uterus, DHT was consistently bound more extensively than testosterone. This is in accordance with the predictions made in the preceding section. Very striking similarities were observed in the apparent K_d values and the ligand specificity of the receptor proteins in the different organs.

A. APPARENT K_d VALUE AND NUMBER OF RECEPTOR SITES IN PROSTATE, KIDNEY, AND UTERUS

The main results of a series of determinations of kinetic characteristics are summarized in Table II. Measurements with both testosterone and DHT yielded reproducible results only in the prostate. In the other tissues, measurements with DHT were hampered by the extremely extensive metabolism of this compound. The apparent K_d of the prostatic receptor for testosterone approximates the corresponding value for DHT. Since these data have not been corrected for metabolism or nonreceptor binding, the real affinity of this receptor for DHT may considerably exceed its affinity for testosterone. The apparent K_d value of the receptor in different tissues for testosterone is similar. It should be noted that in the prostate the number of receptor sites for both ligands is almost identical, suggesting that the same class of binding sites is involved. Comparable kinetic characteristics have been reported for testosterone in rat prostate (Blondeau and Corpéchot, 1974), mouse kidney (Bullock and Bardin, 1974), and rat uterus (Giannopoulos, 1971).

B. THE LIGAND SPECIFICITY OF THE RECEPTOR PROTEINS IN PROSTATE, KIDNEY, AND UTERUS

The ligand specificity of the receptor proteins in different tissues was studied by competition experiments. The ability of more than 20 widely

TABLE II

COMPARISON OF THE APPARENT K_d AND THE NUMBER OF RECEPTOR SITES IN RAT PROSTATE, MOUSE KIDNEY, AND RAT UTERUS

Cytosol	Ligand	Apparent K_d (nM)	Sites (fmoles/mg protein)
Rat prostate	Dihydrotestosterone[a]	1.3	55
	Testosterone[a]	1.5	60
Mouse kidney	Testosterone[a]	1.2	22
Rat uterus	Testosterone	2.0	100

[a] Mean of 4 determinations.

different compounds to compete for [³H]testosterone or [³H]DHT binding was compared in prostate, kidney, and uterus. Some of the results are shown in Table III. The fact that 5 different steroids compete equally well for the testosterone and the DHT binding sites in prostate makes it likely that the same protein is responsible for the binding of these two ligands in this tissue. Moreover, the striking similarity in the apparent K_i values for the different compounds in the three tissues investigated suggests that the androgen receptors in these tissues are very similar if not identical. It should be noted that not only do potent androgens compete efficiently for the binding site, but, in fact, the apparent K_i value for classical antiandrogens such as cyproterone acetate is very close to the corresponding value for testosterone. This proves unambiguously that binding does not necessarily parallel androgenic activity.

In conclusion, our data suggest that a similar "androgen receptor" is present in rat prostate, rat uterus, and mouse kidney. Both testosterone and DHT bind to this protein. Which of these two ligands gets linked to the receptor in one of these tissues is determined not by the specificity of the receptor, but by the steroid which is secreted or administered, by the target cell metabolism, and perhaps by the presence of competing

TABLE III

LIGAND SPECIFICITY OF THE ANDROGEN RECEPTOR PROTEIN IN RAT PROSTATE, MOUSE KIDNEY, AND RAT UTERUS CYTOSOL[a]

Origin of cytosol:	Prostate		Kidney	Uterus
Labeled ligand:	Testosterone	Dihydrotestosterone	Testosterone	Testosterone
Competitor	Apparent K_i value (nM)			
Testosterone	4.0	3.3	1.3	2.0
Dihydrotestosterone	2.0	2.0	4.1	4.3
Epitestosterone	74	33	20	33
5α-Androstane-3α,17β-diol	—	35	26	39
5α-Androstane-3β,17β-diol	—	9.9	10	7.2
17β-Estradiol	—	12	5.3	6.1
17α-Methyl-19-nortestosterone	1.5	0.9	0.2	0.4
Dianabol	2.2	2.0	4.8	3.3
Cyproterone acetate	—	4.1	5.4	2.6

[a] The concentration of the labeled ligands was 1.25×10^{-10} M. The concentration of competitors was varied from 10^{-11} to 10^{-7} M. Values were calculated from logit-log plots.

nonreceptor cytosol binding proteins. Furthermore, the observed dissociation between receptor binding and androgen activity, the finding that, after *in vivo* administration of [³H]DHT, [³H]DHT is very efficiently accumulated in nuclei of "testosterone-responsive" tissues such as the mouse kidney (Bullock and Bardin, 1975), and the fact that for several parameters DHT is considerably more active than testosterone in the same tissues (Ohno *et al.*, 1971; Bardin *et al.*, 1973; Swank *et al.*, 1973) raises the possibility that even in these organs the effects of testosterone are actually mediated by minor amounts of DHT, produced *in situ* or supplied by the blood.

VII. CYTOSOL RECEPTOR PROTEINS AND THE ACTIVITY OF OTHER 5α-REDUCED ACTIVE METABOLITES

Both 5α-androstane-3α,17β-diol and the corresponding 3β-diol bind poorly to the cytoplasmic receptor proteins (Table III). A distinct microsomal binding protein for the 3β-diol has recently been characterized in prostate microsomes (Robel *et al.*, 1974). The relation of the latter binding protein to the activity of this compound remains to be established. The 3α-diol is a particularly active androgen in exorbital lacrimal gland (Cavallero and Ofner, 1967), mouse and rat kidney (Ohno *et al.*, 1971; Bardin *et al.*, 1973; Grossman *et al.*, 1974; Verhoeven, 1974), prostate and seminal vesicles (Dorfman and Dorfman, 1963; Moore and Wilson, 1973). After *in vivo* administration of [³H]3α-diol, however, [³H]DHT was the main androgen identified in rat prostate nuclei (Bruchovsky, 1971), mouse kidney nuclei (Bullock and Bardin, 1975), and human prostate (Becker *et al.*, 1973; Horst *et al.*, 1974). Moreover, it has been demonstrated that those tissues that are particularly responsive to the 3α-diol are able to convert this metabolite into DHT *in vitro*. Their relative ability to catalyze this reaction shows a striking paralellism with the presence of a particular NADH-linked microsomal 3α-hydroxysteroid dehydrogenase (Verhoeven, 1974; De Moor *et al.*, 1975). These data make it likely that the activity of the 3α-diol is largely mediated by DHT.

VIII. ARE TESTOSTERONE–RECEPTOR COMPLEXES ACTIVE MEDIATORS OF ANDROGEN ACTION?

Rigorous proof of hormonal activity of testosterone at the cellular level is still lacking. In most of the tissues where under physiological conditions testosterone is the principal steroid bound to the receptor proteins, mini-

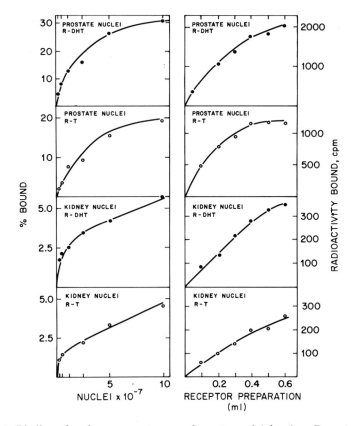

Fig. 1. Binding of androgen-receptor complexes to nuclei *in vitro*. Receptor preparations were obtained by passing cytosol, equilibrated with 10^{-9} M ³H-labeled dihydrotestosterone (DHT) (●——●) or ³H-labeled testosterone (T) (○——○), over a Sephadex G-50 column and collecting the void volume. Purified rat prostate or mouse kidney nuclei were incubated with the homologous cytosol-receptor preparations for 30 minutes at 18°C. In the left panels 0.5 ml of a receptor preparation (containing 2×10^4 cpm/ml) was added to increasing amounts of nuclei. In the right panels various amounts of receptor were added to 2×10^7 nuclei, and the final volume was made up to 0.6 ml with buffer. The incubation was stopped by placing the tubes in melting ice for 5 minutes and centrifugation at 3000 rpm for 10 minutes at 4° C. The nuclear pellets were washed three times with buffer containing Tris-HCl, pH 7.4 (I = 0.01); NaCl, 50 mM; MgCl₂, 5 mM, and EDTA, 5×10^{-5} M; the radioactivity in the nuclei was quantitated by liquid-scintillation counting. Results represent the amount or the fraction of the incubated radioactivity associated with the washed nuclear pellets (G. Verhoeven, unpublished results).

mal amounts of DHT are also bound, and the relative contribution of both steroid-receptor complexes to the final androgen effect is unknown. Androgenic functions that depend on testosterone are rare. In castrated animals DHT can replace the vast majority of the physiological androgen effects. Only the male sexual behavior in the rat requires specifically testosterone. It can be restored, however, by simultaneous administration of DHT and estrogens (Baum and Vreeburg, 1973). Apparently the fact that testosterone can be aromatized (in contrast with its 5α-reduced derivatives) accounts for this exception. Still this is no proof that the effects on male behavior are mediated by testosterone-receptor complexes. The partial masculinization of patients with congenital absence of 5α-reductase activity in male accessory sex tissues is one factor in favor of the contention that testosterone itself is biologically active. Although in some of these patients the circulating level of DHT is quite low (Imperato-McGinley et al., 1974), essentially normal levels have been reported in another patient (Walsh et al., 1974). Accordingly, circulating DHT (arising from direct secretion by the testis or from 5α-reduction in extragonadal tissues as the liver) might account for the partial androgenization observed.

Potent and specific inhibitors of the 5α-reductase would offer another approach to clarify the biological role of testosterone. Using topical application of such an inhibitor (4-androsten-3-one, 17β carboxylic acid), Voigt and Hsia (1973) were able to inhibit the effect of low concentrations of testosterone on the hamster sebaceous gland, whereas DHT remained active. However, the possibility cannot be excluded that these findings reflect only quantitative differences in the relative activity of testosterone and DHT. Direct demonstration of the activity of testosterone-receptor complexes on nuclear processes *in vitro* might be the ultimate way to settle the question of the biological activity of testosterone. Early attempts to demonstrate uptake of testosterone-receptor complexes in prostate nuclei *in vitro* failed (Jung and Baulieu, 1971). Recently, however, we were able to demonstrate that testosterone- and DHT-receptor complexes bind to highly purified rat prostate and mouse kidney nuclei (Fig. 1). The specificity of the nuclear binding process has been questioned, however, and further experiments demonstrating actual activity of the androgen-receptor complexes in this system are required. Davis and Griffiths (1973) offered evidence that DHT-receptor preparations are able to stimulate nuclear RNA-polymerases *in vitro*. Similar data for testosterone–receptor complexes are lacking.

IX. Conclusions

Both DHT and testosterone can be bound to an androgen-receptor protein in rat prostate, rat uterus, and mouse kidney cytosol. The binding of all other natural androgen metabolites to this protein is limited. All available data indicate that the binding site of the receptor in these three tissues is similar or identical. In *in vitro* experiments, metabolism, binding to high-capacity binding proteins, and other technical factors may favor receptor–testosterone or receptor–DHT complex formation. *In vivo* target cell metabolism is probably the main factor that determines which of these ligands is finally bound to the receptor. This metabolism includes not only the 5α-reductase responsible for the formation of DHT, but also several other enzymes, such as the 3α-hydroxysteroid dehydrogenases which may favor or inhibit the accumulation of DHT (Verhoeven, 1974). Differences in the ability of various target tissues to use different precursors for the production of DHT or testosterone merit further investigation, as they might explain the differences in the relative activity of various androgens in different organs. Similar discrepancies in steroid transformation between differentiated cells of a particular tissue might even account for qualitative differences in the androgen responses to different compounds. Whether testosterone itself is an active hormone at the cellular level remains unclear. However, it is tempting to speculate that the predominant binding of an androgen with a higher dissociation rate, such as testosterone, in tissues outside the genital tract is one of the mechanisms that limit the androgen response in these tissues.

ACKNOWLEDGMENTS

G. Verhoeven is Aspirant of the Belgian Research Foundation (NFWO) and recipient of a Biomedical Fellowship of the Population Council of New York. The authors wish to thank Dr. Jean D. Wilson for stimulating discussion of the manuscript.

REFERENCES

Adachi, K., and Kano, M. (1972). *Steroids* 19, 567.
Anderson, K. M., and Liao, S. (1968). *Nature (London)* 219, 277.
Bardin, C. W., Bullock, L. P., Sherins, R. J., Mowszowicz, I., and Blackburn, W. R. (1973). *Recent Progr. Horm. Res.* 29, 65.
Baulieu, E. E., Jung, I., Blondeau, J. P., and Robel, P. (1971). *Advan. Biosci.* 7, 179–191.
Baum, M. J., and Vreeburg, J. T. M. (1973). *Science* 182, 283.
Becker, H., Grabosch, E., Hoffman, C., and Voigt, K. D. (1973). *Acta Endocrinol. (Copenhagen)* 73, 407.
Blaquier, J. A. (1971). *Biochem. Biophys. Res. Commun.* 45, 1076.
Blondeau, J. P., and Corpéchot, C. (1974). *J. Steroid Biochem.* 5, 332 (abstr.).
Bruchovsky, N. (1971). *Endocrinology* 89, 1212.
Bruchovsky, N. (1972). *Biochem. J.* 127, 561.
Bruchovsky, N., and Wilson, J. D. (1968). *J. Biol. Chem.* 243, 2012.
Bullock, L. P., and Bardin, C. W. (1972). *J. Clin. Endocrinol. Metab.* 35, 935.
Bullock, L. P., and Bardin, C. W. (1974). *Endocrinology* 94, 746.
Bullock, L. P., and Bardin, C. W. (1975). *Steroids* 25, 107.

Bullock, L. P., Bardin, C. W., and Ohno, S. (1971). *Biochem. Biophys. Res. Commun.* **44,** 1537.

Castañeda, E., and Liao, S. (1975). *In* "Methods in Enzymology" (B. W. O'Malley and J. G. Hardman, eds.), Vol. 36, p. 52. Academic Press, New York.

Cavallero, C., and Ofner, P. (1967). *Acta Endocrinol. (Copenhagen)* **55,** 131.

Danzo, B. J., Orgebin-Crist, M.-C., and Toft, D. O. (1973). *Endocrinology* **92,** 310.

Davies, P., and Griffiths, K. (1973). *Biochem. Biophys. Res. Commun.* **53,** 373.

De Moor, P., Verhoeven, G., and Heyns, W. (1975). *J. Steroid Biochem.* **6,** 437.

Dorfman, R. I., and Dorfman, A. S. (1963). *Acta Endocrinol. (Copenhagen)* **42,** 209.

Dorfman, R. I., and Shipley, R. A., eds. (1956). "Androgens." Wiley, New York.

Dubé, J. Y., and Tremblay, R. R. (1974). *Endocrinology* **95,** 1105.

Fang, S., and Liao, S. (1971). *J. Biol. Chem.* **246,** 16.

Giannopoulos, G. (1971). *Biochem. Biophys. Res. Commun.* **44,** 943.

Giannopoulos, G. (1973). *J. Biol. Chem.* **248,** 1004.

Giorgi, E. P., Stewart, J. C., Grant, J. K., and Scott, R. (1971). *Biochem. J.* **123,** 41.

Gloyna, R. E., and Wilson, J. D. (1969). *J. Clin. Endocrinol. Metab.* **29,** 970.

Gloyna, R. E., Siiteri, P. K., and Wilson, J. D. (1970). *J. Clin. Invest.* **49,** 1746.

Goldstein, J. L., and Wilson, J. D. (1972). *J. Clin. Invest.* **51,** 1647.

Gonzalez-Diddi, M., Komisaruk, B., and Beyer, C. (1972). *Endocrinology* **91,** 1129.

Grossman, S. H., Kim, K. H., and Axelrod, B. (1974). *Life Sci.* **14,** 567.

Hadjian, A. J., Kowarski, A., Dickerman, H. W., and Migeon, C. J. (1974). *J. Steroid Biochem.* **5,** 346 (abstr.).

Hansson, V. (1972). *Steroids* **20,** 575.

Hansson, V., Djöseland, O., Reusch, E., Attramadal, A., and Torgersen, O. (1973). *Steroids* **22,** 19.

Hasson, V., McLean, W. S., Smith, A. A., Tindall, D. J., Weddington, S. C., Nayfeh, S. N., French, F. S., and Ritzén, E. M. (1974). *Steroids* **23,** 823.

Heyns, W. (1974). *J. Steroid Biochem.* **5,** 347 (abstr.).

Horst, H. J., Dennis, M., Kaufmann, J., and Voigt, K. D. (1974). *Acta Endocrinol. (Copenhagen), Suppl.* **184,** 42 (abstr.).

Huggins, C., Jensen, E. V., and Cleveland, A. S. (1954). *J. Exp. Med.* **100,** 225.

Imperato-McGinley, J., Guerrero, L., Gautier, T., and Peterson, R. E. (1974). *Science* **186,** 1213.

Jouan, P., Samperez, S., and Thieulant, M. L. (1973). *J. Steroid Biochem.* **4,** 65.

Jung, I., and Baulieu, E. E. (1971). *Biochimie* **53,** 807.

Jung, I., and Baulieu, E. E. (1972). *Nature (London), New Biol.* **237,** 24.

Kappas, A., Bradlow, H. L., Gillette, P. N., and Gallagher, T. F. (1972). *J. Exp. Med.* **136,** 1042.

Kato, J., and Onouchi, T. (1973). *Endocrinol. Jap.* **20,** 429.

Kelch, R. P., Lindholm, U. B., and Jaffe, R. B. (1971). *J. Clin. Endocrinol. Metab.* **32,** 449.

Kochakian, C. D. (1946). *Vitam. Horm. (New York)* **4,** 255.

Krieg, M., Steins, P., Szalay, R., and Voigt, K. D. (1974a). *J. Steroid Biochem.* **5,** 87.

Krieg, M., Szalay, R., and Voigt, K. D. (1974b). *J. Steroid Biochem.* **5,** 453.

Lasnitzki, I., Franklin, H. R., and Wilson, J. D. (1974). *J. Endocrinol.* **60,** 81.

Lesser, B., and Bruchovsky, N. (1973). *Biochim. Biophys. Acta* **308,** 426.

Liao, S., and Fang, S. (1969). *Vitam. Horm. (New York)* **27,** 17.

Mainwaring, W. I. P. (1969). *J. Endocrinol.* **45**, 531.
Mainwaring, W. I. P., and Peterken, B. M. (1971). *Biochem. J.* **125**, 285.
Moore, R. J., and Wilson, J. D. (1973). *Endocrinology* **93**, 581.
Naftolin, F., Ryan, K. J., and Petro, Z. (1971). *J. Clin. Endocrinol Metab.* **33**, 368.
Ohno, S., Dofuku, R., and Tettenborn, U. (1971). *Clin. Genet.* **2**, 128.
Ritzén, E. M., Nayfeh, S. N., French, F. S., and Aronin, P. A. (1972). *Endocrinology* **91**, 116.
Robel, P., Lasnitzki, I., and Baulieu, E. E. (1971). *Biochimie* **53**, 81.
Robel, P., Corpéchot, C., and Baulie, E. E. (1973). *FEBS (Fed. Eur. Biochem. Soc.) Lett.* **33**, 218.
Robel, P., Blondeau, J. P., and Baulieu, E. E. (1974). *Biochim. Biophys. Acta* **373**, 1.
Schweikert, H. U., Milewich, L., and Wilson, J. D. (1975). *J. Clin. Endocrinol. Metab.* **40**, 413.
Siiteri, P. K., and Wilson, J. D. (1970). *J. Clin. Invest.* **49**, 1737.
Siiteri, P. K., and Wilson, J. D. (1974). *J. Clin. Endocrinol. Metab.* **38**, 113.
Stern, J .M., and Eisenfeld, A. J. (1969). *Science* **166**, 233.
Sullivan, J. N., and Strott, C. A. (1973). *J. Biol. Chem.* **218**, 3202.
Swank, R. T., Paigen, K., and Ganschow, R. E. (1973). *J. Mol. Biol.* **81**, 225.
Valladares, L., and Minguell, J. (1975). *Steroids* **25**, 13.
Verhoeven, G. (1974). "A Comparative Study of the Androgen Receptor Apparatus in Rodents." Acco, Leuven.
Voigt, W., and Hsia, S. L. (1973). *Endocrinology* **92**, 1216.
Walsh, P. C., Madden, J. D., Harrod, M. J., Goldstein, J. L., MacDonald, P. C., and Wilson, J. D. (1974). *N. Engl. J. Med.* **291**, 944.
Wilson, J. D. (1973). *Endocrinology* **92**, 1192.
Wilson, J. D., and Gloyna, R. E. (1970). *Recent Progr. Horm. Res.* **26**, 309.
Wilson, J. D., and Goldstein, J. L. (1972). *J. Biol. Chem.* **247**, 7342.
Wilson, J. D., and Lasnitzki, I. (1971). *Endocrinology* **89**, 659.
Wilson, J. D., and Walker, J. D. (1969). *J. Clin. Invest.* **48**, 371.

DISCUSSION

E. Diczfalusy: Do you find a testosterone receptor in pituitary tissue?

G. Verhoeven: Personally, we did not investigate the pituitary gland, although this is obviously a very interesting target tissue. P. Jouan, S. Samperes and M. L. Thieulant [*J. Steroid Biochem.* **4**, 65 (1973)] have published evidence for a similar protein in rat hypophysis.

I. Mainwaring: Is there any obvious difference in methodology between your own work and that of G. Giannopoulos [*J. Biol. Chem.* **248**, 1004 (1973)] on the testosterone receptor in rat uterus? Unlike yourself, he finds that cyproterone acetate cannot compete for the high-affinity binding sites in this female reproductive organ.

G. Verhoeven: As I mentioned, this work has been done by Dr. Heyns (*J. Steroid Biochem,* in press) in our laboratory. As far as I know, the methods used were very similar. In any event, he had no difficulty in showing the competitive activity of cyproterone acetate on the rat uterus receptor.

K. B. Eik-Nes: May I ask Dr. Voigt or Dr. Baulieu whether they have observed metabolism of T to DHT and the 3α- and 3β-diols by the levator ani muscle *in vivo* or *in vitro*. We published such conversion in 1972. However, the rate of metabolism of T to DHT was minute in levator ani from rats *in vitro*.

K.-D. Voigt: In levator ani muscle, practically no 5α-reduction of testosterone occurs; i.e., testosterone itself is bound to the receptor [M. Krieg, R. Szalay, and K. D. Voigt, *J. Steroid Biochem.* **5,** 453 (1974)]. In addition, my co-worker Dr. Krieg also has found evidence for an androgen receptor in peripheral muscle.

E. E. Baulieu: I agree completely with the data and conclusions that Dr. Verhoeven has presented. I may add some observations concerning the androgen receptor of skeletal muscle (from the thigh) which was discovered recently by G. Michel in the rat. When incubating androstanolone in skeletal muscle homogenate cytosol, as indeed with levator ani muscle homogenate cytosol, one gets evidence for a rapid conversion of the steroid into androstanediol(s), even in a standard 0.1–4°C 2-hour incubation. Therefore, the same considerations for the study of the reciprocal affinity of testosterone and androstanolone to the receptor as described by Dr. Verhoeven apply to this system. Indeed, the findings published by I. Jung and E. E. Baulieu [*Nature (London), New Biol.* **237,** 24 (1972)] concerning the levator ani in the rat are also relevant to the same considerations.

Androgen Binding and Transport in Testis and Epididymis

E. M. RITZÉN AND L. HAGENÄS

Pediatric Endocrinology Unit, Karolinska Sjukhuset, Stockholm, Sweden

V. HANSSON AND S. C. WEDDINGTON
Institute for Pathology, Rikshospitalet, Oslo, Norway

AND

F. S. FRENCH AND S. N. NAYFEH

Departments of Pediatrics and Biochemistry, and Laboratories for Reproductive Biology, University of North Carolina, Chapel Hill, North Carolina

I. INTRODUCTION

Along with the prostate and the seminal vesicles, the epididymis has long been known to be heavily dependent on androgenic hormones for its normal gross appearance (see review by Hamilton, 1975). The testis, however, being the major source of circulating androgenic hormones, long escaped detection as a major androgen-responsive tissue. The present paper will review some recent evidence indicating that both testis and epididymis are completely dependent on high concentrations of androgens for their normal function and that both contain *intra*cellular receptors, characteristic of androgen responsive tissues. Much of the information on androgen actions in these organs has been uncovered with the aid of a specific product of the Sertoli cells, androgen-binding protein (ABP), which seems to serve as an *extra*cellular carrier of androgenic hormones.

II. The Testis as a Target Organ for Androgens

The observations that most androgenic hormones not only stem from the testis, but also exert direct actions on testicular events, were made during studies on the regulation of spermatogenesis. Walsh *et al.* (1934) noted that large amounts of androgens given to hypophysectomized rats could maintain spermatogenesis in the absence of both interstitial cell-stimulating hormone (ICSH = LH) and follicle-stimulating hormone (FSH). However, spermatogenesis could not be reinitiated in testes that had regressed for some time after hypophysectomy before treatment was begun. Much of the later controversy on this subject depends on the varying, but mostly too small, doses of testosterone administered. It was finally recognized that very large doses must be given to the hypophysec-tomized rat in order to keep the peri- and intratubular concentrations of testosterone up close to the normal. Owing to both the intimate association between the Leydig cells and the seminiferous tubules, and to the presence of androgen concentrating mechanisms in the seminiferous tubules, the rete testis fluid and the testicular lymph contains 10–30 times higher concentrations of testosterone than peripheral plasma. Doses of testosterone that are sufficient to maintain normal weight of accessory sex organs suppress the release of gonadotropins by the pituitary, resulting in inhibited testosterone secretion by the Leydig cells and insufficient androgen concentrations in and around the seminiferous tubules.

Further evidence for the androgen dependence of spermatogenesis may be obtained from studies of the androgen insensitivity syndrome (testicular feminization, Tfm). In humans as well as in rats with this syndrome, spermatogenesis is arrested at the primary spermatocyte level, even if the testes are transplanted from their cryptorchid position (Chan *et al.*, 1969). In rats with this syndrome, radioautographs prepared after injection of ^{3}H-labeled testosterone show no nuclear accumulation of radioactivity in the tubules in contrast to control rats. Also, Tfm rats showed no retention of radioactivity in the Leydig cells (M. Sar, W. E. Stumpf, F. S. French, and V. Hansson, unpublished),

III. The Epididymis as a Target Organ for Androgens

The epididymis is completely dependent on androgenic hormones for its development during fetal life, as well as for its function in the mature male (see the recent reviews by Hamilton, 1975; Orgebin-Crist *et al.*, 1975). Thus, in the androgen insensitivity syndrome, this organ is virtually absent. Also, in the castrated rat, the epididymis has been shown to require more androgenic hormones than other male accessory sex organs to maintain its normal weight and function (Prasad et al., 1973). Orgebin-Crist et al., (1975) have conclusively demonstrated that the process of maturation of spermatozoa in the caput epididymis is strictly dependent on androgenic hormones. These androgens may reach the epididymis in several ways; by way of the arterial blood, by the testicular fluid entering through the efferent ducts, and possibly by the testicular lymph. Judging from the lack of effects of efferent duct ligation on sperm maturation in caput epididymis, Orgebin-Crist et al., (1975) believed that the androgens entering the epididymis via the rete testis fluid are of minor importance. However, there is evidence that the androgens of the testicular fluid may be contributing to the stimulation of the epididymis in states of relative androgen deficiency: Bartke et al. (1975) recently reported that after hypophysectomy the concentration of testosterone in the rat rete testis fluid could be maintained close to normal by administration of pregnenolone. At the same time, the testosterone concentrations in testicular venous and heart blood were grossly subnormal. In these experiments the epididymal weight was significantly higher than in nontreated hypophysectomized rats, while prostate and seminal vesicles were atrophic, indicating a selective stimulation of epididymis through the contents of the testicular fluid. The efferent duct fluid may be an alternative route of "emergency" supply of androgens to the epididymis, securing the function of the epididymis, if other routes go wrong.

IV. Androgen Receptors in Testis and Epididymis

From the above it can be concluded that both testis and epididymis show physiological response to androgenic hormones. Over the last few years, the concept has developed that such cells should also contain androgen receptors, and show translocation and binding of the receptor–hormone complex to the cell nucleus. Both testis and epididymis have proved to contain cytoplasmic as well as nuclear androgen-binding proteins, similar to those found in other androgen-responsive tissues. These so-called receptor molecules should not be confused with the testicular androgen binding protein (ABP) that will be described later in this section. ·

Cytoplasmic and nuclear androgen receptors have been identified in epididydimes of castrated rats (Blaquier, 1971; Tindall et al., 1972, 1975; Blaquier and Calandra, 1973; Hansson et al., 1973b) using several different methods (see Table I). The cytoplasmic receptors show the character-

TABLE I

COMPARISON BETWEEN SOME PHYSICAL CHARACTERISTICS OF THE CYTOPLASMIC
ANDROGEN RECEPTORS IN TESTIS, EPIDIDYMIS, AND PROSTATE WITH
TESTICULAR ANDROGEN-BINDING PROTEIN (ABP)

| Characteristic | Cytoplasmic receptors[a] | | | ABP[a] |
	Testis	Epididymis	Prostate	
Sedimentation coefficient (S)		4 and 7–10		4.6
Stokes radius (Å)		>80		47
Molecular weight		>200,000		~87,000
PAGE, 3.5% gels (R_f)		0.4–0.5		0.75
PAGE, 7.5% gels (R_f)		0.25		0.5
Dissociation rate of bound androgen ($t_{1/2}$)		0° > 2 days		0° ~ 6 min
Heating at 50°, 30 minutes	–	–	–	+
Sulfhydryl agent PCMPS, 1 mM	–	–	–	+
Charcoal	–	–	–	+
Protease	–	–	–	–

[a] –, Binding destroyed; +, binding intact. PAGE, polyacrylamide gel electrophoresis; PCMPS, p-chloromercuriphenyl sulfuric acid.

istic formation of aggregates at low ionic strength, sedimenting at 6–10 S in sucrose gradient centrifugations. It is excluded from G-200 Sephadex gels, but enters as a slow-moving band into 3.5% acrylamide-agarose gels during electrophoresis. It is heat labile and is destroyed by sulfhydryl reagents (Hansson et al., 1973b; Tindall et al., 1972, 1975). All these features are characteristic for the androgen receptor in the prostate, but different from those of ABP (Table I). Also, the receptors show a much slower rate of dissociation of the bound steroid than ABP [$t_{1/2}$ at 0°C more than 24 hours and 6 minutes, respectively (Tindall et al., 1975)]. The slow dissociation of the steroid from the cytoplasmic receptor is consistent with a "receptor function" that requires a stable binding during the translocation into the cell nucleus. It has been shown (Tindall et al., 1972, 1975) that binding of radioactive dihydrotestosterone to cytoplasmic receptors precedes the accumulation of the hormone in the cell nucleus, supporting the functional role of the receptor for nuclear uptake.

As in other androgen target tissues, the nuclear hormone can be extracted as a steroid-protein complex by high ionic strength buffers. The potent antiandrogen cyproterone acetate decreased nuclear uptake of radioactive hormone to the same degree as it inhibited binding to cytoplasmic receptors, also indicating the relationship between cytoplasmic receptors and binding to chromatin (Tindall et al., 1975). After injection of ^{3}H-labeled testosterone, both the unchanged hormone and ^{3}H-labeled dihydrotestosterone are found to be bound to the nuclear receptor. However, from these studies it is difficult to determine the true affinity of the receptor, since the androgen bound may be determined by the prevalent steroid metabolites in the cells.

Since there is abundant physiological and biochemical evidence that the testis is indeed an androgen-responsive tissue, those cells being the targets for androgens should also be characterized by their content of cytoplasmic androgen receptors. This may provide a clue to the identification of which specific cells in the testis are directly responsive to androgenic steroid hormones. An earlier radioautographic study (Appelgren, 1969) seemed to indicate that in the mouse intravenously administered ^{14}C-labeled testosterone was primarily localized to interstitial cells, rather than seminiferous tubules. However, tracers with low specific radioactivity were used, and the resolution of the whole-body radioautography did not permit closer identification of the cells. Later, Sar et al. (1975), using dry-mounting of freeze-dried sections, observed distinct labeling of some nuclei in the seminiferous tubules, the identity of which still has to be confirmed. No such nuclear binding was found in rats of the Stanley— Gumbreck strain (androgen insensitivity syndrome), which lack almost all metabolic effects of androgenic steroid hormones.

The natural high concentrations of testosterone and other androgens in the testis preclude studies of binding of trace amounts of labeled steroids. However, when hypophysectomized and functionally hepatectomized animals were used (to decrease both endogenous testosterone production in Leydig cells and metabolism of injected hormone in the liver), binding of radioactivity to a cytoplasmic soluble protein could be demonstrated by several methods (Hansson et al., 1974a). This binding protein, which showed physical characteristics identical to those of the cytoplasmic receptor of the epididymis and prostate (Table I), could be found in mechanically isolated seminiferous tubules. Purified nuclei from the testis were also shown to contain a salt-extractable steroid-protein complex sedimenting as a single component in sucrose gradients and excluded from Sephadex G-200. When the same study was repeated using the androgen-insensitive rat testis no cytoplasmic or nuclear binding components could be found (French, 1975). Recently Mulder et al. (1974) also showed nuclear binding of androgens in the seminiferous tubules but not in the interstitial tissue. However, injected ^{3}H-labeled testosterone has been found to be retained in Leydig cells of normal but not of Tfm rats using radioautographic methods (M. Sar, unpublished), although a specific receptor molecule is yet to be demonstrated in these cells.

The specific localization of the receptors in the different cell types of the seminiferous tubules is only partly examined. Several different cell types have to be considered—the germ cells, the Sertoli cells, and the peritubular cells. Sanborn *et al.* (1975) have presented data showing nuclear exchange of testosterone in isolated germ cell nuclei. In the uterus such exchange has been shown to represent nuclear receptor proteins (Andersson *et al.*, 1971). There is also other indirect evidence for androgen receptors in germ cells; the testes of "Sertoli-cell-only" rats contain less cytoplasmic receptor than those of germ-cell-containing control testes, when calculated per organ (F. S. French *et al.*, unpublished). Thus, germ cells may be primary targets for androgenic hormones. However, seminiferous tubules from prenatally irradiated rats that later become completely devoid of germ cells (Means and Huckins, 1974) and long-term hypophysectomized rats, where germinal cells at later stages than primary spermatocytes are absent, still contain high concentrations of androgen receptors (Wilson and Smith, 1975; Mulder *et al.*, 1974). This proves that either Sertoli cells or peritubular cells (or both) also contain the receptor molecule. The relative concentrations of receptor in the different cell types are still not established.

The steroid specificity of the androgen receptors in different organs has recently been reviewed (Bardin, 1975). In contrast to what was initially thought, judging from the pioneer work on the prostate (Unhjem *et al.*, 1969; Mainwaring, 1969; Fang *et al.*, 1969), the receptor of some organs (prostate, seminal vesicle, epididymis, preputial gland) preferentially binds dihydrotestosterone, while others bind testosterone (see Bardin, 1975, for review). After injection of ^{3}H-labeled testosterone into the hypophysectomized and functionally hepatectomized rat, both receptor-bound ^{3}H-labeled testosterone and ^{3}H-labeled dihydrotestosterone can be extracted from the testis nuclei. However, this does not *a priori* prove that the receptors are different in different organs, since the spectrum of androgens available for binding may be different. Thus, in the epididymis, there is a very rapid 5α-reduction of testosterone to dihydrotestosterone (Tindall *et al.*, 1972; Djöseland *et al.*, 1973) ; 5 minutes after injection of ^{3}H-labeled testosterone to the rat, most of the epididymal radioactivity is found to be converted to 5α-dihydrotestosterone. In the testis, 5α-reductase is present in both interstitial and tubular fractions (Rivarola and Podesta, 1972; Dorrington and Fritz, 1975; Nayfeh, 1975), although the interstitial compartment may be quantitatively most important (van der Molen, 1975). Among the tubular cells, Dorrington and Fritz (1973) found 5α-reductase activity both in Sertoli cells and spermatocytes, indicating that dihydrotestosterone may be formed from testosterone in either cell type. Furthermore, in the rabbit efferent duct fluid bathing the tubular cells dihydrotestosterone is present at a very high concentration (Guerrero *et al.*, 1975). Consequently, dihydrotestosterone seems to be available for binding by all the tubular cell types. The exact steroid specificity of the receptors has to await studies on partially purified receptors without interference by metabolism or binding to other components.

Concluding the present status of the studies on androgen receptors in the testis, all the specific cells in the tubules seem to be potential androgen target cells—the Sertoli and germ cells both seem to contain receptors. The belief that the Sertoli cell is a target cell for androgens has been supported by studies on the specific Sertoli cell product, ABP, to be reviewed below.

V. Androgen Transport and Retention within the Testis and the Epididymis

There is general agreement that the greater part of the testicular steroid synthesis occurs within the Leydig cells, although isolated seminiferous tubules have been shown to possess many of the enzymes involved in steroid metabolism (see van der Molen, 1975, for recent review). The major product of the Leydig cells is testosterone, which is rapidly released to the interstitial fluid, and then mostly carried away by the blood and lymph. However, steroid hormones also pass into the seminiferous tubules from the interstitial compartment—testosterone readily enters into the tubules, while cholesterol seems to be totally excluded (Parvinen *et al.*, 1970; Setchell, 1975). Furthermore, there seems to be a mechanism in the seminiferous tubules that specifically takes up and retains androgens. Harris and Bartke (1974) found a longer retention of testosterone in rat rete testis fluid than in the peripheral serum after hypophysectomy. Also, in hypophysectomized rats treated with testosterone propionate, testosterone seemed to be actively concentrated in the rete testis fluid, maintaining a high fluid:serum ratio.

VI. Androgen-Binding Protein (ABP) in Seminiferous Fluid and Epididymis

Paradoxically, the testicular androgen binding protein (ABP) was first identified in the epididymis (Ritzén *et al.*, 1971; Hansson and Djöseland, 1972) and only later found to originate in the testis and to be transported to the epididymis by way of the testicular efferent ducts (French and Ritzén, 1973a,b). During its passage through the epididymal tubule ABP is either taken up by the lining cells or degraded in the lumen (French and Ritzén, 1973b; Ritzén and French, 1974; Weddington et al., 1974). However, ABP is not needed for nuclear binding of androgens in the epididymis (Tindall et al., 1972). In the initial segment of the epididymis, there is a very active absorption of fluid from the lumen (Crabo, 1965), causing a further increase in the concentration of the macromulecules and spermatozoa in the lumen. Thus, the initially high concentration of ABP and its bound androgenic hormones in efferent duct fluid (4 to 8×10^{-8} M in the rat, 2.7×10^{-7} M in the rabbit; French and Ritzén, 1973b; Guerrero et al., 1975) may increase further. This is the milieu of the spermatozoa entering the epididymis. It has been shown (Voglmayr, 1971) that such high concentrations decrease the oxygen consumption by isolated spermatozoa. In the rabbit efferent duct fluid, testosterone and dihydrotestosterone are the major androgens present, but androstenedione and dehydroepiandrosterone are also present at high concentrations (Guerrero et al., 1975). A positive correlation was observed between the concentrations of ABP and testosterone and dihydrotestosterone in the individual fluids. Furthermore, there was a selective accumulation of the androgens in the fluid relative to the serum, in the same order as the binding affinities of the various steroids to ABP. This supports the view that ABP is actively influencing the pattern of androgens found in the fluid.

ABP has been characterized in both the epididymal and the testicular 105,000 g supernatants of the rat (Ritzén et al., 1973; Hansson et al., 1973a) and the rabbit (Hansson et al., 1975a), and can be distinctly separated from the cytoplasmic androgen receptors described above (Table I) (Tindall et al., 1975). ABP shows a high binding affinity to dihydrotestosterone > testosterone > 5α-androstane-3α,17β-diol, while there is no binding of androstenedione, DHEA, progesterone, or pregnenolone. Rabbit ABP has recently been purified and found to be a glycoprotein with a molecular weight of 70,000 (Weddington et al., 1975). The physical characteristics are practically identical to those of the serum testosterone-binding globulin (TBG) (Hansson et al., 1975b). In preliminary experiments, antisera raised against purified rabbit ABP cross-react immunologically with TBG (Weddington et al., 1975). This is interesting because ABP and TBG are produced in different cell types [Sertoli cells (Hagenäs et al. (1975) and probably liver] and their respective production rates are regulated in completely different ways (see below).

ABP was found to disappear from the rat testis and epididymis after hypophysectomy but could be reinduced by treatment with FSH (Hansson et al., 1974b; Vernon et al., 1974; Tindall et al., 1974). Since ABP is a specific product of the Sertoli cell, this finding is in agreement with the observations by others that the Sertoli cell seems to be a primary target for FSH in the testis (Castro *et al.*, 1972; Dorrington *et al.*, 1974; Means and Huckins, 1974; Steinberger *et al.*, 1974). For the first time, the effects of FSH can be followed by the production of a specific, biochemically defined end product. This was utilized by Means and Tindall (1975), demonstrating parallel and rapid increases in cAMP formation, RNA polymerase activity, general protein synthesis, and finally ABP synthesis following intravenous injection of FSH into the immature "Sertoli-cell-only" rat.

Testosterone acts synergistically with FSH in stimulating ABP synthesis (Hansson *et al.*, 1974b; Weddington *et al.*, 1975; Elkington *et al.*, 1975). The joint mechanism of action of the two hormones on the Sertoli cell is not yet clear. In a manner similar to the effect of androgens on spermatogenesis, androgens given immediately after hypophysectomy can maintain ABP production, while testosterone given to rats whose testes have regressed after the hypophysectomy is ineffective in stimulating ABP secretion. On the contrary, FSH is always capable of increasing ABP production and secretion, even in the regressed testis. LH, given at sufficiently high doses, also stimulates ABP synthesis, probably indirectly through increased Leydig cell formation of testosterone. Both LH and testosterone stimulate ABP production by whole testicular minces *in vitro* (Ritzén *et al.*, 1975) whereas isolated Sertoli cells in tissue culture apparently do not respond to LH (Fritz *et al.*, 1975).

VII. Conclusions

The testis and epididymis contain two different species of proteins, which both show high binding affinity to androgenic hormones—the mostly *extra*cellular testicular androgen-binding protein (ABP) and the *intra*cellular cytoplasmic androgen receptor. ABP, which is produced by Sertoli cells and then secreted into the lumen of the seminiferous tubules, may serve to increase the supply of androgenic hormones for the germ cells. The cytoplasmic receptor is present in Sertoli cells, but may also be a component of germinal cells, indicating that these cells are natural targets for androgenic hormones. ABP, being hitherto the only well characterized specific product of the Sertoli cells, may be used as an instrument to study the regulation of Sertoli cell function. Thus ABP production is specifically stimulated by FSH, while androgens may maintain Sertoli cell function even after removal of FSH by hypophysectomy, and androgens also potentiate the effects of FSH in the hypophysectomized rat.

The present studies show that secretory proteins may simulate steroid receptors in having both high-affinity and low-capacity steroid hormone-binding activites. In this way, they may facilitate transport from one cell to another and from one organ to another. Whether such extracellular binding proteins exist in other organs remains to be demonstrated.

ACKNOWLEDGMENTS

Supported by grants from the Swedish Medical Research Council (project 3168), WHO (project H9/181/183), the Norwegian Research Council for Sciences and Humanities, Nordic Insulin Foundation, Norwegian Agency for Int. Development, and the NIH (project HDO 4466). Gonadotropins were kindly donated by the NIAAMD.

REFERENCES

Andersson, J., Clark, J. H., and Peck, E. J. (1971). *Biochem. J.* **126**, 561.

Appelgren, L. E. (1969). *Acta Endocrinol. (Copenhagen)* **62**, 505.

Bardin, W. (1975). *In* "Hormonal Regulation of Spermatogenesis" (F. S. French *et al.*, eds.), pp. 237–256. Plenum, New York.

Bartke, A., Harris, M. E., and Voglmayr, J. K. (1975). *In* "Hormonal Regulation of Spermatogenesis" (F. S. French *et al.*, eds.), pp. 197–212. Plenum, New York.

Blaquier, J. A. (1971). *Biochem. Biophys. Res. Commun.* **45**, 1076.

Blaquier, J. A., and Calandra, R. S. (1973). *Endocrinology* **93**, 51.

Castro, A. E., Alonso, A., and Mancini, R. E. (1972). *J. Endocrinol.* **52**, 129.

Chan, F., Allison, J. E., Stanley, A. J., and Gumbreck, L. G. (1969). *Fert. Steril.* **20**, 482.

Crabo, B. (1965). *Acta Vet. Scand., Suppl.* **6**, 5.

Djöseland, O., Hansson, V., and Haugen, H. N. (1973). *Steroids* **21**, 773.

Dorrington, J. H., and Fritz, I. B. (1973). *Biochem. Biophys. Res. Commun.* **54**, 1425.

Dorrington, J. H., and Fritz, I. B. (1975). *Endocrinology* **96**, 879.

Dorrington, J. H., Roller, N. F., and Fritz, I. B. (1974). *In* "Hormone Binding and Target Cell Activation in the Testis" (M.-L. Dufau and A. R. Means, eds.), pp. 237–241. Plenum, New York.

Elkington, J. S. H., Sanborn, B. M., and Steinberger, E. (1975). *Mol. Cell. Endocrinol.* **2**, 157.

Fang, S., Anderson, K. M., and Liao, S. (1969). *J. Biol. Chem.* **244**, 6584.

French, F. S. (1975). *In* "Hormonal Regulation of Spermatogenesis" (F. S. French *et al.*, eds.). Plenum, New York.

French, F. S., and Ritzén, E. M. (1973a). *J. Reprod. Fert.* **32**, 479.

French, F. S., and Ritzén, E. M. (1973b). *Endocrinology* **95**, 88.

Fritz, I. B., Louis, G., Griswold, M., Rommerts, F., and Dorrington, J. H. (1975). *In* "Hormonal Regulation of Spermatogenesis" (F. S. French *et al.*, eds.), pp. 367–382. Plenum, New York.

Guerrero, R., Ritzén, E. M., Purvis, K., French, F. S., and Hansson, V. (1975). *In* "Hormonal Regulation of Spermatogenesis" (F. S. French *et al.*, eds.), pp. 213–222. Plenum, New York.

Hagenäs, L., Ritzén, E. M., Plöen, L., Hansson, V., French, F. S., and Nayfeh, S. N. (1975). *Mol. Cell. Endocrinol.* **2**, 339.

Hamilton, D. W. (1975). *In* "Handbook of Physiology" (Amer. Physiol. Soc., J. Field, ed.), Sect. 7, Vol. V, pp. 259–301. Williams & Wilkins, Baltimore, Maryland.

Hansson, V., and Djöseland, O. (1972). *Acta Endocrinol. (Copenhagen)* **71**, 614.

Hansson, V., Djöseland, O., Reusch, E., Attramadal, A., and Torgersen, O. (1973a). *Steroids* **21**, 457.

Hansson, V., Djöseland, O., Reusch, E., Attramadal, A., and Torgersen, O. (1973b). *Steroids* **22**, 19.

Hansson, V., McLean, W. S., Smith, A. A., Tindall, D. J., Weddington, S. C., Nayfeh, S. N., French, F. S., and Ritzén, E. M. (1974a). *Steroids* **23**, 823.

Hansson, V., Trygstad, O., French, F. S., McLean, W. S., Smith, A. A., Tindall, D. J., Weddington, S. C., Petrusz, P., Nayfeh, S. N., and Ritzén, E. M. (1974b). *Nature (London)* **250**, 387.

Hansson, V., Ritzén, E. M., French, F. S., and Nayfeh, S. N. (1975a). *Mol. Cell Endocrinol.* **3**, 1.

Hansson, V., Weddington, S. C., Naess, O., Attramadal, A., French, F. S., Kotite, N., Nayfeh, S. N., Ritzén, E. M., and Hagenäs, L. (1975b). *In* "Hormonal Regulation of Spermatogenesis" (F. S. French *et al.*, eds.), pp. 323–336. Plenum, New York.

Harris, M. E., and Bartke, A. (1974). *Endocrinology* **95**, 701.

Mainwaring, W. I. P. (1969). *J. Endocrinol.* **44**, 323.

Means, A. R., and Huckins, E. (1974). *In* "Hormone Binding and Target Cell Activation in the Testis" (M.-L. Dufau and A. R. Means, eds.), pp. 145–166. Plenum, New York.

Means, A. R., and Tindall, D. J. (1975). *In* "Hormonal Regulation of Spermatogenesis" (F. S. French *et al.*, eds.), pp. 383–398. Plenum, New York.

Mulder, E., van Beurden-Lamers, W. M. O., DeBoer, W., Mechzelsen, M. J., and van der Molen, H. J. (1974). *FEBS (Fed. Eur. Biochem. Soc.) Lett.* **47**, 209.

Nayfeh, S. N. (1975). *In* "Hormonal Regulation of Spermatogenesis" (F. S. French *et al.*, eds.). Plenum, New York.

Orgebin-Crist, M.-C., Danzo, B. J., and Davies, J. (1975). *In* "Handbook of Physiology" (Amer. Physiol. Soc. J. Field, ed.), Sect. 7, Vol. V, pp. 319–338. Williams & Wilkins, Baltimore, Maryland.

Parvinen, M., Hurme, P., and Niemi, M. (1970). *Endocrinology* **87**, 1082.

Prasad, M. R. N., Rajalakshmi, M., Gupta, G., and Karhwin, T. (1973). *J. Reprod. Fert., Suppl.* **18**, 215.

Ritzén, E. M., and French, F. S. (1974). *J. Steroid Biochem.* **5**, 151.

Ritzén, E. M., Nayfeh, S. N., French, F. S., and Dobbins, M. C. (1971). *Endocrinology* **89**, 143.

Ritzén, E. M., Dobbins, M. C., Tindall, D. J., French, F. S., and Nayfeh, S. N. (1973). *Steroids* **21**, 593.

Ritzén, E. M., Hagenäs, L., Hansson, V., and French, F. S. (1975). *In* "Hormonal Regulation of Spermatogenesis" (F. S. French *et al.*, eds.), pp. 353–366. Plenum, New York.

Rivarola, M. A., and Podesta, E. J. (1972). *Endocrinology* **90**, 618.

Sanborn, B. M., Elkington, J. S. H., and Steinberger, A. (1975). *In* "Hormonal Regulation of Spermatogenesis" (F. S. French *et al.*, eds.), pp. 292–310. Plenum, New York.

Sar, M., Stumpf, W. E., and French, F. S. (1975). *In* "Hormonal Regulation of Spermatogenesis" (F. S. French *et al.*, eds.), pp. 311–320. Plenum, New York.

Setchell, B. (1975). *In* "Hormonal Regulation of Spermatogenesis" (F. S. French *et al.*, eds.), pp. 223–234. Plenum, New York.

Steinberger, A., Tanki, K. J., and Siegal, B. (1974). *In* "Hormone Binding and Target Cell Activation in the Testis" (M.-L. Dufau and A. R. Means, eds.), pp. 177–191. Plenum, New York.

Tindall, D. J., French, F. S., and Nayfeh, S. N. (1972). *Biochem. Biophys. Res. Commun.* **49**, 1391.

Tindall, D. J., Schrader, W. T., and Means, A. R. (1974). *In* "Hormone Binding and Target Cell Activation in the Testis" (M.-L. Dufau and A. R. Means, eds.), pp. 167–175. Plenum, New York.

Tindall, D. J., Hansson, V., McLean, W. S., Ritzén, E. M., Nayfeh, S. N., and French, F. S. (1975). *Mol. Cell. Endocrinol.* **3**, 83.

Unhjem, O., Tveter, K. J., and Aakvaag, A. (1969). *Acta Endocrinol. (Copenhagen)* **62**, 153.

Van der Molen, H. (1975). *In* "Hormonal Regulation of Spermatogenesis" (F. S. French *et al.*, eds.), pp. 3–24. Plenum, New York.

Vernon, R. G., Kopec, B., and Fritz, I. B. (1974). *Mol. Cell. Endocrinol.* **1**, 167.

Voglmayr, J. K. (1971). *Acta Endocrinol. (Copenhagen)* **68**, 793.

Walsh, E. L., Cuyler, W. K., and McCullagh, D. R. (1934). *Amer. J. Physiol.* **107**, 508.

Weddington, S. C. (1975). *In* "Hormonal Regulation of Spermatogenesis" (F. S. French *et al.*, eds.), pp. 433–452. Plenum, New York.

Weddington, S. C., McLean, W. S., Nayfeh, S. N., French, F. S., Hansson, V., and Ritzén, E. M. (1974). *Steroids* **24**, 123.

Weddington, S. C., Hansson, V., French, F. S., Nayfeh, S. N., Ritzén, E. M., and Hagenäs, L. (1975). *Nature (London)* **254**, 145.

Wilson, E. M., and Smith, A. A. (1975). *In* "Hormonal Regulation of Spermatogenesis" (F. S. French *et al.*, eds.), pp. 281–286. Plenum, New York.

DISCUSSION

E. Diczfalusy: Could one attempt to relate your most interesting findings to the concept of the "blood–testis barrier"? What is the testosterone concentration in the tubular fluid in the "Sertoli-cell-only-rat," or in hypophysectomized rats treated with very high doses of testosterone propionate?

M. Ritzen: The findings are compatible with the blood–testis barrier. Actually, Tindall and co-workers have shown that the start of secretion of ABP into the epididymis is temporally correlated with the maturation of the blood–testis barrier. ABP that is produced in the Sertoli cells is not found in testicular lymph or in testicular venous plasma of the rat.

We have no information on the concentration of steroids in the seminiferous fluid of the Sertoli-cell-only rat. Harris and Bartke have shown that when hypophysectomized rats are treated with very large doses of testosterone, the testosterone concentration in the rete testis fluid is still higher than in serum, demonstrating the androgen concentrating mechanism in the seminiferous tubules.

M. B. Lipsett: We have been impressed by the homologies between the granulosa cell and the Sertoli cell and therefore looked for ABP in the rat granulosa cell, and it is there.

G. Verhoeven: Since ABP is regulated both by androgens and by FSH, I wonder whether you have any data on the presence of this protein in the testis of animals with testicular feminization?

M. Ritzén: Yes, ABP is present in the testes of the androgen-insensitive rat (Stanley–Gumbreck strain), but the production rate is hard to measure owing to the lack of epididymis and efferent ducts in these rats. Consequently, the high levels of ABP may be a result of accumulation, even if the rate of ABP production is decreased.

K. B. Eik-Nes: Since FSH and high doses of T will augment ABP, do you have any information on how this increase is brought on mechanistically? You appear to have a most interesting system for investigating the action of a steroid and a peptide hormone on the same cell, giving the same end product—ABP.

M. Ritzén: We are currently working on precisely this problem, but we are not yet ready to offer any explanation.

H. G. Williams-Ashman: Is there any evidence that ABP, in the form in which you isolate it, is comprised of subunits?

M. Ritzén: No, so far we do not have conclusive evidence for ABP subunits, but analysis of purified rabbit ABP, carried out by Drs. Weddington and Hansson, indicate that ABP contains 20% carbohydrates. Studies of purified rabbit ABP have also shown immunological identity with rabbit TBG, while the carbohydrate moieties seem to be different.

Androgen Receptors and Androgen-Dependent Initiation of Protein Synthesis in the Prostate

S. LIAO, J. L. TYMOCZKO, E. CASTAÑEDA, AND T. LIANG

The Ben May Laboratory for Cancer Research and
The Department of Biochemistry, University of Chicago, Chicago, Illinois

I. Introduction

Since 1967, much of our study has been devoted to elucidation of the receptor mechanism involved in the action of 5α-dihydrotestosterone (DHT), an androgen more potent than testosterone in promoting the growth and function of the prostate (Huggins and Mainzer, 1957). Since other participants in this symposium will discuss various aspects of the androgen receptor, this article will be limited to certain selected aspects of our own recent work on this subject and to some of our new findings, which may provide better understanding of the molecular basis of androgen action in the rat ventral prostate. Comprehensive reviews of our earlier work and related topics are available elsewhere (Liao and Fang, 1969; Liao and Liang, 1974; Liao, 1974, 1975a,b).

II. Multiple Forms of Androgen-Receptor Complexes

A. Cellular Localization

The cytosol fraction of ventral prostate contains at least two proteins that bind DHT preferentially over other natural steroid hormones (Fang and Liao, 1971). One of them (β-protein) binds DHT specifically and very tightly (K_a: $> 10^{11}$ M^{-1}). At low concentrations of DHT, the androgen binds exclusively to this high-affinity and low-capacity protein and forms a complex that we have called complex II. If DHT is present in excess at the high-affinity binding sites, the androgen may bind to another low-affinity (K_a: 10^7 M^{-1}) and high-capacity protein (α-protein) and form a complex that we have termed complex I (Liao and Fang, 1970; Fang and Liao, 1971). The low-affinity protein also binds estradiol but not cortisol. These two types of complexes (or proteins) can be separated easily by ammonium sulfate fractionation or by Sephadex gel chromatographic techniques. The most significant difference between the two DHT-binding proteins (Table I) is that only the complex II, but not complex I, can eventually (after undergoing transformation to a new complex, complex II-TR) be retained by the prostate nuclear chromatin. Some of the high-affinity androgen-binding proteins that are fractionated together with complex II are also unable to become the precursor for the nuclear complex. It is not clear whether these are altered forms of complex II or whether they represent another class of biologically important androgen-binding proteins.

The cytoplasmic particulate (microsomal) fraction of the prostate also contains a specific high-affinity and low-capacity DHT-binding protein that can be solubilized by 0.4 M KCl (Liao and Fang, 1970; Liao *et al.*, 1971). The microsomal protein is probably identical with the cytosol β-protein in its steroid specificity, heat sensitivity, sedimentation properties, and ability to be eventually translocated into prostate cell nuclei. This protein may be responsible for the retention of DHT by the microsomal fraction of prostate cells (cf. Kowarski *et al.*, 1969).

The prostate cell nuclei of castrated rats contain very few proteins that can bind steroid hormones (including DHT) specifically and tightly. However, a DHT-protein complex can be detected in the cell nuclei shortly after testosterone or DHT is injected into the castrated rats (Bruchovsky and Wilson, 1968; Anderson and Liao, 1968; Liao, 1968). Several properties of the nuclear complex are very similar to those of the complex transformed from the cytoplasmic complex II (see Section V). Various *in vivo* and *in vitro* cell-free studies have shown that the

TABLE I

5α-Dihydrotestosterone Binding Proteins in Rat Ventral Prostate

Cellular localization	Binding protein	DHT-bound complex	Properties
Cytoplasm Soluble (cytosol)	α-Protein	Complex I, 3.5 S	Binds DHT, testosterone, estradiol, but not cortisol; K_a: 10^7 M^{-1}, stable at 40°C, cannot bind to nuclei or RNP; precipitated by ammonium sulfate at 55–70% saturation
	β-Protein	Complex II, 3.8 S	Binds DHT and some potent synthetic androgens but not androstanediols, estradiol, or cortisol; K_a: 10^{12} M^{-1}, unstable at 40°C, can be converted to nuclear form; precipitated by ammonium sulfate at 0–35% saturation
	β-Protein	Complex II-TR, 3.0 S	Transformed from complex II; all properties similar to complex II; can bind to nuclei and RNP
	β'-Protein	Complex II', 3.0 S	Properties similar to complex II but cannot bind to nuclei or RNP
Membrane-bound (microsomal)	β-Protein	Complex II-TR, 3.0 S	Can be solubilized by 0.4 M KCl; properties similar to the cytosol complex II-TR; can bind to nuclei and RNP
Nucleus Intact	β-Protein	Complex II-TR, 3.0 S	Properties similar to the cytosol complex II-TR; can bind to nuclei and RNP; can be dissociated from chromatin by 0.4 M KCl; probably associated with acidic nuclear protein that can also be extracted by 0.4 M KCl
Disrupted	β-Protein	Complex II-TR, (aggregated)	Some of the complexes bind factitiously to histones and denatured DNA and cannot be dissociated from the chromatin by 0.4 M KCl

nuclear complex originates in the cytoplasm and is transferred into the nucleus only after it interacts and binds DHT (Liao and Fang, 1970; Fang and Liao, 1971).

It is now generally agreed that β-protein has various properties characteristic of a cellular androgen-receptor in a target cell. In accordance with the terminology employed by Jensen *et al.* (1974), who called the uterine estrogen-receptor an *estrophilin*, this prostate androgen-receptor may be called an *androphilin*. The specific DHT-binding protein has been found in many androgen-sensitive tissues and organs, such as seminal vesicles, hair follicles, sebaceous and preputial glands, uterus, kidney, submandibular glands, androgen-sensitive tumors, testis, epididymis, and specific areas of brain (see reviews by Liao, 1974, 1975a,b). There are indications that receptor proteins for testosterone operate in a number of androgen-sensitive tissues, such as the levator ani muscle (Baulieu and Jung, 1972), uterus (Giannopoulos, 1973), and kidney (Ritzén *et al.*, 1972). Furthermore, a receptorlike protein for 3,17-dihydroxylated androstanes (or androstenes) has been found in the cell nuclei of vagina (Shao *et al.*, 1975); erythropoiesis is affected by the 5β-isomer of DHT; and testosterone or its metabolites (other than DHT) are apparently responsible for the androgenlike actions on sexual behavior, anovulatory sterility, and Wolffian ducts in some species of animals (see reviews by Liao, 1974, 1975a,b).

B. SEDIMENTATION PROPERTIES

Gradient centrifugation has been one of the most commonly employed techniques for the study of steroid receptors since its introduction into the field by Toft and Gorski (1966). The prostate cytosol DHT-receptor complex (complex II) carefully prepared at low temperatures can form complexes that sediment as 7–12 S and 3–5 S units. The larger complexes can be transformed to the smaller forms by incubating at 20°–30°C or by bringing the salt concentrations to 0.4 M KCl. The sedimentation properties of the DHT-receptor complex can vary with the changes in pH of the medium. At 0.1 M KCl and a pH lower than 7.5, both the 8 S and 3.5 S complexes gradually aggregate to larger forms. If the pH of the medium is raised from 7 to 9, the amount of aggregates decreases and the 8 S and 3 to 4 S forms emerge (Fig. 1). At pH 9.5, only a 7 S form is clearly observed. The formation of the 8 S form and aggregation obviously involves other cellular materials, since the gradient and hydroxyapatite-purified complex does not aggregate and most of them sediment at about 3 S (Liao and Liang, 1974).

In 0.4 M KCl, the prostate cytosol complex II (3.8 ± 0.3 S) sediments somewhat faster than the nuclear complex (2.9 ± 0.3 S). This difference can be observed even in 2 M urea (Fig. 2). The difference, therefore, may be due to an intrinsic property of the complexes rather than to asso-

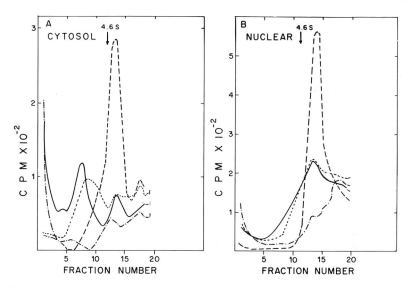

FIG. 1. Effect of pH on the sedimentation pattern of the cytosol complex II (A) and nuclear (B) ³H-labeled dihydrotestosterone(DHT)-receptor complex of rat ventral prostate. The glycerol gradient (10 to 22%) solution contained 1.5 mM EDTA, 20 mM Tris-HCl buffer at the pH shown, with or without 0.4 M KCl. Fractions were collected and numbered from the bottom of the tube. Bovine serum albumin (4.6 S) sedimented at the position shown by the arrow. - - -, pH 6.4–9.5, 0.4 M KCl; · · · ·, pH 9.5, no KCl; ——, pH 8.3, no KCl; . _ . _, pH 6.4, no KCl.

ciation of other macromolecules. At urea concentrations higher than 3 M, DHT is gradually released from the receptor.

Most of the steroid-receptor complexes in crude extracts can sediment at the 8 S region in a medium having a low ionic strength; this provides a convenient method for the detection of the cellular receptor. Since the formation of the 8 S form is dependent on pH, and the level of the 8 S form does not represent the total receptor content in the tissue sample, its usefulness in the quantitative analysis of the receptor is highly questionable. This is particularly so if the microsomal receptor is not taken into account for evaluation.

III. ANDROGEN-RECEPTOR EVALUATION

A. STEROID ENVELOPING AND STRUCTURAL RECOGNITION

We have studied the structural requirements for binding of the androgens to the receptor protein by analyzing a number of androgen analogs

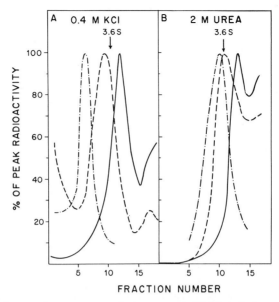

Fɪɢ. 2. Sedimentation patterns of the cytosol ³H-labeled 17β-estradiol receptor complex of calf uterus (·-·-), and of the cytosol (---) and nuclear (——) ³H-labeled dihydrotestosterone (DHT)-receptor complex of rat ventral prostate. The cytosol receptor complex II was obtained by mixing the cytosol with the radioactive steroids. The nuclear receptor was labeled during tissue incubation. The gradient solution contained either 0.4 M KCl (A) or 2 M urea (B). Other conditions were the same as in Fig. 1. Ovalbumin (3.6 S) sedimented at the position shown by the arrows. When the cytosol ³H-labeled DHT-receptor complex was incubated at 20°C for 10 minutes, the complex migrated to the same position as the nuclear complex.

for their ability to bind to the receptor and to be retained by the prostate cell nucleus (Liao et al., 1972, 1973a). These studies have indicated that the bulkiness and flatness of the steroid molecule play a more important role in receptor-binding than the detailed electronic structure or atoms of the steroid nucleus. The role of Δ⁴-3-keto-5α-oxidoreductase in transforming testosterone, a very weak binder, to DHT is not merely to eliminate the double bond of ring A of the steroid, but rather to convert testosterone to a flatter and less bulky molecule with an overall geometry that fits better to the receptor-binding site. In fact potent androgens like 7α,17α-dimethyl-19-nortestosterone and 2-oxa-17β-hydroxyestra-4,9,11-trien-3-one (which have conjugated double bonds extending from ring A and B to C) are very flat molecules, which can bind firmly to the androgen-receptor and probably function without any prior metabolic conversion. Studies with methylated androgens also suggest that the re-

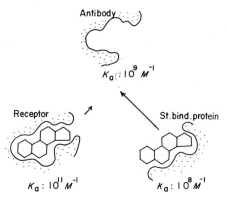

FIG. 3. Differential binding of steroid to the receptor, the nonreceptor steroid-binding proteins, and the antisteroid antibody.

ceptor binds at multiple sites of an androgenic steroid, as though the steroid molecule were being enveloped. This is in marked contrast to steroid-metabolizing enzymes or blood steroid-binding proteins, which generally recognize only a portion of the steroid molecule (Fig. 3).

The concept of steroid "enveloping" implies that it is chiefly the receptor protein, rather than the steroid, which triggers the key event leading to the hormone action, and that the main function of the steroid is to transform the receptor protein to a form that can be recognized by the components involved in the trigger action. The localization of steroid-binding sites well inside the receptor proteins may be responsible for the very-high-affinity constants for the receptor-binding of steroids, the extremely slow rates (many hours) of association and especially dissociation of steroids from the receptor proteins at low temperatures, acceleration of the rates of exchange of unbound steroids with bound steroids by freezing and thawing, and the inability of ethanol (30%) and detergent (2% Triton X-100 or deoxycholate) to free the steroid from the receptors in the cold (Fang and Liao, 1971; Liao 1974).

B. CHARACTERIZATION BY ANTISTEROID ANTIBODY

Additional support for the view of steroid "enveloping" came from our recent study on the ability of antisteroid antibodies to interact with steroids bound to various binding proteins (Castañeda and Liao, 1974, 1975). Various antibodies against DHT and testosterone were found to be effective in removing steroid bound to nonreceptor proteins of blood (including human blood) and prostate, but were not capable of removing DHT bound to the receptor. This property is apparently a general one: We also found that the antibodies for progesterone, estradiol, and dexamethasone can remove the steroids that are initially bound to blood globulins (K_a: 10^8 M^{-1}) and nonreceptor protein of their target tissues, but not the steroids bound to their own receptors.

Based on these observations, we have devised a simple assay method for the qualitative and quantitative characterization of the steroid-receptor complexes. In this assay, the sample solution containing ³H-labeled steroid-receptor complexes is mixed with antisteroid antibody that has the capacity to bind essentially all the ³H-labeled steroid present. The mixture is brought to 0.4 M with respect to KCl and analyzed by gradient centrifugation. Under conditions of the assay, the ³H-labeled steroid molecules, in the free form or attached to nonreceptor proteins, are bound by the antibody and sediment at 8 S, whereas, the receptor-bound ³H-steroid remains at the 3–4 S region and can be measured. The assay method can be simplified considerably by use of the antibody coupled to solid phases such as Sepharose. In this case, the assay mixture is simply centrifuged in a clinical centrifuge to sediment the steroid molecules that were not attached to the receptor originally, but are now bound to the insolubilized antibody. The receptor content can, therefore, be determined directly from the radioactivity of the supernatant (Castañeda and Liao, 1974, 1975).

By using this method, we have been able to show that the cell nuclei and cytoplasm of normal, hyperplastic, and cancerous human prostate contain DHT-receptor complexes that sediment at about 3 S in media with 0.4 M KCl.

IV. Interaction of Dihydrotestosterone-Receptor Complex with Cellular Components

A. Metal Ions

We have studied the effect of various divalent metal ions on the sedimentation properties of the prostate cytosol DHT-receptor complex in the medium containing 0.4 M KCl. In this study, the complex was mixed with a metal ion at 0° or 20°C before it was subjected to gradient centrifugation. $MnCl_2$, $MgCl_2$, or $CaCl_2$ produced no significant effect at concentrations of 1 to 5 mM. $CoCl_2$, however, facilitated aggregation of the complex and reduced the 3.8 S peak significantly. The most striking effect was observed with $ZnCl_2$: Incubation of the complex with 3 mM of Zn^{2+} at 0°C for 20 minutes resulted in a shift of the sedimentation coefficient from 3.8 S to 4.5 S without altering the total ³H-DHT bound to the com-

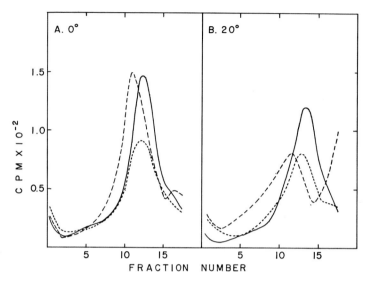

F IG. 4. Interaction of metal ions with ³H-labeled dihydrotestosterone (DHT)-receptor complex of rat ventral prostate. The cytosol complex II was incubated with 3 mM of ZnCl₂, CoCl₂, MgCl₂, or CaCl₂ for 20 minutes at 0°C (A) or 20°C (B) before it was layered on the top of the glycerol gradient (10 to 22%) solution and analyzed by gradient centrifugation. Other conditions were the same as in Fig. 1. Centrifugation was performed at 54,000 rpm for 18 hours. The solid lines represent results with the samples containing no metal ion, or in the presence of MnCl₂, MgCl₂, or CaCl₂ which had no visible effect on the sedimentation patterns; - - -, Zn²⁺; • • • •, Co²⁺. The gradient media had pH of 7.5.

plex. If the incubation was carried out at 20°C, the radioactive peak broadened (5 ± 2S) and a considerable amount of the radioactive androgen dissociated from the receptor and remained near the top of the tube after centrifugation (Fig. 4). This could be due to a Zn²⁺-induced change in the configuration of the receptor protein.

B. MONONUCLEOTIDES

With the expectation that steroid receptor may be involved in certain biochemical reactions involving nucleoside triphosphates (cf. Moudgil and Toft, 1975), we have studied the effect of various mononucleotides on the sedimentation pattern of the cytosol DHT-receptor complex (Tymoczko and Liao, 1975). As shown in Fig. 5, both ATP and GTP can interact and stabilize the DHT-receptor complex. The effect is most clearly observed if the complex preparation is incubated with 1–5 mM of these nucleotides at 20°C for 20 minutes. In the absence of the mono-

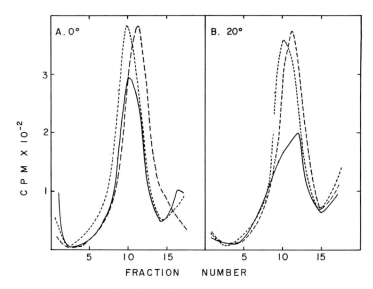

FIG. 5. Interaction of nucleoside triphosphates with ³H-labeled dihydrotestosterone (DHT)-receptor complex of rat ventral prostate. The cytosol complex II was incubated with 4 mM of GTP or ATP for 20 minutes at 0°C (A) or 20°C (B) before it was layered on the top of the glycerol gradient (10 to 20%) solution and analyzed by gradient centrifugation. Other conditions were the same as in Fig. 4, except that centrifugation was performed for 19 hours. The control tube (——) contained no nucleotide; ---, + ATP; ····, + GTP.

nucleotide, the incubation causes a shift in the sedimentation coefficient of the complex from 3.8 S to 3.0 S. If GTP or ATP is present, a small shift in the coefficient can be observed even when the sample is maintained at 0°C. Additional incubation at 20°C does not further change the sedimentation property. CTP and UTP also demonstrate some effect, but this is not as clear as with ATP and GTP. ADP, AMP, and cyclic AMP are not effective. Addition of ATP and GTP to the heat-transformed complex does not result in a significant change in the sedimentation pattern. The phenomenon is clearly not due to the phosphate moiety alone as inorganic mono- or pyrophosphate at these concentrations are not effective. It may be suggested that ATP and GTP can specifically induce a biologically important conformational change of the DHT-receptor complex.

C. POLYNUCLEOTIDES

The prostate DHT-receptor complex can bind to various (but not all) polynucleotides. The radioactive complex was found at 30–80 S with poly(A), poly(G), and poly(U) having sedimentation coefficients of 4 ± 0.5 S, but not with poly(C) and tRNA of liver or *Escherichia coli*. Binding of the complex to the native or heated calf thymus DNA and ribosomal RNA could be demonstrated by gradient centrifugation. The sedimentation patterns of the polymer-bound DHT-receptor complex may be complicated by other proteins in the receptor preparations which also bind to these polymers. A significant portion of the polynucleotide (especially heat-denatured DNA) binding of the DHT-receptor complex appears to be fortuitous and does not occur in the target cells since they are not dissociable from the ternary complex by 0.4 M KCl, which can solubilize virtually all the DHT-receptor complexes retained by the prostate cell nuclei or the cytoplasmic particulated matter *in vivo*.

D. RIBONUCLEOPROTEINS

A major portion of the nuclear RNA exists in protein-bound forms. Some of these ribonucleoprotein (RNP) particles are processed and then utilized in the protein synthesis in the cell cytoplasm. To explore the possibility that some steroid hormones may play a role in the processing and functioning of these RNP particles, we have studied the interaction of the prostate DHT-receptor complex and the nuclear RNP and ribosomal subunit particles (Liao *et al.*, 1973b; Liang and Liao, 1974; Tymoczko, 1973). As shown in Fig. 6, the DHT-receptor complex forms a 60–80 S complex with the nuclear RNP particle of prostate but not liver. The interaction and the formation of the ternary complex can be eliminated by prior heating of the RNP particles at 50°C and above, or by treatment with proteases or RNase (but not with DNase-1). The androgen receptor complex can be dissociated reversibly from the ternary complex by 0.4 M KCl. The receptor-binding sites on the particles can be saturated. From this saturation study, it can be concluded that less than 10% of the nuclear RNP particles can bind the androgen-receptor complex. Apparently, only those RNP particles with certain heat-labile (acceptor) protein factors can bind the androgen-receptor complex. Only about 30–50% of the total cytosol complex II can bind to RNP particles, indicating that other steroid-protein complexes may not be structurally compatible with the acceptor sites.

The cytoplasmic fractions of the prostate contain RNP particles (40 and 60 S) that bind the DHT-receptor complex. Some of these particles prepared from ribosomes can also bind the complex. Most interestingly, the cytoplasmic polysomal or 80 S monosomal forms of ribosomes do not have the receptor-binding ability. DHT itself (in the absence of the receptor protein or in the presence of the heat-denatured receptor prepara-

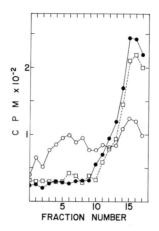

Fɪɢ. 6. Interaction of a ³H-labeled dihydrotestosterone (DHT)-receptor complex of ventral prostate with nuclear RNP particles of ventral prostate and liver. A ³H-labeled complex II preparation, alone (●) or in the presence of nuclear RNP isolated from rat ventral prostate (○) or liver (□), was layered on the top of a centrifuge tube containing sucrose gradient (10 to 30%) solution. The gradient solution and the samples also contained 1.5 mM EDTA and 20 mM Tris-HCl buffer, pH 8.1. Gradient centrifugation was performed at 2°C and 54,000 rpm for 2.3 hours. Fractions were collected and numbered from the bottom of the centrifuge tubes. From Liao et al. (1973b).

tion) is not able to associate with either the nuclear or the cytoplasmic RNP particles under the same conditions. In the absence of DHT, the receptor does not appear to bind tightly to these particles. The receptor-binding activity of the ribosomal subunit particles can be destroyed by heating at 50°C, indicating also the involvement of a heat-labile protein. The latter view is supported by the finding that aurin tricarboxylic acid which can dissociate some proteins from the 40 S ribosomal subunit of the prostate and shift the sedimentation coefficient of the particle to about 30 S, can also eliminate the binding of the DHT-receptor complex to the RNP particles.

E. Nᴜᴄʟᴇɪ ᴀɴᴅ Nᴜᴄʟᴇᴀʀ Cʜʀᴏᴍᴀᴛɪɴ

The ability of the purified prostate cell nuclei to selectively retain DHT-receptor was first demonstrated in our laboratory using cell-free systems (Liao and Fang, 1970; Fang and Liao, 1971). Most important, the receptor is not retained firmly by the prostate cell nuclei unless it interacts and binds DHT. The receptor complex binds tightly to the cell nuclei from the prostate, but not to nuclei from tissues less sensitive to androgens. This observation was confirmed by other investigators using the chromatin fraction of mammalian cell nuclei (Mainwaring and Peterken, 1971; Steggles *et al.*, 1971), although chromatin binding *in vitro* of steroid-receptor complexes might be seriously complicated by nonspecific aggregation of the complex with histones, DNA, and other nuclear components.

V. Receptor Transformation and Nuclear Acceptor Molecules

The DHT-dependent translocation of the cytoplasmic receptor protein to the prostate cell nuclei is temperature dependent. More rapid nuclear retention as seen by radioautography (Sar *et al.*, 1970) and reconstruction of the cellular fractions (Fang *et al.*, 1969; Fang and Liao, 1971; Mainwaring and Peterken, 1971) occurs at 20–30°C than at 0°C. The temperature effect is primarily on the alteration of the cytosol DHT-receptor complex (Liao and Liang, 1974). According to Mainwaring and Irving (1973), this process is accompanied by a change in the isoelectric point of the complex from 5.8 to 6.5. Our study (Fig. 2) has revealed that under the conditions favoring nuclear retention, the cytosol complex II (3.8 S) can be transformed at 20°C to a new complex (complex-TR) that has the same sedimentation coefficient as the nuclear complex (3 S) (Liao, 1975a,b). It is not certain whether such a temperature-dependent receptor transformation is strictly due to a change in the conformation of the receptor molecules, as Jensen and DeSombre (1973) have suggested, or to a proteolytic factor shown by Bresciani *et al.* (1973).

Heating or proteolytic treatment of nuclei can result in the loss of specific binding (but increase in nonspecific association) of the DHT-receptor complex with the aggregated chromatin. Because of this observation and the fact that the prostate nuclear retention of the androgen-receptor is highly tissue-and steroid-specific and the nuclear binding sites can be saturated, we have suggested that certain proteins are involved in the specific interaction of the DHT-receptor complex with the prostate cell nuclei and nuclear chromatin (Liao and Fang, 1970; Liao *et al.*, 1971; Fang and Liao, 1971). The protein(s) we defined as "acceptor" protein(s) appear(s) to be nonhistone nuclear (acidic) protein(s). Using a reconstructed system and employing Millipore membrane filtration, the acceptorlike activity can be assayed by measuring the effectiveness of the fractionated nuclear protein(s) to retain the receptor complex in the presence of the native calf thymus DNA. The acceptor molecule(s) can be extracted from the purified prostate cell nuclei by 0.4 M KCl, fractioned by ammonium sulfate and ethanol, or precipitated from the solution by adjusting the pH to 4.0 to 4.5 (Tymoczko and Liao, 1971). In the acceptor activity assay, heat-denatured DNA and various histones or basic polypeptides (such as polylysine) alone or together, can bind the DHT-receptor complex nonspecifically. The bound form cannot be extracted by 0.4 M KCl and, therefore, no acceptor activity is demonstrated. Poly(A), poly(G), and ribosomal RNA, but not poly(U) or poly(C), are able to substitute for the native DNA in the assay (Tymoczko and Liao, 1971).

O'Malley et al. (1972) have also used the "acceptor" concept to explain the specific retention of the progesterone-receptor complex by the chick oviduct nuclei, and also have isolated an acidic protein fraction that appears to contain an acceptorlike protein. Both the prostate and oviduct acceptor preparations are very crude, and their identity and role in recep-tor binding are obscure. In fact, it is not clear whether there is more than one type of biologically meaningful acceptor site in the cell nuclei of these target tissues. The prostate cell nucleus appears to contain a limited, but not necessarily constant, number (2000–10,000) of the recep-tor binding sites. Since receptor binding to the nuclear RNP particles may also require these acceptor proteins, the number of the nuclear acceptor molecules may vary among cells.

We have estimated that the apparent dissociation constant (K_d) for the binding of DHT-receptor complex to the nuclear acceptor sites is about 0.5 nM. This is similar to that estimated for the nuclear binding of estradiol receptor in uterus (King and Gordon, 1972; Higgins et al., 1973a) and dexamethasone receptor in hepatoma cells (Higgins et al., 1973b) and lung (Ballard, 1972).

VI. Androgen and Gene Expression

A. Gene Transcription

The prostate ribosomes isolated from androgen-injected rats have higher protein-synthesizing activity than those from the control castrates. This effect can be attributed to the androgen-dependent increase in the mRNA content of the ribosomal fractions (Liao and Williams-Ashman, 1962; Liao, 1968) and cell nuclei (Liao, 1965). This conclusion was sup-ported recently by a prudent work of Mainwaring et al. (1974), who studied the aldolase mRNA content of the rat ventral prostate. However, the androgen effects can be clearly observed only after the rats are treated with androgen for 10–20 hours, and apparently reflect the general increase in the synthetic activity induced by androgen in the prostate cells (Fig. 7). Ichii et al. (1974) also suggested that the long-term

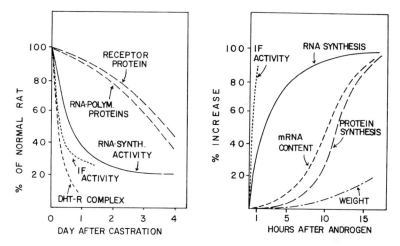

Fɪɢ. 7. Early changes in cellular activities after castration or administration of a single dose of androgen. Biochemical parameters shown are the activity of the initiation factor (IF) that binds methinonyl-tRNA$_f$; RNA synthesizing activity of isolated cell nuclei; mRNA activity of the nuclear and ribosome-bound RNA; protein-synthesizing activity of isolated ribosomes; RNA-polymerase proteins (assayed with external DNA); DHT-receptor complex remaining, receptor protein available for binding DHT; and the fresh weight of the ventral prostate. See text for sources of the data.

(2 days) effect of androgen on protein synthesis may also be due to the increase in the activity of the factors (especially the initiation factor and to some extent the elongation factor) that are associated with the ribosomal particles and are necessary in the protein synthesis.

A much earlier effect of androgen appears to be on the cell nuclei. Within 1 hour after an androgen is administered to castrated rats, the RNA polymerase activity of the isolated cell nuclei is enhanced considerably (Liao *et al.*, 1965). Our biochemical (Liao *et al.*, 1966; Liao and Lin, 1967) and radioautographic (Liao and Stumpf, 1968) studies have shown that this early effect occurs most distinctly at the nucleolar chromatin region that synthesizes rRNA precursors, although mRNA syntheses may also be affected in this early stage of androgen action (Liao and Fang, 1969; Liao, 1975a).

Since the DHT-receptor complex can be retained by the prostate cell nuclei specifically and rapidly, and antiandrogens that inhibit the receptor binding of androgens (Fang and Liao, 1969; Liao *et al.*, 1974; Tymoczko and Liao, 1975) can suppress the androgen effect on RNA synthesis (Anderson *et al.*, 1972), the DHT-receptor complex appears to play a role in the event that leads to the enhancement of RNA synthesis by prostate nuclear chromatin. In cell-free systems, according to Davies and Griffiths (1974), RNA synthesis by the isolated prostate nuclei or chromatin fractions can be stimulated by prostate protein preparations that contain the DHT-receptor complex.

B. POSTTRANSCRIPTIONAL PROCESS

Experimental evidence supporting the view that steroid hormones (and their receptors) act primarily at the level of gene transcription (particularly in cases involving the use of experimental animals starved for these hormones for an extensive period of time and the responsive cells require new RNA synthesis for general cellular activity) is rather overwhelming. Nevertheless, the possible involvement of steroid hormones in the posttranscriptional control of gene expression cannot be excluded at all at this time. For this reason and because we have observed that androgen- and estrogen-receptor complexes can bind to certain nuclear RNP and ribosomal subunit particles *in vitro* and *in vivo* (Liao *et al.*, 1973b; Liang and Liao, 1974), we have in recent years reinvestigated the effect of steroid hormones on the protein-synthesizing machinery of the target tissues.

One of our emphases on this aspect of research has been on the factors that can affect the initiation process required for protein synthesis. We have made a detailed study and found that the initiation process in the prostate is essentially identical with that proposed for bacterial and other eukaryotic systems. The methionyl-tRNA$_f$, the initiator tRNA, first binds to an initiation factor (IF protein) in the presence of GTP. The initiator complex then binds a small ribosomal subunit and forms the [40 S-methionyl-tRNA$_f$] initiation complex. With the assistance of other protein factors the initiation complex binds mRNA and a 60 S ribosomal subunit (Fig. 8) to form an 80 S complex on which the polypeptide synthesis begins.

The first step of the process (IF$_1$ activity) can be assayed, since both

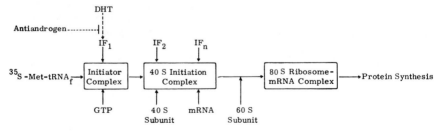

FIG. 8. Initiation steps involved in protein synthesis in the prostate. IF, initiation factor; DHT, dihydrotestosterone.

the IF_1-methionyl-tRNA$_f$ and the 40 S initiation complexes can be retained on a Millipore filter and measured. For this purpose, ^{35}S-methionine is charged onto rat liver tRNA by a bacterial synthetase that acylates *only* the initiator species of tRNA. Comparison is made using the prostate cytosol as the source of the initiation factors. As shown in Fig. 9, the IF activity of the prostate cytosol from normal rats is much higher than that from the control castrate. This loss of the IF activity is prevented by injection of testosterone or DHT to the castrated animals. The IF activity decreases within hours after castration and is reversed within 1 hour after an intraperitoneal injection of DHT. If intravenous injection is used, 5–20 μg/400 gm rat of DHT or testosterone can have a significant effect within 10 minutes. The effect is not due to a differential degradation of GTP or deacylation of ^{35}S-methionyl-tRNA or to the RNA present in the cytosol preparations. The factor involved is heat-labile, undialyzable, and can be fractionated by salt pre-

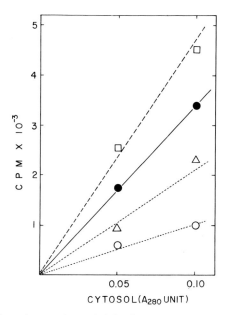

FIG. 9. Effect of an intraperitoneal injection of dihydrotestosterone (DHT) on the cytosol initiation factors. The prostate cytosol fractions were obtained from normal rats (●), rats castrated 19 hours previously (○), and from castrated rats injected with 2.5 mg of DHT immediately after castration (□) or 1 hour before being killed (△). The binding of ^{35}S-methionyl-tRNA$_f$ to the cytosol initiation factor was assayed in the presence of prostate ribosomes. Millipore filters were used to trap the radioactive initiator complex formed. The effect can be demonstrated within minutes after intravenous injection of the androgen. From Liang and Liao (1975).

TABLE II
Very Rapid Enhancement by Steroid Hormones of the Initiation-Factor (IF) Activity Involved in Protein Synthesis in Target Tissues[a]

Target tissue	Effective steroid	Effective antagonist
Ventral prostate	DHT, testosterone	Cyproterone, Flutamide
Uterus	Estradiol	Parke-Davis CI-628
Liver	Dexamethasone	Cortexolone
Skeletal muscle	Testosterone, DHT	Cyproterone

[a] Rats were castrated and adrenalectomized 18 hours before the study. If used, the antagonist (100 μg) was injected intraperitoneally. Steriod hormones were injected intravenously (1 μg for estradiol and 20 μg for other steriods) 10 minutes before the animals were killed. The cytosol fractions were prepared and assayed for the IF activity. Since no ribosomal particle was included in the assay medium, the effect (50 to 100%) was clearly on the IF protein binding of met-tRNA$_f$. The antagonists listed could abolish the hormonal effect *in vivo*. We also found that the IF activity of the thymus cytosol preparations was reduced by dexamethasone treatment of the animals.

cipitation, chromatographic techniques, and gradient centrifugation. This, and the fact that the androgen effect can be observed even when the ribosomal particle is omitted from the assay mixture, clearly show that the factor affected is the IF$_1$ protein that binds the initiator tRNA (Liang and Liao, 1975).

In many of our experiments we found that actinomycin D and cycloheximide, at high concentrations, were not able to suppress the androgen-dependent increase in the IF activity. Therefore, the effect does not appear to be dependent on new synthesis of RNA or protein. Interestingly, cyproterone acetate (an antiandrogen), which can inhibit the receptor binding of DHT, can eliminate *in vivo* the androgen effect.

The very rapid effect described above is apparently a general phenomenon that occurs in the target cells of many steroid hormones. As summarized in Table II, estrogen and glucocorticoids at low concentrations can also stimulate the IF$_1$ activity in their target tissues within minutes, and their effect is inhibited by their antagonists.

C. Dual Regulation

Although the findings from many studies have indicated that a primary role of the steroid-receptor complex is to regulate RNA synthesis in the cell nuclei, the possibility that the steroid and/or its receptor may act at the level of processing and utilization of RNA remains attractive. Our new finding that steroids can significantly augment the activity of the factor involved in the very first step of protein synthesis in the target cells, and that this effect is not dependent on the new synthesis of RNA or protein, indicates strongly that the steroid hormones (and/or their receptors) may function at an extranuclear site.

In some target tissues, steroid hormones may indeed act at both nuclear and extranuclear sites. Such a dual control mechanism may operate independently at the two sites or be performed by a factor that has a dual role in the transcription and translation processes to assure a well-coordinated and efficient regulation of gene expression in the target cells. The latter type of mechanism may be similar to one that appears to exist in some bacterial systems in which certain ribosome-associated proteins are able to function as subunits of RNA synthetase or regulate the genome-dependent RNA synthesis (Leavitt *et al.*, 1972; Groner *et al.*, 1972; Miller and Wahba, 1974).

The simplest explanation for the rapid enhancement of IF activity by the steroid hormones is that the receptor itself provides the increased activity. Our preliminary experiments also appear to indicate the possibility that the steroid hormones and/or their receptors may activate IF activity by interfering with an inhibitor system. A thorough investigation of this aspect may reveal a general mechanism through which the steroid hormones and other cellular regulators or drugs modulate the cellular function and growth in the target tissues.

ACKNOWLEDGMENTS

The authors thank Ms. Linda M. Gluesing and Ms. Pamela A. Chudzinski for their skillful technical assistance in the studies included in this article. Work in our laboratory was supported by research grants from the U.S. Public Health Service (AM-9461, HD-07110) and the American Cancer Society (BC-151).

REFERENCES

Anderson, K. M., and Liao, S. (1968). *Nature (London)* **219**, 277.

Anderson, K. M., Cohn, H., and Samuels, S. (1972). *FEBS (Fed. Eur. Biochem. Soc.) Lett.* **27**, 149.

Ballard, P. L., and Ballard, R. A. (1972). *Proc. Nat. Acad. Sci. U.S.* **69**, 2668.

Baulieu, E. E., and Jung, I. (1972). *Nature (London), New Biol.* **237**, 24.

Bresciani, F., Nola, E., Sica, V., and Puca, G. A. (1973). *Fed. Proc., Fed. Amer. Soc. Exp. Biol.* **32**, 2126.

Bruchovsky, N., and Wilson, J. D. (1968). *J. Biol. Chem.* **243**, 5953.

Castañeda, E., and Liao, S. (1974). *Endocrine Res. Commun.* **1**, 271.

Castañeda, E., and Liao, S. (1975). *J. Biol. Chem.* **250**, 883.

Davies, P., and Griffiths, K. (1974). *Biochem. J.* **140**, 565.

Fang, S., and Liao, S. (1969). *Mol. Pharmacol.* **5**, 420.

Fang, S., and Liao, S., (1971). *J. Biol. Chem.* **246**, 16.

Fang, S., Anderson, K. M., and Liao, S. (1969). *J. Biol. Chem.* **244**, 6584.

Giannopoulos, G. (1973). *J. Biol. Chem.* **248**, 1004.

Groner, Y., Scheps, R., Kamen, R., Kolakofsky, D., and Revel, M. (1972). *Nature (London), New Biol.* **239**, 19.

Higgins, S. J., Rousseau, G. G., Baxter, J. D., and Tomkins, G. M. (1973a). *J. Biol. Chem.* **248**, 5866.

Higgins, S. J., Rousseau, G. G., Baxter, J. D., and Tomkins, G. M. (1973b). *J. Biol. Chem.* **248**, 5873.

Huggins, C., and Mainzer, K. (1957). *J. Exp. Med.* **105**, 485.

Ichii, S., Izawa, M., and Murakami, N. (1974). *Endocrinol. Jap.* **21**, 267.

Jensen, E. V., and DeSombre, E. R. (1973). *Science* **182**, 126.

Jensen, E. V., Mohla, S., Gorrell, T. A., and DeSombre, E. R. (1974). *Vitam. Horm. (New York)* **32**, 89.

King, R. J., and Gordon, J. (1972). *Nature (London), New Biol.* **240**, 185.

Kowarski, A., Shalf, J., and Migeon, C. J. (1969). *J. Biol. Chem.* **244**, 5269.

Leavitt, J. C., Moldave, K., and Nakada, D. (1972). *J. Mol. Biol.* **70**, 15.

Liang, T., and Liao, S. (1974). *J. Biol. Chem.* **249**, 4671.

Liang, T., and Liao, S. (1975). *Proc. Nat. Acad. Sci. U.S.* **72**, 706.

Liao, S. (1965). *J. Biol. Chem.* **240**, 1236.

Liao, S. (1968). *Amer. Zool.* **8**, 233.

Liao, S. (1974). *In* "Biochemistry of Hormones" (H. V. Rickenberg, ed.), p. 154. Medical and Technical Publ. Co., Oxford.

Liao, S. (1975a). *Int. Rev. Cytol.* **41**, 87.

Liao, S. (1975b). *In* "Receptors and Mechanism of. Action of Steroid Hormones" (J. R. Pasqualini, ed.). Dekker, New York (in press).

Liao, S., and Fang, S. (1969). *Vitam. Horm. (New York)* **27**, 17.

Liao, S., and Fang, S. (1970). *In* "Some Aspects of the Aetiology and Biochemistry of Prostate Cancer" (K. Griffiths and C. G. Pierrepoint, eds.), p. 105. Alpha Omega Alpha Publ., Cardiff, Wales.

Liao, S., and Liang, T. (1974). *In* "Hormones and Cancer" (K. W. McKerns, ed.), p. 229. Academic Press, New York.

Liao, S., and Lin, A. H. (1967). *Proc. Nat. Acad. Sci. U.S.* **57**, 379.

Liao, S., and Stumpf, W. E. (1968). *Endocrinology* **83**, 629.

Liao, S., and Williams-Ashman, H. G. (1962). *Proc. Nat. Acad. Sci. U.S.* **48**, 1956.

Liao, S., Leininger, K. R., Sagher, D., and Barton, R. W. (1965). *Endocrinology* **77**, 763.

Liao, S., Barton, R. W., and Lin, A. H. (1966). *Proc. Nat. Acad. Sci. U.S.* **55**, 1593.

Liao, S., Tymoczko, J. L., Liang, T., Anderson, K. M., and Fang, S. (1971). *Advan. Biosci.* **7**, 155.

Liao, S., Liang, T., and Tymoczko, J. L. (1972). *J. Steroid. Biochem.* **3**, 401.

Liao, S., Liang, T., Fang, S., Castañeda, E., and Shao, T. C. (1973a). *J. Biol. Chem.* **284**, 6154.

Liao, S., Liang, T., and Tymoczko, J. L. (1973b). *Nature (London), New Biol.* **241**, 211.

Liao, S., Howell, D. K., and Chang, T. M. (1974). *Endocrinology* **94**, 1205.

Mainwaring, W. I. P., and Irving, R. (1973). *Biochem. J.* **134**, 113.

Mainwaring, W. I. P., and Peterken, B. M. (1971). *Biochem. J.* **125**, 285.

Mainwaring, W. I. P., Mangan, F. R., Irving, R. A., and Jones, D. A. (1974). *Biochem. J.* **144**, 413.

Miller, M. J., and Wahba, A. J. (1974). *J. Biol. Chem.* **248**, 3808.

Moudgil, V. K., and Toft, D. O. (1975). *Proc. Nat. Acad. Sci. U.S.* **72**, 901.

O'Malley, B. W., Spelsberg, T. C., Schrader, W. T., Chytil, F., and Steggles, A. W. (1972). *Nature (London)* **235**, 141.

Ritzén, E. M., Nayfeh, S. N., French, F. S., and Aronin, P. A. (1972). *Endocrinology* **91,** 116.

Sar, M., Liao, S., and Stumpf, W. E. (1970). *Endocrinology* **86,** 1008.

Shao, T. C., Castañeda, E., Rosenfield, R. L., and Liao, S. (1975). *J. Biol. Chem.* **250,** 3095.

Steggles, A. W., Spelsberg, T. C., Glasser, S. R., and O'Malley, B. W. (1971). *Proc. Nat. Acad. Sci. U.S.* **68,** 1479.

Toft D., and Gorski, J. (1966). *Proc. Nat. Acad. Sci. U.S.* **55,** 1574.

Tymoczko, J. L. (1973). Ph.D. Dissertation, University of Chicago, Chicago, Illinois.

Tymoczko, J. L., and Liao, S. (1971). *Biochim. Biophys. Acta* **252,** 607.

Tymoczko, J. L., and Liao, S. (1975). *J. Reprod. Fert.* (in press).

DISCUSSION

D. S. Coffey: Have you tested for androgen induction of the initiation factor in a cell-free system of the prostate? Have you observed this type of induction in androgen-insensitive animals?

S. Liao: In some cell-free experiments we have observed *in vitro* effects, but we would like to understand the effects a little better before we make a definite statement on the nature of these effects. We have not used the androgen-insensitive animal in our study.

F. Neumann: Recently our chemists synthesized Δ^{16}-D-homotestosterone. This steroid is about 100 times as active as testosterone. Does this fit in with your theory of molecular structure and biological activity?

S. Liao: A-homosteroids are very bulky at the A-ring; they are not active and probably do not bind firmly to the DHT receptor. On the other hand, B-homo, C-homo, and D-homo androstanes have the correct dimensions and should be able to bind to the receptor. As you know, they are active androgens.

N. Bruchovsky: If androgen binding is due to clefts in proteins that admit only flat molecules, is it possible that the number of clefts might be proportional to the number and diversity of proteins within the cell? Binding of steroid would then be related to the state of differentiation of the tissue rather than to the presence of a specific receptor protein.

S. Liao: It may be.

J.-G. Forsberg: You spoke about cAMP as structurally similar to steroids. Can you demonstrate any interaction between the androgen receptor and cAMP? Second, is the activation of the initiation factor correlated with any changes in the degree of phosphorylation?

S. Liao: Cyclic AMP does not compete with ^{3}H-labeled DHT for receptor binding. We have not studied protein phosphorylation in the way you mentioned.

D. S. Coffey: Can you separate the initiation factor from the receptor on sucrose density gradient? Have you tested the presence of initiation factor induction in androgen-insensitive tissue?

S. Liao: The ^{3}H-labeled DHT-receptor complex overlaps, but does not coincide with, the initiation complex on sucrose gradient centrifugation. With testosterone we found that the liver was not as sensitive as the ventral prostate.

Androgen *Receptors* in the Rat Ventral Prostate and Their Hormonal Control

J. P. BLONDEAU, C. CORPÉCHOT, C. LE GOASCOGNE, E. E. BAULIEU, AND P. ROBEL

ER 125 Cnrs, Unité de Recherches sur le Métabolisme Moléculaire et la Physio-Pathologie des Stéroïdes de l'Institut National de la Santé et de la Recherche Médicale (Inserm), Département de Chime Biologique, Faculté de Médecine Paris-Sud, Bicêtre, France*

I. INTRODUCTION

The specific binding of androgens to their target organ *receptors* has been investigated mainly in the ventral prostate gland of the castrated adult rat. The discovery of androgen *receptors* followed the observations of Bruchovsky and Wilson (1968) and Anderson and Liao (1968), who found that the nuclear bound radioactivity in the prostate gland of castrated rats is essentially recoverable as androstanolone-^{3}H[†] after the administration of testosterone-^{3}H *in vivo* or incubation of prostate *in vitro* and the demonstration that androstanolone is a very active metabo-

---

* Postal address: Lab Hormones, 94270–Bicêtre, France.

† Abbreviations and trivial names: testosterone, 17β-hydroxy-4-androsten-3-one; androstanolone (dihydrotestosterone), 17β-hydroxy-5α-androstan-3-one; 3α-andros-

319

lite in organ culture (Baulieu *et al.*, 1968). All the currently available evidence suggests that cytoplasmic binding protein(s) are implicated in the specific nuclear binding of androstanolone, along the line originally suggested by Jensen *et al.* (1968) and Gorski *et al.* (1971) for the nuclear binding of estrogens in uterus. Fang *et al.* (1969) have reported the existence of a binding component for 5α-dihydrotestosterone in the cytoplasmic fraction of rat prostate after the administration of testosterone-^{3}H *in vivo*. The ^{3}H-labeled steroid protein complex has a sedimentation coefficient of 3.5 S on linear sucrose gradients. However, other studies have generally demonstrated the existence of a binding protein in the cytoplasm of rat prostate that has a sedimentation coefficient of 8 S (Mainwaring, 1969, Unhjem *et al.*, 1969; Baulieu and Jung 1970; Ritzén *et al.*, 1971).

The use of sucrose or glycerol gradient ultracentrifugation has allowed the study of several properties of the cytoplasmic *receptors:* their proteinaceous nature, sensitivity to heat and to SH-blocking agents, the interconversion of "8–10 S" and "KCl 4–5 S" forms, and the temperature-dependent nuclear transfer of the androstanolone–*receptor* complex. These characteristics have been reviewed by Liao and Fang (1969), Baulieu *et al.* (1971), and King and Mainwaring (1974).

Although gradient ultracentrifugation and several other techniques, such as gel exclusion chromatography or isoelectric focusing, have provided much information on the physicochemical properties of the *receptor* and have suggested a high association constant for androstanolone, they are not convenient for the determination of binding constants and the quantitative assessment of binding inhibition by various androgens, antiandrogens, and other steroid hormones. Since 1974, however, methods have been described for the quantitation of androgen-binding constants in the rat ventral prostate. In Section II they are reviewed and a new technique, based on the principle of *receptor* precipitation by protamine sulfate, is reported. In Section III, the present state of knowledge concerning the regulation of androgen *receptors* is discussed.

---

tanediol, 5α-androstane-3α,17β-diol; 3β-androstanediol, 5α-androstane-3β,17β-diol; androstanedione, 5α-androstane-3,17-dione; androstenedione, 4-androstene-3,17,dione; Δ^5-androstenediol, 5-androstene-3β,17β-diol; dehydroepiandrosterone, 3β-hydroxy-5-androsten-17-one; epitestosterone, 17α-hydroxy-4-androsten-3-one; 19-nortesterone, 17β-hydroxy-4-estren-3-one; 5β-androsterone, 3α-hydroxy-5β-androstan-17-one; R 1881, 17β-hydroxy-17α-methyl-4,9,11-estratrien-3-one; 14-dehydro-19-nortestosterone, 17β-hydroxy-4,14-estradien-3-one; estradiol, 1,3,5(10)-estratriene-3,17β-diol; progesterone, 4-pregnene-3,20-dione; cyproterone acetate, 1,2α-methylene-6-chloro-17α-yl-acetoxy-4,6-pregnadiene-3,20-dione; RU 21270, N(3,4-dichlorophenyl)isobutyramide; RU 21757, N(3,4-dichlorophenyl)-2-hydroxyisobutyramide; R 2956, 17β-hydroxy-2α,2β,17α-trimethyl-4,9,11-estratrien-3-one.

II. METHODS FOR THE QUANTITATION OF ANDROSTANOLONE BINDING CONSTANTS AT EQUILIBRIUM IN RAT VENTRAL PROSTATE EXTRACTS

In most biological samples, any given ligand interacts with several binding components. These components can be separated functionally into two classes. "Specific" binding is characterized by high affinity for the ligand and a small binding capacity, while "nonspecific" binding is characterized by a low affinity and a very large (practically unlimited) capacity. All investigators have shown binding of ^{3}H-labeled steroids in the 3.5–4.5 S region of sucrose gradients, even when androstanolone-^{3}H concentration is low: 1–5 nM; this is due to nonspecific, low-affinity but high-capacity binding components. A much smaller amount of nonspecific binding is observed when uterine cytosol is labeled with the same concentrations of estradiol-[3]H. In addition, with the rat ventral prostate, it is necessary to use very concentrated cytosol (15–25 mg of protein per milliliter), to demonstrate well-shaped 8–10 S binding components.

A. DEXTRAN-COATED CHARCOAL ADSORPTION

1. *Failure to Demonstrate Rat Ventral Prostate Receptor with Conventional Dextran-Coated Charcoal Procedures*

Ritzén *et al.* (1971) have used a procedure derived from Murphy (1967). Whereas a high-affinity binding component ($K_d = 2.4$ nM) was demonstrated in epididymis cytosol, attempts to make comparable studies of androgen-binding components in prostatic cytosol using the dextran-coated charcoal and Sephadex gel methods were unsuccessful. Later it was demonstrated that the epididymis cytosol component is not the intracellular *receptor* but the androgen-binding protein of the testicular and epididymal fluid (Hansson *et al.*, 1973).

We have tried several variants of the dextran-coated charcoal technique, where different concentrations of cytosol proteins and of dextran-coated charcoal were used. We have also used the "differential dissociation" method (Milgrom and Baulieu, 1969), since the apparent dissociation of androstanolone–receptor complex is very slow (Baulieu *et al.*, 1977). None of these variants was successful in demonstrating a specific binding component in rat ventral prostate cytosol.

2. *Improved Dextran-Coated Charcoal Adsorption Methods*

Short exposure of rat ventral prostate androstanolone–*receptor* complex to dextran-coated charcoal does not remove a large amount of nonspecific binding (Blondeau and Robel, 1975). Longer exposure seems to inactivate the specific binding component. Therefore it is necessary to use conditions where the nonspecific binding is quickly dissociated so that a rather short exposure to the adsorbent will be sufficient. Shain *et al.* (1975) have shown the efficient removal of nonspecific binding by incubating the androstanolone-^{3}H–cytosol *receptor* complexes with 2.2 volumes of an ice-cold solution of 5% charcoal, 0.5% dextran, and 1% human γ-globulin, followed after 10 minutes by the addition of 7.8% absolute ethanol and incubation at 0°C for an additional 20 minutes. C. Bonne (personal communication, 1975) has also obtained a rather small contribution of nonspecific binding by adding to the cytosol an equal volume of dextran-coated charcoal (charcoal, 1.25% ; dextran, 0.625%).

B. Gel Filtration

1. *Gel Exclusion Column Chromatography*

Separation of bound and unbound hormone can result from small Sephadex G-25 column chromatography; such separation was successfully used for the assessment of progesterone *receptors* (Milgrom *et al.*, 1972a). With this fast chromatography, nonspecific binding does not dissociate, and therefore such a technique can be used only with very diluted cytosol when the contribution of nonspecific binding sites is limited. This is not the case with rat ventral prostate. Bruchovsky and Craven (1975) have proposed a dual-column system consisting of a precolumn (0.9 × 30 cm) of Sephadex G-25 connected in series with a separating column (0.9 × 100 cm) of Sephadex G-200. In each case the cytosol fraction is pretreated with ammonium sulfate at 80% saturation and the protein precipitate is analyzed by gel-exclusion chromatography. This technique is not suitable for the measurement of the association constant, since the free hormone concentration is unknown.

2. *Thin-Layer Gel Filtration*

Sephadex G-100 layered on a glass plate coated with a cellulose film has been used (Töpert *et al.*, 1974), but no detailed information was given concerning the evaluation of specificity, of ligand dissociation during gel filtration, and of free hormone concentration.

C. Ammonium Sulfate Precipitation

Although it is known that androgen *receptor* proteins of rat prostate cytosol can be precipitated at low concentrations of ammonium sulfate

(Fang and Liao, 1971; Mainwaring and Perterken, 1971), this salt was not used as a tool for quantitative studies until the work of Verhoeven (1974). Separation of *receptor*-bound ligands from unbound ligands and from the major part of the nonspecifically bound ligands is achieved by the gradual addition of an equal volume of 70% saturated solution of ammonium sulfate (adjusted to pH 7.4) at 0°C over a period of 15 minutes, and the solution is allowed to stand for another 30 minutes. After centrifugation at 10,000 *g* for 20 minutes, the supernatant is decanted, and the precipitate is resuspended in homogenization buffer containing 2 mg of bovine albumin per milliliter. The steroid–*receptor* complex is reprecipitated at 35% ammonium sulfate, left for another 45 minutes and centrifuged.

D. PROTAMINE SULFATE PRECIPITATION

Steroid hormone *receptors* are acidic proteins that can be precipitated selectively by protamine (Steggles and King, 1970; Mainwaring, 1969). An application of the principle of protamine sulfate precipitation to rat ventral prostate cytosol is described.

1. *Preparation of the Rat Ventral Prostate Cytosol*

Sprague-Dawley adult male rats weighing approximately 250 gm are bilaterally orchiectomized 24 hours before sacrifice. Ventral prostates are removed, dissected, washed in ice-cold buffer, and minced with scissors. All subsequent operations are performed at 0–4°C. Homogenization is performed in GTEM (Tris-HCl, 10 mM; EDTA, 1.5 mM; mercaptoethanol, 2 mM; glycerol, 15% v/v, pH 7.4) buffer in a Teflon–glass Potter homogenizer with a 4:1 buffer:tissue ratio. After removal of a 800 $g \times$ 10 minute pellet, the high-speed supernatant (cytosol) is prepared by centrifugation at 105,000 g for 90 minutes. The concentration of protein is 5–10 mg/ml. Freshly prepared cytosol is incubated 2 hours at 0°C with androstanolone-^{3}H (40 Ci/mmole) or the same amount of androstanolone-^{3}H plus a 100-fold excess of cold steroid.

2. *Protamine Sulfate Precipitation Step*

Protamine sulfate (protamine sulfate from salmon roe, Koch-Light laboratories) is added to homogenization buffer (1.2 mg/ml). Aliquots (0.25 ml) of labeled cytosol and protamine sulfate solution are thoroughly mixed and allowed to stand at 0–4°C for 15 minutes. The precipitate is filtered on glass fiber paper (Whatman GF/C) under vacuum, rinsed with 30 ml of ice-cold buffer, then transferred into a scintillation vial. Steroid is eluted with 2 ml of absolute ethanol and counted in 10 ml of toluene-based scintillator (Omnifluor 4 gm/liter).

3. *Validation*

The androstanolone-³H dpm precipitated in the presence of an excess androstanolone are subtracted from the androstanolone-³H dpm precipitated in the absence of excess androstanolone, and the difference is considered as representative of specific binding.

The amount of specifically bound androstanolone is dependent on protamine sulfate concentration and shows a maximum between 0.6 and 1 mg/ml (Fig. 1). This optimal value is well below the final 2.5 mg/ml concentration used by Steggles and King (1970) to precipitate rat uterus estradiol *receptor*.

The amount of specific binding precipitated is the same between 5 and 60 minutes and is not changed by volumes of washing buffer between 15 and 60 ml. Therefore, the precipitation time chosen is 15 minutes and the volume of washing buffer is 30 ml. The specific binding in precipitate is proportional to the protein concentration below 15 mg/ml (Table I). It is completely precipitated, since no residual binding is detectable in the supernatant by hydroxyapatite adsorption (Table II) (Erdos *et al.*, 1970). The addition of an SH-blocking agent completely abolishes the differential counts, suggesting again that they correspond to *receptor*-bound androstanolone (Table III). Finally, protamine sulfate precipitation is accurate and reliable, since in three different pools of ventral pros-

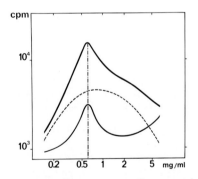

Fɪɢ. 1. Influence of protamine sulfate concentration on androstanolone-³H–receptor complex precipitation. Rat ventral prostate cytosol (15 mg of protein per milliliter) was incubated with 10 nM androstanolone-³H alone (incubation a) or 10 nM ³H-androstanolone-³H + 1 μM androstanolone (incubation b). Upper full line = cpm in precipitate of incubation a; lower full line = cpm in precipitate of incubation b; dashed line = difference between incubations a and b. The abscissa indicates the concentration of protamine sulfate (mg/ml); and the ordinate, the cpm in the precipitate.

TABLE I

INFLUENCE OF CYTOSOL PROTEIN CONCENTRATION ON ANDROSTANOLONE-[3]H *Receptor* COMPLEX PRECIPITATION[a]

Cytosol protein concentration (mg/ml)	Specifically bound androstanolone (dpm/mg of protein)
20	173,571
15	214,716
10	206,732
5	201,000
2.5	205,320

[a] Cytosol was incubated with 10 nM androstanolone-[3]H (B_1) or 10 nM androstanolone-[3]H + 1 μM androstanolone (B_2). The difference $B_1 - B_2$ was taken as the measure of specific binding.

TABLE II

COMPLETE PRECIPITATION OF ANDROSTANOLONE-[3]H *Receptor* COMPLEX BY PROTAMINE SULFATE[a]

	Specifically bound androstanolone (cpm/0.25 ml cytosol)
Protamine sulfate precipitation	1350
Hydroxyapatite adsorption	1380
Hydroxyapatite adsorption of protamine sulfate supernatant	90

[a] Cytosol samples (4 mg of protein/ml) were incubated with 1 nM androstanolone-^{3}H, and the differential counts were determined in the protamine sulfate precipitate. Hydroxyapatite microcolumn adsorption was used, as described by Erdos *et al.* (1970), for whole cytosol and protamine sulfate precipitation supernatant.

TABLE III

PROTAMINE SULFATE PRECIPITATION IS SPECIFIC[a]

	Cpm in precipitate	
Incubations	Without PHMB	With PHMB
(1) Androstanolone-^{3}H, 10 nM	7160	3470
(2) Androstanolone-^{3}H, 10 nM, + androstanolone 1 μM	2150	3800
Difference (1) − (2)	5110	−380

[a] Cytosol samples (16.8 mg of protein per milliliter) were incubated with androstanolone as indicated. The incubations with PHMB contained *p*-hydroxymercuribenzoate, 1 mM. The counts per minute for 0.25 ml of cytosol were determined in the protamine sulfate precipitates.

tate cytosol the total number of specific binding sites has been 102 ± 17 fmoles/mg of protein (mean $\pm$ standard deviation).

E. Other Techniques

Several other techniques are of potential interest for the measurement of androgen-binding constants to target organ specific proteins, such as polyacrylamide gel electrophoresis under steady state conditions (Ritzén et al., 1974), agar gel electrophoresis (Krieg et al., 1974), microelectrofocusing (Katsumata and Goldman, 1974), or the use of steroid antibodies (Castañeda and Liao, 1975).

F. Some Theoretical and Methodological Problems Underlying the Measurement of Specific Binding Constants

The calculation of equilibrium binding constants of any specific protein–ligand interaction requires the exact determination of the unbound ligand concentration and of the specifically bound ligand concentration. These are not directly available experimentally, owing to the contribution of nonspecific binding. The use of two correction terms, kn and f, has been proposed (Blondeau and Robel, 1975); kn is the product of the equilibrium association constant k times the number of binding sites n of the nonspecific binding components; while f is the fraction of the nonspecific binding included in the experimental estimates of bound ligand. These factors are easily measured experimentally. The corrections used for the determination of androstanolone and testosterone binding constants to rat ventral prostate cytosol are

$$U = U_1/[1 + (1 - f)kn]$$

where U_1 is the apparent unbound steroid concentration given by the difference between total steroid concentration and measured bound steroid concentration, and

$$B_S = (B_1 - B_2)[T/(T - B_2)]$$

where B_1 is the concentration of ligand bound after incubation with a concentration T of radioactive ligand, B_2 is the concentration of ligand bound after incubation with the same concentration of radioactive ligand plus a large (100-fold) concentration of nonradioactive ligand, and B_S is the concentration of specifically bound ligand. In the case of binding systems containing more than one specific component, the individual constants have been determined by nongraphical methods, using computer-aided iterative statistical calculations (Blondeau and Robel, 1975).

Rat ventral prostate cytosol is characterized by a large amount of nonspecific binding. Therefore, omission of the above-cited correction factors will result in a large underestimation of the equilibrium association constant, K_a, and an overestimation of the number of specific binding sites, N_s. The errors made will be larger for androstanolone than for testosterone, since the contribution of nonspecific binding is much larger for the former steroid. In addition, rat ventral prostate cytosol contains a very active 3α-hydroxysteroid dehydrogenase (Gore and Baron, 1965) which, even at $0\text{--}4°C$, might reduce the amount of unbound ligand. However, it has been determined that during the 2.5 hours necessary for the completion of protamine sulfate precipitation, the conversion of androstanolone 1 nM into androstanediol is less than 10%.

G. Testosterone and Androstanolone Binding Constants

These determinations were made on Sprague-Dawley male rats 24 hours after castration. The binding curve of androstanolone drawn according to Scatchard (1949), with the use of a statistical curvilinear regression program, is best fitted by assuming one nonspecific binding component plus two categories of specific binding sites (Fig. 2). Testosterone seems also to bind the same two categories of binding sites as androstanolone; but these two binding species cannot be discriminated as easily on the basis of Scatchard curves.

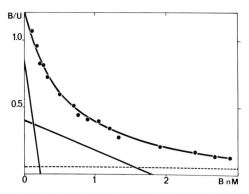

Fig. 2. Binding of androstanolone to cytosol. Protamine sulfate precipitation. Cytosol was prepared from 1-day castrates (16.0 mg of proteins/ml) incubated with increasing concentrations of androstanolone-³H (0.4–60 nM) at $0°C$ for 2 hours. Aliquots (0.25 ml) of each incubation were precipitated with protamine sulfate in GTEM buffer (1.2 mg/ml). The bound radioactivity was measured in the washed precipitates as reported in Section II, D, 2. The curvilinear Scatchard plot was characteristic of two high-affinity low-capacity components (full lines) plus low-affinity large-capacity binding (dashed line), calculated according to Blondeau and Robel (1975). B = bound androstanolone; U = unbound androstanolone.

The values obtained for androstanolone and testosterone binding constants are given in Table IV assuming two categories of specific binding sites, and compared with the values reported by other authors. The case of a single category of specific binding sites has been also considered. Graphical regression gives the following values: androstanolone equilibrium association constant (K_a) = 1.2×10^9 M^{-1} and number of specific binding sites (N) = 50 fmoles/mg of protein; testosterone K_a = 1.0×10^9 M^{-1}, and N = 50 fmoles of protein.

Other possibilities than the presence of two binding components, for instance, negative cooperativity, might explain the curvilinear Scatchard plots. Definitive conclusions should await the physical separation of the two specific components and reassessment of their binding characteristics. Fang and Liao (1971) have demonstrated the presence of two androstanolone-binding species in rat ventral prostate cytosol, called β and α protein, which can be separated by several procedures—in particular by ammonium sulfate fractionation of crude cytosol. Indeed, when 40% ammonium sulfate precipitation was used instead of protamine sulfate, the Scatchard plot obtained demonstrated a single category of binding sites of K_a = 1.2×10^9 M^{-1}, and N = 25.9 fmoles per milligram of protein (Fig. 3). These values are in reasonable agreement with the values obtained for the highest-affinity component of Table IV and with the results of Verhoeven (1974).

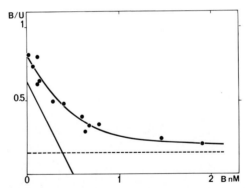

Fig. 3. Binding of androstanolone to cytosol. Ammonium sulfate precipitation. Cytosol (16.3 mg of protein per milliliter) was prepared from 1-day castrates and incubated with increasing concentrations of androstanolone-^{3}H in the same conditions as described in the legend to Fig. 2. Aliquots (0.25 ml) of each incubation were precipitated with ammonium sulfate at 40% saturation. The bound radioactivity was measured in the washed precipitate as reported in Section II, C. The curvilinear Scatchard plot was characteristic of one high-affinity low-capacity component (full line) plus low-affinity large-capacity binding (dashed line), calculated according to Blondeau and Robel (1975). B = bound androstanolone; U = unbound androstanolone.

TABLE IV

ANDROSTANOLONE AND TESTOSTERONE BINDING CONSTANTS TO RAT
VENTRAL PROSTATE CYTOSOL

Reference	Androstanolone[a]				Testosterone[a]			
	K_{a_1}	K_{a_2}	N_1	N_2	K_{a_1}	K_{a_2}	N_1	N_2
Present work:								
2-site hypothesis	3.8	0.22	13	113	3.0	0.08	19	113
1-site hypothesis	1.2	—	50	—	1.0	—	50	—
Töpert *et al.* (1974)	0.36	—	276	—	—	—	—	—
Shain *et al.* (1975)	0.69	—	85.5	—	—	—	—	—
Bruchovsky and Craven (1975)	—	—	174	—	—	—	—	—
Bonne (1975)	0.4–1.6	—	—	—	—	—	—	—
Verhoeven (1974)	0.77	—	54	—	0.68	—	60	—

[a] K_a = equilibrium association constant ($\times 10^9 \ M^{-1}$); K_{a_1}, K_{a_2} = association constant of each specific binding component. N = number of specific binding sites (expressed in androstanolone-binding capacity, fmoles/mg of protein); N_1, N_2 = number of specific binding sites of each specific binding component.

It is not known whether the techniques used by Töpert *et al.* (1974) and Bruchovsky and Craven (1975) will separate both components, whereas obviously the techniques of Shain *et al.* (1975) and Bonne (1975) cannot. Therefore, in addition to the methodological and theoretical reasons discussed previously, failure to discriminate between both components will result in binding constants intermediate between the true values.

Fang and Liao (1971) have reported that the β-protein which is precipitated at 40% ammonium sulfate concentration has an almost exclusive affinity for androstanolone whereas the α-protein, in addition to binding androstanolone, also binds testosterone, progesterone, and estradiol in significant amounts. The high selectivity of the β-protein (the effective component responsible for the nuclear transfer of androstanolone–*receptor* complex), is a very disputed observation. From inhibition studies conducted on the 8–10 S component of glycerol gradients. Baulieu and Jung (1970) reported significant effects of testosterone and estradiol. In the present study, testosterone is bound to both specific binding species of rat ventral prostate cytosol, with affinities only slightly smaller than those of androstanolone.

Binding inhibition studies conducted with a variety of androgens, antiandrogens, and other steroid hormones are reported on Table V. The binding inhibiton curves (not given) show that all competitors are bound

TABLE V

LIGAND SPECIFICITY OF PROSTATE CYTOSOL *Receptor(s)*[a]

Steroid	Relative competition ratio
14-Dehydro-19-nortestosterone	0.66
R 1881	0.71
19-Nortestosterone	0.80
Androstanolone	1.0
Testosterone	1.13
3α-Androstanediol	12.1
Epitestosterone	15.8
Androstanedione	25
Δ^4-Androstenedione	27.5
3β-Androstanediol	28.8
5β-Androsterone	∞
R 2956	3.9
Cyproterone acetate	4.3
Estradiol	8.5
Progesterone	13.2
RU 21270	215
RU 21757	300

[a] Rat ventral prostate cytosol was incubated with androstanolone-^{3}H at 10 nM and with increasing concentrations of inhibitors. Bound radioactivity was measured in the protamine sulfate precipitate. The relative competition ratio is the ratio of the concentration of inhibitor which gives a 50% inhibition of androstanolone-^{3}H binding over the concentration of androstanolone which gives a 50% inhibition of androstanolone-^{3}H binding.

TABLE VI

DECREASING ORDER OF BINDING AFFINITIES OF VARIOUS STEROIDS TO SPECIFIC ANDROGEN BINDING COMPONENTS IN PROSTATE CYTOSOL

Present work	Verhoeven (1974)	Shain and Boesel (1975)
19-Nortestosterone	19-Nortestosterone	19-Nortestosterone
Androstanolone	Androstanolone	Androstanolone
Testosterone	Testosterone	Testosterone
Cyproterone acetate	Cyproterone acetate	Estradiol
Estradiol	Progesterone	Cyproterone acetate
Progesterone	Estradiol	Progesterone
Epitestosterone	Epitestosterone	Epitestosterone
Androstenedione	Androstenedione	Androstenedione
RU 21.270	Flutamide	

to both specific components. The data are expressed in terms of relative competition ratio, i.e., the ratio of competitor concentration over the concentration of androstanolone which brings about the displacement of 50% of the radioactive androstanolone. For some competitors, the K_i of the competitor was also determined (J. P. Blondeau, unpublished results) and is in good agreement with the relative competition ratio. The competition data reported here are in fairly good agreement with those reported by Verhoeven (1974) and Shain and Boesel (1975) (Table VI). The only major discrepancy between the three groups is for the relative positions of cyproterone acetate, estradiol, and progesterone. Contrary to Shain and Boesel (1975), we find that 14-dehydro-19-nortestosterone, a very potent androgen described by Segaloff and Gabbard (1973), has more affinity for the cytosol binders than does androstanolone.

Both 3α-androstanediol and 3β-androstanediol were thought not to compete for androstanolone binding to the 8–10 S rat ventral prostate cytosol receptor (Baulieu and Jung, 1970). It has now been found that these compounds can inhibit androstanolone binding to some extent. Metabolic conversion of 3α-androstanediol into androstanolone might explain, at least in part, the inhibition observed. The inhibition produced by other compounds might also be related to the formation of active metabolites. However, no specific binding can be demonstrated by protamine sulfate precipitation of cytosol incubated with androstanediol-^{3}H, 3β-androstanediol-^{3}H, or estradiol-^{3}H. The binding specificity of the cytosol *receptor* is clearly different from the binding specificity of the component described in rat ventral prostate microsomes (Robel *et al.*, 1974), which has a very high affinity for 3β-androstanediol and for androstanolone, whereas testosterone and 3α-androstanediol are weak competitors and estradiol, progesterone, and cortisol are ineffective.

III. The Control of Androgen *Receptors* in the Rat Ventral Prostate

No investigation had been made up to now of the ontogeny of androgen *receptors* in the prostate. In prepubertal rats, the level of androgen *receptors* is very low (J. P. Blondeau and P. Robel, unpublished observations) and therefore, with the onset of testicular secretions, a concomitant rise of androgen *receptor* in the rat ventral prostate is expected. Indeed, the initial observations dealt with the influence of castration on the level of cytosol *receptor:* when the prostate cytosol of 1, 2, or 3-day castrates was analyzed, a decreased value for the 8–10 S *receptor* peak and more binding in the 4–5 S region of glycerol gradients were observed (Baulieu and Robel, 1970). However, the initial events immediately following castration could not be evaluated owing to the methodogical problems raised by the binding of endogenous hormone to the *receptor* sites.

A. METHODOLOGICAL PROBLEMS

Exchange techniques have been described for the measurement of specific high-affinity binding sites occupied by endogenous hormone (Anderson *et al.*, 1972; Milgrom *et al.*, 1972; Katzellenbogen *et al.*, 1973). Endogenous hormone is exchanged with added radioactive hormone. Owing to the very slow dissociation of hormone at 0°C, heating is necessary to achieve a complete exchange within a reasonable period of time. Unfortunately, in the case of androgen-bound receptors, we were unable to get exchange without a considerable loss of binding sites, owing to the degradation of the *receptor*. Therefore, we propose an alternative technique for the measurement of occupied receptor sites: *the measurement of endogenous hormone by radioimmunoassay after a rigorously specific separation of receptor-bound ligand*. The protamine sulfate precipitation technique used for the measurement of binding constants (see Section II, D, 2) although very selective, still includes some contribution of nonspecific binding which must be subtracted. It has been observed that an additional wash of the precipitate with buffer containing 10% ethanol and 1% Triton X-100 almost completely eliminates the nonspecific binding without change of the specific component (Table VII). In a representative

TABLE VII

SELECTIVE PRECIPITATION OF *Receptor*-BOUND ANDROSTANOLONE
BY PROTAMINE SULFATE[a]

	Dpm in precipitate		
	GTEM	GTEM + ethanol	GTEM + ethanol + Triton X-100
(1) Androstanolone-^{3}H, 10 nM	25,428	22,935	20,578
(2) Androstanolone-^{3}H, 10 nM, +androstanolone 1 μM	5,094	2,543	1,414
Difference (1) − (2)	20,334	20,392	19,164

[a] Cytosol from 24-hour castrated rat ventral prostates was prepared in GTEM buffer (Tris-HCl, 10 mM; EDTA, 1.5 mM; mercaptoethanol, 2 mM; glycerol, 15%, pH 7.4) and incubated with radioactive androstanolone, as indicated, 2 hours at 0°C. Aliquots, 0.25 ml, were precipitated with 0.25 ml of protamine sulfate 1.2 mg/ml. The precipitates were collected on glass paper filters and washed with 3 × 10 ml of GTEM buffer. Eventually the first wash contained 10% ethanol or 10% ethanol + 1% Triton X-100.

control experiment, rat ventral prostate cytosol is incubated with either androstanolone-³H, 10 nM, or androstanolone-³H, 10 nM, plus androstanolone, 1 μM, or with nonradioactive androstanolone, 10 nM (Table VIII). The first two incubations allow the measurement of *receptor* binding sites by the differential approach. The aliquots of the first and of the third incubations are precipitated with protamine sulfate, the precipitates are washed with the ethanol–Triton buffer and resuspended in water. A tracer amount of androstanolone-³H is added to the latter suspension, then both are extracted with ethyl acetate. The extract corresponding to the first incubation is counted for radioactivity, whereas the extract corresponding to the third incubation is chromatographed on a Celite column (Barberia and Thorneycroft, 1974) and the fraction corresponding to androstanolone is measured by radioimmunoassay with an antibody raised against testosterone-3-carboxymethyloxime-BSA (C. Corpéchot and P. Robel, unpublished results). All three procedures give similar results.

A control is used to validate the measurement of nuclear androstanolone–*receptor* complexes. Identical aliquots of rat ventral prostate cytosol are incubated (A) with 10 nM androstanolone-³H, and (B) with 10 nM nonradioactive androstanolone. The crude nuclear pellet is resuspended and is divided into equal portions, which are incubated with (A) and (B) for 30 minutes at 30°C. The incubated nuclei are sedimented at 800

TABLE VIII

"RADIOIMMUNOASSAY" OF CYTOSOLIC ANDROSTANOLONE–*Receptor* COMPLEXES[a]

	Specifically bound androstanolone (pmoles/ml of cytosol)
(1) Androstanolone-³H-*receptor* complex, differential technique	3.11 ± 0.07[b]
(2) Androstanolone-³H-*receptor* complex, ethanol + Triton-washed protamine sulfate	3.13 ± 0.02
(3) Androstanolone-*receptor* complex, ethanol + Triton-washed protamine sulfate, radioimmunoassay	3.13 ± 0.17

[a] Rat ventral prostate cytosol was incubated (a) with androstanolone-³H, 10 nM; (b) with androstanolone-³H, 10 nM, +androstanolone, 1 μM; (c), with androstanolone, 10 nM. Aliquots of (a) and (b) were precipitated with protamine sulfate and the (a) − (b) dpm were converted to picomoles per milliliter of cytosol. Aliquots of (a) and (c) were precipitated with protamine sulfate and washed with 10% ethanol + 1% Triton X-100. These precipitates were resuspended in water and extracted with ethyl acetate. The extract of (a) was counted, the extract of (c) was submitted to radioimmunoassay for androstanolone; the results were again expressed in picomoles per milliliter of cytosol.

[b] Mean ±SEM.

TABLE IX

"Radioimmunoassay" of Nuclear Androstanolone–*Receptor* Complexes[a]

	Nuclear bound androstanolone (pmoles/gm of prostate)
(1) Androstanolone-^{3}H–*receptor* complexes	1.50 ± 0.03[b]
(2) Androstanolone–*receptor* complexes, radioimmunoassay	1.70 ± 0.03

[a] Identical rat ventral prostate cytosol aliquots were incubated (a) with androstanolone^{-3}H, 10 nM, or (b) with androstanolone, 10 nM. The corresponding nuclear pellets were added and incubation was continued for 30 minutes at 30°C. Then the nuclear pellets were resedimented, washed once with buffer containing 10% ethanol and 1% Triton X-100, and twice again with buffer. The final pellets were resuspended in water and extracted with ethyl acetate. The extract of (a) was counted, the extract of (b) was submitted to a radioimmunoassay for androstanolone, and the results were expressed in pmoles per gram of prostate.

[b] Mean ±SEM.

g for 10 minutes, then washed once with GTEM buffer containing 3 mM MgCl$_2$, 3 mM CaCl$_2$, 20 mM KCl, 10% ethanol, and 1% Triton X-100 and twice with the same buffer without ethanol and Triton. The final pellets are resuspended in water, extracted with ethyl acetate, then processed as described above for cytosol (Table IX).

B. Disappearance of Nuclear Androstanolone–*Receptor* Complexes After Castration

Several control experiments (not shown) were made to demonstrate that with the use of the ethanol–Triton wash only specifically bound androstanolone remained in the nuclear pellet. No specifically bound testosterone was found. Therefore the radioimmunoassay of androstanolone extracted from the nuclear pellets so prepared can be considered to be a measurement of nuclear androstanolone–*receptor* complexes, and probably of nuclear *receptor* sites, since empty nuclear *receptor* sites are very few or absent (Jensen *et al.*, 1968; Fang *et al.*, 1969). Data reported in Fig. 4 deal with the disappearance of nuclear androstanolone–*receptor* complexes. Their decrease seems to follow a first-order law with a half-life of approximately 190 minutes. This value is in good agreement with that of 200 minutes reported by Mester and Baulieu (1975) for the rat uterus estrogen *receptor*. The initial value in normal noncastrated rats is 12 pmoles per milligram of DNA or 54,000 sites per nucleus assuming 7.4 pg of DNA per nucleus (Shain *et al.*, 1975). After 6.5 hours, the

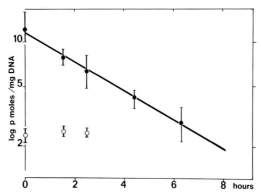

FIG. 4. Nuclear androstanolone–*receptor* complexes and cytosol *receptor* at short-term intervals after castration. The crude nuclear and cytosolic fractions were prepared from individual prostates between 0 and 6.5 hours after castration. Cytosol was incubated with 10 nM androstanolone for 2 hours at 0°C, then precipitated with protamine sulfate (1.2 mg/ml). Nuclei and precipitates were washed with buffer containing 10% ethanol and 1% Triton X-100, to remove all nonspecific binding. Then both fractions were processed for androstanolone radioimmunoassay. Androstanolone is expressed in pmoles per milligram of DNA (mean ± SEM, at least 3 determination). ●, Nuclei; ○, cytosol.

nuclear complexes still represent 2.8 pmoles per milligram of DNA. They are undetectable 21 hours after castration.

C. DEPLETION OF CYTOSOL *Receptor* AFTER CASTRATION

To determine the amount of total cytosol *receptor* in normal noncastrated rats, the cytosol is incubated with 10 nM androstanolone at 0°C for 2 hours, followed by protamine sulfate precipitation and ethanol + Triton wash. The concentration of total cytosol *receptor* is 2.6 pmoles per milligram of DNA, corresponding to approximately 11,500 sites/cell. Approximately 90% of the binding sites are occupied by endogenous androstanolone. In the initial hours after castration and up to hour 24, the concentration of cytosol *receptor* does not vary significantly (Fig. 4). Later on, a steady decrease of cytosol *receptor* occurs until day 4 after castration, when only 25% of the initial amount is left. The half-life of this decrease is 40 hours (Fig. 5). A subsequent increase of cytosol receptor is observed during the following days until a maximum on day 10. This increase is very striking when expressed in pmoles of *receptor* per milligram of protein since the level exceeds that of the noncastrated animal. However, when expressed in picomoles per milligram of DNA, the increase of cytosol *receptor* is less dramatic, although a significant

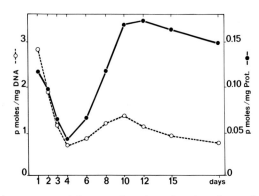

Fig. 5. Cytosol *receptor* activity as a function of various intervals after castration.
The cytosol was prepared from a pool of at least 4 prostates at intervals of 1–20
days after castration. Each cytosol was incubated with 10 nM androstanolone-^{3}H
(incubation a) or 10 nM androstanolone-^{3}H $+$ 1 μM androstanolone (incubation b),
and the total number of specific binding sites was calculated from the difference
between incubations (a) and (b), as described by Blondeau and Robel (1975). Results are expressed in picomoles of androstanolone binding capacity per milligram
of protein or of DNA.

increase occurs after day 8. Then a lightly declining plateau is observed
until day 21 after castration.

D. Discussion

1. *Steady-State Levels of Cytosol and Nuclear Receptors in Intact Rats*

The total amount of androgen *receptor* in the rat ventral prostate that
is measured by radioimmunoassay is 14.6 pmoles per milligram of DNA,
representing approximately 65,000 sites/cell. Slightly more than 80% of
the total sites are represented by nuclear androstanolone *receptor* complexes. Negligible amounts of testosterone are bound either to cytosol
or to nuclear *receptors*. There are very few empty sites in the cytosol
receptor. This is expected, since the concentration of circulating total testosterone in the male rat is in the 10–30 nM range, and then the concentration of free, nonprotein-bound circulating testosterone should be in
the 1 nM range, of the same order or greater than the 0.4 nM K_D of
the *receptor* and should bring about a large occupancy of *receptor* sites.
Therefore, nearly maximum stimulation of the ventral prostate may be
the physiological situation in the normal adult rat.

Few reports deal with the measurement of steroid hormone *receptors*
in intact adult animals. The estradiol-binding capacity of rat uterus
cytosol (Feherty *et al.*, 1970) and of rat uterus nuclei (Clark *et al.*, 1972)

have been investigated during the estrous cycle; maximum values were obtained at proestrus: 5 pmole per milligram of DNA for the cytosol receptor and 1.3 pmole per milligram of DNA for the nuclear *receptor*. The progesterone cytosol *receptor* of guinea pig uterus (Milgrom *et al.*, 1972b) shows also a maximum at proestrus of 41,000 sites/cell; the nuclear *receptors* were not determined but represented a rather small proportion of total *receptor*. Hence, in comparison with the female sex hormone *receptors* in uterus, the ventral prostate *receptors* are more abundant and show a much larger proportion of occupied binding sites, and consequently much larger proportions of the *receptors* are present in the nuclear fraction.

2. *The Decrease of Receptor after Castration*

There is a general agreement that the concentration of cytosol *receptor* declines after castration. This was shown for the 8–10 S receptor by Baulieu and Jung (1970), and confirmed by Mainwaring and Mangan (1973), who have shown a 90% decrease of the high-affinity binding of androstanolone to proteins of mean Stokes radius of 80 Å by gel exclusion chromatography on Sephadex G-200 between the first and fourth day after castration. The comprehensive study of Sullivan and Strott (1973) used the radioactivity of the 8 S regions of sucrose gradients (after incubation with 3 nM androstanolone-^{3}H) as a criterion for the quantitation of the cytosol *receptor*. They have observed a fall of the cytosol *receptor* specific activity to a minimum on day 4 (about 25% of the initial value 24 hours after castration), then a rise to nearly twice its initial level, whereas the size of the prostate and the DNA content per prostate continued to fall. The present study shows that this biphasic phenomenon cannot be attributed to a change in the molecular form of the receptor but to changes of the number of specific binding sites. However, contrary to the findings of Sullivan and Strott (1973), the secondary increase of cytosol *receptor* was less marked when expressed per milligram of DNA, so that the cytosol *receptor* content per prostate and also per cell remained rather low after its early fall after castration. Sullivan and Strott (1973) have also shown that the same phenomenon occurs in animals that were either hypophysectomized or adrenalectomized at the time of castration. This finding indicates that restoration of *receptor* is probably not mediated by adrenal androgens or pituitary hormones.

The rapid and, at least in part, transient disappearance of prostate cytosol *receptor* seems temporally related with the presence of increased proteolytic activity. This is suggested by ultrastructural and cytochemical evidence for increased lysosomal activity and autophagy of epithelial cells after castration (Helminen and Ericsson 1971; Brandes, 1974). This

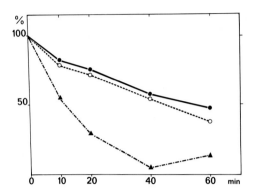

Fɪɢ. 6. Thermal stability of androstanolone-*receptor* complexes. Cytosol samples were prepared from 1, 4 and 10 day castrates and incubated with 5 nM androstanolone-³H (incubation a) or 5 nM androstanolone-³H + 1 μM androstanolone (incubation b) for 2 hours at 0°C. Then both incubations of each cytosol were heated at 37°C; aliquots were removed at the indicated time intervals, chilled, and precipitated by protamine sulfate. The difference between incubations (a) and (b) was calculated and expressed as percentage of control in incubation at 0°C. ●——●, 10-day castrates; ○ - - - - - ○, 1-day castrates; ▲-·-·-▲, 4-day castrates.

might result in greatly decreased *receptor* stability after castration. Indeed, when the cytosol is prepared from 1-day or 10-day castrates and androstanolone-³H-*receptor* complexes are heated at 37°C, about 50% of the complexes remain in the cytosol after 60 minutes, whereas all the binding activity is lost after 40 minutes in 4-day castrates (Fig. 6). A similar observation was made by Bruchovsky and Craven (1975), who made tissue-mixing experiments in which equal amounts of prostate from 1-day and 7-day castrates were incubated and homogenized together, and who observed a loss of binding activity, presumably due to proteolytic enzymes in the 7-day castrate cytosol. A 100% increase in proteolytic activity was also observed by Mainwaring and Mangan (1973) 3 days after castration.

E. Rᴀᴅɪᴏᴀᴜᴛᴏɢʀᴀᴘʜɪᴄ Sᴛᴜᴅɪᴇs ᴏꜰ *Receptor*

Nuclear localization of radioactive hormone can be demonstrated in rat ventral prostate cells by radioautography of freeze-dried sections after injection of testosterone-³H *in vivo* (Tveter and Attramadal, 1969; Sar *et al.*, 1970). These investigators demonstrated the selective retention of radioactive hormone in the epithelial cell nuclei. In the present investigation, 1-, 4-, and 9-day castrates received a subcutaneous injection of 400 μCi (1.3 μg) of testosterone-³H (SA 84 Ci/mmole), 1 hour before decapitation and removal of the ventral prostates. The prostates were fixed in glutaraldehyde (1.6% in phosphate buffer), frozen sections were prepared and processed for radioautography (Fig. 7). It can be seen that the pattern of nuclear labeling gives results similar to the measurement of cytosol *receptor* expressed in picomoles per milligram of DNA (see Fig. 5), i.e., a sharp decrease of nuclear labeling between days 1 and 4, followed by a slight increase at day 9. This experiment allows two conclusions: (1) The early decrease of binding sites does not seem to be an artifact secondary to the intense proteolytic activity in the 4-day castrate cytosol, which might have led to the destruction of *receptor* during the homogenization, ultracentrifugation, and incubation of the cytosol, since similar decrease occurs when all these preliminary steps are omitted. (2) The secondary increase of binding cannot be attributed to nonepithelial prostatic cells (fibroblasts or smooth muscle cells), since these cells are always very poorly labeled.

F. INDUCTION OF ANDROGEN *Receptor* BY TESTOSTERONE

Testosterone injection at the time of castration maintains some of the *receptor* activity (Sullivan and Strott, 1973). Is this effect of testosterone due only to the inhibition of proteolysis which follows castration? It must be stressed that during the first day after castration no increase of proteolysis is yet observed, but nevertheless a dramatic fall in the total cell *receptor* is observed, mainly due to the disappearance of nuclear complexes. It seems reasonable to conclude that most of the nuclear *receptor* is inactivated after the release of bound androstanolone. The question is raised whether testosterone, like estradiol (Sarff and Gorski, 1971), is able to induce the synthesis of its own *receptor*.

1. *Materials and Methods*

Twenty-four-hour castrates have been used throughout this study. Four groups of rats were investigated. Besides controls, the second group received one subcutaneous injection of 75 μg of testosterone in 0.2 ml of ethanol, the third group received in addition 400 μg of cycloheximide per 100 gm body weight, 10 minutes before and 6 hours after testosterone, and the fourth group received cycloheximide alone. This amount of cycloheximide was shown to inhibit protein synthesis in the prostate (cpm per milligram of protein after intraperitoneal injection of 5 μCi of leucine-^{3}H) by 60–62%; amounts of cycloheximide necessary to get more complete inhibition of protein synthesis were lethal. The dose of testosterone injected was calculated so as to get a plasma concentration of testosterone above or within the normal range (5–8.5 pmoles/ml) during the 6 hours after injection. Under such conditions, the ventral prostate con-

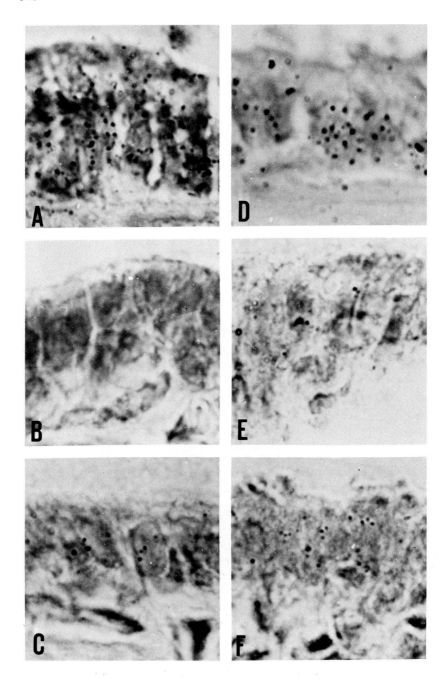

centration of androstanolone fell below the normal value (10 ± 1.8 pmoles/gm, mean $\pm$ SEM; Robel *et al.*, 1973) at 3 hours after castration, then declined slowly between the third and the twelfth hour. All experimental groups (3–10 animals) were killed by decapitation 36 hours after castration, and the "radioimmunoassay" of cytosol receptor and nuclear complexes was made as described.

2. *Results*

In control animals, no nuclear complexes are found, whereas the level of cytosol *receptor* is slightly lower in 36-hour castrates than in 24-hour castrates. In cycloheximide-treated rats, the concentration of cytosol *receptor* is very low, suggesting that continued protein synthesis is necessary to maintain the basal level of cytosolic *receptor*. Twelve hours after the injection of testosterone to 24-hour castrates, the concentration of cytosolic *receptor* was unchanged; however, the nuclear *receptor* was replenished to the level observed in intact animals. Unexpectedly, cycloheximide was without effect on the replenishment of androgen *receptor* produced by testosterone (Table X).

3. *Conclusion: Mechanisms Controlling the Level of Androgen Receptors and Comparison with Other Sex Steroid Receptors*

The control of the prostate *receptor* by testosterone bears some similarities to the control of the estrogen *receptor* in the uterus (Feherty *et al.*, 1970; Sarff and Groski, 1971; Clark *et al.*, 1972; Mester and Baulieu, 1975). In animals exposed to hormone, the level of cytosol *receptor* is larger than in hormone-depleted animals. However, in the case of uterine *receptors*, the replenishment of cytosol *receptor* is obviously blocked by protein synthesis inhibiting agents. In the case of rat ventral prostate, although testosterone induced a very large increase in total *receptor* from

---

Fig. 7. Radioautograms of rat ventral prostate at various intervals after castration. Testosterone-^{3}H (400 μCi/1.34 μg) or androstanolone-^{3}H (400 μCi/0.66 μg) were injected subcutaneously in 0.4 ml of ethanol 1 hour before sacrifice of 1-, 4-, and 9-day castrates. Rats were decapitated; the ventral prostates were quickly removed, chilled, and fixed in 1–6% glutaraldehyde. Frozen sections, 6 μm thick, were made, overlaid with stripping film Kodak AR 10, and exposed for 6 months. The sections were poststained with methyl green pyronine. (A, B, C) testosterone-^{3}H; (D, E, F) androstanolone-^{3}H; (A and D) 1-day castrates, 8–10 grains per epithelial cell per nucleus; (B and E) 4-day castrates, less than 1 grain per nucleus; (C and F) 9-day castrates, 1–3 grains per nucleus. In control experiments, not shown, nuclear grains are not present when thousandfold unlabeled testosterone or dihydrotestosterone is injected together with the radioactive steroid. $\times$2000.

TABLE X

NUCLEAR AND CYTOSOL *Receptors* IN INTACT, CASTRATED, AND TESTOSTERONE-INJECTED RATS[a]

	Nuclei	Cytosol	Total	p^c
(1) Intact	12.0 ± 0.4[b] (6)	2.6 ± 0.4 (3)	14.6	1 versus 5 and 6, NS
(2) 24-Hour castrates[d]	0	2.8	2.8	
(3) 36-Hour castrates[d]	0	2.4	2.4	
24-Hour castrates				
(4) 12-Hour cyclo-heximide	0	0.76 ± 0.02 (3)	0.76	4 versus 6, $p < 0.025$
(5) 12-Hour testos-terone	11.9 ± 1.4 (10)	2.3 ± 0.2 (5)	14.2	5 versus 6, NS
(6) 12-Hour testos-terone + cycloheximide	12.5 ± 1.7 (9)	1.7 ± 0.22 (5)	14.2	

[a] The measurement of nuclear receptor androstanolone complexes and of the cytosol total receptor was made by the radioimmunoassay technique (see text, Section III, A).

[b] Picomoles per milligram of DNA, mean ± SEM. The figures in parentheses give the number of determinations.

[c] Probability (p) of significance between cytosol receptor levels (Student t test). No significant difference (NS) was found between nuclei from experiments 1, 5, and 6.

[d] Values taken from the data reported in Fig. 5.

2.6 to 14.1 pmoles per milligram of DNA, this increase was not prevented by cycloheximide. This failure might be related to the incomplete inhibition of protein synthesis, but other possibilities might be considered, for example, the formation of receptor from a precursor present in the microsomal fraction (Little *et al.*, 1972; Robel *et al.*, 1974) or even from a soluble precursor that does not bind androstanolone with high affinity. The synthesis of progesterone *receptor* is induced by estradiol in the guinea pig uterus (Milgrom *et al.*, 1972b). The effect of estradiol on androgen receptors is not known, but it should be recalled that the presence of estrogen receptors in the rat ventral prostate is doubtful. Once induced by estradiol, progesterone *receptors* have a prolonged half-life. The breakdown of the progesterone *receptor* is accelerated by the injection of progesterone. On the contrary, in the case of the prostate, hormone deprivation is followed by a very important increase of proteolytic activity, which seems to be responsible, at least in part, for the rapid disappearance of the cytosol *receptor*. However, it is very likely that the *receptor* transferred to the nuclei is largely inactivated after the removal of bound hormone, and this situation might be common to all sex steroid *receptors*.

ACKNOWLEDGMENTS

We thank B. Eychenne, F. Delahaye, and M. Pouplet for their skillful technical assistance, Roussel-Uclaf, Schering A.G., and A. Segaloff for the provision of reference compounds, D. Prod'homme and M. Leblondel for the preparation of this manuscript.

REFERENCES

Anderson, J., Clark, J. H., and Peck, E. J. (1972). *Biochem. J.* **126**, 561.
Anderson, K. M., and Liao, S. (1968). *Nature (London)* **219**, 277.
Barberia, J. M., and Thorneycroft, I. H. (1974). *Steroids* **23**, 757.
Baulieu, E. E., and Jung, I. (1970). *Biochem. Biophys. Res. Commun.* **38**, 599.
Baulieu, E. E., and Robel, P. (1970). *In* "Some Aspects of the Aetiology and Biochemistry of Prostate Cancer" (K. Griffiths and C. G. Pierrepoint, eds.), p. 74. Alpha Omega Alpha Publ., Cardiff, Wales.
Baulieu, E. E., Lasnitzki, I., and Robel, P. (1968). *Nature (London)* **219**, 1155.
Baulieu, E. E., Jung, I., Blondeau, J. P., and Robel, P. (1971). *Advan. Biosci.* **7**, 179.
Blondeau, J. P., and Robel, P. (1975). *Eur. J. Biochem.* **55**, 375.
Bonne, C. (1975). Ph.D. Dissertation, Univ. Rene Descartes of Paris, Paris, France.
Brandes, D. (1974). *In* "Male Accessory Sex Organs" (D. Brandes, ed.), p. 184. Academic Press, New York.
Bruchovsky, N., and Craven, S. (1975). *Biochem. Biophys. Res. Commun.* **62**, 837.
Bruchovsky, N., and Wilson, J. D. (1968). *J. Biol. Chem.* **243**, 5953.
Castañeda, E., and Liao, S. (1975). *J. Biol. Chem.* **250**, 883.
Clark, J. H., Anderson, J., and Peck, E. J. (1972). *Science* **176**, 528.
Erdos, T., Best-Belpomme, M., and Bessada, R. (1970). *Anal. Biochem.* **37**, 244.
Fang, S., and Liao, S. (1971). *J. Biol. Chem.* **246**, 16.
Fang, S., Anderson, K. M., and Liao, S. (1969). *J. Biol. Chem.* **244**, 6584.
Feherty, P., Robertson, D. M., Waynforth, H. B., and Kellie, A. E. (1970). *Biochem. J.* **120**, 837.
Gore, M. B. R., and Baron, D. N. (1965). *J. Endocrinol.* **33**, 353.
Gorski, J., Toft, D., Shyamala, G., Smith, D., and Notides, A. (1971). *Recent Progr. Horm. Res.* **24**, 45.
Hansson, V., Djöseland, O., Reusch, E., Attramadal, A., and Torgersen, O. (1973). *Steroids* **22**, 19.
Helminen, H. J., and Ericsson, J. L. (1971). *J. Ultrastruct. Res.* **36**, 708.
Jensen, E. V., Suzuki, T., Kawashima, T., Stumpf, W. E., Jungblut, P. W., and DeSombre, E. R. (1968). *Proc. Nat. Acad. Sci. U.S.* **59**, 632.
Katsumata, M., and Goldman, A. S. (1974). *Biochim. Biophys. Acta* **359**, 112.
Katzenellenbogen, J. A., Johnson, H. J., and Carlson, K. E. (1973). *Biochemistry* **12**, 4092.
King, R. J. B., and Mainwaring, W. I. P., eds. (1974). "Steroid-Cell Interactions," p. 41. Butterworths, London.
Krieg, M., Steins, P., Szalay, R., and Voigt, K. D. (1974). *J. Steroid Biochem.* **5**, 87.
Liao, S., and Fang, S. (1969). *Vit. Horm. (New York)* **27**, 17.
Little, M., Rosenfeld, G. C., and Jungblut, P. W. (1972). *Hoppe-Seyler's Z. Physiol. Chem.* **353**, 231.

Mainwaring, W. I. P. (1969). *J. Endocrinol.* **44**, 323.

Mainwaring, W. I. P., and Mangan, F. R. (1973). *J. Endocrinol.* **59**, 121.

Mainwaring, W. I. P., and Peterken, B. M. (1971). *Biochem. J.* **125**, 285.

Mester, J., and Baulieu, E. E. (1975). *Biochem. J.* **146**, 617.

Milgrom, E., and Baulieu, E. E. (1969). *Biochim. Biophys. Acta* **194**, 602.

Milgrom, E., Perrot, M., Atger, M., and Baulieu, E. E. (1972a). *Endocrinology* **90**, 1064.

Milgrom, E., Atger, M., Perrot, M., and Baulieu, E. E. (1972b). *Endocrinology* **90**, 1071.

Murphy, B. E. P. (1967). *J. Clin. Endocrinol.* **27**, 973.

Ritzén, E. M., Nayfeh, S. N., French, F. S., and Dobbins, M. C. (1971). *Endocrinology* **89**, 143.

Ritzén, E. M., French, F. S., Weddington, S. C., and Nayfeh, S. N. (1974). *J. Biol. Chem.* **249**, 6597.

Robel, P., Corpéchot, C., and Baulieu, E. E. (1973). *FEBS (Fed. Eur. Biochem. Soc.) Lett.* **33**, 218.

Robel, P., Blondeau, J. P., and Baulieu, E. E. (1974). *Biochim. Biophys. Acta* **373**,

Sar, M., Liao, S., and Stumpf, W. E. (1970). *Endocrinology* **86**, 1008.

Sarff, M., and Gorski, J. (1971). *Biochemistry* **10**, 2557.

Scatchard, G. (1949). *Ann. N.Y. Acad. Sci.* **51**, 660.

Segaloff, A., and Gabbard, R. B. (1973). *Steroids* **22**, 99.

Shain, S. A., and Boesel, R. W. (1975). *J. Steroid Biochem.* **6**, 43.

Shain, S. A., Boesel, R. W., and Axelrod, L. R. (1975). *Arch. Biochem. Biophys.* **167**, 247.

Steggles, A. W., and King, R. J. B. (1970). *Biochem, J.* **118**, 695.

Sullivan, J. N., and Strott, C. A. (1973). *J. Biol. Chem.* **248**, 3203.

Töpert, M., Zabel, I., and Ziegler, M. (1974). *Anal. Biochem.* **62**, 514.

Tveter, K. J., and Attramadal, A. (1969). *Endocrinology* **85**, 350.

Unhjem, O., Tveter, K. J., and Aakvaag, A. (1969). *Acta Endocrinol. (Copenhagen)* **62**, 153.

Verhoeven, G. (1974). Ph.D. Thesis, University of Leuven, Belgium.

DISCUSSION

S. Liao: It is important to consider the number of receptor molecules per cell, but I think it is also important to consider what is the actual concentration of the receptor in the cell, because the affinity of the receptor toward the nuclear acceptor may be such that the receptor concentration can be a determining factor. Since both the number of the receptor molecules and the prostate cell size decrease after castration, is it possible that the receptor concentration in the prostate cell may not decrease very much and actually may increase?

P. Robel: No comment.

N. Bruchovsky: Could you clarify a point? Is it correct that you observed a large increase in the number of nuclear receptors during an interval when there was no change in the number of cytoplasmic receptors? Does this mean that the nuclear receptor is not derived from the cytoplasmic receptor?

P. Robel: That is correct. The nuclear receptor went up to the level of intact rats without change of the cytosol receptor. However, during the 12-hour period of testosterone action, synthesis of a large amount of *receptor* might have taken place. Obviously, a time-course study of the reinduction of nuclear *receptor* is desirable. The failure of cycloheximide to prevent the rise in total cell *receptor* might indeed suggest that the nuclear *receptor* derives from a precursor that is not the cytosol *receptor*. The correlation that I have reported between the level of the cytosol *receptor* in 1-, 4-, and 9-day castrates and the amount of the nuclear *receptor* demonstrated by radioautography 1 hour after ^{3}H-labeled testosterone injection *in vivo* does not support such an interpretation.

K. J. Tveter: Have you investigated the amount of cytosol receptor several months after orchiectomy? In animals castrated 3 months previously it is possible to restore completely the fine structure of the prostate in rats.

P. Robel: No, we did not investigate the amount of cytosol *receptor* of rats castrated for more than 3 weeks. However, the *receptor* seems to plateau after the tenth day, and a similar level might be expected in 3-month castrates.

K. B. Eik-Nes: In the experiments with cycloheximide depicted on your last slide, were these animals also adrenalectomized?

P. Robel: This is a good point. The animals were not adrenalectomized, and they were heavily stressed. Possibly this might in part explain the unexpected results of the cycloheximide and testosterone experiment.

M. B. Lipsett: Have you attempted to use the protamine sulfate–*receptor* complex at 23°C to determine, by exchange, total receptor?

P. Robel: No, I did not, but William McGuire (personal communication) has shown that the estradiol *receptor*–protamine sulfate complex from human breast cancer and the dihydrotestosterone *receptor*–protamine sulfate complex from rat ventral prostate are very stable and might be used to set up an exchange technique at 23°C, or perhaps preferably at 30°C. In addition, the disadvantage of hormone metabolism by hydroxysteroid dehydrogenases present in the cytosol is also eliminated, and therefore the procedure of McGuire seems to improve the protamine sulfate precipitation technique.

Round Table Discussion on Prostatic *Receptors*

(*Rapporteur:* E. E. BAULIEU)

The presence of specific high-affinity steroid binding proteins in target cells is largely accepted as an important indicator of their steroid hormones' "receptivity." Even though the concept of the necessary presence of receptors for mediating hormone action has not been verified in prostatic cells, there is no evidence against it. Therefore, a critical evaluation of the binding proteins' specificity and affinity for different agonistic and antiagonistic hormonal compounds, of their abundance in prostatic cells, and of the hormonal and extrahormonal controls of their concentration is of great importance. In recent years, the concept has been substantiated that *receptors* are not "static" components and that their concentrations may change according to specific physiopathological conditions. The regression of the androgen *receptor* in the ventral prostate following castration was one of the earliest observations supporting this view. During this meeting, data showing the induction of androgen *receptors* by androgen have been presented for the first time. It may be of great advantage to be able to quantitatively evaluate *receptors*, in order to estimate hormone sensitivity leading to better hormonal therapeutics of genetic and pathological disorders.

Methodological problems are therefore of great importance. Throughout the meeting and the round table discussion, several difficulties have been reported. In tissue samples and extracts, one should be able to distinguish hormone bound to a specific *receptor* and hormone bound by (a) nonspecific proteins and (b) specific protein(s) of plasma origin, such as sex steroid binding plasma protein (SBP), also referred to as sex hormone binding globulin (SHBG) or testosterone–estradiol binding globulin (TEBG). The ability to differentiate between the high affinity of the receptor and the lower affinity of the nonspecific binding proteins may be possible by the use of isotopic dilution, a procedure of primary importance for future development of this methodology. Physical methods for separating receptors from plasma proteins have been discussed by Dr. De Voogt, using the Wagner agar gel electrophoresis, and by Dr. Robel, who has utilized differential sedimentation on gradients and polyacrylamide gel preparations. The differential binding specificity between steroids may also be used for *receptor* isolation; for instance, 3α-androstanediol has a low binding affinity for SBP, but displaces androstanolone (or dihydrotestosterone) from the *receptor*.

347

Another difficulty in quantitating *receptors* is the possible *aggregation*, which may lead to underestimation in techniques employing charcoal due to sedimentation of the aggregate with the absorbent.

Finally, and probably most important in prostatic tissue, is the problem of *proteolysis*. This contributes to the destruction of the *receptors*, resulting in a decreased amount of measurable *receptor* protein. This point has been discussed by Dr. Ritzén, who emphasized that homogenization leads to the rupture of lysosomes; by Dr. Williams-Ashman, who indicated that lysosomes are associated with acid proteinases and proteolytic enzymes which are under the control of androgens; and by Dr. Tagnon, who described three different proteolytic systems in prostatic cytosol and discussed the use of specific inhibitors (ε-aminocaproic acid soybean inhibitor) that may be useful. This discussion took place after Dr. Bruchovsky's disclosure that there is proteolytic activity during the autophagic response following castration and that there may also be *receptor*-inactivating factor(s), which could contribute to the mechanisms modulating *receptor* activities under various circumstances. This was suggested by the fact that the prostate from 7-day castrated rats treated by androgen for 7 days undergoes regeneration to normal size with normal cell number, but may still contain some *receptor* "inactivating factors."

Another aspect of the discussion was the binding of *different ligands* to androgen *receptors*. It is known that 3α-androstanediol is an active androgen and that it is metabolized to other active compounds, mostly androstanolone. Dr. Verhoeven has indicated that several androgen target organs, including lacrimal glands, kidney, and prostate, show high concentrations of 3α-hydroxysteroid dehydrogenase. The question therefore was raised whether it can be ascertained that 3α-androstanediol acts only through its conversion to androstanolone. Dr. Lipsett stated that 3α-androstanediol is very active in producing BPH in the dog whereas DHT is not. Dr. Voigt believes that 3α-androstanediol is a poor precursor of androstanolone.

The question of the ability of the *receptor* to bind *Flutamide*, an antiandrogen, was discussed by Drs. Neri, Mainwaring, Coffey, and Robel. It appears that even when considering the formation of the hydroxylated metabolite and the well-recognized negative effect of Flutamide on the formation of the nuclear androgen *receptor* in the prostate, the answer is still very unclear. Dr. Pierrepoint posed another interesting question during the discussion of his work with Dr. Evans and Dr. Griffiths at the Tenovus Institute. They found *5α-androstane-3α,17α-diol* to be the active androgen in the dog prostate, and they have evidence of the binding of this "α-diol" to a 4–5 S *receptor* which does not bind other C_{19} steroids. This is also found in perianal adenoma of the dog, a condition that can be treated either with stilbestrol or by surgical castration. Dr. Pierrepoint also stated that the α-diol will stimulate dog prostatic RNA polymerase in a subcellular system similar to the one used by Dr. Davies with rat prostate, whereas androstanolone reduces this activity.

The final discussion was concerned with the *estrogen receptor*. Everyone agreed that estradiol can competitively inhibit androstanolone from binding to the androgen *receptor* in the *rat* prostate. However, evidence for an independent estrogen *receptor* in rat ventral prostate cytosol is not conclusive. Dr. Sandberg remarked that the dog prostate can concentrate estrogen which cannot be readily displaced by androgen. Also in the baboon prostate, as established by Dr. Suffrin in Sandberg's laboratory, there is an estrogen *receptor* that binds estradiol, estriol, and diethylstilbestrol, and the estrogens cannot be displaced by either testosterone or androstanolone. In the *human*, Dr. De Voogt cited a case of carcinoma of the prostate where a specific estrogen *receptor* was identified which was different from the androstanolone *receptor*. Dr. Baulieu stated that in mammary cancer cell cultures, probably representative of one cell type following cloning, there are simultaneously androgen and estrogen *receptors* which are biochemically distinct. As in most target organs, the estrogen *receptor* binds various estrogens, including diethylstilbestrol, but has a very low affinity for androgens. Conversely, the binding of androstanolone to the androgen *receptor* can be competitively inhibited by testosterone, and to a lesser extent by progesterone and estradiol, but not by diethylstilbestrol. A multiplicity of *receptors* that bind the same steroids with different affinities and can distinguish between natural and artificial estrogens was reported.

The implication of prostatic *receptors* responding to hormones of prostatic origin was suggested by Dr. Davies, who discussed the effect of the steroid *receptor* complexes on *transcription* of chromatin and nuclear preparations. Similar stimulation of RNA polymerase activity with rat and human (BPH) components was presented. During the discussion of these results, Dr. Mainwaring remarked that the seminal vesicle might be an interesting tissue to study with regard to specific androgen *receptors*.

In conclusion, following Dr. Tveter's report during the meeting, the discussion centered on *problems* relating to the human prostate. Dr. Robel presented analytical studies clearly discriminating between *receptors* and SBP. He analyzed steroid metabolism in human explants perfused with culture medium containing the plasma proteins human serum albumin and purified SBP. Not only was there a reduction of available testosterone due to protein binding in the medium, but also a specific effect of SBP on androgen metabolism in the explants was reported. Dr. De Voogt reported a study performed on 25 patients, 20 with BPH and 5 with prostatic cancer. (Using agar gel electrophoresis, he obtained interpretable data in prostatic carcinoma even in biopsies between 50 and 100 mg). It is clear, however, that the work with *receptors* in prostatic diseases is at its very beginning.

Regarding *BPH*, it is most important to measure not only the androgen *receptor*, but also the estrogen *receptor*. In addition, the question of the interactions between epithelial and stroma cells, both of which respond to the two hormones, is an important consideration. Dr. Coffey's presentation indicated that it may not be possible to define the hormonal parameters of human BPH in terms of one hormonal action on one specific function of the prostatic cells. In the instance of *cancer*, a primary difficulty is to obtain samples on which the necessary histological and multireceptor analysis can be conducted without problems created by interference due to therapeutics, endogenous hormones, lack of "physiological" normal values, etc.

From the lucid presentations of all participants, it is obvious that many difficulties are still before us. A very precise methodology for the quantitative assessment of tissue steroid *receptors* must be developed. In addition, it was the general consensus that the "rat model" is not necessarily inferior to the dog model, and should be used in addition to other systems for studying hormonal control of the prostate.

Treatment of Prostatic Carcinoma with Various Types of Estrogen Derivatives

G. JÖNSSON, A. M. OLSSON, AND W. LUTTROP

Department of Urology, University Hospital of Lund, Lund, Sweden

AND

Z. CEKAN, K. PURVIS, AND E. DICZFALUSY

*Swedish Medical Research Council, Reproductive Endocrinology Research Unit,
Karolinska Sjukhuset, Stockholm, Sweden*

I. Clinical Results

Endocrine therapy of prostatic carcinoma has been the rule ever since Huggins and Hodges demonstrated the hormone dependence of the prostate. The methods used have varied from time to time and from one hospital to another. Opinions still differ on the mechanisms of the methods used, their suitability, side effects, etc. The therapeutic programs have included orchiectomy, estrogen administration, pituitary ablation, corticosteroid therapy, administration of antiandrogen, etc. Also nonendocrine methods such as radiotherapy as well as treatment with cytostatics have proved useful.

The main purpose of endocrine therapy from the very beginning was to reduce the amount of androgen via inhibition of the secretion of the gonadotropins by the pituitary. The potency of the substances administered was generally estimated from determinations of the steroid substances in the urine. In recent years, however, the mechanisms bringing about the effect of endocrine therapy have proved to be much more complex than was formerly supposed. This has been made clear by recent investigations with technically advanced methods. Among other things, the introduction of radioimmunoassay methods for determining steroidal and polypeptide hormones in the serum as well as demonstration of the action of androgens on the prostate have shed light on certain points previously difficult to understand.

Oral treatment with estrogenic compounds, such as stilbestrol, has several disadvantages in the form of dyspeptic symptoms, sodium retention, edema, cardiovascular complications, etc.

To eliminate the above-mentioned disadvantages we began in 1955 to use a long-acting parenteral drug of low toxicity, Estradurin® (polyestradiol phosphate). The estrogenic effect of an intramuscular injection persists for a couple of months.

In an initial series consisting of 105 patients, 40% had metastases before the beginning of treatment (Jönsson et al., 1963). Many of the patients had had symptoms for a fairly long time before they sought medical advice. In 97 patients it was possible to estimate the interval between the onset of symptoms and the beginning of treatment fairly accurately: the mean interval was 12 months. In all cases the diagnosis had been histologically confirmed by perineal puncture or transurethral resection.

In 47 of the 105 cases the urine was examined in respect to steroids, which included determinations of the total 17-ketosteroids, 17-hydroxycorticosteroids, individual 17-ketosteroid metabolites, such as androsterone (A) + etiocholanolone (E), dehydroepiandrosterone, and estrone, 17β-estradiol, and estriol. The series was divided into two groups according to the dose of Estradurin: 80–120 mg monthly and 150–200 mg monthly in a single injection.

The results of the steroid analysis are given in Table I. The data thus suggest that in the group treated with 80–120 mg of Estradurin per month

TABLE I

URINARY EXCRETION OF 17-KETOSTEROIDS (a), ANDROSTERONE + ETIOCHOLANOLONE (b), DEHYDROEPIANDROSTERONE (c) BEFORE AND AFTER ESTRADURIN THERAPY

	Estradurin dosage (mg)	Before treatment (mg/24 hours)	After 4 months' treatment (mg/24 hours)
a	80–120	4.93	4.86
	160–200	4.72	3.92
b	80–120	2.79	2.86
	160–200	2.69	2.16
c	80–120	0.29	0.28
	160–200	0.20	0.20

the mean excretion value of 17-ketosteroids did not differ significantly from the pretreatment value. On the other hand, in patients treated with 160–200 mg of Estradurin treatment resulted in a probably significant decrease in the excretion of 17-ketosteroids.

Like the urinary total ketosteroids, the excretion of A + E was not decreased after administration of 80–120 mg of Estradurin per month. But treatment with the larger dose of Estradurin produced a probably significant decrease in the elimination of A + E.

Subsequent orchiectomy, however, resulted in a highly significant decrease in the excretion of 17-ketosteroids, androsterone, and etiocholanolone.

Neither Estradurin therapy nor orchiectomy influenced the excretion values of dehydroepiandrosterone significantly.

Although Estradurin is a fairly weak gonadotropin inhibitor, the clinical results were good: 40% of the patients were alive 5 years after the beginning of treatment.

The good clinical results together with the determinations of the steroids suggested that Estradurin has a therapeutic effect directly on the malignant cells. The favorable clinical results obtained in a small group of patients with an initially low excretion of androgen metabolites lend additional support to this view.

In view of the aforementioned results of the determinations of steroids and the clinical response, Estradurin was combined with a stronger gonadotropin inhibitor, e.g. ethynylestradiol, in the next series (Jönsson, 1971).

The material in this series consisted of 126 patients. The age distribution and the frequency of metastases were the same as in the first series. The patients in this series came from the same receiving area, the disease was equally advanced (75% thus belonged to stage III + IV, VACURG classification), and had received the same supplementary therapy besides estrogen therapy. All the patients were reexamined after 3 months and afterward twice a year for at least 5 years.

The estrogen therapy in this series consisted of Estradurin given intramuscularly in a dose of 160 mg per month for 3 months, after which the dose was reduced to 80 mg per month. This treatment was combined with 1 mg of ethynylestradiol a day for 14 days. This was followed by a daily maintenance dose of 150 μg of ethynylestradiol.

The effect of treatment was largely the same as that of estrogen therapy in general: substantial improvement of the patients' general condition, and abatement or disappearance of urinary symptoms and of metastatic pain. In several cases the number and spread of metastases became stationary, and in some cases roentgen examination showed regression.

Of the 126 patients, 78 (62%) survived for more than 5 years. As expected, the 5-year survival rate of patients in stages I and II was high (74%); in stage IV it was 45%. The lower the differentiation, the higher the mortality from the basic disease. The present investigation produced no evidence in support of the assumption of an overmortality from cardiovascular diseases in patients treated with these estrogens, but patients with such diseases before treatment must be regarded as less good risks unless they receive adequate treatment of their cardiovascular complaints.

Irrespective of the type of estrogen treatment given, most patients with prostatic carcinoma sooner or later deteriorate. These patients, like those primarily resistant to conventional estrogen treatment, constitute a serious therapeutic problem.

In these two groups, increasing and sometimes very large doses of estrogen, radiation, corticosteroids, hypophysectomy, antiandrogens, cytostatics, etc., have been tried. In some cases palliation has been achieved, but, on the whole, the results are less encouraging, besides which several of the methods have serious side effects.

It is not known why certain cases do not respond to antiandrogenic treatment or why they first respond but later become unsusceptible. In such cases, changes probably occur in the biological behavior of the carcinoma.

During the last 7 years we have used estramustine phosphate (Estracyt®), a nitrogen mustard derivative of estradiol, in the two abovementioned groups of prostatic carcinoma (Jönsson and Högberg, 1971; Nilsson and Jönsson, 1975). Our own clinical material consisted of 128 patients with advanced prostatic carcinoma. One hundred and seventeen belonged to stage IV (metastases) and 11 to stage III. All patients are followed for more than one year. Ninety patients had previously received some other antiandrogenic therapy (secondary treatment group) but had deteriorated during treatment. Judging from clinical experience, the expected duration of survival of these patients would be less than 6 months. Thirty-eight patients were given Estracyt from the very beginning (primary treatment group). All the patients were admitted to hospital for the treatment. Investigation on admission included histological and cytological examination of the prostate and sometimes of lymph nodes, roentgenological investigation of the skeleton, lungs, and urinary tract, analysis of the blood picture, determination of the acid and alkaline phosphatases, renal and liver function tests, etc. The examinations were repeated at certain intervals. Careful notes were made of the patient's general condition, pain, use of analgetics, difficulty in urination, etc.

The histological and cytological investigation showed that 37 were poorly differentiated, 51 moderately differentiated, and 21 well differentiated; the degree of differentiation of 19 was uncertain. One hundred and seventeen patients had metastases, often in more than one site. The acid phosphatases were increased in 68%. Estracyt was given intravenously in a dose of 300–450 mg/day for about 3 weeks. If the patient responded well, intravenous treatment with 300–450 mg twice a week was continued for a varying period depending on the patient's response. If the patient was symptom free and the disease under control after 2–3 months' treatment, the injections were stopped. In the event of exacerbations, intense treatment with daily injections was resumed. If no effect could be recorded after 3 weeks' daily treatment, the preparation was withdrawn.

We have also used Estracyt by mouth since 1971. The patients have received a dose of 600–900 mg a day either as primary treatment or as secondary maintenance therapy after intravenous treatment.

It is sometimes not easy to assess the results of treatment, because it is difficult to evaluate the patients' symptoms, especially pain. Estimation of the effect of treatment could, however, often be based on objective observations. For instance, previously bedridden patients could sometimes get up and even return to work. A most striking effect was the abatement of the pain and the improvement of the patient's general condition. Regression or disappearance of metastases was noted in 33 of the 128 cases. During treatment the acid phosphatases fell in many cases, sometimes to normal level. There seems to be a close correlation between falling acid phosphatases and improvement of the patient's general condition. Reelevation of the acid phosphatase levels in patients who had responded favorably was usually associated with a new deterioration.

Changes were noted in the prostatic tumor in the form of cellular pycnosis, vacuolization, rupture of cell membranes, squamous epithelial metaplasia, and increased lipofuscin.

On numerical evaluation of the results we found that about half of the patients who had got secondary therapy improved. Of the patients who received Estracyt as primary therapy, 80–90% improved. The results in these series suggest that in the group given secondary treatment the hitherto expected survival of less than 6 months might be prolonged to anything up to 5 years. The primary treatment group was too small to warrant any conclusions regarding the survival time.

The side effects must be regarded as insignificant. There was occasionally thrombophlebitis in patients treated intravenously. Gastrointestinal disturbances, though usually only transient, occurred in some patients treated by mouth. A mild reaction of the liver, allergic reactions, leukopenia, and thrombocytopenia occurred in a few cases.

II. Steroid Levels

A. Methods and Materials

A critical assessment of the endocrine effects of the three types of estrogen treatment discussed above, namely of Estradurin® (polyestradiol phosphate, hereafter PEP), Estradurin + ethynylestradiol (hereafter PEP + EE), and Estracyt® (estramustine phosphate, hereafter EMP) necessitates serial measurements of a number of relevant hormonal parameters in the blood of previously untreated patients. Therefore, patients with histologically and/or cytologically diagnosed prostatic carcinoma and without any previous hormone therapy were allocated randomly to one of the above treatments, and the pretreatment values of a number of circulating steroids and pituitary hormones were then compared with those found monthly during treatment with the three estrogen regimens described.

1. *Clinical Material*

This consisted of 24 patients with prostatic carcinoma stages II to IV (Veterans classification) diagnosed histologically and/or cytologically. The average age of the patients was 72.5 years (range 62–84 years).

2. *Therapeutic Regimens and the Design of the Study*

The patients were randomly allocated to one of the three regimens, consisting of (a) PEP (160 mg im monthly), (b) PEP + EE (PEP 160 mg im monthly; and EE 150 μg per os daily), and (c) EMP (600 mg per os daily). The structural formulas of PEP and EMP are indicated in Fig. 1.

Pretreatment (control) plasma samples were drawn from each patient

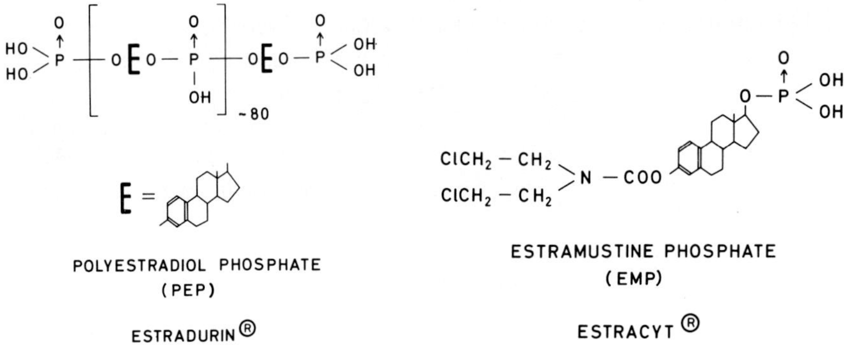

Fig. 1. Structural formulas of polyestradiol phosphate (PEP) and estramustine phosphate (EMP).

on each of three consecutive days. Then treatment was initiated immediately. Plasma samples were then obtained from each subject after 1 and 2 weeks, as well as after 1, 2, 3, 4, 5, and 6 months of treatment. Blood samples of 20 ml were withdrawn on each occasion from the antecubital vein into heparinized test tubes. The collection of plasma samples occurred invariably between 9:00 and 10:00 AM. The blood was centrifuged immediately; the plasma was separated, frozen, and stored at −20°C until analyzed.

3. Hormonal Parameters Studied

The following *unconjugated steroids* were measured: pregnenolone (3β-hydroxy-5-pregnen-20-one), 17-hydroxypregnenolone (3β,17-dihydroxy-5-pregnen-20-one), dehydroepiandrosterone (3β-hydroxy-5-androsten-17-one), 20α-dihydroprogesterone (20α-hydroxy-4-pregnen-3-one), 17-hydroxyprogesterone (17-hydroxy-4-pregnene-3,20-dione), androstenedione (4-androstene-3,17-dione), testosterone (17β-hydroxy-4 androsten-3-one), dihydrotestosterone (17β-hydroxy-5α-androstan-3-one), cortisol (11β,17-dihydroxy-4-pregnene-3,20-dione), estradiol (1,3,5(10)-estratriene-3,17β-diol), and estrone (3-hydroxy-1,3,5(10)-estratrien-17-one). The following immunoreactive *pituitary hormones* were estimated: follicle-stimulating hormone (FSH), luteinizing hormone (LH), and prolactin.

4. Assay Procedures

All steroids except cortisol were measured by radioimmunoassay procedures involving chromatographic purification and separation of steroids as described in detail in previous communications (Brenner *et al.*, 1973; Purvis *et al.*, 1975; Aedo *et al.*, 1976). Cortisol was assayed by the protein-binding method described by Nugent and Mayes (1966). The assays of LH were performed according to Midgley (1966) as modified by Robyn *et al.* (1971), using the Second International Reference Preparation of human menopausal gonadotropin (2nd IRP-HMG) as standard. The measurements of FSH and prolactin were performed by the use of kits purchased from Biodata S.A., Rome, Italy. In the FSH assays an HMG standard calibrated against the 2nd IRP-HMG was used, whereas the results of prolactin assays were expressed in terms of the NIH-1 human prolactin preparation.

5. Calculation and Evaluation of Results

In all calculations, a log normal between-patients distribution of individual values was assumed (Gaddum, 1945). Hence in Figs. 2–14, geometric mean values and 95% confidence limits are indicated.

In order to assess differences between control and treatment values for

---

each treatment group, an analysis of variance was performed and the significance of the differences was computed, using appropriate contrasts. The percentage changes occurring during therapy and their statistical significance are indicated on p. 368 in Table II. Furthermore, differences between control (pretreatment) values of all three groups were tested by an analysis of variance for each steroid or pituitary hormone assayed. If no significant difference was found, another analysis of variance was performed to compare the means of treatment results obtained by various treatment schedules (1–6 months of treatment) for each hormone. The significance of differences between group means was assessed by the q-test (Dixon and Massey, 1969). The results of these computations are shown on p. 369 in Table III.

In the case of the assays of 17-hydroxyprogesterone, estrone, estradiol and prolactin, a significant difference was found in the pretreatment (control) values of the 3 groups. In these instances, every individual measure-

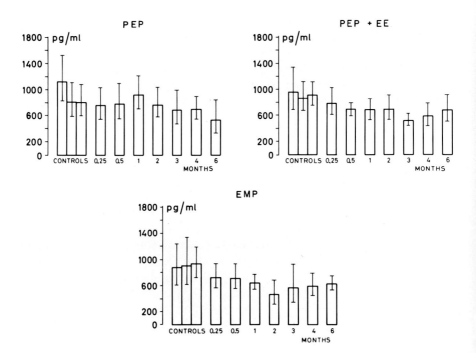

FIG. 2. Circulating levels of pregnenolone in patients with prostatic carcinoma before and during treatment with polyestradiol phosphate (PEP given in monthly injections of 160 mg), polyestradiol phosphate + ethynylestradiol (PEP + EE: 160 mg im monthly and 150 μg per os daily, respectively) and estramustine phosphate (EMP: 600 mg per os daily). Each column represents the geometric mean value of 8 subjects. Vertical bars indicate 95% confidence limits.

ment was transformed to a percentage, and differences between treatment groups were computed using an analysis of variance and the q-test, as indicated above.

B. RESULTS

The results of the assays of three Δ^5-steroids, pregnenolone, 17-hydroxy-pregnenolone, and dehydroepiandrosterone, are indicated in Figs. 2–4. Whereas the decrease in pregnenolone levels during PEP therapy was barely significant (cf. Table II), a highly significant decrease was noted during the administration of EMP or of PEP + EE. The levels of 17-hydroxypregnenolone were reduced by each form of therapy; however the effect of PEP was weaker than that of PEP + EE, or EMP (cf. Table III). Furthermore, whereas PEP did not induce a significant change in circulating dehydroepiandrosterone levels, a highly significant depression was noted in the patients treated with either EMP or PEP + EE. Hence the two latter forms of estrogen therapy appeared to be more powerful inhibitors of these Δ^5-steroids than was PEP.

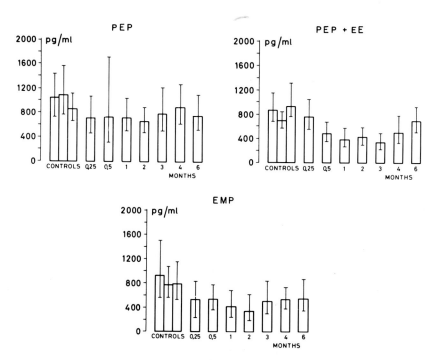

FIG. 3. 17-Hydroxypregnenolone levels in patients with prostatic carcinoma before and during treatment with various estrogen derivatives. For explanation, consult legend to Fig. 2.

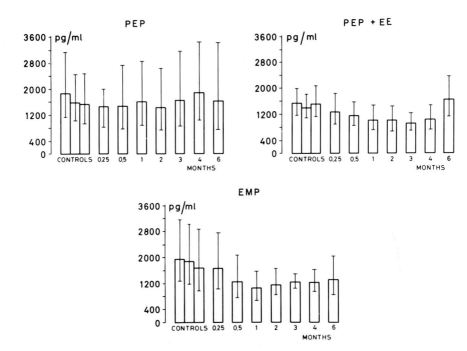

Fɪɢ. 4. Dehydroepiandrosterone levels in patients with prostatic carcinoma before and during treatment with various estrogen derivatives. For explanation, consult legend to Fig. 2.

Closer examination of Figs. 2–4 reveals a more or less conspicuous trend toward an increase in circulating steroid levels between the third and sixth treatment months in patients treated with PEP + EE. Indeed, a regression analysis revealed that this increase was significant in both 17-hydroxypregnenolone ($p < 0.001$) and dehydroepiandrosterone levels ($p < 0.01$). A similar trend has not been observed in patients treated with PEP alone or with EMP.

The plasma levels of 20α-dihydroprogesterone (Fig. 5) were influenced only by PEP + EE and to a limited extent. However, the assay of 17-hydroxyprogesterone revealed a highly significant suppression of this steroid during each therapeutic regimen studied (Fig. 6).

Furthermore, the decrease in 17-hydroxyprogesterone levels was significantly greater during the administration of EMP or PEP + EE than after the administration of PEP alone (cf. Table III).

As far as the levels of androstenedione were concerned, there was a limited (23–33%) but highly significant decrease in every group of patients (Fig. 7). In this respect, there was no difference between the various forms of estrogen treatment.

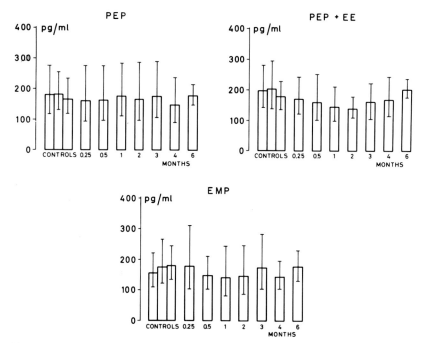

FIG. 5. 20 α-Dihydroprogesterone levels in patients with prostatic carcinoma before and during estrogen treatment. For explanation, consult legend to Fig. 2.

In agreement with the findings shown in Figs. 3 and 4, a highly significant increase ($p < 0.001$) was found between the third and sixth months of treatment in 17-hydroxyprogesterone levels and a significant increase ($p < 0.05$) in androstenedione levels in patients treated with PEP + EE (Figs. 6 and 7). Again, no similar effect was observed during treatment with PEP or with EMP.

The testosterone and dihydrotestosterone levels are shown in Figs. 8 and 9, respectively. All three estrogen regimens caused a highly significant suppression of both testosterone and dihydrotestosterone levels. However, treatment with EMP or with PEP + EE resulted in a much stronger suppression ($p < 0.001$) than did treatment with PEP alone (Table III). The testosterone levels in the latter group were approximately 2.0 ng/ml, whereas in the two other groups the values were in the vicinity of 150 pg/ml. Furthermore, dihydrotestosterone levels were diminished to values of the order of 300 pg/ml in the PEP-treated group, whereas they were approximately 100 pg/ml in the patients treated with PEP + EE or with EMP.

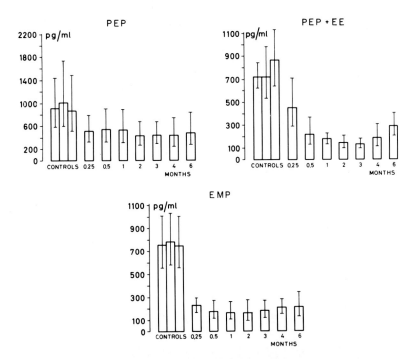

FIG. 6. 17-Hydroxyprogesterone levels in patients with prostatic carcinoma before and during estrogen treatment. For explanation, consult legend to Fig. 2.

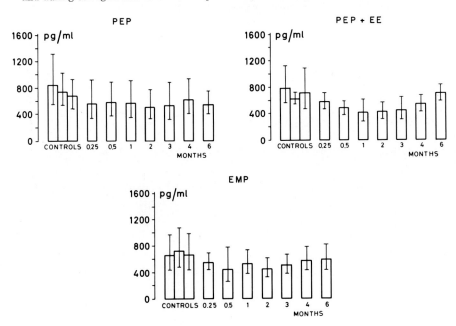

FIG. 7. Androstenedione levels in patients with prostatic carcinoma before and during estrogen treatment. For explanation, consult legend to Fig. 2.

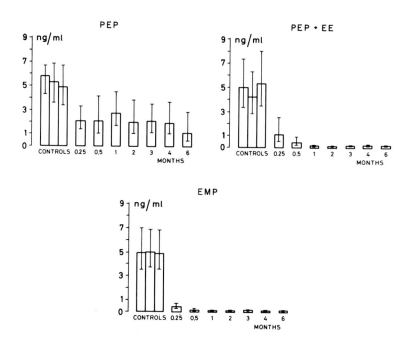

FIG. 8. Testosterone levels in patients with prostatic carcinoma before and during estrogen treatment. For explanation consult legend to Fig. 2.

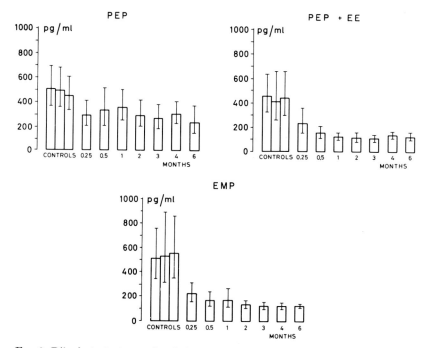

FIG. 9. Dihydrotestosterone levels in patients with prostatic carcinoma before and during estrogen treatment. For explanation, consult legend to Fig. 2.

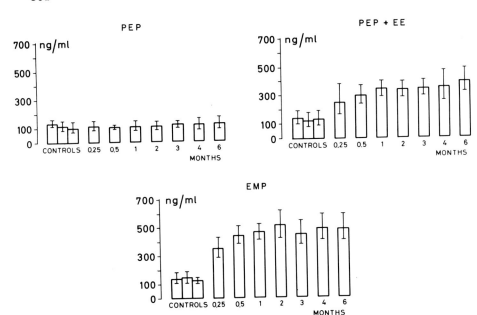

FIG. 10. Cortisol levels in patients with prostatic carcinoma before and during estrogen treatment. $n = 7$. For explanation, consult legend to Fig. 2.

The assay of cortisol revealed major differences, as shown in Fig. 10. Whereas treatment with PEP did not alter circulating cortisol levels, the administration of PEP + EE resulted in a marked elevation $(p < 0.001)$ of cortisol in plasma. The effect of EMP was even more marked; cortisol levels in EMP-treated patients greatly exceeded those found in subjects treated with PEP + EE $(p < 0.001)$.

The results of estrone and estradiol assays obtained during the administration of PEP and of PEP + EE are indicated in Fig. 11.

The higher values seen in the latter group should be viewed in the light of the slight but significant (0.1%) cross-reaction between EE and estradiol or estrone. The data of Fig. 11 indicate a progressive rise in estrone and estradiol values in PEP-treated patients from the first month onward. A regression analysis indicated that this gradual rise was significant $(p < 0.01)$. The same was true also in patients treated with PEP + EE $(p < 0.001)$, suggesting an accumulation of these estrogens and/or of their precursors.

In the plasma samples of subjects treated with daily doses of 600 mg of EMP, the estrone-like immunoreactive material varied between 50 and 100 ng/ml and the estradiol-like material between 5 and 10 ng/ml. Also in these cases there was a highly significant increase in measured levels

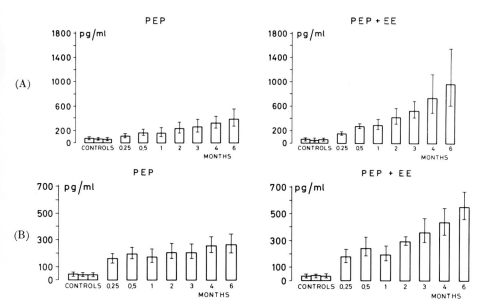

FIG. 11. Estrone (A) and estradiol (B) levels in patients with prostatic carcinoma before and during treatment with PEP and PEP + EE. For explanation, consult legend to Fig. 2.

from the first to the sixth month of treatment ($p < 0.001$). However, when another aliquot of some of these samples was partitioned between toluene and 1 N NaOH prior to chromatography, a considerable amount of this immunological activity remained in the toluene phase. The chemical identity of the immunoreactive estrone- and estradiol-like material is under investigation.

The results of FSH and LH assays are depicted in Figs. 12 and 13. All three therapeutic regimens resulted in a marked reduction of circulating FSH and LH levels ($p < 0.001$) in all instances. However, the gonadotropin-suppressing effect of both PEP + EE and of EMP was much stronger ($p < 0.001$) than that of PEP.

The results of prolactin assays are indicated in Fig. 14. Prolactin assays were performed only on two occasions during the pretreatment period and then 1 and 5 months following the initiation of estrogen treatment. There was no change in prolactin levels in subjects treated with PEP. However, combined treatment with PEP + EE resulted in a significant increase ($p < 0.05$). Moreover, treatment with EMP produced a much more marked ($p < 0.001$) elevation. Indeed, the increase in prolactin levels in the EMP group was higher ($p < 0.01$) than in patients treated with PEP + EE.

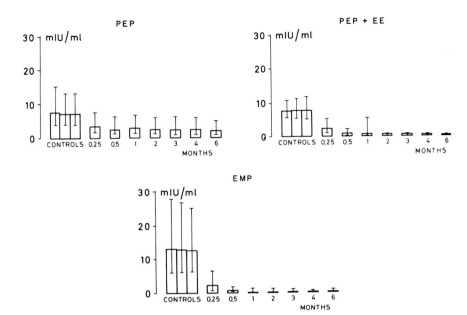

Fig. 12. Immunoreactive follicle-stimulating hormone (FSH) levels in patients with prostatic carcinoma before and during estrogen therapy. $n = 7$. For explanation, consult legend to Fig. 2.

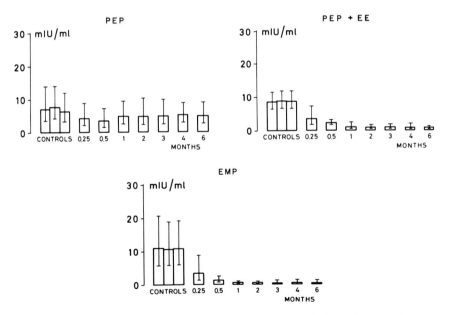

Fig. 13. Immunoreactive luteinizing hormone (LH) levels in patients with prostatic carcinoma before and during estrogen treatment. $n = 7$. For explanation, consult legend to Fig. 2.

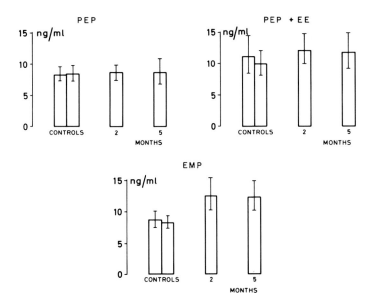

FIG. 14. Immunoreactive prolactin levels in patients with prostatic carcinoma before and during estrogen therapy. For explanation, consult legend to Fig. 2.

Summary of Hormonal Changes

Table II presents the mean percentage change in each of the hormonal parameters studied, which was induced by the various therapeutic regimens administered. In the statistical analysis of these changes, the mean pretreatment values were compared with the mean of the values found 1, 2, 3, 4, and 6 months after the initiation of the therapy, using appropriate contrasts in the analysis of variance. In the case of prolactin assays, the mean pretreatment value was contrasted with the mean of the first and fifth treatment months.

The data of Table II indicate that the different degrees of gonadotropin suppression were closely correlated with similar decreases in testosterone, dihydrotestosterone, and 17-hydroxyprogesterone levels, but were poorly or not at all correlated with androstenedione and 20α-dihydroprogesterone levels. Also the changes observed in prolactin and cortisol levels reflected major differences in estrogenic effect, whereas the three Δ^5-steroids studied represented less-sensitive parameters of testicular endocrine function than testosterone, dihydrotestosterone, and 17-hydroxyprogesterone.

TABLE II

EFFECT OF VARIOUS FORMS OF ESTROGEN THERAPY ON CIRCULATING HORMONE
LEVELS IN PATIENTS WITH PROSTATIC CANCER

Hormones in plasma	Estrogen treatment[g]		
	PEP	PEP + EE	EMP
Pregnenolone	18.7^b	-31.1^d	-37.2^d
17-Hydroxypregnenolone	-23.8^d	-41.4^d	-40.4^d
Dehydroepiandrosterone	$+1.4^a$	-23.7^d	-40.1^d
20α-Dihydroprogesterone	0.0^a	-16.8^c	-4.9^a
17-Hydroxyprogesterone	-50.3^d	-73.5^d	-73.7^d
Androstenedione	-23.4^d	-32.8^d	-23.8^d
Testosterone	-55.0^d	-96.7^d	-96.9^d
Dihydrotestosterone	-37.2^d	-73.0^d	-73.7^d
Cortisol	$+1.6^a$	$+154^d$	$+227^d$
Estrone	$+341^d$	$+966^{d,e}$	$+2.1 \times 10^{5f}$
Estradiol	$+443^d$	$+931^{d,e}$	$+2.1 \times 10^{4f}$
FSH	-55.7^d	-91.9^d	-98.6^d
LH	-30.7^d	-87.6^d	-95.4^d
Prolactin	$+3.0^a$	$+13.9^b$	$+46.9^d$

[a] Not significant.
[b] $p < 0.05$.
[c] $p < 0.01$.
[d] $p < 0.001$.
[e] 0.1% Cross-reaction between EE and estrone or estradiol.
[f] Chemical identity not definitely established.
[g] Figures indicate percentage changes during therapy. PEP, polyestradiol phosphate; EE, ethynylestradiol; EMP estramustine phosphate; FSH, follicle-stimulation hormone; LH, luteinizing hormone.

In Table III the significance of differences between treatment groups is assessed.

The administration of PEP alone resulted in a significantly lower degree of suppression of circulating gonadotropin and steroid levels than treatment with either PEP + EE or with EMP. This was especially true in the case of testosterone, dihydrotestosterone, and 17-hydroxyprogesterone, 17-hydroxypregnenolone, and dehydroepiandrosterone. An exception was androstenedione, which showed approximately the same degree of suppression in the different treatment groups. Also the cortisol and prolactin levels indicated a highly significant difference between the endocrine effect of PEP and of the two other regimens. Finally, the effect of EMP significantly exceeded that of PEP + EE as far as their effect on cortisol and prolactin levels is concerned.

TABLE III

SIGNIFICANCE OF DIFFERENCES IN HORMONAL CHANGES INDUCED
BY DIFFERENT FORMS OF ESTROGEN THERAPY

	Contrasts[c]		
Hormones in plasma	PEP vs PEP + EE	PEP vs EMP	PEP + EE vs EMP
Pregnenolone	NS	$p < 0.01$	NS
17-Hydroxypregnenolone	$p < 0.001$	$p < 0.001$	NS
Dehydroepiandrosterone	$p < 0.001$	$p < 0.001$	NS
20α-Dihydroprogesterone	NS	NS	NS
17-Hydroxyprogesterone	$p < 0.001$	$p < 0.001$	NS
Androstenedione	NS	NS	NS
Testosterone	$p < 0.001$	$p < 0.001$	NS
Dihydrotestosterone	$p < 0.001$	$p < 0.001$	NS
Cortisol	$p < 0.001$	$p < 0.001$	$p < 0.001$
Estrone	$p < 0.001^{a}$	$p < 0.001^{b}$	$p < 0.001^{a,b}$
Estradiol	$p < 0.001^{a}$	$p < 0.001^{b}$	$p < 0.001^{a,b}$
FSH	$p < 0.001$	$p < 0.001$	NS
LH	$p < 0.001$	$p < 0.001$	NS
Prolactin	NS	$p < 0.001$	$p < 0.001$

[a] 0.1% Cross-reaction between EE and estrone or estradiol.

[b] Chemical identity of the estrone- and estradiol-like immunoreactive material in the plasma of EMP-treated subjects not established definitely.

[c] NS, not significant; PEP, polyestradiol phosphate; EE, ethynylestradiol; EMP estramustine phosphate; FSH, follicle-stimulating hormone; LH, luteinizing hormone.

III. DISCUSSION

It is recognized that the hormonal changes induced by the administration of estrogens to men are complex and the effects manifold. Estrogens affect not only the steroidogenic function of the testicles and the pituitary feedback mechanisms; they may also alter the function of other endocrine glands, as well as the metabolic disposition and binding of several steroids by their ability to increase the quantity of certain enzymes and steroid-binding proteins. Hence the interpretation of changing plasma levels of a single steroid may easily become naive and simplistic. Nevertheless, bearing in mind these limitations, a few findings reported in this paper seem to deserve comments.

In view of obvious problems with cross reactions when estrogen radioimmunoassays are carried out in the presence of huge excesses of potentially interfering estrogen derivatives and a variety of their metabolites, the estrone and estradiol assays in the present investigation were considered *a priori* to represent parameters of limited diagnostic value, especially in the case of EMP-treated subjects. During treatment with daily doses of 600 mg of EMP, 50–100 ng/ml quantities of immunoreactive estrone-like and 5–10 ng/ml of estradiol-like material were detected in the plasma. These excessively high levels were of considerable interest in view of the lack of severe estrogen side effects in subjects treated with massive doses of EMP. Indeed, when the same plasma extracts were subjected to a classical phenolic partition prior to the radioimmunological determination, the amounts of estrone and estradiol found were greatly reduced. Hence large amounts of ether-soluble estrone- and estradiol-like immunoreactive material measured in the plasma samples of EMP-treated subjects were not identical with unconjugated estrone and estradiol, respectively. Experiments are now in progress to elucidate the chemical nature of the estrone- and estradiol-like immunoreactive material. However, regardless of the chemical nature of the estrogen circulating in such subjects, it can be concluded, on the basis of the results of prolactin and cortisol assays, that in the doses administered the estrogenic activity of EMP exceeded that of PEP + EE.

The results reported in this investigation indicate that PEP significantly reduced, but did not completely suppress, FSH and LH levels.

This condition was also reflected by the incompletely suppressed testosterone, dihydrotestosterone, and 17-hydroxyprogesterone levels. On the other hand, treatment with PEP + EE or EMP virtually eliminated circulating gonadotropin levels and induced a most dramatic reduction in the endocrine activity of the testes, as reflected by a variety of circulating steroids.

Did those two regimens completely eliminate testicular androgen synthesis? The data presented in this paper support this contention. The blood production rate of testosterone in normal men is estimated to be 7.0 mg/24 hours and the testicular secretion 6.9 mg/24 hours (Lipsett, 1974). Thus, 98–99% of the circulating testosterone appears to be of testicular origin, a figure which comes very close to the 97% reduction observed in the present paper. It seems likely that the residual 3% testosterone (some 150 pg/ml) is of adrenal origin. It is more difficult to make a similar calculation for dihydrotestosterone, since a considerable part of this steroid arises as an extragonadal metabolite to testosterone. Approximately one-third of the blood production rate is supposed to represent testicular secretion (Lipsett, 1974). In the present study, a suppression of 75% is reported. This seems to suggest that one-third of circulating dihydrotestosterone is not derived from testosterone of testicular origin. Furthermore, according to Strott *et al.* (1969), the testicular secretion of 17-hydroxyprogesterone (1.5 mg/24 hours) is approximately 78–79% of the blood production rate (1.9 mg/24 hours), a figure that is in close agreement with our finding of 74% decrease in the circulating levels of this steroid during maximal (or near maximal) estrogen suppression. Hence the serial estimation of testosterone, dihydrotestosterone, and 17-hydroxyprogesterone seems to offer an efficient tool for monitoring testicular endocrine function.

The role of the three Δ^5-steroids measured appears to be less clear. It is generally believed that the bulk of these steroids in the plasma is of adrenal origin (Lipsett, 1974), although suggestive evidence is available indicating that some 17-hydroxypregnenolone (McKenna et al., 1974) and dehydroepiandrosterone (Lipsett, 1974) is secreted by the human testis. Further studies will be needed to elucidate whether the significant reduction in pregnenolone, 17-hydroxypregnenolone, and dehydroepiandrosterone levels in patients treated with PEP + EE or with EMP is due to alterations in testicular, or adrenal steroidogenesis. Also, the significance of the changes in androstenedione levels remains to be established. Levels of this steroid were reduced by some 25% in each of the three groups. This reduction was unrelated to circulating gonadotropin or steroid levels. These findings do not support the concept according to which androstenedione is an immediate precursor of testosterone in the biogenetic pathway. Furthermore, the gradual rise in circulating 17-hydroxypregnenolone, 17-hydroxyprogesterone, androstenedione, and dehydroepiandrosterone levels during therapy with PEP + EE is of considerable interest. Since they were not associated with similar alterations in testosterone and dihydrotestosterone levels, these changes seem to reflect an alteration in adrenal function. Whether the rise in steroid levels is due to an increase in secretion or in protein-binding remains to be seen. These changes suggest, however, that adrenal function—especially adrenal androgens—should be regularly monitored in patients with prostactic carcinoma. On the other hand, it is more than likely that the elevated cortisol levels are attributable to increased levels of corticosterone-binding globulin, induced by estrogens in a dose-related fashion (Sandberg and Slaunwhite, 1959; Musa et al., 1965). Also the prolactin levels seem to reflect a dose-effect relationship with the estrogens administered.

The results of this study raise some rather fundamental questions as to the rationale of hormonal therapy in prostatic cancer. What is the smallest amount of circulating androgen sufficient to stimulate growth of the neoplastic tissue? Should one attempt to eliminate the residual testosterone and 17-hydroxyprogesterone and dihydrotestosterone levels of presumably adrenal origin? What is the significance of elevated prolactin levels? Should one try to reduce those levels by the administration of a prolactin inhibitor such as 2-bromoergocryptin? It has been demonstrated in animal experiments that the specific binding of prolactin to the ventral prostate is stimulated by androgens and reduced by castration (Kledzik *et al.*, 1975), and that prolactin accentuates the effect of androgens on the prostate (Farnsworth, 1972). Would the concurrent administration of antiandrogen and estrogen be beneficial? Carefully designed studies may provide answers to some of these questions. At any rate, the data presented in this paper indicate that the endocrine effects of estrogen therapy can be quantitated rapidly and effectively. It seems to be possible, therefore, to establish the minimal dose of any estrogen regimen which will cause near maximal suppression of the pituitary–gonadal axis. Other methods will be needed for the verification of specific therapeutic effects at the tissue level.

IV. CONCLUDING REMARKS

Although the clinical assessment of PEP and PEP + EE was not carried out simultaneously, the 5-year survival figures strongly suggest that PEP + EE (Estradurin + Etivex®) is superior in its therapeutic effect to PEP (Estradurin) alone. The observation time on the effect of EMP (Estracyt) is too short to allow any definite conclusions concerning the survival time. However, improvement in a high proportion of desolate cases which became unresponsive to other types of estrogen therapy seems to suggest that the use of EMP offers definite advantages in the treatment and management of advanced prostatic cancer.

On the basis of their inhibitory effect on (1) circulating gonadotropin levels, (2) circulating steroid levels, and stimulatory effect on (3) plasma prolactin and cortisol levels, both EMP and PEP + EE possess stronger estrogenic effects than PEP. Furthermore, a comparison of these effects on prolactin and cortisol levels indicates that, in the doses administered, the estrogenic effect of EMP exceeded that of PEP + EE.

ACKNOWLEDGMENTS

We are indebted to Dr. P. Eneroth, Stockholm, for performing the prolactin assays. The expert technical assistance of Miss Marianne Ekwall and Miss Sara Ohlsson is also gratefully acknowledged.

The expenses of the investigations reported were defrayed by a Research Grant from the Leo Research Foundation, Helsingborg, Sweden.

REFERENCES

Aedo, A. R., Landgren, B. M., Cekan, Z., and Diczfalusy, E. (1976). *Acta Endocrinol (Copenhagen)* (In press).
Brenner, P. F., Guerrero, R., Cekan, Z., and Diczfalusy E. (1973). *Steroids* **22**, 775.

Dixon, W. J., and Massey, F. J., Jr. (1969). "Introduction to Statistical Analysis." McGraw-Hill, New York.

Farnsworth, W. E. (1972). *In* "Prolactin and Carcinogenesis" (A. R. Boyns and K. Griffiths, eds.), p. 217. Alpha Omega Alpha Publ., Cardiff, Wales.

Gaddum, J. H. (1945). *Nature (London)* **15,** 463.

Jönsson, G. (1971). *Scand. J. Urol. Nephrol.* **5,** 97.

Jönsson, G., and Högberg, B. (1971). *Scand. J. Urol. Nephrol.* **5,** 103.

Jönsson, G., Diczfalusy, E., Plantin, L. O., Röhl, L., and Birke, G. (1963). *Acta Endocrinol. (Copenhagen), Suppl.* 83.

Kledzik, G. S., Marshall, S., Gelato, M., and Meites, J. (1975). No. 56 presented at the *57th Annu. Meet. Endocrine Soc., 1975* Abstract No. 56, p. 78 (1975).

Lipsett, M. B. (1974). "The Endocrine Function of the Human Testis" (V. H. T. James, M. Serio, and L. Martini, eds.), Vol. II, p. 1. Academic Press, New York.

McKenna, T. J., Di Pietro, D. L., Brown, R. D., Strott, C. A., and Liddle, G. W. (1974). *J. Clin. Endocrinol. Metab.* **39,** 833.

Midgley, A. R. (1966). *Endocrinology* **79,** 10.

Musa, B. U., Seal, U. S., and Doe, R. P. (1965). *J. Clin. Endocrinol. Metab.* **25,** 1163.

Nilsson, T., and Jönsson, G. (1975). *Cancer Chemother. Rep., Part 1* **59,** 229.

Nugent, C. A., and Mayes, D. M. (1966). *J. Clin. Endocrinol. Metab.* **26,** 1116.

Purvis, K., Brenner, P. F., Landgren, B.-M., Cekan, Z., and Diczfalusy, E. (1975). *Clin. Endocrinol.* **4,** 237.

Robyn. C., L'Hermite, M., Petrusz, P., and Diczfalusy, E. (1971). *Acta Endocrinol. (Copenhagen)* **67,** 417.

Sandberg, A. A., and Slaunwhite, W. R., Jr. (1959). *J. Clin. Invest.* **38,** 1290.

Strott, C. A., Yoshimi, T., and Lipsett, M. B. (1969). *J. Clin. Invest.* **48,** 930.

DISCUSSION

L. Andersson: Recently a survey has been made of the publications on estramustine phosphate in carcinoma of the prostate. This compilation includes 466 patients; 402 of them had had previous antiandrogenic therapy of some other kind but had either been nonresponsive or had developed so-called secondary resistance. Sixty-four patients were given estramustine phosphate as primary treatment. In the first group, good clinical effect was reported in 55% of the patients, whereas 88% of the patients in the second group were said to respond favorably to estramustine phosphate.

Based on more preliminary evidence of this difference in effect, we had already earlier started a study in Stockholm concerning the effect of oral estramustine phosphate as the primary treatment in prostatic carcinoma. This is done with the cooperation of all the Urology Departments in Stockholm.

To randomly selected patients with carcinoma of the prostate we administer either estramustine phosphate in a dose of 840 mg per day or intramuscular polyestradiol phosphate, 80 mg once per month plus oral ethynylestradiol, 150 μg per day.

In another randomized series of patients with anaplastic prostatic carcinoma without known dissemination of the tumor, we give local high-voltage irradiation to the primary tumor plus either estramustine phosphate or polyestradiol phosphate, the aim of the hormonal therapy being to influence a possible component of highly differentiated tumor.

At present these studies have been running for only 8 months. It is therefore still too early to have any conception of the results.

H. J. Tagnon: In any comparison of Estracyt and ordinary 17β-estradiol one should be careful that patients are randomized between the two treatments and that each group receives the two compounds in equivalent amounts of estradiol content or activity. This is to eliminate the possibility that a superior effect of Estracyt could be due just to an increased estrogen administration. The need for a controlled trial is now becoming urgent and the lack of it is doing harm to a possibly excellent compound. Also, it is not legitimate to compare a present-day series of patients with a series of patients treated 20 years ago, because circumstances have changed in 20 years, supportive treatment has improved, etc.

A control series of patients is not a series of patients left untreated (this is ethically not permitted); it is a series of patients treated by the best classical treatment, to which the new treatment is being compared.

L. Denis: Of the patients on secondary treatment (Dr. Jonsson, 90; Dr. Andersson, 264), how many had previous castration, and of these, how many were in relapse or reactivation?

G. Jönsson: In the series from Lund, all patients in the secondary treatment group (the patients had hormonal treatment before) were in relapse before EMP treatment. None of the patients had an orchiectomy before EMP treatment.

L. Andersson: On the whole, at present orchiectomy is not often performed in prostate carcinoma patients in Sweden.

M. B. Lipsett: Professor Tagnon has suggested that it would be appropriate to use functionally equivalent amounts of estrogen in groups receiving different therapies. But this is hardly possible. What would one measure? TBG, which is a good measure of estrogen effect on liver, or gonadotropins for a pituitary effect? We have no generally available assessments of estrogen effect. Thus, comparisons of Estracyt and various estrogens will always suffer from this problem.

K. Griffiths: A study similar to that reported by Dr. Diczfalusy is underway in Britain. The Tenovus Institute is responsible for the hormone assays. After 1 month, FSH, LH, and testosterone concentrations had fallen to low levels in patients treated with small doses of diethylstilbestrol or with Honvan (300 mg/day), the diethylstilbestrol diphosphate. Plasma estradiol also decreased with treatment. Prolactin levels increased especially in patients on Honvan, and growth hormone concentrations were elevated in only some of the patients. As Dr. Diczfalusy said, a routine monitoring of plasma hormones should provide the necessary data to allow us to recommend dosage regimes. The small baseline levels of testosterone, under 100 ng/100 ml, are apparently of adrenal origin since administration of deamethasone to the patient being treated for carcinoma results in a marked decrease in these concentrations.

Also worth mentioning is the fact that CB154 (Sandoz) administration to patients on diethylstilbestrol therapy will decrease the plasma prolactin to extremely low levels. Obviously, if prolactin has any trophic action on the prostate, or possibly an effect on adrenal androgen secretion, then it would seem preferable to offer treatment that does not result in high prolactin concentrations.

A. A. Sandberg: The elevated DHT levels, relative to those of testosterone, can possibly be explained by the increased binding of DHT by the greatly elevated concentrations of TBG (and transcortin?), both proteins having a higher affinity for DHT than for testosterone. This same parameter explains the very high levels of cortisol observed, due to the greatly elevated concentrations of transcortin.

We have studied the fate of labeled Estracyt, and it appears that in the human about 20% of the Estracyt is hydrolyzed in the liver and the released estradiol is then metabolized almost identically to administered estradiol. Most of the Estracyt is probably excreted in the bile, probably as an intact molecule.

The lack of severe estrogenic effects in patients receiving Estracyt can possibly be explained by the hydrolysis of the Estracyt almost exclusively in the liver, at which site it is conjugated and/or metabolized without the estradiol having a chance to reach the circulation, thus possibly explaining the lack of severe estrogenic effects. The rises in the transcortin levels can be explaned by the effects of the estradiol (from the hydrolyzed Estracyt) producing an effect in the liver cells *in situ*, resulting in increased transcortin synthesis by the liver cells.

E. E. Baulieu: To Dr. Sandberg: You may have both "local" hydrolysis in liver and even pulmonary, hypothalamic, and differential sensitivity to hormones of different range systems.

To Professor Diczfalusy: Are the hormone levels of prostatic cancer patients normal (vs control healthy people) with respect to adrenal and testicular functions?

E. Diczfalusy: We have no corresponding control material of the same age group, but we have published normal values in the blood plasma of middle-aged, apparently healthy, men. Those values are compared in Table A with the pretreatment values obtained in the present study. Estradiol levels are significantly higher, and the levels of a number of other steroids significantly lower, in the present study compared to those reported earlier. Whether these differences are due to aging alone or also to prostatic carcinoma remains to be established.

TABLE A

GEOMETRIC MEANS AND 95% CONFIDENCE LIMITS OF STEROID LEVELS IN THE PERIPHERAL PLASMA OF 21 MIDDLE-AGED, APPARENTLY HEALTHY MEN[a] AND 24 ELDERLY MEN WITH RECENTLY DIAGNOSED UNTREATED PROSTATIC CARCINOMA[b]

Steroid	Age 20–51 years (pg/ml)	Age 62–84 years (pg/ml)	Significance
Pregnenolone	1390 (1210–1600)	901 (773–1050)	$P < 0.001$
17-Hydroxypregnenolone	2300[c]	875 (741–1030)	—
Dehydroepiandrosterone	5500 (4520–6690)	1650 (1320–2050)	$P < 0.001$
20α-Dihydroprogesterone	210[c]	180 (150–215)	—
17-Hydroxyprogesterone	1510[c]	816 (757–879)	—
Androstenedione	1260 (1100–1440)	707 (587–851)	$P < 0.001$
Testosterone	6460 (5660–7360)	5010 (4180–6000)	$P < 0.05$
Dihydrotestosterone	672 (610–738)	482 (394–588)	$P < 0.01$
Estrone	48.5 (43.7–53.8)	52.8 (46.2–60.4)	NS[d]
Estradiol	22.2 (19.3–25.5)	33.8 (28.2–40.5)	$P < 0.001$

[a] Purvis *et al.* (1975) *Clin. Endocrinol.* **4,** 237.

[b] Present paper.

[c] Provisional values obtained by measurement of a plasma pool collected from 8 men (32–45 years of age).

[d] NS, not significant.

K. D. Voigt: Did you compare the starting levels of prolactin and LH in so-called normal volunteers with those obtained in patients with prostatic cancer? And do you have any biological data on blood prolactin content?

E. Diczfalusy: The prolactin results are as yet preliminary, and we have no representative values for our normal male population. We do not have a bioassay method in our laboratory, but I understand that you have; it would certainly be of interest to do some comparative assays.

K. J. Tveter: Will these different estrogens, at certain levels at least, increase the level of ACTH? If so, might increased ACTH, leading to increased synthesis of adrenal androgens in combination with elevated prolactin levels, be responsible for reactivation of some prostatic cancers?

E. Diczfalusy: We have not measured ACTH in the present study. I agree that it will be important to monitor carefully and during a prolonged period of time the prolactin and androgen levels (and gonadotropins as well) in patients treated with various doses of estrogens.

K. Griffiths: On the problem of adrenal activity of patients on estrogen therapy, some of our recent results are worth reporting. Explants of human adrenal tissue have been cultured for periods up to 72 hours with and without ACTH and also prolactin. Prolactin will stimulate testosterone and androstenedione synthesis by this tissue, but in most instances not as well as does ACTH. Of course, in the patient with carcinoma and on estrogen therapy, the responsiveness of the adrenal to prolactin may well be different from this *in vitro* situation.

The Nonsurgical Treatment of Prostatic Carcinoma

G. D. CHISHOLM AND E. P. N. O'DONOGHUE

Institute of Urology and St. Peter's, St. Paul's and St. Philip's Hospitals; Royal Postgraduate Medical School and Hammersmith Hospital, London, England

I. INTRODUCTION

In 1922, Bumpus wrote, "The average duration of cancer of the prostate if untreated is 3 years." At that time, the aim of treatment for this disease consisted only of the relief of urinary obstruction and symptomatic treatment for pain due to bony metastases; direct radiation treatment, introduced by Pasteau and Degrais (1913), was later abandoned because of the poor results (Widman, 1934).

The rationale for primary endocrine therapy was first presented by Dr. Charles Huggins in a series of articles in which he described how his laboratory studies had shown that both adult prostatic epithelium and carcinomatous prostatic tissue (and metastases) had a high acid phosphatase content. It was suggested that malignancy represented an overgrowth of adult prostatic epithelium and, since a reduction in androgens was known to produce atrophy of this epithelium, then a reduction

377

in androgenic hormones by castration or estrogen therapy should reduce the malignant activity (Huggins and Hodges, 1941; Huggins *et al.*, 1941).

There can be little doubt that both the clinical and biochemical effects in some patients are profound; not only does the tumor shrink, the serum acid phosphatase decrease, and the anemia disappear but the patient may have a striking subjective improvement. However, more than 30 years later, the precise role of endocrine therapy in the management of prostatic carcinoma especially for early stage tumors has become less certain. Not all patients respond equally, some show little response, others relapse after a variable length of treatment; the treatment itself can produce its own morbidity and mortality.

This uncertainty has led to renewed efforts to establish the exact hormonal relationships in prostatic carcinoma. In addition, alternative approaches to antiandrogen therapy are under continuous assessment, while methods for more precise diagnosis and tumor staging have revived the possibility that local nonendocrine therapy should be considered, and advances in external irradiation techniques are now being applied.

II. Presentation of Prostatic Carcinoma

Because of its hidden position in the body, carcinoma of the prostate often remains undetected until it causes either obstructive urinary symptoms or symptoms due to distant spread, usually pain. The terms clinical, latent, and occult are used to describe these various presentations. Thus, the *clinical* tumor presents with symptoms of obstruction or pain, and rectal examination reveals an obvious tumor; the *latent* tumor is that focus of tumor found at prostatectomy or autopsy with no other evidence of the disease; an *occult* tumor becomes manifest by its metastases for there is little or no local abnormality.

The average age at presentation (Bumpus, 1926) is 65 years, approximately 50% occurring between 60 and 70 years. In our own experience, the mean age at presentation for all stages of the tumor was approximately 70 years. The tumor is rare under the age of 50, becomes increasingly frequent with age, but after the age of 80, the clinical tumor becomes less common and the latent cases are more common so that most men by 80–90 years have a lesion varying from a microscopic focus to a macroscopic nodule.

The most common symptoms associated with carcinoma of the prostate are either obstructive (65%) or pain (25%) in the back, thighs, or perineum. Approximately 10% of patients present with either hematuria or general debility. Bony symptoms rarely correlate with the extent of the disease as shown by either radiological or scanning techniques; widespread bone involvement may be entirely asymptomatic. Lymphatic spread is also difficult to assess without resorting to biopsy or lymphangiography (see later).

The incidence of latent tumors is known only with respect to autopsy material and from prostatectomy specimens, and figures range from 5 to 16%. In a series of random perineal prostatic biopsies in 688 virtually asymptomatic men aged 50–69, Hudson (1957) found localized carcinoma in one in ten. The detection rate for asymptomatic tumors increases where well-person screening is practised, and in one series more than half of the tumors were found as part of a routine clinical examination (Kimbrough, 1956).

III. Natural History

Information concerning the natural history of untreated carcinoma of the prostate is available only from studies carried out prior to the introduction of hormone therapy. In a review of a thousand cases, Bumpus (1926) reported that in 485 cases in which no treatment was given, the average survival from the first symptom to death was approximately 31 months, and only 4 patients in this untreated group lived more than 3 years; when metastases were evident at the initial presentation 60% of these patients died within 9 months. In a group of 125 patients in whom cystostomy was carried out for outflow tract obstruction, the average survival was 57 months, and this represented the best "treatment" group.

A collected series of 795 untreated patients formed the so-called control group against which Nesbit and Baum (1950) compared their early experience with hormone therapy. The 5-year survival for the untreated group with no metastases at the time of admission was 10%; it was 6% if metastases were present.

The uncertain character of the disease and its varied natural history indicated to Franks (1956, 1967) that there were two types of prostatic cancer: one behaved as an active tumor and eventually killed the patient; the other, a latent tumor, was usually an incidental finding at autopsy. Histologically these tumors appear identical, but their behavior is very different. Franks found that latent tumors could be large or small, well differentiated or anaplastic. Recently, a detailed study of autopsy material by McNeal (1969) has led him to challenge this view. He has concluded that rather than two types of tumor with different biological responses, there is a single type that has a slow rate of growth with a logarithmic progression.

The importance of histological grade has yet to be resolved. Franks *et al.* (1958) found no correlation between tumor grade and survival, whereas Schirmer *et al.* (1965) have given strong support to the view that grade is important in determining the incidence of metastases and the prognosis. Indeed, Scott (1973) believed that had Nesbit and Baum (1950) considered the tumor grade in addition to the stage, then it is almost certain that they would have shown that the well differentiated cancers fared better than the poorly differentiated—irrespective of stage.

There is debate as to whether there is any association between benign prostatic hyperplasia and cancer of the prostate (Armenian *et al.*, 1974; Greenwald *et al.*, 1974). The data are conflicting, but it is suggested that there is an indirect association through certain epidemiological factors that affect the natural history of benign prostatic hyperplasia.

The relevance of the presentation and the natural history of the disease has become of major importance because of the mortality and morbidity that can occur when estrogen therapy is given to a patient with early-stage tumor (Byar, 1973). *Pari passu* with the increased knowledge of the physiology of the prostate, there has been an increasing controversy over the choice and timing of treatment; these uncertainties can be resolved only by more detailed investigation of the patient in relation to clinical staging and the use of prospective controlled clinical trials.

IV. INVESTIGATION IN RELATION TO STAGING

A. TUMOR STAGING

The investigation of a patient with prostatic cancer must be considered with particular reference to staging of the tumor. Accurate staging is a prerequisite for the formulation of a rational treatment policy and can best be established by the use of an orderly sequence of investigations. Although several staging systems are available, our preference is for the T, N, M system of the Union Internationale Contre Le Cancrum (Wallace *et al.*, 1975), which allows a full description of the tumor in terms of the primary tumor mass (T), lymphatic spread (N), and distant metastases (M). The following are the minimum requirements for assessment of the T, N, and M categories. If these cannot be met, the symbol, TX, NX, or MX is used.

> T categories: Clinical examination, urography, endoscopy, and biopsy (if indicated) prior to definitive treatment.
> N categories: Clinical examination, lymphography, and/or urography.

M categories: Clinical examination, chest X-ray, skeletal studies, and determination of the acid phosphatase level on two or more occasions.

B. Clinical Examination

Prostatic carcinoma occurs with increasing frequency with age, and therefore predominantly at a time of life when other disease processes such as vascular degeneration or diabetes may directly affect the life expectancy of an individual patient. A full clinical evaluation is therefore mandatory and may indicate the need for further investigation of other systems.

1. *Rectal Examination*

An attempt should always be made to allocate a T category for each lesion on presentation, by careful rectal examination. Particular attention is paid to any evidence of invasion outside the prostatic capsule, into the seminal vesicles or into the urogenital diaphragm. There are six categories to describe the primary tumor (T).

TX Minimum requirements for assessment cannot be met.
T0 No tumor palpable.
T1 Intracapsular tumor surrounded by palpably normal gland.
T2 Tumor confined to the gland. Smooth nodule deforming contour but lateral sulci and seminal vesicles not involved.
T3 Tumor extending beyond capsule.
T4 Tumor invading neighboring structures.

2. *Lymphatic Examination*

Lymphatic spread is a common feature of prostatic carcinoma and occurs with increasing frequency as the primary tumor stage progresses (Arduino and Glucksman, 1962; Paxton *et al.*, 1975). The regional nodes lie along the iliac vessels and cannot be assessed clinically. In advanced disease, there may be evidence of metastases to superficial nodes in the groins, axillae, and supraclavicular fossae. Massive metastases to regional pelvic nodes may on occasion be evident clinically as a suprapubic mass.

3. *Distant Metastases to Other Organs*

Bone is the most frequent and important site of distant metastases. However, despite extensive involvement of the skeleton, there are frequently no clinical manifestations. On occasion, bone pain, paraplegia, and pathological fracture may be the presenting symptoms and so provide clinical evidence of metastatic disease. Hepatic metastases occur less commonly as a result of blood-borne invasion via the prostatic plexus and its communication with the portal system. Varkarakis et al. (1975) have suggested that bone is the primary site of distant organ metastases and that further spread occurs by cascade dissemination from bone. Certainly in the terminal stages of the disease there may be clinical evidence of widespread tumor dissemination. Mental confusion or specific neurological signs such as an oculomotor palsy may signify underlying cerebral metastases, and cutaneous nodules denote multiple deposits in the skin.

C. Laboratory Investigations

1. Biopsy

A tissue diagnosis must always be included in the initial assessment of a patient. The specimen may be obtained with a biopsy needle (via the perineal or transrectal route), by transurethral resection, or by transrectal aspiration.

2. Renal Function

Estimation of the blood urea or creatinine affords a rough index of renal function, and elevation of either of these values provides presumptive evidence of extraprostatic spread with bilateral ureteric obstruction.

3. Serum Acid and Alkaline Phosphatase

Nesbit and Baum (1950) reported that the total acid phosphatase was elevated in 65% of cases with distant metastases and in only 20% of those confined to the prostatic area. There may be some advantage in estimating total and tartrate labile fractions, as there is evidence that the latter represent true prostatic activity (Abul-Fadl and King, 1949). False positive elevations of serum acid phosphatase activity may occur after rectal examination or operative manipulation of the prostate, and blood sampling should always be done prior to such procedures (Marberger et al., 1957). False negative results are of greater importance, and a normal serum acid phosphatase result is of no value in assessing tumor stage. Alkaline phosphatase levels reflect bone metabolic activity, and raised values indicate bone metastases in the absence of other metabolic bone disorders or obstructive liver disease.

4. *Hematology*

The minimum hematological investigations are hemoglobin and packed cell volume determinations. Anemia is a frequent occurrence in advanced disease and is a useful indicator of dissemination (Williams *et al.*, 1974). Examination of bone marrow aspirates for malignant cells has been studied as a staging investigation in a number of centers. Nelson *et al.* (1973) studied 556 bone marrow aspirates in 449 patients with histologically confirmed prostatic cancer and concluded that it was of little value as a routine procedure. Only 21% of 103 patients with proven distant metastases had positive bone marrow aspirates, but 10% of patients had a positive marrow despite normal skeletal surveys and normal serum acid phosphatase levels.

D. Radiological and Radioisotopic Investigations

1. *Intravenous Urography*

Evidence of upper tract obstruction is the most useful indication of tumor stage on an intravenous urogram. Extravesical ureteric obstruction may be caused by direct extension of tumor in the rectovesical plane or by extrinsic compression from secondary lymphatic deposits. It is usually possible to differentiate extravesical ureteric obstruction from bladder outlet obstruction by the examination of postmicturition films.

2. *Metastatic Screening*

A chest X-ray and a radiological skeletal survey constitute the initial screening procedures. Pulmonary deposits are rarely seen except in advanced disease, but there may be bone metastases in up to 50% of patients on presentation (Whitmore, 1973). Prostatic metastases in bone are typically osteoblastic, but osteolytic lesions also occur. Radioisotope bone scanning offers increased sensitivity in the detection of bone metastases but is relatively nonspecific; increased uptake of isotope occurs in such conditions as Paget's disease, eosinophilic granuloma of bone, healing fractures, and osteomyelitis as well as metastatic bone disease. Strontium 85 and 87 were the original isotopes used, but in many cases the quality of the scan pictures was poor. Fluorine-18, a cyclotron-generated isotope, is in many respects an ideal material, but its short half-life restricts its application (Roy *et al.*, 1971; Chisholm *et al.*, 1973). Technetium-labeled polyphosphates and, recently, diphosphonate are more convenient to handle and the quality of these scans is comparable to fluorine scans (Shearer *et al.*, 1974; Merrick, 1975). Our further experience with fluorine-18 scans has recently been reviewed by Buck *et al.* (1975).

Early bone lesions were detected in 25% of patients with no radiological evidence of metastases. Furthermore, on follow-up it was shown that scan abnormalities preceded radiological changes by one to two years. In this study of 74 patients there were no false negative results.

3. *Lymphography*

Histological studies following pelvic lymphadenectomy have shown a high incidence of regional lymph node metastases (Arduino and Glucksman, 1962; McCullough *et al.*, 1974). Moreover, there is a definite relationship between the incidence of lymphatic spread and the primary tumor stage. Assessment of pelvic and paraaortic nodes by bilateral pedal lymphography has revealed a very similar picture (Grossman *et al.*, 1974; Castellino *et al.*, 1973; Paxton *et al.*, 1975). The use of pedal lymphography remains controversial. Lymphography can opacify the external iliac, common iliac, and paraaortic nodes but provides no information concerning the internal iliac, obturator, and midsacral groups. Moreover, there is some doubt concerning the accuracy of interpretations. Reactive hyperplasia, lymphadenitis, or fatty replacement may be the cause of false positive results, and microscopic metastases without distortion of the nodal architecture may lead to false negatives. The accuracy rate of lymphography when compared to the histological findings after lymphadenectomy in a small series of 18 patients was reported to be 89% (Castellino *et al.*, 1973). There is a great need for further controlled studies, which are now in progress in several centers. Although lymphography is a time-consuming procedure and pulmonary oil embolism may be a hazard to patients with diminished respiratory reserve, the available evidence indicates that it is the most acceptable method for the assessment of lymphatic spread. Paxton *et al.* (1975) have reported that 46.9% of new cases without evidence of skeletal metastases and 48% of new cases with normal serum acid phosphatase values had lymphographic evidence of node spread.

E. SURGICAL STAGING METHODS

A true pathological stage can only be determined either by histological examination of a radical prostatectomy specimen or by postmortem examination. Open perineal biopsy of the posterior surface of the prostate is probably the most accurate biopsy technique, but is rarely practised except as a prelude to radical perineal prostatectomy (Culp and Meyer, 1973) or prior to open perineal cryosurgery (O'Donoghue *et al.*, 1975).

Despite the fact that it can provide an apportunity for assessing capsular invasion, this approach has not won general acceptance as a staging procedure.

1. *Cystourethroscopy*

Cystourethroscopy is of little value in staging early lesions owing to the predominantly peripheral and posterior site of the lesion, but in more advanced disease it can reveal invasion of the bladder neck and trigone as well as the membranous urethra. Endoscopy is a minimal requirement for the category in a T, N, M classification.

2. *Examination under Anesthesia*

Rectal examination under anesthesia with adequate muscular relaxation can be a useful adjunct in staging and permits a better assessment of extraprostatic spread, particularly in the region of the seminal vesicles.

3. *Staging Laparotomy*

Staging laparotomy has to date been the most accurate assessment of lymphatic spread. However, there may be an appreciable morbidity from a complete laparotomy and biopsy of abdominal and paraaortic nodes (W. R. Fair, personal communication, 1975). Most authors have related the incidence of lymphatic deposits to primary tumor stage, and it is evident that there is a high incidence of lymphatic spread in T3 and T4 lesions (Table I). However, there is a considerable discrepancy in the reported incidence of lymph node metastases with T1 and T2 (or stage B) lesions. It may be that errors in staging the primary tumor explain these discrepancies: careful histological studies of radical prostatectomy speci-

TABLE I

INCIDENCE OF PELVIC NODE METASTASES RELATED TO TUMOR STAGE

Reference	T1 and T2 (B)	T3 (C)	(D)
Flocks et al. (1959)[a]	7%	38%	—
Arduino and Glucksman (1962)[a]	32%	91%	—
Whitmore and Mackenzie (1959)[a]	0%	45%	—
McCullough et al. (1974)[a]	25%	51%	82%
Castellino et al. (1973)[a,b]	44%	55%	—
Paxton et al. (1975)[b]	41%	60%	92%

[a] Histological assessment.
[b] Lymphographic assessment.

mens have revealed that clinical evaluation of the prostate frequently underestimates the true pathological stage (Jewett, 1975).

V. Endocrine Therapy

A. Rationale for Treatment

A variety of endocrine manipulations have been used since Huggins and Hodges (1941) recommended the reduction of the level of androgenic hormones for the treatment of prostatic carcinoma. The choice consists of either the removal of androgen sources by castration (and adrenalectomy) or the suppression of androgen activity by the administration of estrogens, progestogens, or antiandrogens or by pituitary ablation.

Suppression of luteinizing hormone, and hence the suppression of testosterone production by Leydig cells, remains the principal mechanism affected by estrogens. However, there is a risk that current interest concerning levels of serum testosterone may overshadow a direct effect of estrogen on the prostate.

Earlier studies have shown that estrogen inhibits both prostatic growth and secretions. More recently, Shimazaki *et al.* (1965) and Farnsworth (1969) have presented evidence for a direct and suppressive effect of estrogens on prostatic metabolism of testosterone *in vitro*. It has since been shown that stilbestrol can inhibit DNA polymerase (Harper *et al.*, 1970) and 5-reductase activity (Shimazaki *et al.*, 1971; Altwein *et al.*, 1974), although the dose of estrogen used in both studies was in excess of therapeutic dosages. In addition, both estrogen and androgen cytoplasmic receptors have now been demonstrated in the prostate, and it may be that prostate growth is, in part, regulated by estrogens (Jungblut *et al.*, 1971). The relevance of these observations to the dosage of estrogen is unknown, but it would appear that pituitary-mediated androgen suppression is only one of the factors controlling the growth (and overgrowth) of prostatic tissue.

B. Estrogens

The drug used to suppress androgen production is usually stilbestrol (diethylstilbestrol, DES). No estrogenic substance has been demonstrated to produce a more complete or lasting suppression of pituitary activity in man or a more adequate suppression of prostatic tumor cell growth than synthetic stilbestrol. There is little objective evidence upon which the decision to use other drugs can be made, and there is little evidence that either a change in dose or a change in drug has any useful effect after a patient has relapsed on estrogen therapy.

The synthetic estrogen chlorotrianisene (Tace) was introduced because it was suggested that adrenal hyperplasia did not occur as with other estrogens and that other side effects of dyspepsia, edema and gynecomastia were less. However, this substance is much less effective in lowering serum testosterone levels than other estrogens; indeed Shearer *et al.* (1973) showed no substantial suppression.

Estradiol phosphate (Estradurin) is an injectable preparation whose effects last for 4 weeks after one injection. Since it has only a weak effect on gonadotropin and yet has a satisfactory clinical response, it has been suggested that the action may be mainly by a direct effect on the tumor cells (Jönsson *et al.*, 1963). As with chlorotrianisene, the main role of this drug is as an alternative to stilbestrol, especially when the patient is either unable to take tablets or orchiectomy has been refused.

1. *Dose of Estrogen*

The majority of dose schedules used to achieve androgen suppression have been in the range of 1–5 mg DES orally each day. The variations in dosage were often little more than random attempts to find the optimum *clinical* response. Baker (1953) found that as little as 0.25 mg of DES intramuscularly per day would produce a remission. Birke *et al.* (1954) measured the urinary excretion of androgenic steroids (androsterone, etiocholanolone, and total 17-ketosteroids) in relation to several dose schedules and found that the most rapid and effective response was with 30 mg of stilbestrol per day for 5 days. With a dose of 10–15 mg of stilbestrol per day the reduction in urinary androgenic steroids took 15–21 days, and with 5 mg per day the effect was even slower.

Fergusson (1963, 1967) has recommended 100 mg of stilbestrol per day, and this has been widely used in the United Kingdom. Usually the dose is reduced to 15 mg per day either within 2–3 months or when breast discomfort is evident. Apart from an apparently better survival at 6 months there was no other objective evidence to favor a high dose. During the past decade the Veterans Administration Cooperative Urological Research Group (V.A.C.U.R.G.) has carried out clinical trials that have emphasized the cardiovascular risks from estrogens, and the results from their Study II have shown that 1.0 mg of DES is just as effective as 5.0 mg (Byar, 1973; Chisholm, 1974).

Recent studies have attempted to determine the minimal effective dose of estrogen by measuring plasma testosterone levels. It has been shown that the same reduction of plasma testosterone is achieved within about 7 days using doses of stilbestrol varying from 100 mg three times daily to 1 mg three times daily (Robinson and Thomas, 1971; Shearer *et al.*, 1973). It was also shown that natural conjugated estrogens from pregnant mare's urine (2.5 mg three times a day) and ethynylestradiol (0.05 mg twice daily) suppressed plasma testosterone levels equivalent to 3 mg of stilbestrol per day. Thus, if plasma testosterone is acceptable as an index of clinical chemical castration, then 1 mg three times a day is the minimum effective dose. However, Bracci and Di Silverio (1973) have shown that the suppression of plasma testosterone following castration is more effective than after estrogen therapy.

C. CASTRATION

In the report by Nesbit and Baum (1950), it appeared that survival following castration-estrogen therapy was better than the survival following either therapy alone, and especially for those patients without metastases on the first admission. Nevertheless, this combination has not always been the favored primary treatment, and some urologists have found orchiectomy alone to be the most reliable initial treatment while others, often for esthetic reasons, or because of patient choice, have preferred to reserve castration for the patient who has "escaped" from estrogen control. Orchiectomy has remained the primary treatment for a patient with cardiovascular disease or for a patient who is unable to take the tablets regularly.

In those patients treated by estrogen alone, the escape from estrogen control is usually determined by a rise in serum acid phosphatase, extension of bony metastases (by X-ray or scan), and the onset of pain. A more precise measure of tumor escape is needed by the clinician, and it may be that serum hormone measurements will be the source of this information. It has been shown that men with metastatic carcinoma of the prostate who have late reactivation of symptoms after bilateral orchiectomy have normal levels of plasma androstenedione, dehydroepiandrosterone, and testosterone (Walsh, 1975). It has also been suggested that changes in prolactin and growth hormone may be correlated with the clinical progress of the disease M. E. Harper, personal communication, 1975).

D. OTHER METHODS

1. *Cytotoxic Drugs*

There are two compounds whose formulation is designed to produce a direct local effect on the tumor cell, in one by a high concentration of estrogen and in the other by releasing nor-nitrogen mustard. The former, stilbestrol diphosphate (Honvan) is a phosphorylated synthetic estrogen formed by the substitution of a phosphate complex for the hydroxy grouping at each end of the stilbestrol molecule. It is almost inactive unless broken down by the enzyme phosphatase. This reaction results in the liberation of free stilbestrol from the phosphorylated compound and is believed to occur mainly in prostatic tumor tissue, including metastases, where the concentrations of phosphatase are high and the requisite pH is present. Efforts to demonstrate that a high local concentration occurs have been inconclusive (Segal *et al.*, 1959; Fergusson, 1961). However, the drug is well tolerated and is of particular value when a rapid response is required because of metastatic pain or urinary retention (Lambley and Ware, 1967).

Estramustine phosphate (Estracyt) consists of a nor-nitrogen mustard which is linked to a phosphorylated estradiol. (A detailed discussion of this drug is presented in this volume.) Estramustine acts by using the phosphorylated estradiol to carry the compound to the tumor tissue where enzymic breakdown releases the nor-nitrogen mustard. The exact mode of action is not known, but it appears to be more effective in depressing the activity of acid phosphatase and β-glucuronidase than estrogen alone (Nilsson and Müntzing, 1973). Clinical experience has shown that this drug is valuable for palliation, but it should not replace conventional antiandrogenic treatment unless the patient presents with an advanced, poorly differentiated tumor.

Few of the conventional chemotherapeutic agents have been adequately tested in prostatic cancer. Their use is usually restricted to the patient who has relapsed and failed to respond to more orthodox endocrine measures (The management of such patients is discussed in this volume by Murphy.) A controlled clinical trial of cyclophosphamide and 5-fluorouracil compared with standard therapy in patients with advanced prostatic cancer was established by the National Prostatic Cancer Project (NPCP) in the United States in 1973. The use of other drugs, such as adriamycin, strepozotocin, and Mithramycin, either as single agents or in sequential or combined chemotherapy, are also under assessment, but no specific recommendations can be made until the results of these controlled studies are made available (Schmidt, 1975).

2. *Progestogens and Other Drugs*

The advantage of a drug that has a significant effect on plasma testosterone but does not produce feminization has led to the investigation of a variety of drugs that are known to inhibit androgen synthesis.

There have been several reports of favorable results with the use of chlormadinone acetate (Chlormadinone), hydroxyprogesterone caproate (Delalutin), and cyproterone acetate (Androcur). Only relatively few patients have been treated with each drug, and many of these have been treated only after the tumor has escaped estrogen control (Walsh, 1975). Medroxyprogesterone (Provera) has been included in the V.A.C.U.R.G. Study III.

Clinical experience with two other drugs that inhibit androgen synthesis—aminoglutethamide (Shearer *et al.*, 1973) and spironolactone (Walsh, 1975) showed only little suppression of plasma testosterone with aminoglutethamide but a 90% suppression with spironolactone.

Apart from any effect on circulating androgen, chlormadinone acetate and cyproterone acetate may both suppress tumor growth, though through their peripheral antiandrogenic effect. A nonsteroidal antiandrogen has been developed (SCH 13521, Flutamide) which is nonprogestational and does not suppress plasma testosterone levels (Neri *et al.*, 1972).

Interest in this range of drugs has led to the development of laboratory methods for assessing their relative effect prior to clinical use (These methods are reviewed in this volume by Sandberg, see p. 155.)

3. *Adrenalectomy and Hypophysectomy*

The place of either of these methods to achieve endocrine control of prostatic carcinoma and its metastases has always been limited to the patient who has relapsed after a period of conventional estrogen-castration therapy. Because there is no standard method of treatment for such a patient, there have been many uncontrolled studies of new antiandrogens, adrenal suppressive agents as well as chemotherapeutic agents. Eventually, such patients have been considered for either adrenalectomy or hypophysectomy in such a random manner as to make their evaluation difficult.

There is now little justification for bilateral adrenalectomy. Not only is this major surgical procedure associated with a significant operative mortality but also the mean survival is usually less than one year (Mahoney and Harrison, 1972; Bhanalaph *et al.*, 1974).

Although the survival following hypophysectomy may not appear very different from the adrenalectomy results, the subjective improvement is generally better; 70 of the 100 patients reported from the Institute of Urology by Fergusson and Hendry (1971) had a subjective improvement following this procedure. Smaller series have had more variable proportions of improvement in symptoms, but in all series the mean survival was less than one year. It may be concluded that the principal indication for hypophysectomy is the relief of *widespread* bony pain.

VI. RADIOTHERAPY

A. EXTERNAL IRRADIATION

Interest in the use of external irradiation for localized prostatic malignancy has increased rapidly since Del Regato (1967) pointed out that these tumors were not necessarily radioresistant but regressed slowly with radiation.

The application of supervoltage radiotherapy techniques allows a uniformly high dose to a precise area within the pelvis. The dose to the prostate by current techniques varies from 3500–5500 rads using cobalt-60 (McLoughlin et al., 1975) to 7000–75000 rads using either the betatron or linear accelerator (Mollenkamp et al., 1975). The precision with which the dose can be given has minimized the complications, and although most patients have some rectal, bladder, or urethral irritation, this is usually transient and resolves within a month. A few patients may develop increasing bladder neck obstructive symptoms and require a transurethral resection either during or after radiotherapy. The incidence of severe persistent rectal and urinary symptoms is approximately 10% (Ray et al., 1973). Potency has been maintained in some 70% of patients though this may decline during the first year after treatment.

Radiotherapy has been given to patients in all stages of the disease with apparently good results. For example, Ray et al. (1973) have reported 5- and 10-year survival rates (uncorrected) of 72% and 48%, respectively, for localized cancer and 48% and 30%, respectively, for extracapsular cancer. However, neither this nor other radiotherapy series has a control group, and interpretation of these data is further handicapped by the fact that a high proportion of patients have received pre-radiation hormonal therapy.

In addition, there is doubt about both tumor staging and the follow-up. Carlton et al. (1972), who have recommended retropubic exploration for surgical staging, reported that 30% of stage C patients were found to be stage D at exploration. The assessment of response after radiotherapy by Ray et al. (1973) was by rectal examination only. Recently, serial transrectal biopsy follow-up has been used to determine the response and has shown that there is a high proportion (65%) with residual tumor at one year (Sewell et al., 1975); but even this observation must be interpreted with caution, for the malignant cells appear to be nonviable (Mollenkamp et al., 1975).

Although external irradiation has gained wide acceptance, follow-up has revealed the need for accurate clinical staging before considering this form of treatment. The use of extended radiation fields to include regional lymph nodes has yet to be evaluated.

B. Local Implantation

Earlier experience with radium implantation was eventually abandoned because of poor results and local complications (Widman, 1934). In 1973, Flocks reviewed his experience with the interstitial injection of radioactive gold (^{198}Au). The technique consisted of multiple injections either alone or in combination with prostatectomy. However, it is difficult to assess the true value of the procedures since most patients had received, or later received, other forms of treatment. However, using combined treatment there was a 27.5% 15-year survival for stage C tumors without node involvement. A more recent technique of retropubic implantation of ^{125}I seeds is both safe and simple, but the use of supplementary treatment again makes interpretation of results difficult to assess (Whitmore et al., 1972).

C. Systemic Radioactive Therapy

The rationale for the use of radioactive phosphorus (^{32}P) is based on the fact that it is localized in active bone and therefore in new bone associated with metastases. It has been claimed that the addition of testosterone increases the effectiveness of ^{32}P, but there is little evidence for this (Smart, 1965). Parathyroid hormone has been used to produce a withdrawal effect that results in an increased deposition of ^{32}P in active bone; dramatic relief of severe pain has been reported by Tong (1971).

VII. Summary and Treatment Protocol

In view of the inaccuracy of a clinical evaluation of carcinoma of the prostate by the T category, it is now evident that the main emphasis in tumor staging should lie in the detection of extraprostatic disease. This is of particular practical importance when curative therapy either by radical prostatectomy or by external irradiation is being considered for early disease. Radioisotope bone scanning has now been established and is widely used; if the accuracy of pedal lymphography in controlled studies proves to be acceptable, this will be a valuable addition in tumor staging. The 1974 T, N, M classification can be related to a widely used ABCD staging, but it is evident that since the T, N, M requires a fuller assessment it adds more precision to the description of the tumor.

It is not possible to present an unqualified treatment policy for carcinoma of the prostate based on controlled clinical data. However, so much information has become available in the past decade that the evaluation of this material now provides a consensus of opinion (Chisholm, 1974; Blackard, 1974):

T0 N0 M0 (or A)	The management of incidentally diagnosed local disease consists of regular follow-up, but no specific treatment.
T1 T2 N0 M0 (or B)	Opinions differ widely over the management of a malignant nodule. The choices are external irradiation, low dose estrogen (or castration) therapy, radical prostatectomy, and no treatment. In general, a more aggressive policy is recommended in a fit patient under the age of 70.
T3 T4 N0 N1 M0 (or C)	A locally extensive tumor with or without lymph node involvement should be treated by low dose estrogen (or castration) therapy. An alternative, to withold treatment until the patient develops symptoms (other than obstruction), has received support from V.A.C.U.R.G., but this has not been universally accepted.
T0–T4, N1 M1 (or D)	The management of these patients is similar to that described for the previous group; the V.A.C.U.R.G. data for this stage showed a better survival for the treated patients.

Our management policy relies on a detailed preliminary assessment including the collection of baseline serum hormone data. There are two treatment groups based on the N and M categories:

Group I. N0 M0. The treatment for this small proportion of cases is allocated randomly into two groups:

a. External irradiation to the prostate only

b. No treatment

Group II. N1 and/or M1. If there is a past history of cardiovascular disease, treatment is randomized between orchiectomy and cyproterone acetate; in the absence of cardiovascular disease, treatment is randomized between stilbestrol (1 mg three times daily) and cyproterone acetate. If there is subsequent progression of the disease as judged by symptoms or investigations, the treatment is changed to estramustine phosphate.

If symptoms persist, we favor irradiation to local painful sites and hypophysectomy for extensive bony pain.

REFERENCES

Abul-Fadl, M. A. M., and King, E. J. (1949). *Biochem. J.* **45**, 51.

Altwein, J. E., Orestano, F., and Hohenfellner, R. (1974). *Invest. Urol.* **12**, 157.

Arduino, L. J., and Glucksman, M. A. (1962). *J. Urol.* **88**, 91.

Armenian, H. K., Lilienfeld, A. M., Diamond, E. L., and Bross, I. D. J. (1974). *Lancet* **2**, 115.

Baker, R. (1953). *Ann. Surg.* **137**, 29.

Bhanalaph, T., Varkarakis, M. J., and Murphy, G. P. (1974). *Ann. Surg.* **179**, 17.

Birke, G., Franksson, C., and Plantin, L. O. (1954). *Acta Endocrinol. (Copenhagen)* **17**, Suppl., 1.

Blackard, C. E. (1974). *Brit. J. Hosp. Med.* **11**, 357.

Bracci, U., and Di Silverio, F. (1973). *Proc. Int. Congr. Urol., 16th, 1973* Vol. 2, p. 265.

Buck, A. C., Chisholm, G. D., Merrick, M. V., and Lavender, J. P. (1975). *Brit. J. Urol.* **47**, 287.

Bumpus, H. C. (1922). *Amer. J. Roetgenol.* [N. S.] **9**, 269.

Bumpus, H. C. (1926). *Surg., Gynecol. Obstet.* **43**, 150.

Byar, D. P. (1973). *Cancer* **32**, 1126.

Carlton, C. E., Jr., Dawoud, F., Hudgins, P., and Scott, R., Jr. (1972). *J. Urol.* **108**, 924.

Castellino, R. A., Ray, G., Blank, N., Govan, D., and Bagshaw, M. (1973). *J. Amer. Med. Ass.* **223**, 877.

Chisholm, G. D. (1974). *In* "The Treatment of Prostatic Hypertrophy and Neoplasia" (J. E. Castro, ed.), pp. 121–146. M.T.P., Lancaster.

Chisholm, G. D., Buck, A. C., Merrick, M. V., and Lavender, J. P. (1973). *Proc. Int. Congr. Urol., 16th, 1973* Vol. 2, p. 86.

Culp, O. S., and Meyer, J. J. (1973). *Cancer* **32**, 1113.

Del Regato, J. A. (1967). *Radiology* **88**, 761.

Farnsworth, W. E. (1969). *J. Invest. Urol.* **6**, 423.

Fergusson, J. D. (1961). *Brit. J. Urol.* **33**, 442.

Fergusson, J. D. (1963). *Proc. Roy. Soc. Med.* **56**, 81.

Fergusson, J. D. (1967). *Trans. Med. Soc. London* **83**, 92.

Fergusson, J. D., and Hendry, W. F. (1971). *Brit. J. Urol.* **43**, 514.

Flocks, R. H. (1973). *J. Urol.* **109**, 461.

Flocks, R. H., Culp, D., and Porto, R. (1959). *J. Urol.* **81**, 194.

Franks, L. M. (1956). *Lancet* **271**, 1037.

Franks, L. M. (1967). *Trans. Med. Soc. London* **83**, 101.

Franks, L. M., Fergusson, J. D., and Murnaghan, G. F. (1958). *Brit. J. Cancer* **12**, 321.

Greenwald, P., Kirmss, V., Polan, A. K., and Dick, V. S. (1974). *J. Nat. Cancer Inst.* **53**, 335.

Grossman, I., von Phul, R., Fitzgerald, J. P., Masih, S., Turner, A. F., Kurohara, S. S., and George, F. (1974). *Amer. J. Roentgenol., Radium Ther. Nucl. Med.* [N. S.] **120**, 673.

Harper, M. E., Fahmy, A. R., and Pierrepoint, C. G., and Griffiths, K. (1970). *Steroids* **15**, 89.

Hudson, P. B. (1957). *J. Amer. Geriat. Soc.* **5**, 338.

Huggins, C., and Hodges, C. V. (1941). *Cancer Res.* **1**, 293.

Huggins, C., Stevens, R. E., and Hodges, C. V. (1941). *Arch. Surg. (Chicago)* **43**, 209.

Jewett, H. J. (1975). *Urol. Clin. N. Amer.* **2**, 105.

Jönsson, G., Diczfalusy, E., Plantin, L. O., Röhl, L., and Birke, G. (1963). *Acta Endocrinol. (Copenhagen)* **44**, Suppl. 83, 1.

Jungblut, P. W., Hughes, S. F., Görlich, L., Gowers, U., and Wagner, R. K. (1971). *Hoppe-Seyler's Z. Physiol. Chem.* **352**, 1603.

Kimbrough, J. C. (1956). *J. Urol.* **76**, 287.

Lambley, D. G., and Ware, J. W. (1967). *Brit. J. Urol.* **39**, 147.

McCullough, D. L., and Prout, G. R., and Daly, J. J. (1974). *J. Urol.* **111**, 65.

McLoughlin, M., Hazra, T., Schirmer, H. K. A., and Scott, W. W. (1975). *J. Urol.* **113**, 378.

McNeal, J. E. (1969). *Cancer* **23**, 24.

Mahoney, E. M., and Harrison, J. H. (1972). *J. Urol.* **108**, 936.

Marberger, H., Segal, S. J., and Flocks, R. H. (1957). *J. Urol.* **78**, 287.

Merrick, M. V. (1975). *Brit. J. Radiol.* **48**, 327.

Mollenkamp, J. S., Cooper, J. F., and Kagan, A. R. (1975). *J. Urol.* **113**, 374.

Nelson, C. M. K., Boatman, D. L., and Flocks, R. H. (1973). *J. Urol.* **109**, 667.

Neri, R., Florance, K., Koziol, P., and Van Cleave, S. (1972). *Endocrinology* **91**, 427.

Nesbit, R. M., and Baum, W. C. (1950). *J. Amer. Med. Ass.* **143**, 1317.

Nilsson, T., and Müntzing, J. (1973). *Scand. J. Urol. Nephrol.* **7**, 18.

O'Donoghue, E. P. N., Milleman, L. A., Flocks, R. H., Culp, D. A., and Bonney, W. W. (1975). *Urology* **5**, 308.

Pasteau, O., and Degrais, J. (1913). *J. Urol. Med. Chir.* **4**, 341.

Paxton, R. M., Williams, G., and McDonald, J. S. (1975). *Brit. Med. J.* **1**, 120.

Ray, G. R., Cassay, J. R., and Bagshaw, M. A. (1973). *Radiology* **106**, 407.

Robinson, M. R. G., and Thomas, B. S. (1971). *Brit. Med. J.* **4**, 391.

Roy, R. R., Nathan, B. E., Beales, J. S. M., and Chisholm, G. D. (1971). *Brit. J. Urol.* **43**, 58.

Schirmer, H. K. A., Murphy, G. P., and Scott, W. W. (1965). *Urol. Dig.* **4**, 15.

Schmidt, J. D. (1975). *Urol. Clin. N. Amer.* **2**, 185.

Scott, W. W. (1973). *Cancer* **32**, 1119.

Segal, S. J., Marberger, H., and Flocks, R. H. (1959). *J. Urol.* **81**, 474.

Sewell, R. A., Braren, V., Wilson, S. K., and Rhamy, R. K. (1975). *J. Urol.* **113**, 371.

Shearer, R. J., Hendry, W. F., Sommerville, I. F., and Fergusson, J. D. (1973). *Brit. J. Urol.* **45**, 668.

Shearer, R. J., Constable, A. R., Girling, M., Hendry, W. F., and Fergusson, J. D. (1974). *Brit. Med. J.* **2**, 362.

Shimazaki, J., Kurihara, H., Ito, Y., and Shida, K. (1965). *Gunma J. Med. Sci.* **14**, 313.

Shimazaki, J., Horaguchi, T., and Ohki, Y. (1971). *Endocrinol. Jap.* **18**, 179.

Smart, J. G. (1965). *Brit. J. Urol* **37**, 139.

Tong, E. C. K. (1971). *Radiology* **98**, 343.

Varkarakis, M., Murphy, G. P., Nelson, C. M. K., Chehval, M., Moore, R. H., and Flocks, R. H. (1975). *Urol. Clin. N. Amer.* **2**, 197

Wallace, D. M., Chisholm, G. D., and Hendry, W. F. (1975). *Brit. J. Urol.* **47**, 1.

Walsh, P. C. (1975). *Urol. Clin. N. Amer.* **2**, 125.

Whitmore, W. F., Jr. (1973). *Cancer* **32**, 1104.

Whitmore, W. F., and Mackenzie, A. R. (1959). *Cancer* 12, 396.
Whitmore, W. F., Jr., Hilaris, B., and Grabstald, H. (1972). *J. Urol.* 108, 918.
Widman, B. P. (1934). *Radiology* 22, 153.
Williams, G., Wallace, D. M., and Bloom, H. J. G. (1974). *Brit. J. Urol.* 46, 61.

DISCUSSION

D. S. Coffey: I congratulate you on a very informative presentation of this most complex problem, your emphasis on the misleading nature of many earlier clinical evaluations of hormone therapy.

In your suggested protocol for testing antiandrogens and Estracyt, I would caution that you are testing these drugs under conditions where the tumor may have already become insensitive to hormonal therapy. Under these conditions, tumors may not be expected to respond. However, if these drugs were compared with standard estrogen therapy earlier in the disease process, it is possible that they could be as effective and maybe without some of the adverse effects of estrogen. Of course, this would need to be established; nevertheless, it would be a fairer comparison than that of treating advanced or relapsing patients.

G. D. Chisholm: I agree that by recommending antiandrogens for failed estrogen cases we could be treating some who are hormone insensitive; but these patients form the largest part of any study and there are not many treatment options to offer them.

L. Andersson: For the choice of therapy and to compare various kinds of treatment, it is important to know that, even in patients in whom we believe the tumor to be localized, there is lymph node dissemination in a high percentage. In my experience it is difficult to visualize the pelvic nodes on lymphography. What is your opinion on the most satisfactory technique for lymphography in these patients?

G. D. Chisholm: Pedal lymphography is the technique most widely used—but it is well recognized that nodes in the internal iliac (obturator) areas are not visualized. It is for this reason that we have to consider surgical staging as well.

M. B. Lipsett: In patients who relapse after estrogen therapy and have a subsequent response to orchiectomy, does the acid phosphatase fall again? What percentage of estrogen-relapse patients respond to subsequent orchiectomy?

G. D. Chisholm: The acid phosphatase does fall again in those that respond. I do not know the percentage.

K. Griffiths: In relation to Dr. Coffey's comment that antiandrogen therapy will be of little value in the relapsed patient, is it not true that a large proportion of patients who have responded well to estrogen therapy but have relapsed will subsequently respond again to orchiectomy?

G. D. Chisholm: Yes, it is worthwhile to carry out an orchiectomy on relapsed patients because they may respond.

M. B. Lipsett: It seems from Nesbit's old data and those of others that estrogen therapy is no better than orchiectomy. Since estrogen in these doses causes severe functional depression of testicular function as well, there is no evidence for an additional "cytotoxic" effect of estrogen.

I do not think you should look to the endocrinologist to predict relapse. It is clear that relapse can occur with complete suppression of pituitary and gonadal function. You will need something akin to CEA or α-fetoprotein.

G. D. Chisholm: The second point first: the measurement of CEA and α-fetoprotein in carcinoma of the prostate has not been helpful: data from several Centers have been similar and discouraging.

I agree that there is no good supporting evidence for a cytotoxic effect.

T. Nilsson: de Byar within the Veterans Administration study group now announces that he is not so sure any longer that 1 mg of DES is as good as he previously thought, in the light of further experience within the VA study. Of those patients with negative lymphagiography, 20% had positive nodes along the obturator nerve; these, of course, do not show up on the X-ray.

G. D. Chisholm: Thank you. These are both important points.

N. Bruchovsky: I wish to draw attention to the observation that a significant percentage of hormone-unresponsive tumors lack cytoplasmic receptor and fail to incorporate steroids into the nucleus. Perhaps the pharmaceutical industry should attempt to develop agents that would render the nuclear membrane more permeable to the passage of steroid hormone into the nucleus. With such agents it might be possible to activate homeostatic constraint mechanisms and produce the highly desirable carcinostatic or carcinocidal changes associated with tissue involution.

G. D. Chishlom: I believe the permeability of the nuclear membrane could be relevant in explaining the effect of, e g., Honvan in failed estrogen-treated patients.

H. J. de Voogt: I would like to comment on the cytotoxic effect of estrogenic compounds. Perhaps we should, as clinicians and endocrinologists, invite the pathologists and cytologists again. There are some very well conducted trials in Germany on the effect of estrogens on prostatic cancer cells in aspiration cytology; effects that were, for instance, different from the effects of antiandrogens.

L. Denis: Commenting on Dr. Lipsett's remark; after endocrine treatment, a situation of relapse with serum acid phosphatase probably means good response to bilateral orchiectomy.

G. D. Chisholm: Yes.

I. Lasnitzki: A comment relating to the question of direct hormonal effects on the cytology of prostatic carcinomas: We found that estrogens and antiandrogens certainly affect prostatic epithelium at the cellular level. In organ cultures of rat ventral prostate, estradiol-17β, cyproterone acetate, and stilbestrol induce atrophy of the epithelial cells and also inhibit the effect of added testosterone. In organ cultures of human BPH, estradiol-17β and stilbestrol cause cellular degeneration.

K. J. Tveter: Estrogens are very potent carcinogens and may give rise to a variety of tumors in experimental animals. What is the implication of this fact when discussing endocrine treatment of prostatic tumors, especially reactivated carcinomas?

G. D. Chisholm: An interesting thought! If it was remotely possible I believe we should have seen tumors elsewhere in the body—as well as reactivated prostatic tumors.

Management of Reactivated Prostatic Cancer*

G. P. MURPHY

*Roswell Park Memorial Institute, New York State Department of Health,
State University of New York at Buffalo, Buffalo, New York*

I. SCOPE OF THE PROBLEM

Adenocarcinoma of the prostate as we know it in the United States and elsewhere is a generalized disease in which most patients have metastases at the time of presentation (Murphy, 1974; Williams *et al.*, 1974). It is not infrequent that patients exhibit anemia associated with this metastatic disease, although some of the anemias can be corrected (Williams *et al.*, 1974). The probability of developing clinical carcinoma of the prostate increases with age, and death rates appear to be higher in the United States in white married men, ages 54 to 74 years, than in single men (Murphy, 1974). There is also some suggestion in Western culture that in certain population groups, mortality rates are rising faster in nonwhite males than in white males (Murphy, 1974).

Because of the situation of advanced stage D or advanced classification of disease by TNM or any other system, many patients are treated with hormonal palliation therapy involving estrogen, orchiectomy, or estrogens plus orchiectomy. Regardless of the clinical stage of the disease, even if it is limited or localized to the prostate, patient survival is not long and remissions are of short duration (Schoonees *et al.*, 1972a). Clinical survival in stage C carcinoma using the classification of Whitmore (Schoonees *et al.*, 1972a) at our own institution has an average of slightly under four years. State D patients survive for an average of 1.7 years.

It is important to note that, despite primary treatment such as orchiectomy or castration and orchiectomy in stage C or D cases, the cause of death is generally prostatic carcinoma in 50–65% of instances (Scho-

* This paper was supported in part by United States Public Health Service grant Nos. 55-05648-08 and RR-00262-09, of The National Institutes of Health.

onees *et al.*, 1972a). Postmortem studies at our own Institution corroborate the findings of others that the actual survival of patients with metastatic disease with palliative therapy is not significantly altered from those who receive no treatment (Schoonees *et al.*, 1972a). Thus one is faced with an important clinical dilemma in the management of patients who have been given hormonal treatment whether in a developing stage of metastases or in a presenting stage of metastases. These patients, when they progress further have had, until now, little to afford them clinical relief and present a clinical dilemma.

The purpose of this presentation is to review possible objective criteria associated with additional techniques for beneficial management of patients in these situations.

II. The Basis for Hormonal Therapy

The basis for manipulation of the hormonal milieu of patients with prostatic cancer is based upon sound experimental evidence from the laboratories of Dr. Huggins (1947) and others (Schoonees *et al.*, 1972b). For example, marked differences in the composition of resting and pilocarpine-stimulated canine prostatic fluid have been described (Huggins, 1947). The volume and acid phosphatase concentration of pilocarpine-stimulated canine prostatic fluid have been proved to be reliable indices of androgenic stimulation of the prostate in experimental situations (Schoonees *et al.*, 1972b). The role of zinc concentration in the prostate and in its secretions has also been suggested to have an associated hormonal relationship (Schoonees *et al.*, 1972b). Surprisingly, certain alterations in the mature prostatic tissue of the dog can be effected by castration (Varkarakis *et al.*, 1973). For example, depleting such animals of testosterone increases the avidity of the prostate equally for dihydrotestosterone and for estriol (Varkarakis *et al.*, 1973). In experimental situations such studies emphasize again that there may well be species differences. The fact that the dog apparently can concentrate administered radiolabeled estriol and possibly diethylstilbestrol to an equal degree as dihydrotestosterone, suggests that following castration other basic hormonal relationships of the prostate gland may be altered. To what degree this is applicable in a clinical situation, is unknown. We suspect that it is important, when considering further hormonal manipulation in a patient who has relapsed following orchiectomy and/or estrogens.

Understandably, in ongoing work further studies are necessary before the nature of the conjugated steroids present in prostatic fluid can be further established in experimental situations (Varkarakis *et al.*, 1972a).

However, a detectable relationship in aging males with benign prostatic hyperplasia was not demonstrable in carefully conducted studies (Schoonees *et al.*, 1971a). By no means, however, may the same situation be present in adenocarcinoma of the prostate in man.

Antiandrogens are also known to have demonstrable effects on various species, including the canine, in terms of various criteria of prostatic function (Schoonees *et al.*, 1973). Similar results have been found when antiandrogens have been employed to treat prostatic carcinoma in man (Schoonees *et al.*, 1971b). However, in our hands, such agents have not been of marked benefit when used following relapse after conventional hormonal palliative therapy for advanced clinical carcinoma of the prostate in man (Murphy, 1973a). For this reason at the present time, as well as in the past, other surgical steps have been undertaken in an effort, in selected instances, to produce a remission in a patient following castration and estrogen treatment who is in a state of relapse in the presence of advanced clinical disease.

III. Further Hormonal Manipulations in Relapsing Metastatic Prostatic Cancer

Hypophysectomy for advanced prostatic carcinoma as described by W. W. Scott and associates has been utilized in selected instances since 1952 (Scott, 1953). In review of such series, although significant palliation has been achieved for periods of 1–2 years on the average, the open hypophysectomy has proved to be a hazardous procedure with a considerable morbidity and operative mortality (Murphy *et al.*, 1969, 1971). Ablation of the anterior pituitary and its subsequent control over other hormonal factors associated with widespread prostatic cancer has been the basis for the utilization of hypophysectomy. However, open procedures have been generally found not to be associated with entire ablation of all pituitary cells (Scott and Schirmer, 1962).

In 1969 in our own clinic, we approached the possibility of using a functional assessment of a degree of ablation of the anterior pituitary (Murphy *et al.*, 1969, 1971). These studies were conducted in order to assess whether by transsphenoidal cryosurgical hypophysectomy significant destruction of the anterior pituitary could be achieved, in comparison to the open conventional procedure (Murphy *et al.*, 1969). As an end point in measurement, growth hormone levels were assayed in various patients before and after surgery. The levels were provoked by insulininduced hypoglycemia. This technique has now been utilized in a series of well over 50 such patients who have had repeat measurements in fol-

low-up periods extending as long as three years. The measurement of
the growth hormone levels in the presence of insulin-induced hypoglycemia has been achieved without any untoward episode but always with
a physician in attendance.

Pre- and postoperative measurements of growth hormones exhibit a
typical flat curve following open hypophysectomy (Fig. 1). Such flat
curves are maintained for an indefinite period. West and Murphy (1973)
studied an additional group of patients who had undergone adenohypophysectomy by either open craniotomy in 8 instances or by stereotaxic
cryohypophysectomy in 19 patients. All these patients had multiple
growth hormone assays performed during insulin-induced hypoglycemia
in the preoperative control period and at least twice during the postoperative experimental period, which lasted up to and including an average
of one year.

Figure 2 shows the close correlation, before and after surgery with open
hypophysectomy, between the levels of growth hormone and the depression of blood glucose. To our surprise, we also learned that such similar
levels of depressions were observed following cryosurgical hypophysectomy (Fig. 3).

Such studies performed in a careful and chronological fashion have
established that the anterior pituitary can be destroyed to an equal de-

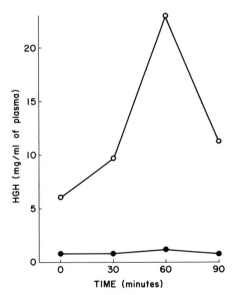

FIG. 1. Typical flat curve for human growth hormone (HGH) seen after open
hypophysectomy (●——●) in advanced metastatic prostatic cancer in man.
○——○, preoperative.

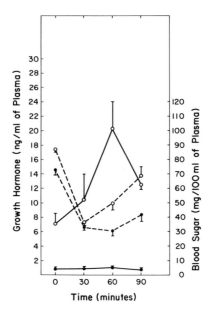

FIG. 2. Concentrations of plasma growth hormone associated with blood glucose depression plotted as a function of time following the intravenous infusion of insulin. Each point represents a mean value with a standard error for 8 to 16 determinations on eight patients. ●, After open hypophysectomy; ○, before surgery; ——, growth hormone; ---, blood sugar.

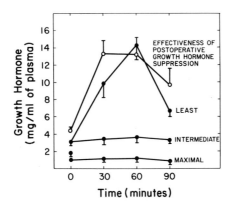

FIG. 3. Concentrations of plasma growth hormone plotted as a function of time after start of insulin infusin. Each plotted point represents mean values with standard error of mean (vertical half bars) for ten or more determinations from five or more patients in each group designated. ●, After cryohypophysectomy; ○, before surgery.

gree by either cryosurgical or open procedure (Murphy *et al.*, 1969, 1971; West and Murphy, 1973). These observations have similarly established that growth hormone levels under insulin-induced provocation are suitable criteria for the degree of ablation of the anterior pituitary (Murphy *et al.*, 1971; West and Murphy, 1973).

The criteria for response to hypophysectomy regardless of the technique, involved both objective and subjective signs (Murphy *et al.*, 1969). The common criteria that have been found of benefit both by ourselves and others are the subjective responses as follows: (1) pain relief; (2) sense of well being; (3) improved appetite. The criteria for objective response similarly have been as follows: (1) decrease in serum acid phosphatase level; (2) sustained decrease in serum alkaline phosphatase level; (3) weight gain; (4) improved radiological and radioisotopic appearance of osseous metastases; (5) improvement of anemia defined as an increase in relative hematocrit or by stability of hematocrit readings at 30 volumes percent or greater. Naturally the sixth criterion is survival. This may be difficult to measure in such patients who are under prior

TABLE I

REMISSION AND SURVIVAL PERIODS[a]

	Operative Procedures			
	Stereotaxic cryosurgical adenohypophysectomy (effectiveness of GH suppression[b])			Craniotomy with adenohypo- physectomy
Criterion	Least	Inter- mediate	Maximal	
Number of patients	7	5	7	8
Age (years)	70.40	65.0	67.14	58.09
	(± 1.76)	(± 1.78)	(± 2.40)	(± 1.30)
Duration of remission (months)				
Subjective	0.87	10.25	7.54	5.11
	(± 0.52)	(± 3.84)	(± 2.22)	(± 1.48)
Objective	0.12	7.60	6.25	6.78
	(± 0.05)	(± 3.04)	(± 2.55)	(± 2.62)
Survival following adenohypophysectomy (months)	4.80	13.58	13.57	10.88
	(± 1.3)	(± 3.0)	(± 2.83)	(± 2.36)

[a] Following adenohypophysectomy for disseminated prostatic carcinoma; values tabulated represent means ($\pm$SEM).

[b] Categories of least, intermediate, and maximal effectiveness of GH suppression refer to similar categories designated in the text; GH indicates growth hormone.

palliative therapy and, of course, have a dire prognosis. Such responses have been found in our hands to be reproducible with cryohypophysectomy to an equal degree as with an open procedure. To this date in 1975, we have not had any morbidity or mortality using this procedure (Table I). The degree of benefit to the patient with cryosurgical hypophysectomy can be measured in terms of the depression of growth hormone. A quantitative separation is possible. Based on such results, we have repeated the cryosurgical procedure in selected cases until a suitable level of depression of growth hormone is seen. In such instances, both objective and subjective signs of improvement have been uniformly observed. As shown in Table II, the degree of depression of the anterior pituitary can be expressed in terms of the index of ablation. Over 90% of the tissue is destroyed by the open procedure (Table II). However, with cryosurgical hypophysectomy, when maximal reduction is achieved as measured by growth hormone levels, a similar degree of ablation is noted. Patients with intermediate reduction have clinical remissions. Thus the fact that

TABLE II

HUMAN GROWTH HORMONE (GH) RESPONSES TO
INSULIN-INDUCED HYPOGLYCEMIA[a]

Procedure	Integrated average GH level, over 90-minute period (mg/ml of plasma)		Index of adeno-hypophyseal ablation (%)[b]
	Preoperative	Postoperative	
Craniotomy with hypophysectomy	**8/8** 15.6 (±0.9)	**8/16** 0.94 (±0.03)	93.9
		7/14 1.3 (±0.12)[c,f]	90.3
Stereotaxic cryohypophysectomy	**19/19** 13.5 (±1.8)	**5/10** 3.6 (±0.6)[d,f]	73.3
		7/14 10.5 (±0.8)[e,f]	22.2

[a] Data tabulated represent mean values ($\pm$SEM) for the number of determinations indicated in boldface (number of patients/number of determinations). All patients underwent GH assay once preoperatively and twice in the postoperative period.

[b] Based on GH suppression; mean differences between respective preoperative and postoperative values are significant at the level of $P < 0.001$ and are expressed as percent decrease from preoperative values.

[c] Maximal reduction.

[d] Intermediate reduction.

[e] Least reduction.

[f] Significance of mean difference between adjacent postoperative values at the level of $P < 0.001$.

70% reduction in growth hormone levels can be associated with objective clinical responses proves that destruction of the entire anterior pituitary is not necessary in this group of patients. This knowledge should be further applied to other individuals, as the technique can be performed under local anesthesia in less than an hour. Immediate relief is characteristically evident (Murphy et al., 1969, 1971; West and Murphy, 1973).

The initial reduction of androgenic hormone by bilateral orchiectomy and/or estrogen therapy has been noted to produce a regression of advanced prostatic carcinoma (Huggins and Hodges, 1941). Measurement of the 24-hour excretion of urinary 17-ketosteroids correlates well with the relapse of the disease and can be decreased following bilateral adrenalectomy (Bhanalaph et al., 1974). Since cortisone has become available, adrenalectomy has been used to a limited extent following relapse of advanced carcinoma of the prostate. Previous investigators have agreed that bilateral adrenalectomy produced a remarkable degree of subjective improvement (Table III). It has been unclear in the minds and opinion of some, however, whether increased survival with objective response could be obtained to a satisfactory degree. In our own studies, which have now exceeded 50 patients, we have found this to be true (Bhanalaph et al., 1974; Reynoso and Murphy, 1972; Schoonees et al., 1972c; Merrin et al., 1974) (Fig. 4).

As shown in Table IV, in a series of 26 patients with proven disseminated reactivated prostatic carcinoma, subjective improvement was achieved in most instances. In the presence of prior castration and hypophysectomy, however, a significant degree of improvement was not noted (Table IV). Following bilateral adrenalectomy, serum acid phosphatase levels are usually decreased within 1 month. They are increased again, however, in association with a demonstrable clinical relapse (Bhanalaph et al., 1974). Mean plasma testosterone levels after adrenalectomy generally exhibit no significant change (Bhanalaph et al., 1974). This is not unremarkable, as such levels, although generally low, have not been found to be helpful in following patients who have been hypophysectomized (Murphy et al., 1971). The 24-hour urinary excretion of total 17-ketosteroids in previously castrated or hypophysectomized patients is sometimes slightly higher before adrenalectomy (Bhanalaph et al., 1974). However, a marked decrease of the 11-deoxy-17-ketosteroids is consistently noted in previously castrated patients (Bhanalaph et al., 1974). This has been noted in follow-up periods extending up to 1 year and beyond (Merrin et al., 1974) and is associated with clinically evident and suitable signs of subjective and objective response. The major cause of death following adrenalectomy is disseminated disease (Bhanalaph et al., 1974). Such studies demonstrate the 24-hour urinary ketosteroid ex-

TABLE III

RESULTS OF BILATERAL ADRENALECTOMY FOR ADVANCED PROSTATIC CARCINOMA FROM A REVIEW FROM THE LITERATURE

Author	Number of patients	Subjective improvement[a]		Objective improvement[b]	Immediate postoperative death	Longest survival
		Good	Fair			
Huggins and Scott (1945)	4	1	2	—	3	115 Days
Huggins et al. (1952)	7	3	2	—	1	?
Baker (1953)	10	7	1	—	—	6 Months
Scardino et al. (1953)	3	1	1	1	—	9 Months
Taylor et al. (1953)	6	5	—	1	—	7 Months
Whitmore et al. (1954)	17	6	5	2	1	330 Days
Fergusson (1954)	17	9	3	—	2	10 Months
Pyrah (1954)	3	2	—	—	—	—
Morales et al. (1955)	20[c]	4/10	5/10	1	2	24 Months
MacFarlane et al. (1960)	13	9	—	1	—	46 Months
						(mean 13 months)

[a] Judged according to pain and sense of well-being.
[b] Judged according to growth regression (no bone improvement).
[c] Only ten patients had pain before adrenalectomy.

TABLE IV

SUBJECTIVE IMPROVEMENT AFTER BILATERAL ADRENALECTOMY IN DISSEMINATED PROSTATIC CARCINOMA IN ROSWELL PARK SERIES

Conditions of patient at the time of bilateral adrenalectomy	N^b	Patients still alive	Period of subjective improvement[a]			Mean period of subjective improvement	Mean survival time[c]
			Up to 3 months	>3–12 Months	>12 Months		
Previous castration with relapse	16	5	10 Cases (62.5%)	1 Case	4 Cases (25%)	4.8 Months	8.2 Months
No relapse[d]	5	4	—	1 Case	4 Cases (80%)	18.0 Months	20.8 Months
Previous castration and hypophysectomy with relapse	5	—	2 Cases (40%)	1 Case	—	1.6 Months	6.8 Months

[a] Period of subjective improvement after adrenalectomy in months.
[b] N = Number of patients who had bilateral adrenalectomy.
[c] Mean survival time in months after adrenalectomy.
[d] Castration 2–4 months after adrenalectomy.

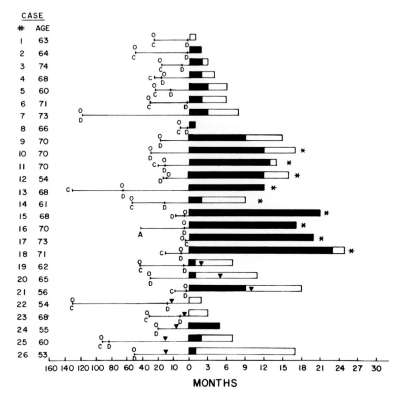

FIG. 4. The survival and remission rates for a Roswell Park Memorial Institute prostatic cancer adrenalectomy series. Time course of 26 patients with advanced prostatic carcinoma after bilateral adrenalectomy. ■, Period of subjective improvement; □, period of nonresponse or relapse after treatment. O, Orchiectomy; A, D, C, clinical stage of prostatic carcinoma; ▼, hypophysectomy; *, alive.

cretion, particularly that associated with the androgenic fraction (11-deoxy) is also a good index and prognostic indicator in the presence of hypophysectomy (Bhanalaph *et al.*, 1974) or after hypophysectomy. Those patients who respond to hypophysectomy or adrenalectomy show a persistent and significant decrease in 11-deoxy-17-ketosteroid 24-hour excretion rates (Murphy *et al.*, 1969; West and Murphy, 1973; Bhanalaph *et al.*, 1974) (Table V). Widespread use of adrenalectomy remains limited, as patients who are candidates for adrenalectomy are generally younger and must have the ability to withstand a more formidable operative procedure.

We have found that such patients who have previously shown a response to endocrine therapy, whether it be orchiectomy or exogenous es-

TABLE V

Twenty-Four Hour Urinary Ketosteroid Excretion after Bilateral
Adrenalectomy in Advanced Prostatic Carcinoma Patients with
Prior Castration (Mean Value ±SEM)

Ketosteroid	Before adrenalectomy	After adrenalectomy		
		2 Weeks	1 Month	2–3 Months
Total 11-deoxy-17-Keto-steroids	2.56 (0.60)	1.30 (0.17)[a]	1.59 (0.34)[b]	1.32 (0.54)[b]
N^c	15	17	7	8
Total 11-oxy-17-Keto-steroids	1.48 (0.30)	4.39 (0.95)[a]	4.97 (1.66)	4.27 (1.22)
N	15	17	7	8
Total 17-ketosteroids	4.04 (0.71)	5.66 (0.97)	6.61 (1.8)	5.60 (1.72)
N	15	17	7	8

[a] $P < 0.01$.
[b] $P < 0.05$.
[c] N = Number of observations.

trogens, generally will do well following adrenalectomy (Bhanalaph et al., 1974; Merrin et al., 1974). A similar situation has been generally but not uniformly true in the case of hypophysectomy by either route (Murphy et al., 1971; West and Murphy, 1973). We do not recognize that adrenal suppression and androgen excretion can be achieved to a significant degree by present chemical or nonoperative means despite claims to the contrary (Robinson et al., 1974). Such studies have failed to show the essential urinary depression in androgenic excretions as described in this presentation. In advanced prostatic cancer patients, following relapse, radiotherapy similarly has not proved to be of superior advantage (Varkarakis et al., 1972b). However, there has been some suggestion, in the hands of others, that hormonal therapy combined with megavoltage radiation therapy may provide some increased palliation and improved survival (Tsuya et al., 1974). We have not found this in our own experience (Varkarakis et al., 1972b).

IV. Newer Agents

Estracyt, a chemical ester of a nitrogen mustard with estradiol-17β, has been tested for its effects on the prostate in various species (Kirdani et al., 1974) and is further discussed in this symposium. Oral or parenteral estracyt was shown to have clinical activity in the early studies or Jönsson and Högberg (1971). Swedish and other investigators in Europe as well as in the United States (Müntzing *et al.*, 1974) have used the compound in the presence of advanced carcinoma of the prostate resistant to conventional therapy. The oral agent has been given with minimal toxicity at a generally effective therapeutic dose of 15 mg/kg daily in three divided doses (Müntzing *et al.*, 1974). Any toxicity when noted is mild and exclusively gastrointestinal. We have not seen any objective evidence of estrogen effects following the administration of this agent for prolonged periods (Müntzing *et al.*, 1974). There is good evidence that Estracyt is specific for human prostatic carcinoma (Tritsch *et al.*, 1974). In a recent series of 32 patients with stage D carcinoma of the prostate treated at a therapeutically effective dose (Mittelman *et al.*, 1975a,b), objective remission, which included decreases in soft tissue masses, lymph nodes, and prostatic masses, were noted in 25%, that is, 8 of 32 patients. Subjective responses, which included relief of pain, weight gain, sense of well-being, and improved performance status occurred in all the objective responders and 7 other patients with stable disease for a rate of 47%, or 15 out of 32 patients. Nonhematologic or hepatic or renal toxicity was observed. Transient nausea occurred early in half the patients, and in only 2 patients in this particular series was nausea and vomiting dose-limiting. Oral Estracyt is thus well tolerated and worthy of further clinical use (Mittelman *et al.*, 1975a,b). We feel that this agent, on the basis of both phase I and II trails (Müntzing *et al.*, 1974; Mittelman *et al.*, 1975a,b) in the United States may be a preferable alternative to hypophysectomy or adrenalectomy. In fact, a recent review evaluated the survival rates in such relapsed patients following the various forms of palliation including bilateral adrenalectomy, hypophysectomy, combination hypophysectomy and adrenalectomy, or chemotherapy with Estracyt (Welvaart *et al.*, 1974). Good long-term palliative responses were achieved with bilateral adrenalectomy, hypophysectomy, or Estracyt. However, because of ease of administration, effectiveness, and lack of toxicity, oral Estracyt may be considered the method of choice in such cases for failures following conventional hormonal therapy (Welvaart *et al.*, 1974). Such observations must necessarily be repeated by others, but if valid will provide an easier means of initial management of a relapsed patient with advanced disease. Hypophysectomy and adrenalectomy still have their roles but may be utilized in more selective instances.

Thus far, other more conventional chemotherapy has also not been fully evaluated (Murphy, 1973b). The National Prostatic Cancer Project in the United States is currently demonstrating that 5-fluorouracil or cytoxan may provide both objective and subjective responses in patients with advanced metastatic disease who have relapsed following conventional therapy (Murphy, 1973b). At the present time, a variety of cooperative groups in the United States are evaluating the effectiveness of cyclophosphamide, methotrexate, 5-fluorouracil, vincristine, actinomycin, adriamycin, and procarbazine. That single agent chemotherapy can be given to patients in this age group with dose adjustments with minimal toxicity is indeed important to note (Murphy, 1973b). Single agent or multiple agent chemotherapy may well, in the future, have a role in the management of reactivated prostatic carcinoma following conventional therapy. At the present time, it appears in the National Prostatic Cancer Project that 5-fluorouracil and cytoxan are superior to conventional chemotherapeutic agents used in such circumstances (Murphy, 1973b).

Although initial pilot studies altering the immune status of the advanced prostatic cancer patient are underway, there is no immediate projection that such therapy will become routine in an adjuvant manner (Merrin *et al.*, 1973). However, results have been noted and cannot be dismissed lightly. With the development of other means of measuring progression of disease, including biological markers and so forth, further exploration of other therapies will doubtless be fruitfully pursued. At the present time the management of the patient with advanced prostatic carcinoma following relapse from conventional therapy is thus hardly in a state of hopelessness nor necessarily one of confusion. Multiple agents and operative procedures are available and can be safely used with a reasonable hope for palliation, subjective improvements, and, to a surprising degree, increased survival.

V. Summary and Conclusions

The management of a patient with metastatic relapsing prostatic carcinoma following conventional therapy has been a clinical dilemma. Earlier endeavors in this limited field have been devoted toward hormonal manipulation. In view of the fact that the majority of the patients in the United States present with metastatic disease, and that their palliation may be limited for a short period, other forms of management have been sought by various clinical investigators over the years. Hypophysectomy through the open route has been somewhat hazardous with a significant operative mortality rate. It has been found in recent times that cryosurgical transsphenoidal hypophysectomy can achieve both objective and subjective response rates equal on occasion to that of open hypophysectomy. Moreover, with the cryosurgical technique, it has also been determined that growth hormone levels under insulin-induced hypoglycemia are an accurate index of the degree of pituitary ablation necessary for a subjective and objective clinical response. Such responses can be achieved by either route of hypophysectomy with a minimal ablation of 70% of the anterior pituitary. In view of this and in view of the absence of morbidity and mortality in our hands, transsphenoidal cryosurgical hypophysectomy appears to be the route of choice for such patients in whom hypophysectomy is selected. Bilateral adrenalectomy, similarly, for younger patients has provided a suitable means of subjective and objective improvement following relapse after conventional therapy. In both types of patients, the daily 24-hour measurement of 11-deoxy-17-ketosteroids in the urine has provided a better assay of the degree of androgenic ablation following either endocrine procedure or their combination. When such objective measurements are made for long periods following the initial procedure, a persistent decrease is associated with a good clinical course.

Estracyt, a new oral, nonsteroidal agent has been found to be of superior benefit compared to radiation therapy or antiandrogens. Moreover, in ongoing studies reported in this presentation, it is of equal benefit to patients after adrenalectomy or hypophysectomy. The agent has been found to have minimal toxicity in phase I and II studies with response rates of a significant degree that have lasted for over one year in our own hands. The evaluation of chemotherapy with such agents as 5-fluorouracil and cytoxan is currently underway. However, such agents at the present time can be administered to such patients with minimal toxicity and offer significant hope for improvement in objective remission. Immune manipulation with BCG injection is in its earliest clinical trails. In the face of these variations, it is thus possible to provide additional modes of management to the patient who has reactivated prostatic cancer.

REFERENCES

Baker, W. J. (1953). *J. Urol.* **70**, 275.
Bhanalaph, T., Varkarakis, M. J., and Murphy, G. P. (1974). *Ann. Surg.* **179**, 17.
Fergusson, J. D. (1954). *Proc. Roy. Soc. Med.* **47**, 1007.
Huggins, C. (1947). *Harvey Lect.* **42**, 148.
Huggins, C., and Bergenstal, D. M. (1952). *Proc. Nat. Acad. Sci. U.S.* **38**, 73.
Huggins, C., and Hodges, C. V. (1941). *Cancer Res.* **1**, 293.
Huggins, C., and Scott, W. W. (1945). *Ann. Surg.* **122**, 1031.
Jönsson, G., and Högberg, B. (1971). *Scand. J. Urol. Nephrol.* **5**, 103.
Kirdani, R. Y., Müntzing, J., Varkarakis, M. J., Murphy, G. P., and Sandberg, A. (1974). *Cancer Res.* **34**, 1031.
MacFarlane, D. A., Thomas, L. P., and Harrison, J. H. (1960). *Amer. J. Surg.* **99**, 562.
Merrin, C., Han, T., Klein, C., and Murphy, G. P. (1973). *Urology* **2**, 651.
Merrin, C., Murphy, G. P., Chu, T. M., and Mittelman, A. (1974). *Urology* **3**, 223.
Mittelman, A., Shukla, S. K., and Murphy, G. P. (1975a). *J. Urol.* (in press).

Mittelman, A., Shukla, S. K., Welvaart, K., and Murphy, G. P. (1975b). *Cancer Chemother. Rep.* **59**, 219.

Morales, P. A., Brendler, H., and Hotchkiss, R. S. (1955). *J. Urol.* **73**, 399.

Müntzing, J., Shukla, S. K., Chu, T. M., Mittelman, A., and Murphy, G. P. (1974). *Invest. Urol.* **12**, 65.

Murphy, G. P. (1973a). *In* "Perspectives in Cancer Research and Treatment" (G. P. Murphy, D. Pressman, and E. A. Mirand, eds.), pp. 1–24. Alan R. Liss, Inc., New York.

Murphy, G. P. (1973b). *Cancer* **32**, 1089.

Murphy, G. P. (1974). *Cancer* **24**, 282.

Murphy, G. P., Boctor, Z. N., Gailani, S., and Belmusto, L. (1969). *J. Surg. Oncol.* **1**, 81.

Murphy, G. P., Reynoso, G., Schoonees, R., Gailani, S., Bourke, R., Kenny, G., Mirand, E. A., and Schalach, D. S. (1971). *J. Urol.* **105**, 817.

Pyrah, L. N. (1954). *Proc. Roy Soc. Med.* **47**, 1002.

Reynoso, G., and Murphy, G. P. (1972). *Cancer* **29**, 941.

Robinson, M. R. G., Shearer, R. J., and Fergusson, J. D. (1974). *Brit. J. Urol.* **46**, 555.

Scardino, P. L., Prince, C. L., and McGoldrick, T. A. (1953). *J. Urol.* **70**, 100.

Schoonees, R., Bender, M. A., Schalch, D. S., and Murphy, G. P. (1971a). *Cur. Top. Surg. Res.* **3**, 233.

Schoonees, R., Schalach, D. S., and Murphy, G. P. (1971b). *Invest. Urol.* **8**, 635.

Schoonees, R., Palma, L. D., Gaeta, J. F., Moore, R. H., and Murphy, G. P. (1972a). *N.Y. State J. Med.* **72**, 1021.

Schoonees, R., Reynoso, G., and Murphy, G. P. (1972b). *J. Surg. Oncol.* **4**, 169.

Schoonees, R., Schalch, D. S., Reynoso, G., and Murphy, G. P. (1972c). *J. Urol.* **108**, 123.

Schoonees, R., Reynoso, G., DeKlerk, J. N., and Murphy, G. P. (1973). *Invest. Urol.* **10**, 434.

Scott, W. W. (1953). *Trans. Amer. Ass. Genitourin. Surg.* **44**, 101.

Scott, W. W., and Schirmer, H. K. A. (1962). *In* "On Cancer and Hormones: Essays in Experimental Biology," pp. 175–204. Univ. of Chicago Press, Chicago, Illinois.

Taylor, S. G., III, Li, M. C., Eckles, N., Slaughter, D. P., and McDonald, J. H. (1953). *Cancer* **6**, 997.

Tritsch, G. L., Shukla, S. K., Mittelman, A., and Murphy, G. P. (1974). *Invest. Urol.* **12**, 38.

Tsuya, A., Kawai, T., Fukushima, S., Shida, K., Shimazaki, J., Matsumoto, K., and Seto, T. (1974). *Strahlentherapie* **148**, 24.

Varkarakis, M. J., Kirdani, R. Y., Murphy, G. P., and Sandberg, A. A. (1972a). *J. Surg. Res.* **13**, 39.

Varkarakis, M. J., Webster, J., Bhanalaph, T., and Murphy, G. P. (1972b). *J. Surg. Oncol.* **4**, 520.

Varkarakis, M. J., Kirdani, R. Y., Abramczyk, J., Murphy, G. P., and Sandberg, A. A. (1973). *Invest. Urol.* **11**, 106.

Welvaart, K., Merrin, C. E., Mittelman, A., and Murphy, G. P. (1974). *Urology* **4**, 283.

West, C. R., and Murphy, G. P. (1973). *J. Amer. Med. Ass.* **225**, 253.

Whitmore, W. F., Jr., Randall, H. T., Pearson, O. H., and West, C. D. (1954). *Geriatrics* **9**, 62.

Williams, G., Wallace, D. M., and Bloom, H. J. G. (1974). *Brit. J. Urol.* **46**, 61.

DISCUSSION

E. E. Baulieu: Concerning the correlation between hormonal response and presence of receptor, which may have an implication in the prediction of hormone-responsive cancer, I would like to state in a simplified manner the following considerations. From several pieces of work with different sorts of cells in culture, and also from the experience gained by estrogen-receptor analysis in experimental tumors and in human breast cancer, one can say that (a) when there is no receptor, there is no corresponding hormonal effect; (b) when there is no effect, in a surprisingly high proportion of cases, say 80%, one does not find a receptor, this leaving 20% of cases where there are specific binding sites, but the abnormality must be elsewhere, for instance, at the level of receptor transfer or at the acceptor or any other piece of the cellular machinery; (c) when there is effect of hormone, there is always a receptor; (d) when there is receptor, there is either effect or no effect. Statement (d) is in a way a reciprocal of the (b) statement, and the question is now to evaluate the percentage of the responsive and nonresponsive cases. In human breast cancer, I believe that a large proportion of the cases (more than 50% probably) of receptor-containing tumors have been found to be responsive to hormone.

However, there are two very serious limitations from the theoretical viewpoint, even if we also neglect the difficulty of obtaining appropriate samples of tumor. Since at the present time receptors are determined only by specific steroid binding, the first problem is to establish the limit above which receptors are considered as positive and under which receptors are considered as absent or negligible. In the case of human cancers, it is probably only possible to obtain such information empirically, after much work. The other problem is that it seems that there are at least two receptors, one for androgen and one for estrogen, in the human prostate and that estrogen can interact with both of them; therefore both should be determined, a further complication at the technical level.

M. B. Lipsett: Although the data are not available for prostate cancer, there are many data for breast cancer. There is no correlation between grade of the cancer and receptor content, a finding that one would not have predicted *a priori*.

Androgen Metabolism in Patients with Benign Prostatic Hypertrophy

K.-D. VOIGT, H.-J. HORST, AND M. KRIEG

Department of Clinical Chemistry, Medical Clinic, University of Hamburg, Hamburg, Federal Republic of Germany

I. INTRODUCTION

The last comprehensive review on the metabolism of androgens in human prostate was by Peter Ofner (1968) in *Vitamins and Hormones*. Since then the growing interest is best reflected by the increasing number of symposia devoted to the topic. The purpose of this review is to discuss recent findings on the metabolism of androgens in human patients with benign prostatic hypertrophy (BPH). It will concentrate on the possible influence of specific steroids and their binding properties in plasma and prostate on the development of the disease and on endogenous levels and metabolites of various androgens in human prostatic adenoma.

Methodological progress which has enabled precise and sensitive measurement of androgens in various biological tissues revealed that the process of aging has a considerable impact on androgen production, androgen binding in blood, and androgen metabolism. For this reason the discussion of androgens in BPH should be preceded by a short survey of our present knowledge concerning the influence of aging on androgen balance. The fact that BPH is a very common disease in elderly males but quite unusual in men below 40 years old gives further support to this concept. It should also be stressed that human males over 60 who have no clinical

417

symptoms of BPH are rare. Any "normal group" of comparable age range differs from a group of patients with BPH probably only by the fact that the latter has a clinically apparent disease, whereas the former does not show the respective symptoms.

It is not the aim of our review to fully account for the recent data on androgen binding in human prostatic tissue. However, a short discussion of the "state of the art" seems necessary for the understanding of specific metabolic events. Studies on skeletal muscle as a so-called non-target organ for androgens have also been included which add further information on the question whether a binding protein which has been demonstrated in target organs is organ specific or not and to what extent plasma contamination influences the metabolite pattern obtained.

II. Androgens in Biological Fluids: Influence of Aging and Benign Prostatic Hypertrophy (BPH)

A. Endogenous Concentrations

Data on testosterone and 5α-dihydrotestosterone (5α-DHT) concentrations in peripheral blood are summarized in Table I. It is apparent that no significant decrease in blood testosterone concentration occurs before the seventh age decade. Unfortunately, in spermatic vein blood only few results are available relating age and testosterone concentration. According to Hollander and Hollander (1958), a decrease with advancing age is evident. With regard to the physiological significance, an interpretation of the results obtained is difficult as only three men younger than 40 have been studied and in the older age group patients with prostatic carcinoma and patients who have been treated with estrogens are included.

Testosterone excretion in urine exhibits a clear-cut age dependency (Schmidt, 1968). Highest values are observed between ages 25 and 30, after which a continuous decrease of the mean values is seen until the seventh age decade, thereafter the excretion remaining practically unaltered. While androgen concentrations in biological fluids decrease with advancing age a reverse tendency is found regarding estrogens (Pincus et al., 1954; Kaufmann, 1968), leading in consequence to an elevated estrogen:androgen ratio in urine with increasing age. Similarly in plasma an increase in this ratio of about 2-fold was observed when comparing young males to males in their seventh age decade (Kley et al., 1974; Pirke and Doerr, 1973). Rubens et al. (1974) obtained a smaller but still significant increase.

In patients with BPH only normal values have been reported in the literature (Table II), with the exception of Farnsworth (1970, 1971),

TABLE I

PLASMA CONCENTRATION OF TESTOSTERONE, 5α-DIHYDROTESTOSTERONE (5α-DHT), AND ESTRADIOL-17β (E₂) IN NORMAL MALES ACCORDING TO AGE

Age range	Testosterone (ng/ml)									5α-DHT (ng/ml)	E₂ (pg/ml)
20–30	6.35[a]	6.16[b]	6.77[c]							0.64[c]	
30–40	5.60	6.34	6.81	6.50[d]						0.64	16.6[g]
40–50	4.70	6.40	7.71		7.4[e]	7.42[f]	5.45[g]	4.92[h]	7.9[i]	0.81	19.75[j]
50–60	5.90	5.82	6.12							0.65	
60–70	5.90	4.62	6.03	5.0	4.35	6.07	4.59			0.61	25.6
70–80	6.50	3.73	5.22					2.81	6.6	0.46	28.75
>80	2.80	2.45	5.40							0.64	

[a] = Kent and Acone (1966).
[b] = Vermeulen et al. (1972).
[c] = Mahoudeau et al. (1974).
[d] = Coppage and Cooner (1965).
[e] = Frick (1969).
[f] = Nieschlag et al. (1973).
[g] = Pirke and Doerr (1973).
[h] = Rubens et al. (1974).
[i] = H.-J. Horst, unpublished data.
[j] = Kley et al. (1974).

TABLE II

PLASMA CONCENTRATIONS OF ANDROGENS IN BENIGN PROSTATIC HYPERTROPHY

Age range	n	T^a (ng/ml)	n	$5\alpha\text{-DHT}^a$ (ng/ml)	Authors
62–73	7	5.80	—	—	Gandy and Petersen (1968)
60–79	3	4.20	—	—	Isuguri (1967)
58–78	10	1.09	—	—	Farnsworth (1971)
55–86	10	5.46	5	0.82	Becker et al. (1972)
51–81	29	5.13	29	0.52	Mahoudeau et al. (1974)
72 ± 5.5	25	5.80	—	—	H.-J. Horst, unpublished data

[a] T = testosterone; 5α-DHT = 5α-dihydrotestosterone.

who found significantly lower plasma testosterone and dehydroepiandrosterone concentrations. A systematic study of the urinary testosterone excretion in patients with BPH has been performed by Kaufmann (1968), who found in patients from 60 to 70 years significantly lower values than in "normal" men, although no differences in testosterone excretion both in younger and older groups could be demonstrated. Regarding estrogen levels, we could not find systematic studies in blood for patients with BPH. In urine, to the best of our knowledge, the only extensive study of estrogen excretion under such circumstances is also by Kaufmann (1968). Estrone (E_1) and estradiol-17β (E_2) concentrations in 24-hours urine did not differ from values obtained from control groups.

B. METABOLITE PATTERN

The effect of age on testosterone and estradiol metabolism has been studied in detail by Vermeulen and his co-workers (Vermeulen et al., 1972; Rubens et al., 1974). From their investigations in 14 subjects with a mean age of 68 years, the results of which were compared to those for 6 males between 20 and 50 years, they concluded that "testosterone metabolism in male senescence is essentially characterized by a relative increase of the importance of 5β-metabolites over 5α-metabolites and . . . by a fall in diol formation" (Vermeulen et al., 1972). It is of interest to note that these changes lead to a metabolic picture very similar to that observed in normal females (Mauvais-Jarvis, 1966; Mauvais-Jarvis et al., 1968), hypogonadic males (Horton and Tait, 1966), and males after treatment with estrogens (Vermeulen et al., 1971). Such clinical conditions are characterized by a drop in the blood level of 5α-androstane-3α,17β-diol (3α-diol) which correlates positively with the free testosterone fraction and negatively with testosterone binding in serum. Since 3α-diol arises mainly from extrahepatic metabolism of testosterone (Mauvais-Jarvis et al., 1970), the theory that this age-dependent change could reflect the decreased testosterone metabolism in target organs (Vermeulen et al., 1972) seems quite convincing.

Regarding estrogen levels, it is known that under physiological conditions plasma estradiol and estrone originate only partly from direct testicular and adrenal cortical secretion, respectively. A considerable fraction of both estrogens derives from peripheral interconversion of either testosterone or androstendione. The positive correlation between absolute amounts of estradiol and testosterone within any age group (Rubens et al., 1974), offset by the age-dependent rise in estradiol:testosterone ratio, suggest an increased peripheral conversion of androgens to estrogens in senescence.

Comparatively few studies have been devoted to the peripheral interconversion of potent androgens in normal males and in patients with BPH. Ito and Horton (1970) observed that plasma 5α-DHT in normal males is derived from testosterone, whereas in females the main precursor seemed to be androstenedione. Mahoudeau et al. (1971) carefully examined this question on a quantitative basis and reported that 4% of plasma testosterone is converted to the reduced compound. Very recently Mahoudeau et al. (1974) have shown that in patients with BPH plasma 5α-DHT was higher in prostate vein blood than in peripheral veins, thus resembling the situation in dogs (Eik-Nes, 1971/1972). Therefore, the prostate may be regarded as a tissue which adds to total extrahepatic peripheral 5α-DHT production from androgenic precursors, specifically testosterone and androstenedione. However, prostatectomy did not lead to a decrease of blood 5α-DHT concentration (Mahoudeau et al., 1974). Furthermore, they show that the conversion of 5α-DHT and testosterone to 3α-diol was higher in males than in females corresponding to results obtained in urine by Mauvais-Jarvis et al. (1968, 1970). Regarding the conversion of 5α-DHT to both diols the 3α isomer is the preferred metabolite. From a kinetic point of view (Kinouchi and Horton, 1974) the steroid 3α-diol is rather exceptional: whereas its inner pool volume, e.g., plasma + liver, is similar to that of testosterone and 5α-DHT, its calculated outer pool is very large. This is reflected by a high metabolic clearance rate, which is due largely to extrahepatic metabolism.

Concerning our own in vivo studies on androgen metabolism (Becker et al., 1972; Horst et al., 1975), tritiated testosterone, 5α-DHT, 3α-diol, or 5α-androstane-3β,17β-diol (3β-diol) was injected intravenously into patients undergoing prostatectomy. After 30 minutes the hypertrophic prostate and a sample of blood and rectus abdominis muscle were removed. The metabolites found are summarized in Table V. After testosterone injection, approximately 5% of the extracted radioactivity in plasma was found as 5α-DHT. This agrees very well with the aforementioned finding regarding normal men (Mahoudeau *et al.*, 1971). Furthermore, 6% was present as 5α-androstanediols. The preferred metabolites of 5α-DHT in plasma investigated in two patients, were 3α- and 3β-diol, the ratio being 3:1. It seemed very interesting to us, therefore, to examine the metabolism of injected 3α-diol and to compare it with 3β-diol. In plasma the main metabolite from 3α-diol was 5α-DHT followed by 3β-diol, the ratio between 3α- and 3β-diol again being 3:1. Regarding 5α-DHT and 3α-diol, the significance of the data of Mahoudeau *et al.* (1971) and Kinouchi and Horton (1974) is reflected by our findings. In plasma 3β-diol remained largely unaltered after its injection, the most significant metabolite again being 5α-DHT. The only other compound exceeding 3% was epiandrosterone. No comparable data on blood metabolites from 3β-diol are available in the literature. In human urine after 3β-diol injection a large amount of 3α-diol conjugates were found (Mauvais-Jarvis *et al.*, 1970), which were believed to be the product of α/β isomeration. Because up to now no experimental proof for a 3β-hydroxysteroid dehydrogenase isomerase (Payne and Jaffé, 1972) exists, the urinary 3α-conjugates could also be regarded as the result of a 5α-DHT pathway.

C. Binding to Plasma Proteins

In blood the active androgens, testosterone, 5α-DHT, and the two 5α-androstane-3,17β-diols as well as the potent estrogen E_2, are attached to various proteins. Regarding physicochemical characteristics, all of them are bound with high affinity but low capacity to a specific protein called sex hormone-binding globulin (SHBG). It is known from studies of Kato and Horton (1968) that this binding requires an unhindered 17β-ol and a 3-ol or 3-one configuration. Other proteins in blood, especially albumin, demonstrate a low affinity but high capacity for the above-named substances. A minor part of total androgens appears not to be bound to plasma proteins. This so-called "apparent free testosterone concentration" (AFTC) (Vermeulen *et al.*, 1971) seems to be the biologically active form. Taking into account the very low SHBG concentration (Table III) compared to the other plasma proteins, the greater part of the hormones in question will be attached to proteins with high capacity and low affinity. However, according to Vermeulen and Verdonck (1972), changes in the concentration of SHBG should influence the AFTC. Various authors observed an increase in the mean SHBG concentration or binding capacity and concomitantly a decrease in the mean AFTC

TABLE III

ANDROGEN BINDING IN BLOOD: INFLUENCE OF AGING[a]

Age range	Percent free steroid			Percent specifically bound steroid		Percent totally bound T	Absolute amounts of free steroid			SHBG concentration (capacity) in plasma	Authors
	T	5α-DHT	E₂	T	5α-DHT		T (pg/ml)	5α-DHT (pg/ml)	E₂ (pg/ml)		
20–50	2.08	—	—	—	—	—	—	—	—	—	Vermeulen et al. (1972)
50–70	1.68	—	—	—	—	—	—	—	—	—	Vermeulen et al. (1972)
70–90	1.36	—	—	—	—	—	—	—	—	—	Vermeulen et al. (1972)
20–50	—	—	—	—	—	—	—	—	—	$5.2 \times 10^{-8}\ M$	Vermeulen et al. (1971)
70–85	—	—	—	—	—	—	—	—	—	$8.9 \times 10^{-8}\ M$	Vermeulen et al. (1971)
22–61	2.24	1.17	2.49	—	—	—	122	5.78	0.42	—	Pirke and Doerr (1975)
67–93	1.65	0.83	2.31	—	—	—	69	4.29	0.56	—	Pirke and Doerr (1975)
22–61	—	—	—	—	—	—	—	—	—	14.4 ng/ml	Pirke and Doerr (1973)
67–90	—	—	—	—	—	—	—	—	—	20.5 ng/ml	Pirke and Doerr (1973)
17–50	—	—	—	—	—	91.4	—	—	—	—	Kley et al. (1974)
51–89	—	—	—	—	—	93.6	—	—	—	—	Kley et al. (1974)
30–35	—	—	—	4.3	54.8	—	—	—	—	—	Horst et al. (1974)
42–67	—	—	—	8.5	60.2	—	—	—	—	—	Horst et al. (1974)

[a] T = testosterone; 5α-DHT = 5α-dihydrotestosterone; E₂ = estradiol-17β; SHBG = sex hormone-binding globulin.

fraction with advancing age (Table III). The cause of the age-dependent increase in SHBG is still not exactly known. From the high positive correlation between E_2 and SHBG found under various physiological and pathological conditions (Ritzén et al., 1974; Wagner and Rüffert, 1974; Vermeulen and Verdonck, 1972), one can conclude that blood levels of estrogens are the main reason for changes in the concentration of this protein. Increased thyroid hormone concentration also results in higher androgen binding whereas testosterone correlates negatively with SHBG (Dray et al., 1969; Clark et al., 1971; Braverman and Ingbar, 1967).

In order to investigate the significance of the observed rise of the SHBG concentration with age we tried to correlate the percent SHBG-bound androgens with the occurrence of BPH. In a first experimental series we found an age-dependent significant increase of percentage of SHBG-bound testosterone and a slight increase in percentage of bound 5α-DHT in normal males (Table III). In patients with BPH (Table IV) higher values were measured when compared to the older normal group; however, the differences in the mean age probably account for this further increase. We also investigated the percentage binding of 3α- and 3β-diol to SHBG (Table IV), but in spite of the speculative role of both diols in the etiology of BPH no further information could be gained. It must be mentioned additionally that the percentage binding of the four androgens to SHBG reflects closely their relative binding affinities (Vermeulen and Verdonck, 1968; Kato and Horton, 1968).

Several authors (Clark et al., 1973; Farnsworth, 1971; Fisher et al., 1974; Vermeulen et al., 1972) have speculated that the amount of free

TABLE IV

PERCENT SPECIFICALLY (SHBG) BOUND ANDROGENS IN HUMAN MALES WITH
BENIGN PROSTATIC HYPERTROPHY[a]

Age range	T (n)	5α-DHT (n)	3α-Diol (n)	3β-Diol (n)
60–69	14.6	79.3	31.4	48.8
	(7)	(7)	(4)	(4)
70–79	16.0	69.4	39.3	51.0
	(9)	(9)	(3)	(3)
>79	10.9	79.4	17.6	33.1
	(7)	(7)	(2)	(2)

[a] T = testosterone; 5α-DHT = 5α-dihydrotestosterone; 3α-diol = 5α-androstane-3α, 17β-diol; 3β-diol = 5α-androstane-3β, 17β-diol; SHBG = sex hormone-binding globulin.

and bound plasma androgen should influence the steroid concentration in a given cell. In fact, a high accumulation of testosterone and 5α-DHT can be observed in prostates of rats, which do not possess any significant amount of a comparable sex hormone-binding in plasma. In organ culture (Lasnitzky and Franklin, 1975) serum of several species with a specific binding protein largely prevented the entry of androgens into the prostate cells of rats. In our laboratory we investigated the influence of androgen binding in plasma on androgen uptake in human prostatic tissue. Uptake of labeled androgens into the prostate correlated with the percentage of easily available testosterone fraction ($r = 0.7$, $p < 0.05$), indicating for the first time direct evidence of the role of SHBG bound or unbound testosterone on androgen supply to the human prostate (Horst, H.-J., unpublished data).

Under physiological conditions the concentrations both of SHBG and of testosterone may influence the percentage of specifically bound testosterone to SHBG in blood. Since the quantities of steroids involved remain practically constant (Table II) but the concentrations of specific binding protein in plasma rises (Table IV), a more or less drastic reduction of testosterone entry into the target organ cells should be the result. However, this fact could not explain the finding of Siiteri and Wilson (1970), who showed that prostate adenomas contain much more 5α-DHT than the normal gland. One could speculate that other factors influence androgen uptake in prostate adenoma, for example, an elevated receptor protein content.

III. Androgens in Prostate Tissue and Skeletal Muscle

A. Endogenous Tissue Pattern

Data on endogenous tissue androgen patterns in BPH are extremely scanty. No real differences could be demonstrated by Siiteri and Wilson (1970) when comparing levels of testosterone and of androstenedione in normal and hypertrophic prostatic tissue. Regarding 5α-DHT, however, on average a 5-fold higher concentration was seen in hypertrophic adenomatous glands. Furthermore Siiteri and Wilson (1970) found a 2- to 3-fold increase in 5α-DHT content in the periurethral glands when related to the outer zone of the prostate. The authors tentatively concluded that the accumulation of 5α-DHT in human prostate could be causally related to BPH on the basis of the following evidence: (1) the positive correlation between prostatic size and 5α-DHT content, (2) its well-known action as a potent stimulator of prostatic growth, (3) the possible induction of prostatic adenomas in dogs by the hormone, and (4) the fact that early castration prevents prostatic hypertrophy.

Farnsworth (1970) compared in ten patients with BPH the concentrations of testosterone, androstenedione, and dehydroepiandrosterone in blood with prostatic tissue. With all three androgens measured, he obtained on average 5 times higher tissue concentrations, whereas no correlation between concentration and tissue structure, i.e., nodules or stroma, could be demonstrated.

B. Metabolism *in Vivo* and *in Vitro*

1. *Testosterone and 5α-Dihydrotestosterone*

Numerous investigators have shown that 5α-DHT is the main metabolite of testosterone both in human and in animal prostates (Baulieu *et al.*, 1968; Becker *et al.*, 1972; Briggs and Briggs, 1973; Bruchovsky and Wilson, 1968; Buric *et al.*, 1972; Harper *et al.*, 1974; Jenkins and Mc-Caffery, 1974; McMahon *et al.*, 1974; Nozu and Tamaoki, 1973; Robel *et al.*, 1971; Tveter and Aakvaag, 1969; for previous literature, see Ofner, 1968). Furthermore, androstenedione, androstanedione, and 17β-hydroxy-5α-androstenediols have been found. Up to now no evidence has been presented for the occurrence of either 5β-ol or 17α-ol derivatives. Our own *in vivo* studies in patients with BPH are summarized in Table V, confirming that 5α-DHT is the main metabolite of testosterone. After the injection of 5α-DHT the major part of radioactivity was recovered as 5α-DHT, the main metabolites being 3α-diol and 3β-diol. In peripheral muscle, testosterone remains practically unmetabolized, confirming previous studies in animal experiments and the findings of Shimazaki *et al.* (1965) for humans. The metabolic pattern resembles closely that found in plasma. Since we know from experiments in rats (Anderson and Liao, 1968; Bruchovsky and Wilson, 1968; Fang *et al.*, 1969; Tveter and Attramadal, 1968) that androgen target organs accumulate injected sex steroids when compared to skeletal muscle, we undertook similar investigations in the human, taking the activity found in the skeletal muscle as reference. We found (Table V) that the human prostate also accumulates radioactivity after the injection of labeled testosterone and 5α-DHT. It is of interest to note that the relative accumulation depended on the type of tissue prevailing, being highest in adenomatous tissue (Becker *et al.*, 1972). The conversion rate of testosterone to 5α-DHT depended also on the tissue type, with a predominance in adenomatous (Becker *et al.*, 1972) and epithelial (Harper *et al.*, 1974) cells. Probably due to SHBG, radioactivity in human blood always exceeds that found in prostate

TABLE V

METABOLIC PATTERN AFTER *in Vivo* APPLICATION OF ANDROGENS TO HUMAN MALES WITH BENIGN PROSTATIC HYPERTROPHY (BPH)[a]

Compound injected	Tissue	Compound found (%)								Accumulation quotient prostate:muscle
		T	5α-DHT	3α-Diol	3β-Diol	An	Epi-An	Δ4-Dion	A-dion	
T[b]	BPH	13.3	56.2		24.1	—	—	3.5	3.1	
	SM	74.7	4.4		5.5	—	—	7.3	8.3	1.9
	Pl	85.7	4.6		6.0	—	—	3.3	<3.0	
5α-DHT[b]	BPH	—	53.0	21.5	12.7	6.0	4.3	—	<3.0	
	SM	—	24.9	39.5	12.1	16.7	3.9	—	<3.0	2.2
	Pl	—	60.9	25.5	8.1	3.0	<3.0	—	<3.0	
3α-Diol[c]	BPH	<3.0	53.9	16.1	9.2	4.8	3.6	<3.0	3.8	
	SM	<3.0	22.7	42.2	8.6	4.9	<3.0	<3.0	<3.0	2.0
	Pl	<3.0	43.0	31.6	9.5	3.9	<3.0	<3.0	<3.0	
3β-Diol[c]	BPH	<3.0	29.2	4.7	53.0	<3.0	6.7	<3.0	<3.0	
	SM	<3.0	7.7	5.2	74.4	<3.0	3.0	<3.0	5.4	1.1
	Pl	<3.0	9.4	<3.0	82.7	<3.0	3.7	<3.0	<3.0	

[a] SM = skeletal muscle; Pl = plasma; T = testosterone; 5α-DHT = 5α-dihydrotestosterone; 3α-Diol = 5α-androstane-3α,17β-diol; 3β-Diol = 5α-androstane-3β,17β-diol; An = androsterone; Epi-An = epiandrosterone; Δ4-Dion = androstenedione; A-dion = androstanedione.

[b] Becker *et al.* (1972).

[c] Horst *et al.* (1975).

adenoma. This is in contrast to similar experiments in rats which do not possess a sex hormone-binding protein. Therefore, the accumulation factors in human males were always substantially smaller than in male rats.

2. *5α-Androstane-3α,17β-diol and 5α-Androstane-3β,17β-diol*

Special interest in the metabolic fate of both diols arose from findings of Baulieu's group (Baulieu *et al.*, 1968; Robel *et al.*, 1971; Levy *et al.*, 1974). The authors observed in rat prostate organ cultures a considerable hypertrophy and enhanced secretory activity of the cells but no apparent proliferation after adding 3β-diol to the culture medium, whereas 3α-diol only induced a weak proliferation. Extensive studies in our laboratory (Becker *et al.*, 1973; Schmidt *et al.*, 1973) and elsewhere (Bruchovsky, 1971) on the mode of action and metabolism of both diols *in vivo* in rat prostates and seminal vesicles allowed the assumption that 3α-diol mediates its biological effect by conversion to 5α-DHT whereas 3β-diol might have its own specific action. These findings prompted us to investigate the metabolism of both diols under *in vivo* conditions in patients with BPH (Horst *et al.*, 1975). After 3α-diol in man more than 50% of the extractable radioactivity in prostatic tissue could be identified as 5α-DHT (Table V). About 15% remained unchanged as the compound administered while 10% and 5% were converted to 3β-diol and androstenedione, respectively. After 3β-diol injection most of the radioactivity (55%) in the prostatic tissue remained unchanged. Two main metabolites could be isolated: About 30% 5α-DHT and 7% epiandrosterone. The metabolic pattern obtained from skeletal muscle differs markedly from that in prostate. The significant conversion of 3α-diol to 5α-DHT agrees well with the respective data after 5α-DHT injection and confirms the easy interconversion of the two substances (Bruchovsky, 1971).

As shown in Table V, the accumulation quotient, i.e., the ratio between radioactivity content in prostate and skeletal muscle after 3α-diol injection is very similar to that seen after 5α-DHT and testosterone application. After 3β-diol injection no accumulation occurred. In principle, the same results could be obtained in rats, although the accumulation ratio was distinctly higher. The metabolite pattern obtained in human prostatic tissue correlated well with our findings in the rat prostate. From a comparison between *in vivo* and *in vitro* binding in castrated male rats, we could conclude furthermore that only that part of the respective diol which has been converted to 5α-DHT will be bound to the specific receptor protein (Becker *et al.*, 1973; Krieg *et al.*, 1974).

Summarizing, it is tempting to speculate on the biological significance of the findings: 3α-diol should accordingly exert its biological effects by conversion to 5α-DHT. If 3β-diol would not be metabolized to 5α-DHT, its biological action must be interpreted as directly related to the compound itself. As our metabolic studies demonstrate, however, a small but still significant conversion in prostates of rats and humans, the substance must act at least partly via 5α-DHT. The question remains still open whether the different biological effects seen after both diols are only due to different velocities of their conversion to 5α-DHT or whether there exist unidentified receptor proteins for 3β-diol in defined cell fractions (Baulieu et al., 1971; Robel et al., 1974).

3. Androstenedione and Dehydroepiandrosterone

Acevedo and Goldzieher (1965) reported that human prostatic tissue metabolized androstenedione to testosterone and to various 5α-reduced compounds but not to 5α-DHT. In rat prostate organ culture Roy et al. (1972) could demonstrate a remarkable conversion of androstenedione to 5α-DHT. As the diketone and in addition dehydroepiandrosterone (DHEA) may be regarded as adrenal androgen precursors in androgen target organs, Harper et al. (1974) investigated the problem anew. In one experimental series either testosterone, androstenedione or DHEA sulfate were injected into patients with BPH 30 minutes prior to the removal of the prostatic adenoma. Furthermore adenomatous tissue was incubated in vitro with these steroids and in addition free DHEA. In vivo administration yielded a substantial conversion of androstenedione and a small conversion of DHEA sulfate to 5α-DHT. Whereas the overall metabolism of DHEA sulfate was very low, androstenedione was converted mainly to epiandrosterone and to androsterone. The metabolite pattern obtained from prostatic tissue under in vitro conditions differed markedly from that found in vivo. Conversion of androstenedione to 5α-DHT now was in the 2% region as opposed to about 10% in the in vivo experiments. As data on the metabolite pattern in blood have not been reported the possibility of a contamination by metabolites derived from systemic metabolism cannot be ruled out. DHEA and its sulfate merit special attention from another point of view, i.e., from the comparatively high blood levels. Farnsworth (1973) could show that the concentration of the free compound, which he regards as the active metabolite, is regulated on the prostatic level by a specific enzyme, dehydroepiandrosterone sulfate sulfatase. Its activity is inhibited by testosterone, 5α-DHT, and 3α-diol and also by stilbestrol and 17α-hydroxyprogesterone. He found a significantly higher specific activity in glands that exhibited benign epithelial hyperplasia and speculated on the potential influence of testicular depletion on DHEA sulfate mobilization, counteracting the beneficial effects of castration in patients with prostate carcinoma. Further investigations supporting the new concept would be very valuable.

C. 5α-DIHYDROTESTERONE BINDING IN HUMAN PROSTATE TISSUE

Using different methodological procedures various authors (Fraser *et al.*, 1974; Geller and Worthman, 1973; Hansson and Tveter, 1971; Hansson *et al.*, 1971; Mainwaring and Milroy, 1973; Reed and Stitch, 1973; Wagner *et al.*, 1975) have demonstrated androgen-binding proteins, but criteria for specificity of the binding in human prostatic tissue were hard to elaborate. In a previous paper (Steins *et al.*, 1974) we failed to discriminate definitely between the 5α-DHT binding in the BPH and plasma, due to the high affinity of 5α-DHT to plasma SHBG, which contaminated the BPH cytosol. However, we could calculate that 5α-DHT is bound in BPH cytosol to a greater extent than could be expected from plasma contamination. This prompted us to modify our *in vitro* binding assay:

In Fig. 1 a typical 5α-DHT binding in the BPH cytosol is presented, as analyzed by agar gel electrophoresis according to Wagner (1972). In our opinion this method allows the best and most easily obtained separation of SHBG from cytosolic receptor proteins. Three binding peaks are found: peak 1 represents SHBG, peak 2 the specific receptor protein, and the activity in peak 3 is bound to a protein with high capacity and low affinity to 5α-DHT. The radioactivity in slices Nos. 20–28 represents the unbound fraction. A 100-fold excess of unlabeled 5α-DHT incubated together with ^{3}H-labeled 5α-DHT displaces the "SHBG" (1) and "receptor" peak (2), while the binding in sclices Nos. 7–11 (3) remained unaffected or even increases. On the other hand, cyproterone acetate displaces in a 1000-fold excess the "receptor" peak (2) completely, while the "SHBG" peak (1) is less affected. In muscle only a well defined "SHBG" peak (1) is obtained. In plasma the binding pattern depends considerably upon the dilution used. Besides the SHBG peak, only one peak in the anodic part in slices Nos. 7–11 is found, which nearly completely disappeared after charcoal treatment of the incubated plasma. We therefore attempted to define peak 2 as the receptor protein in the BPH cytosol which binds 5α-DHT with high affinity and low capacity. This is in agreement with the findings of Wagner *et al.* (1975). The high-capacity, low-affinity 5α-DHT binding peak in slices Nos. 7–11 might be partly due to plasma contamination, or, alternatively, this peak could partly represent the "storage receptors" which were postulated by Giorgi *et al.* (1971) in prostatic adenomas.

Summarizing the binding studies, it becomes obvious that 5α-DHT is bound in BPH cytosol and nuclei. It must be stated that an understanding of the etiology of BPH can be achieved only if one compares the results in normal human prostate tissue, taking into account the high

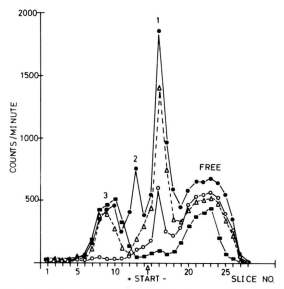

FIG. 1. Binding *in vitro* of ³H-labeled 5α-dihydrotestosterone (5α-DHT) in the cytosol of the benign prostate hypertrophy (BPH) (●——●) and muscle (m. rectus abdominis) (○——○). Homogenates, 1:2 buffer diluted, were incubated with 4.3 × 10⁻⁸ moles of ³H-labeled 5α-DHT per liter for 24 hours at 0°C. In the displacement studies the BPH homogenates were incubated with a 100-fold excess of unlabeled 5α-DHT (■——■) or a 1000-fold excess of cyproterone acetate (△---△) added together with ³H-labeled 5α-DHT. After the incubation the homogenate was centrifuged with 35,000 rpm to obtain the 100,000 *g* cytosol. The cytosol was treated with dextran-coated charcoal (11 mg per milliliter of cytosol) for 1–2 minutes to remove the excess of unbound steroids. After the separation of the dextran-coated charcoal from the cytosol by centrifugation at 3000 rpm, the cytosol was analyzed by agar gel electrophoresis at low temperature. Forty microliters were applied between slices Nos. 14 and 15 (start). The anode is left and the cathode is right from the start. After the run the gel was cut into 28 slices and radioactivity was measured in counts per minute per slice. See text for other details.

endogenous levels of testosterone and/or 5α-DHT within the prostate (Gloyna *et al.*, 1970). It seems that normal human prostatic tissue does not differ qualitatively in binding 5α-DHT specifically (Mainwaring and Milroy, 1973; Wagner *et al.*, 1975). Giorgi *et al.* (1971), on the other hand, found that the quantity of "storage receptors" might differ between normal and hypertrophied prostates.

D. ASPECTS OF HORMONAL TREATMENT

It is not the purpose of our review to deal with the present knowledge of conservative treatment of BPH. However, a short comment on the question of the influence of various drugs on androgen metabolism in BPH seems justified.

Estrogens or substances which possess potent estrogenic activities have long been used in the treatment of prostatic diseases. Their negative feedback action on the pituitary gonadal axis is well known and need not to be discussed here. The interest today focuses on the mode of action at a cellular level on human prostatic tissue and on their possible influence on protein binding of circulating androgens. As far as the first point is concerned the bulk of evidence favors the assumption that estrogens in human prostatic tissue inhibit 5α-reductase, which then in turn should lead to a significant drop in absolute and relative amounts of 5α-DHT and other 5α-reduced androgens. Recent data by Altwein et al. (1974) and by Jenkins and McCaffery (1974) tend to raise some doubt whether this assumption is really valid under in vivo conditions. According to these authors concentrations of estrogens needed to obtain a significant inhibition of 5α-reductase are far beyond the levels which may be achieved in vivo.

The gestagens belong to the group of compounds which cause, also under in vivo conditions, a potent inhibition of 5α-reductase activity (Altwein et al., 1974), this then resulting in a delayed testosterone metabolism. Whether or not this accounts for the therapeutic effect still remains open, as it has been shown that testosterone itself can be bound to the cytoplasmic receptor and stimulate growth in androgen target organs, e.g., rat bulbocavernosus levator ani muscle (Krieg et al., 1974b).

In contrast to estrogens and gestagens, which inhibit 5α-reductase activity at the cellular level, the classic antiandrogen, cyproterone acetate, acts at least partly by displacing 5α-DHT from the cytoplasmic and nuclear receptor protein (Fang and Liao, 1969, Belham and Neal, 1971; Walsh and Korenman, 1971; Krieg et al., 1974a). The androgen metabolism remains unaffected. However, the displacement alone, cannot fully account for the antiandrogenic activity of cyproterone acetate. In biological experiments performed by our group in which castrated rats were treated with a dose relation of cyproterone acetate:5α-DHT of 1:1 the expected androgen actions on prostate and seminal vesicles were completely abolished (Szalay et al., 1975). On the other hand, in a ratio of 10:1 only a 20–30% displacement of 5α-DHT from the cytosolic receptor occurred (Krieg et al., 1974a). Finally, the work done by Giorgi et al. (1971, 1972, 1974) should be mentioned. Using a superfusion technique the authors were able to differentiate between entry, uptake or retention, metabolism, release, and tissue clearance of testosterone and 5α-DHT. By adopting the method for the superfusion of human prostatic adenoma with and without adding either estrogens or antiandrogens to the perfusion medium, they arrived at the conclusion that estrogens or cyproterone acetate increased entry and modified uptake and metabolism of the androgens.

IV. CONCLUSIONS

Looking at the data presented in the foregoing sections one is tempted to put them together under three aspects:

1. A wealth of evidence favors the assumption that the chain of metabolic events in prostatic tissue at a cellular level does not differ between man and other species. The androgen metabolite pattern in human prostatic tissue is quite comparable to that in the respective glands of animals so far investigated. Accumulation in the prostate always affords the conversion of a given compound to 5α-DHT. Human prostatic tissue, too, possesses a specific cytoplasmic and nuclear receptor protein, as has been demonstrated in prostates of all species investigated so far.

2. On the other side, however, many data are available that point to a specific situation in human beings, especially when compared to the most frequently used laboratory animal, the rat: Endogenous androgen concentrations in biological fluids demonstrate a typical age dependency resulting in a decrease of testosterone blood levels and in an increase of the respective E_2 concentrations. The same holds true for changes in androgen metabolism in males, which in senescence approaches the situation in females. The dependence of androgen uptake in human prostate from the specific plasma binding together with the significant increase of SHBG with advancing age is not found in rats. Peculiar findings in human prostate adenoma are the dependence of androgen uptake and metabolism on the histological composition, i.e., whether epithelial, stromal, or muscular cells are prevailing and the occurrence of comparatively high amounts of unspecific "storage protein" besides the specific androgen receptor.

3. It must be stated that etiology and pathogenesis of BPH are still unknown. Owing to the high incidence of BPH in males older than 60 years, the gathering of normal tissue including blood offers serious difficulties. Nevertheless control data from a real "normal" group are badly needed. Therefore the question whether or not disease-specific factors in blood and/or in prostatic tissue lead to BPH or whether it develops as a consequence of "normal" aging processes in human males cannot be answered at the moment.

ACKNOWLEDGMENTS

Our work was supported by the DFG, Sonderforschungsbereich 34 "Endokrinologie." We wish to express our appreciation to Mrs. U. Werber and Mr. M. Dennis for painstaking care in translating, assembling, and typing the manuscript.

REFERENCES

Acevedo, H. F., and Goldzieher, J. W. (1965). *Biochim. Biophys. Acta* **97**, 564.
Altwein, J. E., Rubin, A., Klose, K., Knapstein, P., and Orestano, F. (1974). *Urologe A* **13**, 41.
Anderson, K. M., and Liao, S. (1968). *Nature (London)* **219**, 277.
Baulieu, E. E., Lasnitzki, I., and Robel, P. (1968). *Nature (London)* **219**, 1155.
Baulieu, E. E., Jung, I., Blondeau, J. P., and Robel, P. (1971). *Advan. Biosci.* **7**, 179.
Becker, H., Kaufmann, J., Klosterhalfen, H., and Voigt, K. D. (1972). *Acta Endocrinol. (Copenhagen)* **71**, 589.
Becker, H., Grabosch, E., Hoffmann, C., and Voigt, K. D. (1973). *Acta Endocrinol. (Copenhagen)* **73**, 407.
Belham, J. E., and Neal, G. E. (1971). *Biochem. J.* **125**, 81.
Braverman, L. E., and Ingbar, S. H. (1967). *J. Clin. Endocrinol. Metab.* **27**, 389.
Briggs, M. H., and Briggs, M. (1973). *J. Clin. Endocrinol. Metab.* **36**, 600.
Bruchovsky, N. (1971). *Endocrinology* **89**, 1212.
Bruchovsky, N., and Wilson, J. D. (1968). *J. Biol. Chem.* **243**, 2012.
Buric, L., Becker, H., Petersen, C., and Voigt, K. D. (1972). *Acta Endocrinol. (Copenhagen)* **69**, 153.
Clark, A. F., Calandra, R. S., and Bird, C. E. (1971). *Clin. Biochem.* **4**, 89.
Clark, A. F., Carson, G. D., DeLory, B., Clemov, M. E., and Bird, C. E. (1973) *Clin. Endocrinol.* **2**, 361.
Coppage, W. S., and Cooner, A. E. (1965). *N. Eng. J. Med.* **273**, 902.
Dray, F., Mowszowicz, I., Ledru, M. J., Crepy, O., Delzant, G., and Sebaoun, J. (1969). *Ann. Endocrinol. (Paris)* **30**, 223.
Eik-Nes, K. B. (1971/1972). *Gynecol. Invest.* **2**, 239.
Fang, S., and Liao, S. (1969). *Mol. Pharmacol.* **5**, 428.
Fang, S., Anderson, K. M., and Liao, S. (1969). *J. Biol. Chem.* **244**, 6584.
Farnsworth, W. E. (1970). *In* "Some Aspects of the Aetiology and Biochemistry of Prostatic Cancer" (K. Griffiths and C. G. Pierrepoint, eds.), p. 3. Alpha Omega Alpha Publ., Cardiff, Wales.
Farnsworth, W. E. (1971). *Invest. Urol.* **8**, 367.
Farnsworth, W. E. (1973). *Steroids* **21**, 647.
Fisher, R. A., Anderson, D. C., and Burke, C. W. (1974). *Steroids* **24**, 809.
Fraser, H. M., Mitchell, A. J. H., Anderson, C. K., and Oakey, R. E. (1974). *Acta Endocrinol. (Copenhagen)* **76**, 773.
Frick, J. (1969). *Urol. Int.* **24**, 481.
Gandy, H. M., and Peterson, R. E. (1968). *J. Clin. Endocrinol. Metab.* **28**, 949.
Geller, J., and Worthman, C. (1973). *Acta Endocrinol (Copenhagen), Suppl.* **177**, 4.
Giorgi, E. P., Stewart, J. C., Grant, J. K., and Scott, R. (1971). *Biochem. J.* **123**, 41.
Giorgi, E. P., Stewart, J. C., Grant, J. K., and Shirley, I. M. (1972). *Biochem. J.* **126**, 107.

Giorgi, E. P., Moses, T. F., Grant, J. K., Scott, R., and Sinclair, J. (1974). *Mol. Cell. Endocrinol.* **1**, 271.

Gloyna, R. E., Siiteri, P. K., and Wilson, J. D. (1970). *J. Clin. Invest.* **49**, 1746.

Hansson, V., and Tveter, K. J. (1971). *Acta Endocrinol. (Copenhagen)* **68**, 69.

Hansson, V., Tveter, K. J., Attramadal, A., and Torgersen, O. (1971). *Acta Endocrinol. (Copenhagen)* **68**, 79.

Harper, M. E., Pike, A., Peeling, W. B., and Griffiths, K. (1974). *J. Endocrinol.* **60**, 117.

Hollander, N., and Hollander, V. P. (1958). *J. Clin. Endocrinol. Metab.* **18**, 966.

Horst, H.-J., Becker, H., and Voigt, K. D. (1974). *Steroids* **23**, 833.

Horst, H.-J., Dennis, M., Kaufmann, J., and Voigt, K. D. (1975). *Acta Endocrinol. (Copenhagen)* **79**, 394.

Horton, R., and Tait, J. F. (1966). *J. Clin. Invest.* **45**, 351.

Isuguri, K. (1967). *J. Urol.* **97**, 903.

Ito, T., and Horton, R. (1970). *J. Clin. Endocrinol. Metab.* **31**, 362.

Jenkins, J. S., and McCaffery, V. M. (1974). *J. Endocrinol.* **63**, 517.

Kato, T., and Horton, R. (1968). *J. Clin. Endocrinol. Metab.* **28**, 1160.

Kaufman, J. (1968). *Z. Urol.* **61**, 229.

Kent, J. R., and Acone, A. B. (1966). *Proc. Symp. Steroid Horm. 2nd, 1965 Int. Congr. Ser. No. 101*, p. 31.

Kinouchi, T., and Horton, R. (1974). *J. Clin. Invest.* **54**, 646.

Kley, H. K., Nieschlag, E., Bidlingmaier, F., and Krüskemper, H. L. (1974). *Horm. Metab. Res.* **6**, 213.

Krieg, M., Steins, P., Szalay, R., and Voigt, K. D. (1974a). *J. Steroid Biochem.* **5**, 87.

Krieg, M., Szalay, R., and Voigt, K. D. (1974b). *J. Steroid Biochem.* **5**, 453.

Krieg, M., Horst, H.-J., and Sterba, M.-L. (1975). *J. Endocrinol.* **64**, 529.

Lasnitzki, I., and Franklin, H. R. (1975). *J. Endocrinol.* **64**, 289.

Levy, C., Marchut, M., Baulieu, E. E., and Robel, P. (1974). *Steroids* **23**, 291.

McMahon, M. J., Butler, A. V. J., and Thomas, G. H. (1974). *Acta Endocrinol. (Copenhagen)* **77**, 784.

Mahoudeau, J. A., Bardin, C. W., and Lipsett, M. B. (1971). *J. Clin. Invest.* **50**, 1338.

Mahoudeau, J. A., Delassalle, A., and Bricaire, H. (1974). *Acta Endocrinol. (Copenhagen)* **77**, 401.

Mainwaring, W. I. P., and Milroy, E. J. G. (1973). *J. Endocrinol.* **57**, 371.

Mauvais-Jarvis, P. (1966). *C. R. Acad. Sci.* **262**, 2753.

Mauvais-Jarvis, P., Bercovici, J. P., and Flock, H. H. (1968). *Rev. Fr. Etud. Clin. Biol.* **14**, 159.

Mauvais-Jarvis, P., Bercovici, J. P., and Gauthier, F. (1970). *J. Clin. Invest.* **49**, 31.

Nieschlag, E., Kley, K. H., Wiegelmann, W., Solbach, H. G., and Krüskemper, H. L. (1973). *Med. Wochenschr.* **98**, 1281.

Nozu, K., and Tamaoki, B. (1973). *Acta Endocrinol. (Copenhagen)* **73**, 585.

Ofner, P. (1968). *Vitam. Horm. (New York)* **26**, 237.

Payne, A. H., and Jaffé, R. B. (1972). *Biochim. Biophys. Acta* **279**, 202.

Pincus, G., Romanoff, L. P., and Carlo, J. (1954). *J. Gerontol.* **9**, 113.

Pirke, K. M., and Doerr, P. (1973). *Acta Endocrinol. (Copenhagen)* **74**, 792.

Pirke, K. M., and Doerr, P. (1975). *Acta Endocrinol. (Copenhagen), Suppl.* **193**, 57.

Reed, M. J., and Stitch, S. R. (1973). *J. Endocrinol.* **58**, 405.

Ritzén, E. M., French, F. S., Weddington, S. C., Nayfeh, S. N., and Hansson, V. (1974). *J. Biol. Chem.* **249**, 6597.

Robel, P., Lasnitzki, I., and Baulieu, E. E. (1971). *Biochimie* **53**, 81.

Robel, P., Blondeau, J. P., and Baulieu, E. E. (1974). *Biochim. Biophys. Acta* **373**, 1.

Roy, A. K., Baulieu, E. E., Feyel-Cabanes, C., Le Goascogne, C., and Robel, P. (1972). *Endocrinology* **91**, 52.

Rubens, R., Dhont, M., and Vermeulen, A. (1974). *J. Clin. Endocrinol. Metab.* **39**, 40.

Schmidt, H. (1968). *Acta Endocrinol. (Copenhagen), Suppl.* **128**, 7.

Schmidt, H., Giba-Tziampiri, O., von Rotteck, G., and Voigt, K. D. (1973). *Acta Endocrinol. (Copenhagen)* **73**, 599.

Shimazaki, J., Kurihara, H., Ito, Y., and Shida, K. (1965). *Gunma J. Med. Sci.* **14**, 100.

Siiteri, P. K., and Wilson, J. D. (1970). *J. Clin. Invest.* **49**, 1737.

Steins, P., Krieg, M., Hollmann, H. J., and Voigt, K. D. (1974). *Acta Endocrinol. (Copenhagen)* **75**, 773.

Szalay, R., Krieg, M., Schmidt, H., and Voigt, K. D. (1975). *Acta Endocrinol. (Copenhagen)* **80**, 592.

Tveter, K. J., and Aakvaag, A. (1969). *Endocrinology* **85**, 683.

Tveter, K. J., and Attramadal, A. (1968). *Acta Endocrinol. (Copenhagen)* **59**, 218.

Vermeulen, A., and Verdonck, L. (1968). *Steroids* **11**, 609.

Vermeulen, A., and Verdonck, L. (1972). *J. Steroid Biochem.* **3**, 421.

Vermeulen, A., Stoica, T., and Verdonck, L. (1971). *J. Clin. Endocrinol. Metab.* **33**, 759.

Vermeulen, A., Rubens, R., and Verdonck, L. (1972). *J. Clin. Endocrinol. Metab.* **34**, 730.

Wagner, R. K. (1972). *Hoppe Seyler's Z. Physiol. Chem.* **353**, 1235.

Wagner, R. K., and Rüffert, W. (1974). *Acta Endocrinol. (Copenhagen), Suppl.* **184**, 84.

Wagner, R. K., Schulze, K. H., and Jungblut, P. W. (1975). *Acta Endocrinol. (Copenhagen), Suppl.* **193**, 52.

Walsh, P. C., and Korenman, S. G. (1971). *J. Urol.* **105**, 850.

DISCUSSION

G. D. Chisholm: Changes in the prostate begin at 40–50 age group, but blood changes come much later. Surely they should show up earlier.

K.-D. Voigt: This is an additional difficulty when looking into the etiology of BPH. Possibly we are too late with our investigations. On the other hand, those adenomas probably have a tendency to grow, which could mean that the same factors are still there.

H. G. Williams-Ashman: I would like to raise the question as to whether chronological age may not always be the most meaningful criterion when one measures various parameters of steroid dynamics in relation to the development of BPH or prostate cancer in the human male. In other words, is it possible to distinguish between age in the sense of birth dates and any quantitative criteria of *aging* of the organism in these sorts of correlative studies on sex hormones in tissues and body fluids?

K.-D. Voigt: This is a very relevant question, but at the moment I cannot see a way to solve the problem.

N. Bruchovsky: Commenting on Dr. Williams-Ashman's question about markers of aging, Hayflick has shown that the division potential of cells is reduced with increasing age, and I wonder whether it might be possible to detect any similar change in prostatic epithelial cell proliferation with increasing age of the human.

I. Lasnitzki: A comment relating to the influence of serum albumin and TBG in uptake and metabolism of testosterone: The uptake and metabolism of testosterone was measured in rat prostate glands in organ culture kept in serum-free medium and in medium containing male serum and pregnancy serum, in which the amounts of TBG are considerably increased. The uptake was highest in explants kept in serum-free medium and fell steeply in those kept with the two human sera. But at the same concentration it was significantly higher in explants kept with the male serum as compared with those with pregnancy serum. The formation of 5α-dihydrotestosterone and androstanediol followed the same pattern. The effect of testosterone on the maintenance of the prostatic epithelium was directly related to the uptake of testosterone. It was expressed as the percentage of secretory columnar cells formed. In the absence of serum, this number approximated that of the organ *in vivo;* in explants kept with the male serum it was lower, though still substantial, but in explants kept in the pregnancy serum it was extremely low. The results suggest that the uptake and biological action of testosterone depend on the amounts of free testosterone and are inversely related to the amounts of TBG. The uptake and metabolism of testosterone were also determined in similar explants incubated with serum from patients with BPH and prostatic carcinoma. They were similar with the two sera and also of the same order as in explants kept with serum from normal men of the same age group. These results suggest that there is no difference in the amounts of TBG in the three groups of serum tested.

P. Robel: Constant-flow organ culture of normal and hyperplastic human prostate allows one to investigate testosterone metabolism; the results obtained are identical in normal and hyperplastic samples and in complete agreement with those reported by Dr. Voigt after intravenous injection of ³H-labeled testosterone to humans.

HSA reduces testosterone uptake as a function of free testosterone fraction in the superfusion medium. With SBP, the reduction of testosterone uptake is larger than would be expected from the reduction of free testosterone fraction, and the relative amount of unmetabolized testosterone is increased. These data are compatible with a limited selective uptake of SBP (TBG) by the prostate, resulting in a reduced uptake and metabolism of testosterone.

E. Diczfalusy: I wonder whether you have had an opportunity to search for steroid conjugates, since we found that in human seminal plasma the concentrations of testosterone glucuronide, 5α-dihydrotestosterone sulfate, Δ⁵-pregnenolone sulfate, dehydroepiandrosterone sulfate, and estradiol sulfate vastly exceed those of their unconjugated forms [K. Purvis *et al.* (1975) (to be published)].

K-D. Voigt: No, we did not look into the conjugate fraction. There are always polar components that remain at the starting line, but we did not analyze them.

K. J. Tveter: In the rat, about 10% of the total radioactivity in the epididymis is in the form of conjugated compounds after injection of ³H-labeled testosterone *in vivo.* In the dorsal prostate, about 8% of the total radioactivity is represented by conjugated compounds, while in the ventral prostate and the seminal vesicle, almost 100% of the activity is in the free fraction.

Dr. Voigt, what is your experience with the Wagner technique for studying specific androgen receptors in human prostate tissue? It appears that some people have had difficulties in using this technique.

K.-D. Voigt: In our hands, this method proved to be very efficient in separating SHBG from the specific receptor protein. We also employ sucrose gradient ultracentrifugation, but in human prostatic tissue we arrived at clearer results with agar-gel electrophoresis according to Wagner (1972).

Nonsurgical Treatment of Human Benign
Prostatic Hyperplasia

W. W. SCOTT AND D. S. COFFEY

*Departments of Urology, Pharmacology and Experimental Therapeutics,
and Oncology, The Johns Hopkins Hospital, Baltimore, Maryland*

I. HUMAN BENIGN PROSTATIC HYPERPLASIA

A. INCIDENCE

Benign nodular hyperplasia of the prostate is undoubtedly the most common neoplastic growth in man. Many publications support this statement; among them are those of Moore (1942), Franks (1954a), Lundberg and Berge (1970), and Harbitz and Haugen (1972). For example, Harbitz and Haugen in a study of 206 consecutive autopsies performed on men over 40 years of age found an overall incidence of 80.1% (165/206). This increased with age reaching a maximum of 95.5% (64/67) in the eighth decade (Fig. 1). Figure 1 also includes the incidence of carcinoma of the prostate. However, the frequency of benign hyperplasia in prostates with carcinoma was not different from that to be expected to occur from pure coincidence. In addition, Greenwald *et al.* (1974), have reported in an age-matched study involving groups of 800 patients that the pres-

439

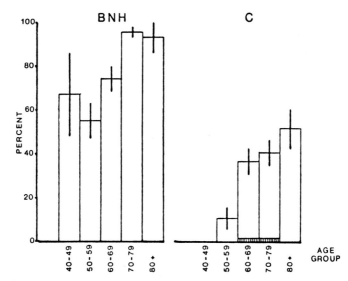

FIG. 1. Prevalence ratio (± standard error of the percentage) of benign nodular hyperplasia (BNH) and carcinoma (C) of the prostate in 206 consecutive autopsies. Hatched parts of columns denote clinically manifest carcinoma. From Harbitz and Haugen (1972), with permission.

ence of benign prostatic hyperplasia (BPH) does not increase the risk of prostatic cancer.

B. HISTOLOGY AND CHARACTERISTICS

The histologic nature of benign prostatic enlargement has been the subject of many studies. Franks (1954b) recognized five different types: stromal, fibromuscular, muscular, fibroadenomatous, and fibromyoadenomatous. Pure adenomatous nodules occur, too. The exact frequency of each type is unknown, but most pathologists agree that the fibromyoadenomatous type is the most common. This is of some importance, for as yet it is not known whether epithelial hyperplasia or stromal hyperplasia are both under the same hormonal control, or which appears first in the developmental process (Pradhan and Chandra, 1975). However, it does appear clear that benign hyperplasia arises in the "inner prostate" in contrast to carcinoma, which arises in the "outer prostate" (Loeschke, 1920; Adrion, 1922; Franks, 1954a; Scott, 1963), and that such zones may be under different hormonal control (Fig. 2). W. L. Valk (personal communication, 1974), in a review of transurethral resection of the prostate for outlet obstruction for two consecutive 3-year periods, 1965–1971, stated that the cause of obstruction was BPH in 70%, contracture of

External on prostatic glands proper
Urethral or mucosal glands
Submucosal glands

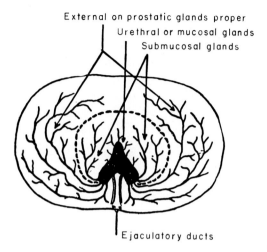

Ejaculatory ducts

Fig. 2. Diagram showing the anatomy of the normal prostate gland, according to Loeschke (1920) and Adrion (1922). Dotted line indicates "a definite fibrous capsule." From Young and Davis (1926), with permission.

the vesical neck in 15%, and carcinoma in 15%. The benign hyperplastic glands were not broken down into types or the frequency of such types, and, to our knowledge, no one has done this for surgical or autopsy specimens. This points up the need of careful morphometric studies, which will be discussed subsequently.

C. Symptomatology and Surgical Treatment

The results of surgical treatment for BPH are good with a low mortality, a modest number of complications, obtainment of a good functional result and with little effect on potentia. However, some candidates are poor surgical risks and must be treated by catheter drainage, a situation that leaves much to be desired.

Urologists recognize that benign nodular hyperplastic prostates—the apparent cause of acute or chronic urinary retention in most men—may become large, even huge, and yet not result in outlet obstruction, and yet it is reasonable to speculate that the basic cause of outlet obstruction is prostatic enlargement. The excellent functional results following surgical removal of the benign enlargement where the "inner prostate" is literally shelled-out from the "outer or true prostate" not only attests to the importance of removing this benign tissue in the relief of outlet obstruction, but suggests that the enlargement itself is the cause of the obstruction.

D. Therapeutic Evaluation

As we progress in an attempt to evaluate nonsurgical methods of treatment, we will discuss and evaluate various parameters, both subjective and objective, which have been used in order to determine whether improvement has occurred following treatment. Most of us are aware of the difficulties involved. There follows a verbatim summary of a control series from a study by Clarke (1937).

(1) A number of theories have been devised to explain prostatic hypertrophy on an endocrine basis. None of these have been proved.

(2) A number of endocrine preparations are in use in an attempt to replace surgery.

(3) Such therapy is still in the experimental stage, and as in other experimental work, accurate controls are desirable.

(4) A series of 93 cases of prostatic obstruction, treated by neither prostatectomy nor endocrines, is presented.

(5) These cases had been followed over an average period of over four years.

(6) A large number showed a sustained improvement after instrumentation alone.

(7) This series may be regarded, (a) as a control series, (b) as a brief summary of the variability of the course of the disease without prostatectomy and as a reminder of the frequent apparent "cure" after minimal instrumentation.

(8) Conclusions as to the efficacy of endocrine or other new methods of treatment are only valid if cases are followed up for a considerable period of time.

(9) The period suggested is five years.

As noted, this author observed sustained improvement in a large number of patients followed over an average of 4 years after instrumentation alone, i.e., catheterization, urethral sounding, and cystoscopy, and believes that valid conclusions concerning nonsurgical therapy can be drawn only if the follow-up is long.

At this juncture, we wish to refer to a quotation from a publication entitled "The Effect of Castration on Benign Hypertrophy of the Prostate in Man," by Charles Huggins and Roland Stevens in 1940: "Whether benign hypertrophy of the prostate is under endocrine control or not is a problem of immediate interest, since not all workers are agreed on this point. Determination of the effect of castration on this disease is one of the most critical ways to settle this problem, but contradiction of opinion exists at the present time as to the effect of removal of the gonads on enlargement of the prostate gland."

E. Effects of Castration

Largely as the result of the efforts of White (1895), deliberate castration was performed on some 200 men between 1893 and 1895, in the treatment of urinary obstruction secondary to "benign hypertrophy of the prostate." In his summary of 111 cases, White wrote: "The theoretical objections which have been urged against the operation of double castration have been fully negatived by clinical experience, which shows that in a very large proportion of cases (thus far in approximately 87.2%), rapid atrophy of the prostatic enlargement follows the operation; and that disappearance or great lessening in degree of long-standing cystitis (52%); more or less return of vesical contractility (66%); and a return of local conditions not far removed from normal (46.4%), may be expected in a considerable number of cases."

In 1896, Cabot presented a longer follow-up in 61 cases: "In twenty-seven cases retention, which existed at the time of the operation, afterward disappeared. In seven of these cases, the retention was acute—that is, had existed for less than a month—while in the other twenty the retention was of long standing"; and "Reducing these facts to percentages we find that these cases show 9.8% failure; 6.6% moderate improvement; and 83.6% of substantial or very great improvement."

In the light of recent studies in which rigid controls were used, it seems evident that these early studies of White and Cabot are exceedingly difficult to interpret. Excluding for the moment the relief of retention in some cases which may have been attributable to passing a catheter, reductions in residual urines and a decrease in the palpable size of the gland, let us examine briefly the evidence for and against "histological atrophy" following castration. In his report, White reproduces the description of the microscopic findings of a patient who died 18 days following castration for prostatic enlargement. This description by Griffiths is also presented in detail with figures in a separate article (1895). "In short, the cell elements first proliferate, and ultimately disappear, leaving a comparatively small amount of fibrous connective tissue in their place. . . . The gland, whether enlarged or normal, undergoes certain degenerative changes after removal of the testicles which lead to its conversion into a small, tough fibrous mass in which there are only remains of the glandular tubules and ducts."

However, in his report, Cabot takes issue with the interpretations of Griffiths as follows: "The changes thus described (by Griffith for the enlarged glands of patients who have not been castrated) are so closely similar to those which he thinks he has found in a case of castration, examined after eighteen days, that there might well be doubt whether the condition which he thought due to the effect of castration might not have been one of degeneration already started before castration was done." Also, "Albarran, who has made microscopical study of prostates after castration, is unwilling to accept White's and Griffiths's observations as evidence of atrophic changes, and says that he has seen similar conditions to those pictured by Griffiths in cases that have never been castrated."

These reports were quickly followed by other publications of failure of relief of prostatic enlargement following castration, and some 30 to 40 years elapsed before Deming and his associates (1935a,b) revived the subject. In their first paper, they report no effect of castration on prostatic enlargement in one patient who was castrated initially and whose failure to improve necessitated open prostatectomy about 1 month later; in their second paper, they present a second patient in their argument against castration. This 74-year-old man had grossly atrophic testes resulting from injury to each at ages 18 to 21 years, and had developed benign prostatic enlargement which required open prostatectomy. However, the authors' suggestion that this enlargement had developed in the presence of testicular atrophy is probably not tenable, because histological examination of one testis removed at the time of prostatectomy showed sheets of interstitial cells which were quite likely functional from a hormonal standpoint. Certainly, this man was not a castrate, as he has been quoted as being.

As indicated heretofore, Huggins and Stevens reexamined the problem in 1940. Three patients were studied. In case 1, no change was noted in the number of acini, their diameter, nor the height of their epithelial cells in a period of 29 days following castration (Figs. 3A and 3B). In case 2, histological examination of prostatic tissue obtained 86 days after castration revealed an increase in the number of acini, these acini being smaller and lined with cuboidal epithelium, when compared with prostatic tissue obtained before castration (Table I and Figs. 4A and 4B). This patient also had disseminated (stage D) prostatic cancer. In case three, no histological sections were reproduced, but they were described: "Section of prostate 91 days after castration: Most of the tissue consists of fibromuscular stroma with relatively infrequent small acini. The acinous epithelium is cuboidal and is stratified in layers of two and three cells. The epithelium resembles the postorchiectomy specimen in case two." Their conclusions were: "Epithelial atrophy was not present 29 days after castration but appeared plainly 86 and 91 days after the operation. . . . The evidence derived from castration on benign prostatic hypertrophy in man supports the view that the prostatic epithelium at least is under control of the testes."

Believing that more data are necessary to draw conclusions between established BPH and the testes, and recognizing that purposeful castration of a large number of men with this condition is not feasible, Wendel et al. (1972), compared the histology of benign hyperplasia in patients with prostatic carcinoma who had been treated by castration and estrogen

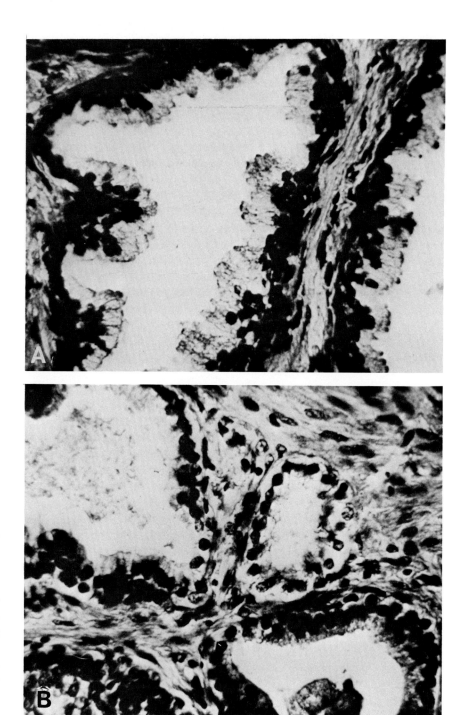

FIG. 3. (A) Benign hypertrophy of prostate before castration. (B) Section of adenomatous prostate from same patient 29 days after castration. Both ×550. From Huggins and Stevens (1940), with permission. © 1940 The Williams & Wilkins Co., Baltimore.

TABLE I

MEASUREMENTS OF EPITHELIUM IN PROSTATIC HYPERTROPHY IN 50
NONCASTRATED CASES, AS WELL AS BEFORE AND AFTER
CASTRATION IN 3 MEN[a]

Measurement	Number of acini per microscopic field ($\times$ 100)	Diameter of acini (mm)	Height of epithelial cells (μm)
Average measurements in 50 non-castrated cases with probable error	24.9 $\pm$ 10.4	0.46 $\pm$ 0.12	14.4 $\pm$ 2.3
Case 1, before castration	32	0.38	11.8
Case 1, 29 days after castration	29	0.33	11.8
Case 2, before castration	19	0.64	14
Case 2, 86 days after castration	34	0.20	8
Case 3, 91 days after castration	18.4	0.24	8.8

[a] From Huggins and Stevens (1940), with permission. © 1940 The Williams & Wilkins Co., Baltimore.

therapy with the histology of benign hyperplasia in patients with prostatic cancer who were not treated. Their conclusions were: "The benign prostatic hyperplasia present in patients with carcinoma of the prostate treated with orchiectomy and estrogens is of a lower grade than in those patients not having this treatment. Infolding of the acinar epithelium and the secretory phase are virtually absent in the group having orchiectomy and estrogens (Figure 5A), as compared to their presence in patients not having this treatment (Figure 5B). The findings in patients with occult or untreated prostatic cancer suggest that the differences are correlated with orchiectomy and estrogens and not with the presence of carcinoma itself. These observations support the concept that cells of benign prostatic hyperplasia are subjected to continuing stimulation by the testes."

Studies such as this are helpful in our approaches to hormonal regulation of benign prostatic growth, but many questions remain unanswered. Thus, the role of testicular estrogens in such growth is not as yet resolved, nor is the effect of castration on the fibromuscular stroma clear.

However, one of us (Scott, 1953) removed the hyperplastic portion of a prostate from a man aged 60 which was causing urinary retention. This man had been castrated at age 28. Figures 6A and 6B are portions of the surgical specimen, A showing typical hyperplasia and B showing classic squamous metaplasia, considered by some to be androgenic and estrogenic effects, respectively.

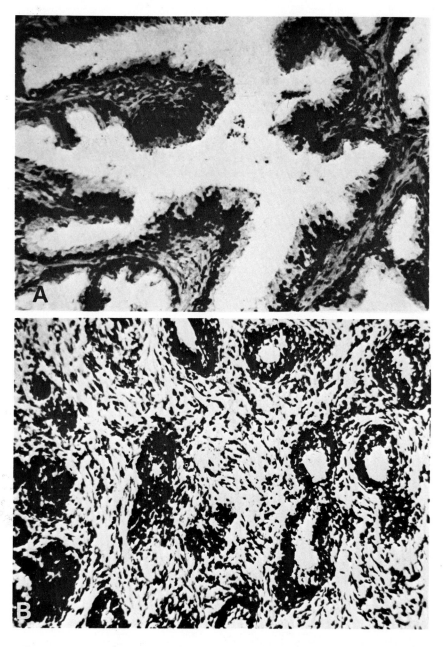

FIG. 4. Case 2. (A) Benign hypertrophy of prostate before castration. (B) Section of prostate 86 days after castration. This section showing epithelial atrophy is typical of most of the gland. Both ×235. From Huggins and Stevens (1940), with permission. © 1940 The Williams & Wilkins Co., Baltimore.

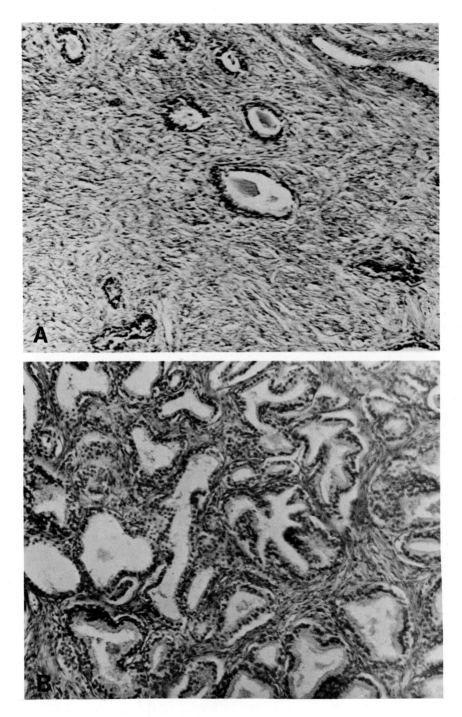

FIG. 5. (A) Photomicrograph of prostatic tissue in patient treated with orchiectomy and estrogen. (B) Photomicrograph of prostatic tissue in patient with untreated prostatic cancer. Both reduced from ×100. From Wendel *et al.*, (1972) with permission. © 1972 The Williams & Wilkins Co., Baltimore.

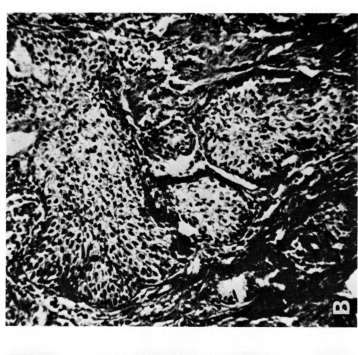

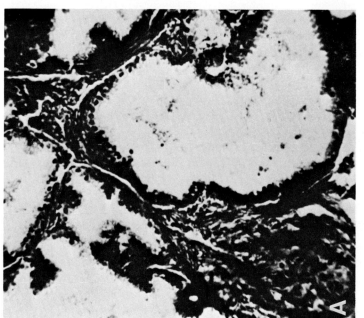

Fig. 6. Sections from prostate gland of a man, aged 60 years, whose testes were removed at the age of 28 years because of tuberculous epididymitis and orchitis. A shows typical benign prostatic hyperplasia; B shows classic squamous metaplasia. Both ×150. From Scott (1953), with permission. © 1953 The Williams & Wilkins Co, Baltimore.

This is not the time or the place to present a chronological, historic review of the multitudinous efforts to control prostate hyperplasia in man by the administration of hormones. Rather, it seems more important to examine the results of the most recent efforts to do this, in light of an appreciation of rigid controls, prospective studies, randomization of patients, the use of placebos, crossover studies, biopsies, etc.

F. Estrogen Therapy

There are a few reports concerned with the use of estrogens alone, and most lack controls. Peirson (1946) used an X-ray balloon catheter technique to determine prostatic size before and after stilbestrol therapy. Whereas he reported some reduction in prostatic diameter in 10 of 13 cases, he concluded that, "The general use of stilbestrol therapy is not, at the present time, warranted in benign prostatic hypertrophy." There are numerous reports, however, which indicate that estrogens administered in sufficient dosage will reduce levels of circulating testosterone.

G. Androgen Therapy

Testosterone has been administered by a number of clinicians in the treatment of benign hyperplasia, but there are no controlled studies. The findings of Lesser et al. (1955) are of some interest. These authors compared the incidence of BPH in 100 men over 45 years of age who had received testosterone propionate in the treatment of either "angina pectoris or the male climacterium" with the incidence in 100 age-matched controls. Testosterone propionate had been administered to these patients intramuscularly in doses of 25–75 mg per week for periods varying from 3 months to 4 years. "Twenty-seven treated patients showed prostatic hypertrophy, but 34 control subjects also had an enlarged prostate." From this study, and within the limitations of the therapy, it would appear that testosterone administration did not alter the incidence of BPH.

H. Androgen–Estrogen Combination

Kaufman and Goodwin (1959) have reported on the results of combined androgen–estrogen treatment in 42 patients; a mixture of 25 mg of testosterone propionate and 2.5 mg of diethylstilbestrol was administered intramuscularly to each patient three times weekly for 6 months. This was not a controlled study. They reported an appreciable amelioration of symptoms in the majority of patients, improvement of voiding velocity in most, reduction of residual urine in a few, histological changes in about one-half, and some apparent reduction in size of the gland, determined by palpation in about one-third. They concluded that, "These features were too inconstant and unpredictable to warrant absolute conclusions."

I. ANTIANDROGENS AND PROGESTATIONAL AGENTS

1. *Spironolactone*

The most recent double-blind, controlled clinical trial of spironolactone by Castro *et al.* (1971), showed this to be better than a placebo for the short-term treatment of BPH, but this advantage was not maintained over a longer period of time and there was a considerable response to placebo. They presented no data on the histology of these glands before and after treatment.

2. *Progestins*

In 1965, Geller and his associates were the first to report on the use of progestational agents in the treatment of benign hyperplasia in man. Their later report appeared in 1969. In the earlier series of 10 patients, hydroxyprogesterone caproate was given in a dosage of 1.5 mg intramuscularly, biweekly. Two of the 10 received dexamethasone in addition. This earlier series lacked controls. In the later series of 11 patients, 8 were treated with hydroxyprogesterone caproate and three with chlormadinone acetate. The revised protocol provided better controls, and in terms of symptomatic improvement, favorable results were obtained.

In an effort to answer the criticisms of some pathologists that needle biopsies are inaccurate because of the selectivity and sampling error, artifacts are produced by the needle, and inadequate tissue for evaluation is obtained at times, Geller and his associates in their later study performed suprapubic prostatectomy in three patients who had received hydroxyprogesterone caproate for 2 months. Hence, the entire specimens were available for histologic comparison with corresponding specimens from untreated patients, but *not* with biopsy material from the same patient before treatment. Figures 7A and 7B are reproduced from their study and are intended to convey a reduction in acinar size, less "interacinar papillation" and a change from columnar to cuboidal epithelium following 2 months of treatment with hydroxyprogesterone caproate. Changes in the fibromuscular stroma are not discussed.

3. *Cyproterone Acetate*

Our studies (Scott and Wade, 1969), using cyproterone acetate, were exploratory ones; they were devoid of adequate controls, but were carefully conducted in terms of patient selection, urine flow rates, residual

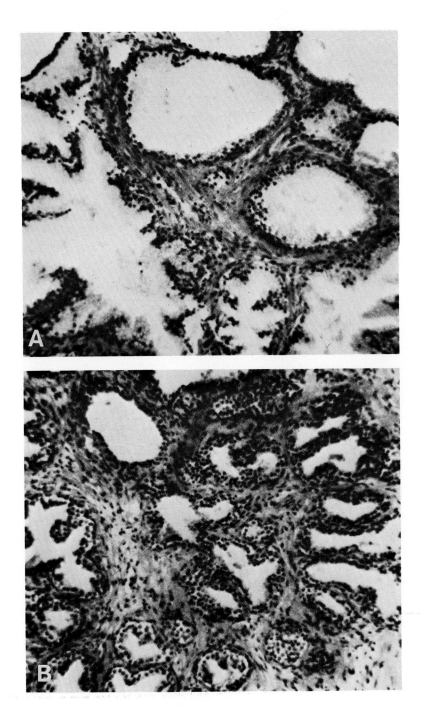

urine determination, serum testosterone levels, and in terms of histological observations of the adenomas before and during the administration of the drug.

At the time of our report in 1969, 13 patients with significant benign prostatic obstruction had received 50 mg of cyproterone acetate orally daily for periods ranging to 15 months. Urinary obstructive symptoms were judged to have lessened in 11 patients, remained unchanged in 1, and worsened in 1. Urine flow rates increased in 9 patients, remained essentially the same in 2 and were reduced in 2. Measured volumes of residual urine decreased in 8 patients, remained the same in 2 and increased in 3. All but 1 patient showed a fall in serum testosterone during treatment. This patient probably did not take the drug regularly and was one of 3 patients who showed an increase in prostatic epithelial height. Epithelial height decreased in 8 of 11 patients when measured and was especially profound in 1 patient (Figs. 8A and 8B). Prostatic size, estimated by digital palpation, decreased in 7 patients and remained unchanged in 6.

4. Medrogestone

In 1971, Rangno et al. reported their studies of 24 patients with established BPH who were treated at random in a double-blind manner with one or two drug schedules: 50 mg medrogestone twice daily for 24 weeks followed by placebo for 24 weeks, or the reverse order.

In summary, "Each of the 5 subjective measurements of frequency, nocturia, hesitancy, intermittency, and force and size of urine stream showed major improvement during medrogestone therapy, the improvement being most significant for force and size of stream. Frequency, nocturia and force and size of stream also showed continued improvement when placebo followed medrogestone. Three objective measurements, prostate size, cystogram and cystoscopy each showed improvement during medrogestone therapy. Further reduction in prostatic size was observed during the placebo period. The reduction in the residual urine for both groups during both treatment periods were not different. Repeated residual urine volumes by this technique showed extremely wide variation."

FIG. 7. (A) Appearance of untreated human benign prostatic hyperplasia at intermediate zone in nodule. Acini are medium in size and lined by simple, tall, columnar epithelium. Note intra-acinar papillation. (B) Similar cells treated with hydroxyprogesterone show small acini lined by cuboidal epithelium with subapical or midzonal nuclei. Basal cells are prominent in places. Hematoxylin and eosin; slightly reduced from ×150. From Geller et al. (1969). Reprinted from the Journal of the American Medical Association, November 24, 1969, Volume 210. Copyright 1969. American Medical Association.

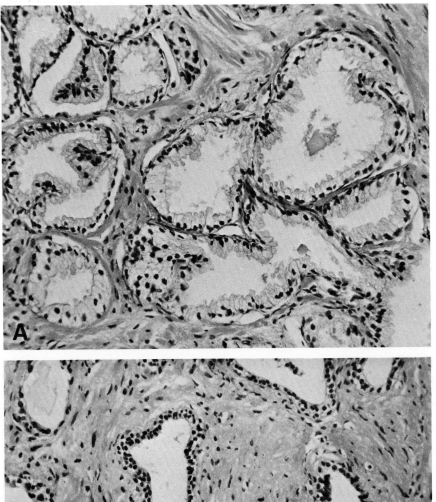

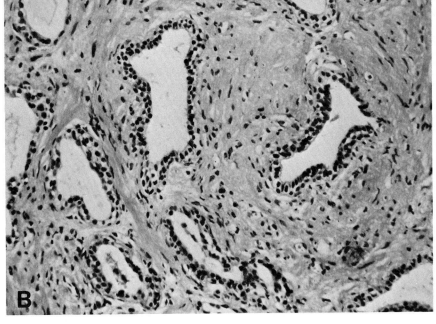

Continuing, "Striking constant histologic changes were observed after medrogestone therapy. There was absence of acinar fronds. The epithelium was flat and broken and lytic fragments filled the lumen. There were no consistent changes in the stroma or excretory ducts. In those patients who received medrogestone during the first 24 weeks, we observed a complete reversal of the lytic changes to normal by the end of the placebo period which followed."

Subsequently, Paulson and Kane (1975) engaged in a study quite similar to that of Rangno *et al.*, except that the dosage of medrogestone was markedly reduced from 50 mg to 7.5 mg twice daily for 15 weeks in one group and to 15.0 mg twice daily for 15 weeks in another.

No significant differences in improvement were reported for medrogestone when compared with placebo except, "Patients treated with 15 mg medrogestone twice a day showed a significant increase in peak urine flow, mean urine flow, and total volume of urine voided during micturition." However, subsequent analysis of these data by R. E. Rangno (personal communication, 1974) suggested no difference in these measurements.

5. *Flutamide, Nonsteroidal Antiandrogen*

Whereas there are several reports on the use of Flutamide (Sch 13521) in the treatment of prostatic cancer, to the best of our knowledge only one report is in press describing the results of the use of this compound in the treatment of BPH, this by Caine *et al.* (1975). Thirty of 31 patients with significant BPH and appreciable residual urine received either 100 mg of Flutamide orally three times daily for 12 weeks or a placebo. Randomization resulted in 15 patients receiving the active compound and 15 receiving placebo. The potency of the compound was manifest by the large number of patients developing nipple tenderness and/or gynecomastia. Whereas subjective effects may have favored the use of Flutamide, the only objective evidence favoring the active compound was a significant improvement in urine flow rate. No differences were found in residual urines, gross prostatic size, and histological changes in prostatic biopsies.

J. Polyene Macrolides

Since Gordon and Schaffner (1968) first showed that orally administered candicidin and other polyene macrolides will reduce the size of the

---

Fig. 8. Patient 8. Histological appearance of prostatic tissue obtained by needle biopsy before (A) and after (B) treatment with cyproterone acetate. Hematoxylin and eosin; ×275. From Scott and Wade (1969), with permission. © 1969 The Williams & Wilkins Co., Baltimore.

prostate glands of older dogs, sporadic efforts have been made to determine the clinical effectiveness of such drugs in the treatment of BPH in men. Regarding amphotericin B, Texter and Coffey (1969) reported a marked reduction in prostatic secretion in dogs with prostatic fistulas and a reduction in the epithelial component of the prostate in 1 month after the oral administration of 200 mg per day. However, it must be emphasized that these observations could not be duplicated by them when other lots of amphotericin were tested.

Our unreported clinical results with candicidin were disappointing. We noted, as did Keshin (1973), that most of our patients who received candicidin experienced extreme nausea and vomiting, and in addition, that a modification of formulation resulted in the microcapsule passing through the entire gastrointestinal tract and appeared unchanged.

A careful review of Keshin's study, in which he reports significant improvement in 92 of 120 patients treated with 300 mg of candicidin by activity per day for 5 months with an 18-month follow-up, reveals no adequate controls. Furthermore, he does not discuss the unreliability of such "objective" indices as estimation of prostatic size, residual urine determinations, and prostatic biopsies.

II. Canine Benign Prostatic Hyperplasia

A. Description and Comparison

The medical management of human BPH has been hindered by the absence of an adequate animal model to elucidate the etiology of this disease and to evaluate the pharmacological effectiveness of new therapeutic modalities. A high incidence of this disease is thought to be prevalent only in the aging human and canine (Zuckerman and Groome, 1937), although complete pathological development of the aging prostate has not been resolved in many species including the higher primates. Nearly all canines with functioning testes exhibit abnormal prostatic growth with advancing age. The occurrence is rare in dogs under 4 years of age (Kracht-Palejeff, 1910), while 80% of the dogs over 8 years of age are reported to present some degree of benign hyperplasia (Moore, 1944). In a normal adult dog the prostate gland weight is in the range of 5–10 mg, and when the weight exceeds 0.7 gm per kilogram of body weight the prostate usually exhibits some abnormal pathology (Schlotthauer and Bollman, 1936). Berg (1958) has proposed a canine prostatic weight index of 15 gm as the minimal criterion for diagnosing benign prostatic hyperplasia; however, the diagnosis always should be confirmed by histological examination.

Unfortunately, the canine model differs in many characteristics from human BPH, and these have been adequately reviewed (Ofner, 1968). The canine prostatic enlargement is due primarily to hyperplasia of the epithelial components with papillary ingrowth, producing dilation of the acini and cystic formation (Goodpasture and Wislocki, 1916; Goodpasture, 1918; Smith, 1919). Even in the dog more than one type of hyperplasia may be defined. Zuckerman and Groome (1937) and Smith and Jones (1966) described the two main types as glandular hypertrophy, which is strictly an increase in hyperplasia of the glandular epithelium, and cystic hyperplasia, characterized by cystic degeneration of the glandular acini. In the canine, both types of growth are usually diffuse and involve the entire gland, and urinary obstruction is not as prevalent as is associated with the human disease, where the lesion is usually of a fibroadenomatous nature originating in the periurethral region of the gland.

B. Hormone Sensitivity

Other important differences may be apparent when human and canine prostatic hyperplasia are compared, particularly with respect to their hormone sensitivities. As discussed in preceding sections, there is no compelling evidence at present to establish the effectiveness of castration, estrogen, or antiandrogen therapy in controlling the human growth. In contrast, the classical studies of Huggins and Clark (1940) clearly indicate the sensitivity of canine BPH to androgen deprivation through castration or estrogen therapy. More recently, antiandrogens have proved effective in reducing the size of canine BPH. For example, Neri and his associates (1968) reported that the administration of cyproterone acetate (SH-714) to four intact old dogs, at a daily dose of 10 mg for 6 weeks, reduced the total gland size of canine prostatic hyperplasia by an average of 73%. The epithelial cell height and the average diameter of the acini were reduced by 72% and 59%, respectively. In addition, a nonsteroidal antiandrogen, Flutamide (Sch 13521) has been reported by Neri and Monahan (1972) to be effective in the treatment of canine BPH. Oral administration of 5 mg or more of Flutamide per kilogram to 12 intact old dogs for 6 weeks reduced the hyperplastic gland size by an average of 80%, and the epithelial cell height by 87%. With both of these antiandrogens the treatment abolished the pathological evidence of canine BPH, and this was maintained for one year with continuous Flutamide therapy. However, when long-term antiandrogen therapy was terminated after 8 weeks, the canine prostate quickly reverted to the original hyperplastic condition with respect to prostate size, epithelial cell height, and

histology (Neri and Monahan, 1972). This is similar to the earlier observation of Huggins and Clark (1940), who reported that castration abolished canine BPH, and subsequent administration of testosterone propionate restored the pathological condition.

C. Etiological Factors

All the above studies would appear to implicate the availability of
testosterone either directly or indirectly in the maintenance of the hyperplastic condition in the dog prostate; however, the role, if any, of testosterone in the etiology may be far more complex. For example, a prepubertal castrate dog that was treated many years later with 10 mg of
testosterone per day for 88 days developed a large (20.1 gm) normal prostate, and cystic hyperplasia was not observed in this gland (Huggins and
Clark, 1940). Huggins and Sommers (1953) also reported that treating
young castrate dogs for 30 days with small and large doses of either testosterone propionate or diethylstilbestrol, or the combination of both the
androgen and estrogen, produced large prostates but no cystic hyperplasia. Wilson and his associates (1975a,b) have confirmed these original
conclusions by castrating 1.5- to 2-year-old dogs and treating them thereafter for 2 years with injections of testosterone, 75 mg/week. Of four
castrate animals receiving this testosterone treatment, none developed
cystic hyperplasia while two of the four animals in the intact noncastrated control group developed large prostates with cystic hyperplasia.
None of the four castrate controls developed BPH.

In summary, all the above findings tend to indicate that the administration of testosterone to *castrate* dogs will not produce cystic hyperplasia; however, *once* the disease has developed, castration ablates the
disease, and this can be reversed with the administration of testosterone
to the castrated dog. This would appear to indicate the necessity of other
factors from the testes in the etiology of canine BPH. To our knowledge,
only one report is available concerning the treatment with exogenous testosterone of old dogs with *normal* prostates and *not* castrated, and the
subsequent development of canine BPH. Neri and his colleagues (1968)
treated three old (6–10 years) intact dogs, with normal prostates, with
25 mg of testosterone propionate per day for 6 weeks. The prostate weight
and epithelial cell height increased 3-fold and the animals developed histological evidence of cystic hyperplasia. Whether the difference in Neri's
observation and those of Huggins or Wilson and their associates can be
explained on the basis of the presence or the absence of testes remains
conjectural at the present time.

Interest is presently being focused on other etiological factors, such as a variety of androgen metabolites (Wilson, 1975b). The classic experiments of Wilson and his associates regarding the role of dihydrotestosterone (DHT) in canine prostatic hyperplasia (Gloyna *et al.*, 1970) and human BPH (Siiteri and Wilson, 1970) are being further resolved (Wilson *et al.*, 1975a,b). Their observations that DHT was in higher concentration in the BPH lesions in both dog and man motivated a study of the long-term effects of the administration of DHT on canine prostatic growth in castrate dogs. After 9 months of DHT therapy (Gloyna *et al.*, 1970), biopsies of the prostate suggested the appearance of canine hyperplasia, but extension of DHT therapy over 2 years now indicates that neither the histology nor the size of the gland increase relative to that observed in the noncastrated and untreated controls, half of which (2 of 4) developed cystic hyperplasia (Wilson *et al.*, 1975a,b). In addition, their studies of the prostatic tissue concentrations of DHT were similar in both the DHT-treated castrates, which did not develop BPH, and the nontreated intact controls, which did develop benign hyperplasia.

From these observations it would appear that the presence of DHT alone is not sufficient to produce canine prostatic hyperplasia. Therefore, Wilson and his colleagues scrutinized other types of androgen metabolites for their potential etiology in the development of canine BPH in castrate animals in anticipation that this information might provide new insight into this perplexing problem. Walsh and Wilson (1975) provided a preliminary report of their recent findings at the Workshop on Benign Prostatic Hyperplasia held at the National Institutes of Health in Bethesda, Maryland on February 20–21, 1975. In a small group of castrate dogs treated for 2 years with 5α-androstane-3α,17β-diol, the prostates developed into large glands, fulfilling Berg's criterion for the requirement for hyperplasia. Furthermore, the histological analysis of these prostates indicated that the 3α-androstanediol had induced canine prostatic hyperplasia in these castrated dogs. When estrogen therapy was combined with the 3α-androstanediol treatment, the prostates were even larger, and the glands developed additional stromal components, which more closely resembled the type of BPH observed in humans. We all await the full report of these interesting new observations, which may provide new impetus and direction to our understanding of the development of canine BPH.

D. Considerations

In the ensuing period since the report of Huggins and Clark (1940), only a minimal number of experiments involving canine BPH have been reported, and these have involved very small groups of animals. Many of these studies were done on animals of unknown age, and the hormonal treatments have been for various times and often under vastly different conditions. For example, in Huggins and Clark's original study (1940), 12 of the 29 dogs with BPH also presented with testicular tumors, which are common in old dogs. Subsequent studies have not discussed the testicular pathology of the dogs prior to treatment. A large controlled study of nonmongrel dogs, age-matched and with chronic administration of appropriate hormones, is an expensive and time-consuming endeavor. However, with proper biochemical and histological indices, these types of studies may resolve many of the important leads suggested by the recent studies of Wilson and his colleagues. The medical management for the prevention and control of human BPH has required a more definitive animal model for evaluating the parameters of therapies and modalities, and it now appears that progress is being made in this direction.

New biochemical and morphometric analyses are now being developed (deKlerk and Coffey, 1975), which will permit quantitative evaluation of the hormonal and therapeutic responses in individual cell types in the various lobes and components of the prostate gland. These correlations and patterns of cellular development and alteration with the aging process, coupled with a more complete understanding of testicular secretions and hormone metabolism in the prostate tissue, may soon provide a sound basis for a rational approach to the medical management of this disease.

Once again one should caution that the hormonal response of the developed canine prostatic hyperplastic gland appears to be markedly different from that of human BPH and this may indicate important differences in the two disease processes. Therefore, more knowledge on the incidence of abnormal prostatic growth in aging higher primates should be actively pursued in order to establish alternative model systems.

Quantitative information is also needed on the hormonal control and responsiveness of the stromal elements of the prostate gland and how these components might modulate epithelial function and growth.

Recent studies by Dr. Daniel deKlerk in our laboratory have provided interesting information on the effects of several important androgens and estrogens on various cellular components of the rat ventral prostate (Table II) (deKlerk and Coffey, 1975). Combining morphometric analysis of histological sections with biochemical analysis of DNA content in the prostate and nuclei provides a quantitative determination of the effects of hormones on various cell types and number. Castration caused a dramatic decrease of 93% of total epithelial cells and only 22% of total stromal cells. Thus, castration reduces the ratio of epithelial to stromal cells by 10-fold. The administration of hyperphysiological (5 mg/day) doses of DHT to the *castrate* for 10 days restores the total

TABLE II

EFFECT OF STEROID HORMONES ON CELLULAR CONTENT IN THE RAT VENTRAL PROSTATE[a]

Condition	Treatment	Total cells		Stromal cells		Epithelial cells		Ratio cells epithelial:stromal
		Total number (10^7)	Relative number	Total number (10^7)	Relative number	Total number (10^7)	Relative number	
	5 mg/day × 10							
Normal	—	6.85 ± 0.4	100 ± 5	1.23 ± 0.1	100 ± 5	5.62 ± 0.3	100 ± 5	4.54
Castrate	—	1.39 ± 0.2	20 ± 2	0.97 ± 0.1	78 ± 9	0.42 ± 0.1	7 ± 1	0.43
Castrate	Testosterone	5.21 ± 0.6	76 ± 9	1.46 ± 0.2	118 ± 13	3.75 ± 0.4	67 ± 8	2.57
Castrate	Dihydrotestosterone	8.32 ± 1.8	121 ± 27	2.45 ± 0.5	198 ± 44	5.87 ± 1.3	104 ± 29	2.40
Castrate	5α-Androstane-3α,17β diol	5.84 ± 0.9	85 ± 13	2.06 ± 0.3	166 ± 25	3.78 ± 0.6	67 ± 10	1.84
Castrate	5α-Androstane-3β,17β diol	2.30 ± 0.5	33 ± 7	0.95 ± 0.2	77 ± 16	1.35 ± 0.3	24 ± 5	1.42
Castrate	(1 mg/day × 10) 17β-Estradiol	2.13 ± 0.2	31 ± 2	0.99 ± 0.1	81 ± 6	1.14 ± 0.1	20 ± 2	1.14

[a] From deKlerk and Coffey (1975), with permission.

number of epithelial cells to normal levels, but increases the number of stromal cells to almost twice the original in the *normal* ventral prostate gland. Therefore, stromal cells are less sensitive to androgen deprivation than the epithelial cells; however, hyperplasia can be induced in these stromal cells with certain androgens.

Androgen deprivation decreases not only the total number of epithelial cells, but also the cell size and ratio of cytoplasmic to nuclear volume. With castration, these indices of individual cell size decrease by 78% in the epithelial cells of castrates and by only 24% in stromal cells. DHT restores both types of cells to normal size.

The stromal components are now being further resolved in a quantitative manner, and these biomorphometric techniques are being expanded to human and canine prostatic hypertrophy and to other sex accessory tissues.

III. CONCLUSIONS

A review of the medical management of human BPH clearly indicates the need for more precise and controlled clinical trials. Although therapies using estrogens, androgens, antiandrogens, and castration have been proposed and have received limited clinical trials, it is nevertheless apparent that compelling evidence is not presently available to fully assess their potential or efficacy. The effects of these treatments may vary with the type of BPH and the method and duration of therapy. Evaluation of these treatments and the accompanying histological changes in the lesion and prostate gland of humans has often been limited or superficial.

Medical treatment of human BPH should be conservative, since only 10% of these patients ultimately require surgical intervention, and the morbidity and mortality of the standard surgical procedures are low when performed by an adequately trained and experienced urologist. However, patients who are poor surgical risks might receive benefit from medical management.

As more understanding is forthcoming on the etiology of this disease, our major contribution may be in prevention rather than cure. Many avenues of investigation have not been traveled, and such obvious approaches as antiestrogen therapy and the combination of steroids and antihormones which function through different sites of inhibition may be rewarding.

Our knowledge of the development of the human prostate and the specific requirements of hormones at specific times of growth is essentially at the beginning phases. The functional differences of the various lobes of the prostate, and biochemical comparison to other sex accessory tissues may explain why abnormal growth of sex accessory tissues in humans is limited primarily to the prostate gland.

The increased tempo of investigation of abnormal prostatic growth has been very evident at this meeting. This will surely hasten our ultimate goal of prevention and medical management of neoplastic growths in the human prostate.

REFERENCES

Adrion, W. (1922). *Beitr. Pathol. Anat. Allg. Pathol.* **70,** 179.

Berg, O. A. (1958). *Acta Endocrinol. (Copenhagen)* **27,** 140.

Cabot, A. T. (1896). *Ann. Surg.* **24,** 265.

Caine, M., Perlberg, S., and Gordon, R. (1975). *J. Urol.* **114,** 564.

Castro, J. E., Griffiths, H. J. L., and Edwards, D. E. (1971). *Brit. J. Surg.* **58,** 485.

Clarke, R. (1937). *Brit. J. Urol.* **9,** 254.

deKlerk, D. P., and Coffey, D. S. (1975). *In* "Workshop on Benign Prostatic Hyperplasia," Nat. Inst. Health Monogr. (in press).

Deming, C. L., Jenkins, R. H., and van Wagenen, G. (1935a). *J. Urol.* **33,** 388.

Deming, C. L., Jenkins, R. H., and van Wagenen, G. (1935b). *J. Urol.* **34,** 678.

Franks, L. M. (1954a). *Ann. Roy. Coll. Surg. Engl.* **14,** 92.

Franks, L. M. (1954b). *J. Pathol. Bacteriol.* **68,** 716.

Geller, J., Bora, R., Roberts, T., Newman, H., Lin, A., and Silva, R. (1965). *J. Amer. Med. Ass.* **193,** 121.

Geller, J., Angrist, A., Nakao, K., and Newman, H. (1969). *J. Amer. Med. Ass.* **210,** 1421.

Gloyna, R. E., Siiteri, P. K., and Wilson, J. D. (1970). *J. Clin. Invest.* **49,** 1746.

Goodpasture, E. W. (1918). *J. Med. Res.* **38,** 127.

Goodpasture, E. W., and Wislocki, G. B. (1916). *J. Med. Res.* **33,** 455.

Gordon, H. W., and Schaffner, C. P. (1968). *Proc. Nat. Acad. Sci. U.S.* **60,** 1201.

Greenwald, P., Kirmss, V., Polan, A. K., and Dick, V. S. (1974). *J. Nat. Cancer Inst.* **53,** 335.

Griffiths, J. (1895). *Brit. Med. J.* **1,** 579.

Harbitz, T. B., and Haugen, O. A. (1972). *Acta Pathol. Microbiol. Scand., Sect. A* **80,** 756.

Huggins, C., and Clark, P. J. (1940). *J. Exp. Med.* **72,** 747.

Huggins, C., and Sommers, J. L. (1953). *J. Exp. Med.* **97,** 663.

Huggins, C., and Stevens, R. (1940). *J. Urol.* **43,** 705.

Kaufman, J. J., and Goodwin, W. E. (1959). *J. Urol.* **81,** 165.

Keshin, J. G. (1973). *Int. Surg.* **58,** 116.

Kracht-Palejeff, P. (1910). *Arch. Tierheilk.* **37,** 299.

Lesser, M. A., Vose, S. N., and Dixey, G. M. (1955). *J. Clin. Endocrinol. Metab.* **15,** 297.

Loeschke, (1920). *Muenchen. Med. Wochenshr.* **67,** 302.

Lundberg, S., and Berge, T. (1970). *Scand. J. Urol. Nephrol.* **4,** 93.

Moore, R. A. (1942). *In* "Problems of Aging. Biological and Medical Aspects" (E. V. Cowdry, ed.), 2nd ed., pp. 495–517. Williams & Wilkins, Baltimore, Maryland.

Moore, R. A. (1944). *Surgery* **16**, 152.

Neri, R. O., and Monahan, M. (1972). *Invest. Urol.* **10**, 123.

Neri, R. O., Casmer, C., Zeman, W. V., Fiedler, F., and Tabachnick, I. I. A. (1968). *Endocrinology* **82**, 311.

Ofner, P. (1968). *Vitam. Horm. (New York)* **26**, 237.

Paulson, D. F., and Kane, R. D. (1975). *J. Urol.* **113**, 811.

Peirson, E. L. (1946). *J. Urol.* **55**, 73.

Pradhan, B. K., and Chandra, K. (1975). *J. Urol.* **113**, 210.

Rangno, R. E., McLeod, P. J., Ruedy, J., and Ogilvie, R. I. (1971). *Clin. Pharmacol. Ther.* **12**, 658.

Schlotthauer, C. F., and Bollman, J. L. (1936). *Cornell Vet.* **26**, 343.

Scott, W. W. (1953). *J. Urol.* **70**, 477.

Scott, W. W. (1963). *Nat. Cancer Inst., Monogr.* **12**, 111.

Scott, W. W., and Wade, J. C. (1969). *J. Urol.* **101**, 81.

Siiteri, P. K., and Wilson, J. D. (1970). *J. Clin. Invest.* **49**, 1737.

Smith, H. A., and Jones, T. C. (1966). "Veterinary Pathology." Lea & Febiger, Philadelphia, Pennsylvania.

Smith, L. W. (1919). *J. Med. Res.* **40**, 31.

Texter, J. H., and Coffey, D. S. (1969). *Invest. Urol.* **7**, 90.

Walsh, P. C., and Wilson, J. D. (1975). (Submitted for publication).

Wendel, E. F., Brannen, G. E., Putong, P. B., and Grayhack, J. T. (1972). *J. Urol.* **108**, 116.

White, J. W. (1895). *Ann. Surg.* **22**, 1.

Wilson, J. D., Gloyna, R. E., and Siiteri, P. K. (1975a). *J. Steroid Biochem.* **6**, 443.

Wilson, J. D., Walsh, P. C., and Siiteri, P. K. (1975b). *In* "Worskhop on Benign Prostatic Hyperplasia," Nat. Inst. Health Monogr. (in press).

Young, H. H., and Davis, D. M., eds. (1926). "Young's Practice of Urology," Vol. I. Saunders, Philadelphia, Pennsylvania.

Zuckerman, S., and Groome, J. R. (1937). *J. Pathol. Bacteriol.* **44**, 113.

DISCUSSION

A. Mittelman: We have been discussing the effects of hormones on tissue that responds in terms of morphology and function. Neoplasia may arise from cells that are atrophied or injured and seemingly not affected by hormones. The atrophic lobe of the mouse thymus develops leukemia. The posterior lobe of the prostate, frequently atrophic when examined, is the most common site of origin of prostatic cancer. Has the tissue ever been under hormonal control? If it has, it may no longer be so.

I. Lasnitzki: We have some evidence that the smooth muscle in human BPH is hormone sensitive. In organ culture, the incorporation of ^{3}H-labeled uridine in the cells of the smooth muscle is increased by testosterone and dihydrotestosterone.

M. B. Lipsett: I agree with your comments about the action of testosterone on rat and human prostate. We do know in man (and do not know in the rat) that aging is associated with increasing production of estrogens from androgens and higher plasma estrogen levels. This may be significant for the problem of stromal hyperplasia.

[End of Symposium articles]

Thiaminases and Their Effects on Animals

W. CHARLES EVANS

Department of Biochemistry and Soil Science
University College of North Wales, Bangor, Gwynedd, Wales

I. INTRODUCTION

Thiaminases are enzymes that act on thiamine in such a way that the products formed no longer possess the biological activity of the vitamin in animal nutrition, i.e., in the intact animal. They were discovered almost by accident, because of the consequences to animal health of incorporating certain uncooked foodstuffs in the diet.

The inclusion of raw fish, e.g., carp viscera, in diets fed to silver foxes on the ranch of J. S. Chastek of Glencoe, Minnesota, resulted in these animals developing a fatal paralyzing disease called Chastek paralysis. Green *et al.* (1941) proved that the affected animals showed all the manifestations of avitaminosis B_1, and in 1942 they described its pathology in detail. That the active agent in the carp viscera was an enzyme system capable of inactivating thiamine *in vitro* was demonstrated by Woolley (1941), Sealock *et al.* (1943), and Krampitz and Woolley (1944). The enzyme was named "thiaminase" by Sealock and White in 1949. Meanwhile, the presence of thiaminase was recorded in many freshwater and saltwater fish—notably the Cyprinidae and Atlantic herring. It also transpired that Japanese nutritionists had discovered a similar enzyme, which they termed "aneurinase," in many shellfish and crustaceans (Fujita and Numata, 1942). The ways in which the Chastek paralysis factor was finally associated with the newly discovered enzyme, thiaminase, has been well documented by Yudkin (1949).

In 1946, Weswig *et al.* found that when green bracken (*Pteridium aquilinum*) was quickly dried, powdered, mixed with a complete diet, and fed to rats, neurological symptoms developed that responded to thiamine therapy. These workers surmised that the factor concerned was unlikely to be an enzyme because of its relative heat stability. However, W. C. Evans *et al.* (1950) demonstrated that a thermolabile system which inactivated thiamine could be extracted from the bracken plant; this "plant" thiaminase behaved in a similar manner to the carp enzyme. They also showed that autoclaving the bracken powder before incorporating it in the diet rendered it incapable of producing thiamine deficiency in animals. Somogyi (1949) claimed that the sole "antithiamine" factor in bracken was thermostable, whereas Fujita *et al.* (1951) concluded that this plant contained both thermolabile and thermostable thiamine-decomposing factors. A survey of the occurrence of thiaminase revealed that the pteridophytes were almost unique in the plant kingdom apart from cockscomb (*Celosia crista*), in possessing this enzyme; this conclusion was supported by animal experiments as the final proof that the vitamin had been destroyed by a thermolabile agent (Jones, 1950, 1952).

Yet another source of thiaminase was discovered in Japan when Matsukawa and Misawa (1949) isolated from human feces certain bacteria which elaborated enzymes capable of destroying thiamine. These were two aerobes, *Bacillus thiaminolyticus* and *Bacillus aneurinolyticus,* and an anaerobe, *Clostridium thiaminolyticum* (Kimura and Aoyama, 1951; Kimura *et al.,* 1952). The culture fluid of all these spore-bearing bacteria were shown to contain a thiaminase, and patients suffering from "thiaminase disease," a form of hypothiaminosis, carried an intestinal flora heavily contaminated by these microbial species. Since then, the list of microorganisms that synthesize a thiamine-destroying enzyme has increased somewhat, extending to the yeastlike fungi *Trichosporon aneurinolyticum* (Aoki, 1955; Yoshioka, 1958), *Candida aneurinolytica* (Nishio, 1957) and to fungi, e.g., *Lentinus edodes* (Ono and Kawasaki, 1968).

By 1954, when Fujita reviewed the subject, considerable progress had been made in characterizing and elucidating the mode of action of the thiamine-decomposing enzymes. It transpires that there are, in fact, two distinct enzymes: thiaminase I, which is the more common, and thiaminase II, the rarer, and only found hitherto among a few microorganisms. The nature of the thermostable "antithiamine" factor of bracken fern, which Somogyi maintained was the only thiamine-decomposing factor present, remained unclear. It had been realized for some time that many plants including bracken (Ågren, 1945; Fujita, 1954) contained thermostable substances that interfered with chemical methods of estimating thiamine. W. C. Evans *et al.* (1950; Evans and Jones, 1952), however, could find no evidence that they were involved in the induction of thiamine deficiency in animals.

In recent years considerable progress has been made in the chemical identification of the so-called thermostable "antithiamine" factors of plants and the ways in which they may react with thiamine. The role of thiaminases in the etiology of some naturally occurring diseases of livestock has also been clarified, but the physiological significance of thiaminases within the living organisms in which they are found is still unclear.

II. THERMOLABILE THIAMINE-INACTIVATING SYSTEMS

A. THIAMINASE I

The main sources of this enzyme (thiamine:base 2-methyl-4-aminopyrimidine-5-methenyltransferase, EC 2.5.1.2) are carp viscera, the bracken fern, and *Bacillus thiaminolyticus*.

Thiaminase I catalyzes the decomposition of thiamine (I) by a base-exchange reaction, involving a nucleophilic displacement on the methylene group of the pyrimidine moiety (Scheme 1).

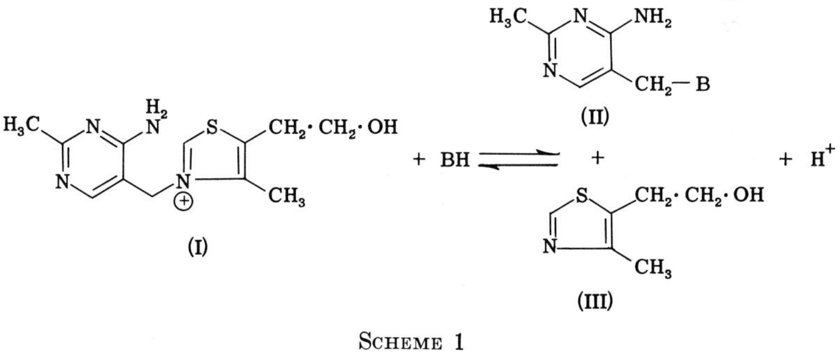

SCHEME 1

It will be noted that a "cosubstrate" is required for this reaction to occur; this is usually a base (certain primary, secondary, or tertiary amines), but can also be a sulfydryl or sulfinic acid.

1. *Properties*

The enzyme protein has been purified from a variety of sources and crystallized by Murata *et al.* (1961a,b) from *Bacillus thiaminolyticus* cultures. Table I records the properties of the pure enzyme from two laboratories. Wittliff and Airth (1968) reported that the maximum velocity of the thiaminase I reaction at pH 5.8 and 25°C is 6.4 mg of thiamine decomposed per minute per milligram of protein. Table II gives a list of some naturally occurring cosubstrates which participate, and the type of pyrimidine analog formed, and also two examples of synthetic bases that proved to be good cosubstrates, very useful in assay determinations during enzyme purification. It will be noted from Table II that some of the pyrimidine analogs formed could have the properties of a thiamine antagonist, depending on the naturally occurring cosubstrate present in a particular environment.

2. Assay Methods

Initially, measurement of thiaminase activity depended on chemical methods that had been developed for estimating thiamine, for example, the colorometric method of Melnick and Field (1939) using diazotized p-aminoacetophenone (the Prebluda–McCollum reaction, 1939) or fluorometrically using the thiochrome reaction (Harris and Wang, 1943; Ågren, 1946). Until the mechanism of thiaminase I action was clarified by

TABLE I
PROPERTIES OF THIAMINASE I[a]

Author	Source	MW	UV	K_m
Ebata and Murata (1961)	BMM[b]	40,000	λ_{max} 280 nm	0.9×10^{-3} M[c] for thiamine at pH 6.5, 30°C
			λ_{min} 250 nm	1.0×10^{-3} M for pyridine[d]
Wittliff and Airth (1968)	BMM	44,000	λ_{max} 277 nm	8.7×10^{-6} M for thiamine at pH 5.8, 25°C
			λ_{min} 252 nm	2.9×10^{-3} M for aniline[d]

[a] Substrate specificity: Specific for thiamine, thiamine pyrophosphate, and other thiamine derivatives with the 4-amino group of the pyrimidine ring intact; e.g., pyrithiamine but not oxythiamine is a substrate. Activators and inhibitors: Many aromatic amines, heterocyclic amines, and sulfydryl compounds; the enzyme is inactive toward thiamine in the absence of a cosubstrate. Both p-chloromercuribenzoate and iodoacetate (10^{-4} M) are potent inhibitors, indicating an SH-group-dependent enzyme. pH optimum: For BMM enzyme, 5.8–6 8; fish viscera enzyme, 5 0–6.0; bracken enzyme, 7.0–8.0. Effect of temperature: Optimum for BMM enzyme, 37°–40°C; shellfish and fern enzymes, 55°–60.0C. All enzymes are destroyed within 10 minutes at 100°C.

[b] BMM = Bacillus thiaminolyticus (Matsukawa et Misawa).

[c] Kuratani (1955) obtained a value of 0.37×10^{-6} M with an impure enzyme preparation.

[d] Cosubstrates.

TABLE II
PYRIMIDINE ANALOGS FORMED AND COSUBSTRATES OF THIAMINASE I

Pyrimidine analog	Cosubstrate	Authors
a. Naturally occurring[a]		
H_3C—pyrimidine ring with NH_2; CH_2—$\overset{O}{\underset{O}{S}}$·$CH_2$·$CH_2$·$NH_2$ **Icthiamine**	Hypotaurine (NH_2·CH_2·CH_2·SO_2H) (carp thiaminase)	Barnhurst and Hennessy 1952)
H_3C—pyrimidine ring; $N(CH_2)$ ring with CH_2, CH_2, CH·CO_2H (proline-type)	Proline (bracken thiaminase)	Thomas (1954); Thomas et al. (1955)
H_3C—pyrimidine ring with NH_2; CH_2—S·CH_2·CH·CO_2H with NH_2	Cysteine (BMM[b] thiaminase)	Murata et al. (1961a,b)
H_3C—pyrimidine ring; CH_2—$\overset{\oplus}{N}$ pyridine ring with CO_2H	Nicotinic acid (BMM thiaminase)	Murata et al. (1968)
b. Synthetic bases[c]		
H_3C—pyrimidine ring; CH_2—$\overset{\oplus}{N}$ pyridine ring **Heteropyrithiamine**	Pyridine (bracken thiaminase)	Fujita et al. (1951), Kenten (1957), Ebata and Murata (1961)
H_3C—pyrimidine ring with NH_2; CH_2—$\underset{H}{N}$—phenyl ring	Aniline (BMM thiaminase)	Hasegawa and Veda (1953), Wittliff and Airth (1968)

[a] These naturally occurring cosubstrates participated when thiamine was added to tissue extracts containing thiaminase I; they also illustrate the different types of pyrimidine analogs formed.

[b] BMM = *Bacillus thiaminolyticus* (Matsukawa et Misawa).

[c] These synthetic bases were used as "artificial" cosubstrates during purification of the enzyme from various sources. An exhaustive list is given by Fujita (1954) and Murata (1965).

Krampitz and Woolley (1944) and Sealock and Davies (1949), the results were uncertain, since the necessity for a cosubstrate was not appreciated, as crude extracts were purified.

A manometric method of thiaminase assay was developed by Kenten (1958) and W. C. Evans *et al.* (1958) based on the fact that the cleavage of one molecule of thiamine is accompanied by the release of a proton (see Scheme 1); this is made to liberate CO_2 from a bicarbonate–carbon dioxide buffer in the presence of a suitable cosubstrate (e.g., aniline, pyridine, or proline).

Thiaminase I activity was measured by Fujita (1954) by determining the thiamine remaining in the reaction mixture by the thiochrome method; Kenten (1957) measured the product, heteropyrithiamine, formed when pyridine is used as cosubstrate; Wittliff and Airth (1968) employed aniline as the base in the exchange reaction, and the product was measured spectrophotometrically by an increase in optical density at 248 nm.

When [2-¹⁴C]thiazole-labeled thiamine became available (The Radiochemical Centre, Amersham, England), a much more convenient method of thiaminase assay was developed by Edwin and Jackman (1970, 1974)—especially for screening biological fluids. Thiaminase activity (I or II) is assayed by extracting labeled 4-methyl-5-hydroxyethylthiazole (III) released by the enzyme into ethyl acetate, in which thiamine itself is insoluble, and measuring the radioactivity of the ethyl acetate solution in a scintillation counter. Nicotinic acid is used as cosubstrate. The radiochemical assay is carried out in the author's laboratory as follows: The sample for assay (plant powder, rumen liquor, feces, or microbial culture), is extracted with citrate–phosphate buffer (0.1 M, pH 6.4) in a ratio of 1 gm/5ml for 24 hours in a refrigerator and centrifuged to give the thiaminase extract. The substrate solution is composed of hot thiamine (200 μg) labeled with 1 μg of radioactive thiamine (55.6 nCi) and nicotinic acid (95 μg) in 1 ml of the same buffer. Each assay involves the following tubes.

Tube a. The thiaminase extract (1 ml) is mixed with substrate solution (1 ml) and incubated for 1 hour at 37°C. Ethyl acetate (4 ml) is added and the mixture is well shaken and centrifuged (2500 rpm, 5 minutes); 0.5 ml of the ethyl acetate layer is withdrawn and mixed with 10 ml of scintillator fluid (butyl PBD, 5gm in toluene, 1 liter), and the radioactivity is counted (cpm = x).

Tube b. A boiled thiaminase extract is substituted for the thiaminase extract in Tube a; this is to check that the activity is thermolabile.

Tube c. Citrate–phosphate buffer is substituted for the thiaminase extract in Tube a; this is to measure any destruction of thiamine due to the incubation conditions alone. The ethyl acetate count of this incubate $= y$ cpm. The aqueous phase gives the total count due to thiamine itself, which is available for the enzyme to act upon (z cpm); for this measurement, the scintillation fluid was composed of butyl PBD (8 gm), naphthalene (100 gm) dissolved in 1,4-dioxan (1 liter).

Tube d. Background count, using scintillation fluid alone, $= \beta$ cpm. Thiaminase activity is calculated as follows. Let

cpm test ethyl acetate (x) $-$ cpm citrate–phosphate
blank ethyl acetate (y) $= a$
cpm blank, aqueous phase (z) $-$ cpm background (β) $= b$.

Then,

Thiaminase activity $= a/b \times 8/4 \times 201/60 \times$
Vol. buffer (5)/Wt. sample (1)

in micrograms of thiamine destroyed per minute per gram.

B. THIAMINASE II

The only sources of this enzyme (thiamine hydrolase, EC 3.5.99.2) known at present are certain microorganisms, notably *Bacillus aneurinolyticus* (Murata, 1965). Thiaminase II catalyzes the hydrolysis of thiamine, according to Scheme 2.

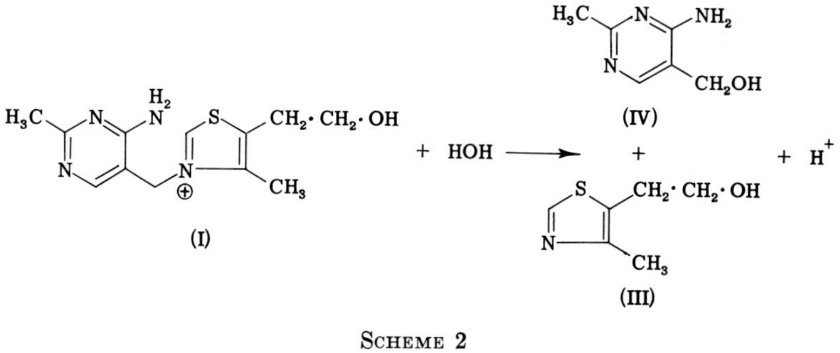

SCHEME 2

Properties

As this enzyme is not a base-transfer enzyme, cosubstrates are not required; the enzyme activity can be measured by determining the amount of thiamine decomposed by a dialyzed enzyme preparation under specified conditions using the thiochrome method or the radiochemical assay procedure. It was purified and obtained crystalline by Ikehata (1960) from the culture fluid of *Bacillus aneurinolyticus*. The molecular weight was 100,000, the Michaelis constant was K_m 3×10^{-6} M at pH 8.6 and

37°C (decomposing 1.3 mg of thiamine per minute per milligram of protein), and it had an absorption maximum at 276 nm and a minimum at 252 nm. The enzyme will hydrolyze thiamine and derivatives with the side chain intact at the 5-position of the thiazole moiety; it will not hydrolyze thiamine pyrophosphate. Thiaminase II is activated by cysteine and EDTA, inhibited by aromatic and heterocyclic amines (i.e., those that act as cosubtrates for thiaminase I), heavy metal ions, and p-chloromercuribenzoate, suggesting that, like thiaminase I, it is an SH-dependent enzyme. The pH and temperature optima of thiaminase II prepared from different microbial species varied; for example, that from *Bacillus aneurinolyticus* showed rather a broad pH optimum between pH 7.0 and 8.6, with a temperature optimum of 60°C; that from some of the yeasts and fungi (*Candida aneurinolyticus, Trichosporon aneurinolyticum*) had a pH optimum of 6.8–7.0 and a temperature optimum between 30° and 40°C. The enzyme from all sources was inactivated in solution within 10 minutes at 100°C.

It will be noted that one of the products of this reaction is the pyrimidine alcohol (IV), toxopyrimidine, which has a structural similarity to pyridoxamine and behaves as an antagonist of the vitamin B_6 group of coenzymes; for example, in the appropriate dose it causes epileptiform fits in small animals (Makino *et al.*, 1954) and even in ruminants (W. C. Evans *et al.*, 1958).

III. Thermostable Factors That React with Thiamine

It is important to be clear at the outset, when using the emotive words "antithiamine" or "thiamine-decomposing" factors what meaning they are intended to convey. Williams (1935), who first isolated and synthesized thiamine, reported its ready degradation by sodium sulfite, giving a pyrimidine sulfonic acid salt (V) and the thiazole moiety (III) (Scheme 3).

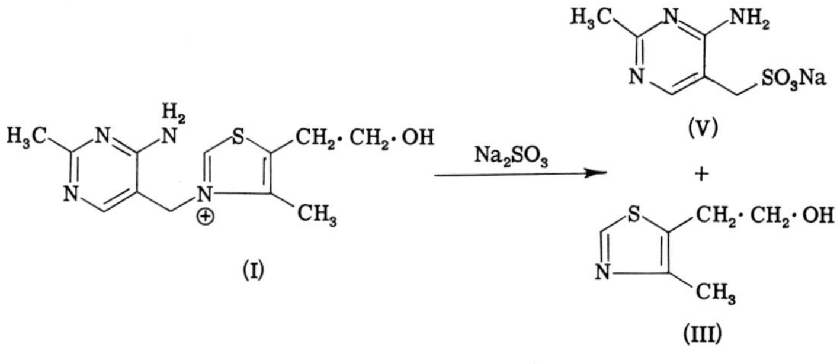

Scheme 3

The products formed were unable to replace thiamine in animal nutrition, and the vitamin is said to be "destroyed" by this procedure. Similarly, when thiaminase I or II act on thiamine, the consequences are duly revealed by using a homogastric animal as the test organism, when a state of thiamine deficiency ensues. These two examples illustrate what the author means by "thiamine-decomposing" or "thiamine-destroying" factors—whether they be thermolabile or thermostable.

Matsukawa and Yurugi (1952) discovered that when thiamine was allowed to react with a garlic extract at pH 8 the product no longer gave the thiochrome reaction—the standard chemical method of estimating thiamine by its oxidation to thiochrome (VI), which fluoresces and can be measured (Scheme 4).

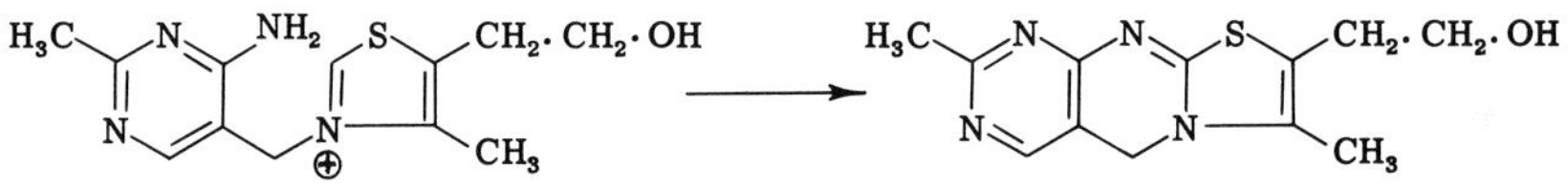

(I) → (VI)

SCHEME 4

The garlic extract contains "alliin" (VII), which is converted by an enzyme allinase (also present in the plant) into "allicin" (VIII) when making the extract (Scheme 5).

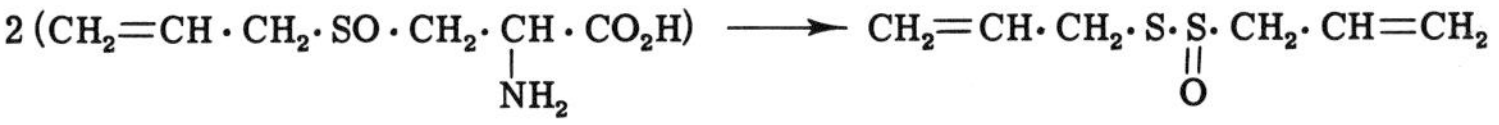

$$2\,(CH_2{=}CH \cdot CH_2 \cdot SO \cdot CH_2 \cdot \underset{\underset{NH_2}{|}}{CH} \cdot CO_2H) \longrightarrow CH_2{=}CH \cdot CH_2 \cdot S \cdot \underset{\underset{O}{\|}}{S} \cdot CH_2 \cdot CH{=}CH_2$$

(VII)   (VIII)

SCHEME 5

Allicin (VIII) reacts readily with thiamine in the thiol form (IX) in alkaline solution to give allithiamine (X) (Scheme 6).

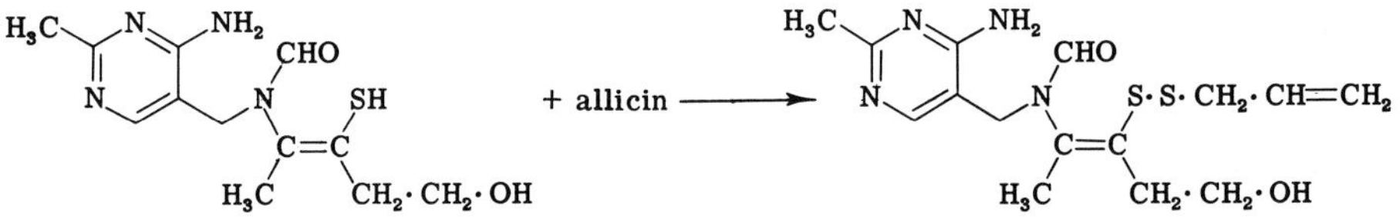

(IX) + allicin → (X)

SCHEME 6

If allithiamine is fed to thiamine-deficient rats, it is equally as effective as thiamine itself in curing the avitaminosis B_1. The Japanese workers found that allithiamine is readily reduced by cysteine (XI) and other biological reducing agents to give the thiol form of thiamine; in the case of cysteine, the other product formed in S-allylmercaptocysteine (XII) (Scheme 7).

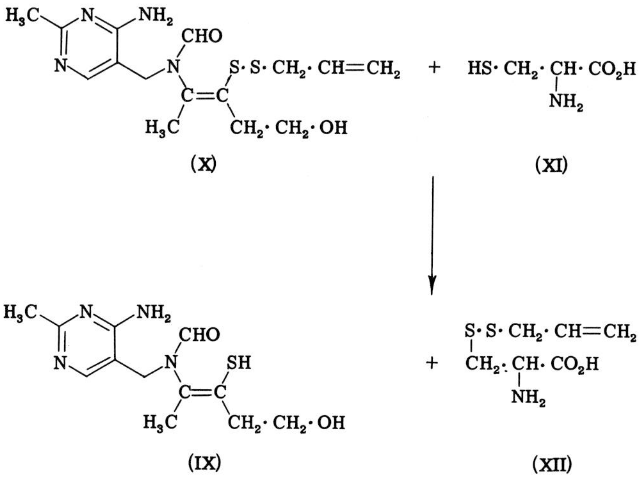

SCHEME 7

This is an example, therefore, of the occurrence in a plant of a thermostable factor that reacts with thiamine to give a product incapable of giving the thiochrome reaction, but still displays the unique physiological properties of thiamine in an animal bioassay, because the mammalian organism can reverse the process. The factor does not destroy thiamine, but merely changes its structure to another form equally active in animal nutrition.

The existence in many plants of thermostable factors that interfere in the chemical methods used for estimating thiamine (either the method of Melnick and Field or the thiochrome reaction) was emphasized by the work of Ågren and his collaborators (Lieck and Ågren, 1944; Ågren, 1945, 1946). Aqueous extracts of aspen and bracken were found to be particularly rich in these substances; they were finally associated with the polyphenolic components of the plants. At the time, they were regarded more as a nuisance and had to be removed from plant extracts before the actual stage of color or fluorescence development was carried out. Whether these phenolic substances reacted with thiamine in such a manner as to destroy the biological activity of the vitamin in animal nutrition was not determined.

Bhagvat and Devi (1944) reported that thiamine was inactivated by the ragi plant (*Eleusine coracana*), rice polishings, bajra (*Pennisetum typhoideum*), wheat germ, green gram (*Phaseolus radiatus*), soy bean, cow pea, mustard seed, cotton seed, linseed, and other plants. Their findings were as follows.

1. Disappearance of the thiochrome reaction when thiamine was incubated with ragi extract. This effect was also obtained with boiled extracts, thus apparently eliminating the involvement of thiaminase.

2. With larvae of a mosquito, *Aedes* (*stegomyia*) *albopictus,* used for bioassay, they obtained inconclusive results; the reaction products of thiamine treated with ragi extract (and with carp extract as a control) supported growth.

3. In the pigeon opisthotonus test, 66% of the birds on ragi extract developed the symptoms.

4. Using rats (on a thiamine-deficient diet) showing thiamine deficiency symptoms, thiamine after incubation with ragi extract was incapable of alleviating the avitaminosis B_1.

These workers seemed to have shown that boiled ragi extract was capable of destroying the usefulness of thiamine in animal nutrition. However, a closer look at their experimental procedure showed that they incubated thiamine (1 mg) for 24 hours at 37°C in a *suspension* of powdered ragi (5 gm) in acetate buffer (25 ml, 0.1 *M*, pH 5.6) which had previously been autoclaved for 15 minutes at 15 psi. The whole was then centrifuged and the clear filtrate *only* was tested for thiamine activity. It is possible that the thiamine would have become adsorbed on the powdered plant material under these conditions; a similar phenomenon had been encountered in the early work on thiaminase. The conclusions of Bhagvat and Devi therefore appear doubtful; the authors themselves commented that the plant materials they investigated had never been known to cause thiamine deficiency in animals, including humans. Nevertheless, they referred to these thermostable components alleged to inactivate thiamine as "antithiamine" factors. Jones (1952) and Watkin (1955) working in the authors' laboratory with the Indian foodstuff green gram and thiamine-deficient rats as the test organisms, could not confirm the work of Bhagvat and Devi.

IV. The "Antithiamine" Factors in Bracken Fern

A. The Thermolabile Thiamine-Destroying System

The importance of understanding the mechanisms involved in the destruction of thiamine by components of the bracken fern (*pteridium aquilinum*) arose when the present author and his collaborators embarked on researches to attempt to elucidate the causative agents of bracken poisoning in farm animals. The following facts were established:

1. Rats fed a complete diet mixed with low temperature-dried green bracken frond powder developed thiamine deficiency (Weswig et al., 1946); this observation was confirmed (Thomas and Walker, 1949; W. C. Evans and Evans, 1949).

2. The naturally occurring disease called "bracken staggers" in the horse was reproduced experimentally by Roberts et al., (1949) (see also E. T. R. Evans et al., 1951) by feeding a dried bracken frond–hay diet; it proved to be an induced thiamine deficiency and responded to thiamine therapy.

3. The ability of bracken extracts to destroy thiamine, with the meaning that it was no longer active as a vitamin in animal nutrition, was shown by W. C. Evans et al. (1950) to be due to a thermolabile plant thiaminase I, and the mechanism of the reaction was partially elucidated. It was also demonstrated that autoclaving the plant abolished this capacity for inducing avitaminosis B_1 in experimental animals.

4. Bracken poisoning in pigs was reproduced by I. A. Evans et al. (1963) by feeding a balanced diet, which also contained some low-temperature dried bracken rhizome powder. The symptoms were those of avitaminosis B_1, and the animals were cured by thiamine therapy.

The above effects are adequately explained by the presence in fresh bracken of a powerful thiaminase I enzyme, and it became of interest to ascertain its distribution and seasonal variation; Fig. 1 illustrates the results obtained (Evans et al., 1975). During the winter months, the rhizomes possess a high level of activity, which begins to fall from January to April to about one-third this value. The very young frond-buds, which emerge in late April, also show a high level of activity; this drops precipitously, however, during early May as the aerial parts of the plant unfold. During the photosynthetic period, the rhizome quickly recovers its high thiaminase content, reaching a peak by August–September. The fact emerges that bracken rhizomes ploughed up in the autumn and winter months usually contain 20–40 times as much thiaminase I per unit weight compared with green fronds harvested in June–July; this observation has recently been utilized for the induction of thiamine deficiency in sheep (W. C. Evans et al., 1975).

B. Thermostable "Antithiamine" Factors

That bracken along with other plants contains water-soluble, heat-stable components which, when incubated with thiamine, especially at

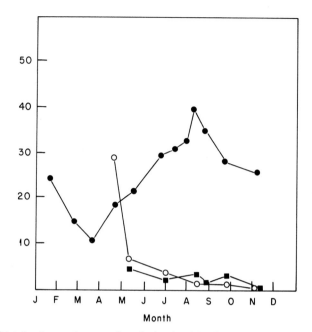

FIG. 1. Distribution and seasonal variation in thiaminase activity of bracken fern: rhizome (●——●), frond (○——○), stem (■——■). Fresh tissue (20 gm) was homogenized in citrate–phosphate buffer (100 ml, pH 6.5, 0.1 M), left overnight at 0°–4°C, filtered through muslin, and centrifuged. Clear extract was assayed by radiochemical method for thiaminase. Results are expressed (ordinate) as micrograms of thiamine destroyed per minute per gram dry weight of tissue.

pH > 7 caused some change in the thiamine molecule resulting in the failure of the thiochrome reaction subsequently to detect the vitamin in the reaction mixture, is generally agreed upon, by all workers. W. C. Evans and his collaborators (1950; Evans and Jones, 1952) asserted that whatever these thermostable factors did to thiamine, the products were still capable of behaving as thiamine in the intact animal; this conclusion was based on extensive experimentation using thiamine-deficient animals for bioassays.

The Japanese workers, Fujita (1954) and Hasegawa et al. (1956) isolated certain flavanoids from bracken (e.g., isoquercitrin, rutin, and an astragalin-type flavanol glucoside), which behaved as thermostable antithiamine substances in the thiochrome method of estimating thiamine. Dihydroxyphenols, e.g., catechol, hydroquinone, and DOPA were also very active. Attempts were made to isolate the products of reaction, and crystals tentatively called "rutinothiamine," etc., were obtained; a reassessment of this work supports the opinion that all these crystalline products are one and the same compound, thiamine disulfide (XIII) (Scheme 8) (Hasegawa *et al.*, 1956). Animal experiments, using lovebirds (*Uroloncha domestica*) showed that the products of the incubations had biological activities practically the same as those of the thiamine originally added. Although Fujita in 1954 referred to the thermostable antithiamine factor in bracken as "thiamine-decomposing," he withdrew this later on the grounds that it was not reasonable (1972).

Somogyi (1952, 1960) believes that the *chief* antithiamine activity of bracken fern is thermostable in nature, and has recently (Beruter and Somogyi, 1967) isolated caffeic acid (3,4-dihydroxycinnamic acid), the most active component present. His criteria are as follows:

1. Interference with the thiochrome method of estimating thiamine.

2. Microbiological assay: Using *Lactobacillus fermenti*, which in synthetic media has an obligate growth requirement for the intact thiamine structure. This assay appears to have been done by a collaborator of Somogyi (the last Professor Bönicke), and no details were given (Somogyi and Bönicke, 1969).

3. Action on a single nerve fiber of the frog: von Muralt (1939) suggested that thiamine plays an important role in nerve conduction in connection with the sodium transport system (von Muralt, 1958, 1962). If one bathes a node of Ranvier with neopyrithiamine (a thiamine antagonist), an almost immediate decrease in the action potential is observed. Petropulos (1960) showed that the thermostable antithiamine factors of Somogyi caused a similar phenomenon to occur. On adding thiamine to these factors prior to their application onto the nerve fiber, no action was noted. It was concluded that the blocking of the Na^+ transport system is specifically connected with the inactivation of thiamine.

Somogyi (1971) has compared the relative efficiency of several naturally occurring phenolic compounds as "antithiamine" factors in an endeavor to correlate the effect with a particular chemical grouping. The experiments were carried out at 37°C and pH 7.8, and the molecular relationship of thiamine to the phenolic derivatives was 1:3. The degree of inactivation of thiamine was measured after 16–24 hours' incubation, using the thiochrome method and microbiologically with *L. fermenti;* the following interesting results were obtained:

1. There was good agreement between the chemical and microbiological methods of assessing the inactivation of thiamine, as judged by these criteria.

2. *o*-Dihydroxyphenols were the most active antithiamine agents; caffeic acid (1 mg) accounted for about 1200 μg of thiamine. Catechol itself and many of its derivatives were as active; monophenols were inactive.

3. The activity was pH and temperature dependent, being much higher at pH 7.8 than 6.0.

4. The course of the reaction was biphasic; the initial fast reaction was independent of molecular oxygen, whereas the second-phase reaction did not take place under anaerobic conditions (see Fig. 2).

5. The initial phase was independent of the hydrogen ion concentration between pH 4.5 and 7.8; the second phase, however, took place only above pH 6.5. Temperature did not seem to affect the fast reaction, whereas the slow reaction did not take place below 20°C.

6. Significantly, cysteine and ascorbic acid (or other reducing substances) partially reversed the first reaction, whereas under the experimental conditions used the second phase was irreversible.

7. One mole of o-dihydroxyphenol inactivated several moles of thiamine.

A discussion of these results will be deferred until later.

C. INTERACTION OF THIAMINE WITH o-DIHYDROXYPHENOLS

Davies and Evans (1974) have recently investigated the products formed when thiamine labeled in the thiazole ring is incubated with caffeic acid, catechol, protocatechuic acid, and 4-methylcatechol, i.e.,

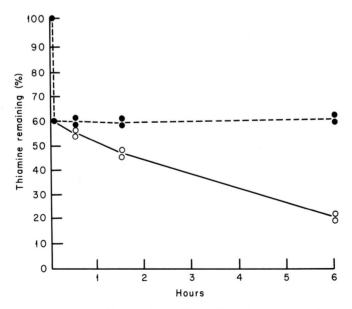

FIG. 2. Inactivation of thiamine by caffeic acid under aerobic (O——O) and anaerobic (●---●) conditions, 37°C and pH 7.5.

some of the most active thermostable antithiamine compounds, according to Somogyi (1971).

S^{35}-labeled thiamine (164 μg, radioactivity 10 μCi/ml) and the alleged "antithiamine" compound were mixed in phosphate buffer (pH 7.8, 0.1 M) to give a molar ratio of 1:3, respectively, as recommended by Somogyi (1971), and the tubes 1–4, together with a control tube (5) of thiamine and buffer alone, were incubated at 37°C for 60 hours. Samples were spotted on Cellulose (Whatman and Merck) coated thin-layer chromatography (TLC) plates (20 × 20 cm, and 5 × 20 cm), developed for 3–4 hours in n-butanol:glacial acetic acid:water (120:30:50 v/v/v), and then dried in warm air. The 20 × 20 cm TLC plates were left in contact with Kodirex X-ray films in the dark for 24 hours, and developed, and the films were examined. The plates were afterward sprayed with iodoplatinate reagent (Stahl, 1969). The 5 × 20 cm plates were examined for radioactivity in a Packard Scanner, and then sprayed with iodoplatinate. Scanner results revealed three radioactive areas in all the tubes except the control, which had only two; the R_f values of these spots are summarized in Table III.

Radioautography agreed with the Scanner results given in Table III. The contents of each tube was concentrated separately to a small volume and rechromatographed along with a marker spot, thiamine disulfide (XIII) (m.p. 177°) prepared by the method of Zima and Williams (1940); the iodoplatinate spray gave a pattern on the TLC plate illustrated by Fig. 3.

Our interpretation of the chromatogram is as follows: Spot (a) was given by all the tubes, including the control, but it was not present in authentic thiamine disulfide. It is a substance, as yet unidentified, formed from thiamine under alkaline conditions. Spot (b) represents some residual unchanged thiamine. Spot (c) moved in an identical manner to

TABLE III

THE R_f OF THE RADIOACTIVE COMPONENTS PRESENT WHEN ^{35}S-LABELED THIAMINE WAS INCUBATED WITH VARIOUS O-DIHYDROXYPHENOL DERIVATIVES

Tube No.	Antithiamine compound	R_f of radioactive areas		
		(a)	(b)	(c)
1	Caffeic acid	0.12	0.38	0.70
2	Catechol	0.11	0.38	0.69
3	Protocatechuic acid	0.13	0.37	0.65
4	4-Methylcatechol	0.08	0.33	0.71
5	None	0.15	0.41	Nil

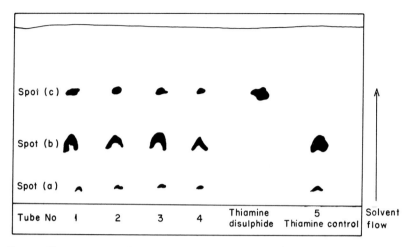

FIG. 3. Chromatogram of reaction products after incubating thiamine with *o*-dihy-droxyphenol derivatives at pH 7.8 and 37°C. Spot (a) is unidentified but appears in the thiamine control; spot (b) is thiamine; spot (c) corresponds with authentic thiamine disulfide.

authentic thiamine disulfide; a variety of different solvent systems failed to resolve the material contained in spot (c) from thiamine disulfide. We tentatively conclude, therefore, that the main product of incubation of thiamine with a number of Somogyi's "antithiamine" substances, under the conditions which he described, is one and the same, thiamine disulphide (XIII).

It is established that the thiazole ring of thiamine undergoes cleavage in alkaline solution to produce the "thiol" form (X), (Williams, 1938; Asahi, 1960) and that *o*-dihydroxyphenols (XIV) are reducing substances, easily autoxidized in air, giving *o*-quinones (XV) that can undergo further polymerization reactions, especially under alkaline conditions. It is conceivable that the thiol and *o*-quinones form an oxidation–reduction system, resulting in the production of thiamine disulfide (XIII) (Scheme 8).

Recently, Murata *et al.* (1974) reported that they could not confirm the biphasic nature of the reaction (Somogyi, 1971). They found that with most plant phenolics (e.g., flavonoids), the reaction was partially reversed by cysteine, indicating that some thiamine disulfide was formed. However, with other dihydroxyphenols (e.g., caffeic acid, catechol) there also occurred a breakdown of the thiazole moiety resulting in the formation of 2,methyl-4-amino-5-aminomethylpyrimidine (XVI), detected by chromatography; the other products of this reaction are thought to be γ-aceto-γ-mercaptopropanol and formic acid. Matsukawa

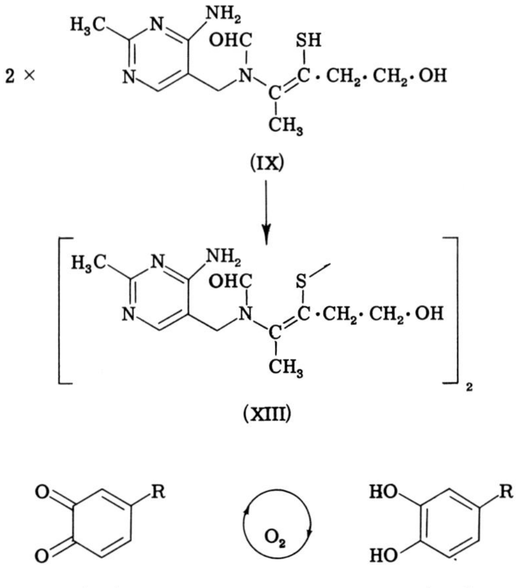

(IX) (XIII) (XV) (XIV)

SCHEME 8

et al. (1951) has already shown that these products appeared when thiamine hydrochloride is boiled in aqueous solution for some time. Our current knowledge regarding the ways which thermostable "antithiamine" factors occurring in plants modify the thiamine molecule is depicted in Scheme 9.

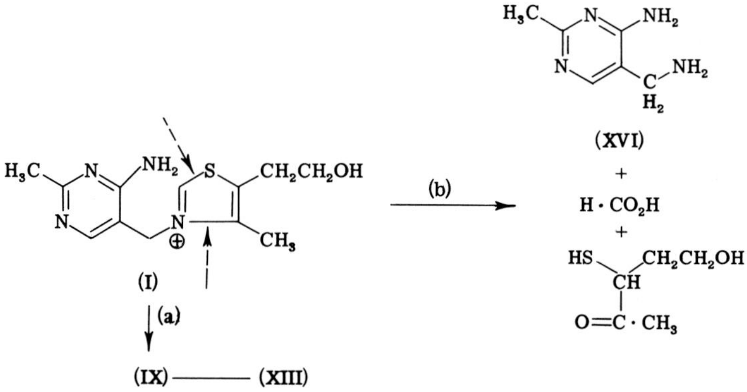

(I) (IX) (XIII) (XVI)

SCHEME 9

NOTE: The extent to which (a) and (b) occur depends on the nature of the plants polyphenols and the conditions of the reaction.

A previous claim (Matsukawa and Kawakami, 1955; Fujita et al., 1955) that some thiochrome (VI) was also formed in this reaction seems not to have been substantiated in recent years. The transformations which dihydrothiamine can undergo (Matsukawa et al., 1957) illustrate that the situation may even be more complex than that shown above, especially with some plant phenolics, e.g., dopa.

If it is accepted that Somogyi's "antithiamine" compounds change thiamine partly into thiamine disulfide (XIII) and the Grewe diamine (XVI), comments on his results recorded on pp. 480–481 may be made as follows:

The thiochrome reaction fails because it is not given by either product (XIII and XVI). If the *Lactobacillus fermenti* strain used had an obligate requirement for the intact thiamine molecule, Banhidi (1960) has shown that thiamine disulfide is inactive in this microbiological test in the absence of reducing agents, e.g., cysteine or ascorbic acid. Similarly, the diamine (XVI) will not replace thiamine as a growth factor for this organism. While not questioning the experimental finding regarding the effect of thermostable plant "antithiamine" factors on the single nerve fiber of the frog, its significance is difficult to evaluate. That the course of the alleged thiamine inactivation is biphasic is also difficult to understand; about 40% of the thiamine could not be accounted for by the thiochrome reaction within a few seconds of the addition of caffeic acid. In the presence of cysteine this fast reaction did not occur; on the other hand, Murata et al. (1974) could not confirm this phenomenon. One plausible explanation is that some samples of caffeic acid and other o-dihydroxyphenol derivatives in aqueous solutions, especially at alkaline pH and with trace amounts of certain metallic ions, quickly autooxidize giving an equilibrium mixture containing some quinonoid forms of these molecules; these could immediately convert the thiol form of thiamine (IX) into thiamine disulfide (XIII). The dependence of the second slower phase of the reaction on pH, temperature, and supply of oxygen is to be expected if indeed the catechol derivatives act as oxidation–reduction catalysts in this reaction.

While conceding that the products formed when thiamine is incubated with boiled aqueous extracts of some plants are of academic interest, these so-called thermostable "antithiamine" factors appear to have little nutritional significance to an animal maintained on a diet containing these plant materials. Evans and his collaborators (1950, 1952, 1975) have shown that steaming abolishes the ability of bracken fern to induce thiamine deficiency in animals; this treatment also inactivates thiaminase I in the plant. The implication is that under these physiological conditions no "antithiamine" activity remains that is capable of denying the vitamin supply to the animal.

It is pertinent to recall that saliva is alleged to contain an enzyme that acts on thiamine in such a way as to give negative results in the thiochrome reaction; the product is thiamine disulfide (XIII) according to Miura *et al.* (1950) and Yasuda (1953). This thiol oxidase (Thiol:oxygen oxidoreductase, EC 1.8.3.2) has an optimum pH of 8 and temperature of 70°C; if the reaction product is incubated at pH 5 with cysteine, thiamine is recovered. Molecular oxygen is an obligate requirement for the reaction (Scheme 10).

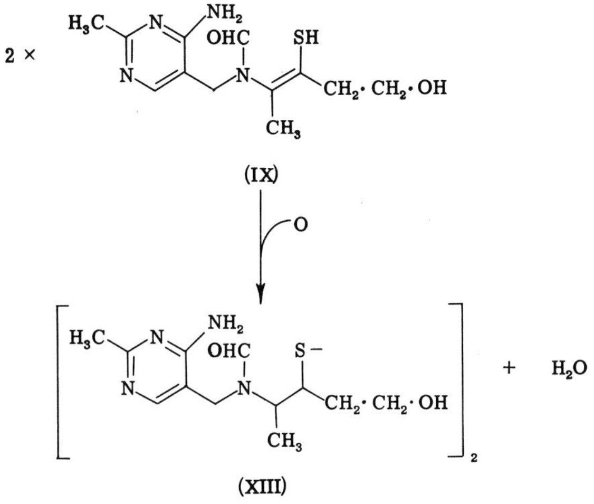

SCHEME 10

V. EFFECTS OF THIAMINASES ON ANIMALS

The history of the discovery, isolation, synthesis, and mode of action of vitamin B_1 in animal nutrition has been told by some of the "dramatis personae" themselves, e.g., Williams (1961), Peters (1967), and Krampitz (1969, 1970): there remained many unsolved problems connected with thiamine in 1962 (Furness, 1962). In thiamine deficiency, the biochemical reactions catalyzed by thiamine pyrophosphate (TPP cocarboxylase) dependent enzymes are impaired; these are reflected in abnormal blood chemistry called "biochemical lesions" by Peters (1963), which can be measured. The commonly used biochemical indicators of thiamine deficiency are an elevated blood pyruvate and a lowered thiamine value; or a sensitive TPP-dependent enzyme, e.g., erythrocyte transketolase measurement (Brin *et al.*, 1960; Warnock, 1970). Accompanying these are the sequence of clinical symptoms of anorexia, incoordination, opisthotonus, and death. The avitaminosis B_1 syndrome usually responds dramatically to thiamine administration provided the condition is not too far advanced. At postmortem, the diagnostic lesions are found in the nervous system when examined microscopically and also in the heart.

Since thiaminase I and II are enzymes which destroy thiamine, and the former thiamine pyrophosphate as well, incorporation of naturally occurring sources of these enzymes in the diet of mammals results in an induced thiamine deficiency—in spite of the fact that, initially, the ration may have contained very adequate amounts of the vitamin. Thiaminase I in fact, is probably the most efficient way of rendering a mixed diet devoid of thiamine, and this enzyme is a valuable tool in nutritional research. Some naturally occurring diseases of livestock, previously of obscure etiology, have in recent years also been shown to be due *either* to the ingestion of foodstuffs containing the enzyme or because their alimentary tract harbors bacteria that elaborate it. These advances in our knowledge have been of value in animal health and of economic benefit to agriculture; they will now be briefly outlined.

1. *Chastek Paralysis*

This disease in silver foxes was the first to be recognized as acute thiamine deficiency brought about by thiaminase I in a component of the diet [carp viscera (spleen, kidney), but not muscle]. C. A. Evans *et al.* (1942) found that sections of the brain and spinal cord revealed small spotlike hemorrhages that could usually be seen by the naked eye. Microscopically, the changes appeared to be vascular—small blood vessels had undergone irregular dilatation and vast proliferation of their endothelium. The lesions involved only some of the paraventricular nuclei, but were commonly found in the inferior olive and the cortex of the splenial gyrus. They were not encountered in the white substance. The brain lesions of Wernicke's disease in man due to chronic alcoholism have been shown by Alexander *et al.* (1941) to be almost identical.

There have been recorded in the literature other examples of thiamine deficiency resulting from the inclusion of raw fish offal in the diet, e.g., when fed to mink and other small animals; the food industry is now well aware of the phenomenon and of the necessity of inactivating the enzyme by a heat process.

2. *Thiaminase Disease of Microbial Origin*

a. General. Matsukawa and Mosawa (1949) first discovered thiaminase-elaborating bacteria because aqueous suspension of human feces from patients with beriberi or hypothiaminosis (subacute thiamine deficiency) showed thiaminase activity. Subsequently, the Japanese workers recognized "thiaminase bacillary carriers," i.e., normal individuals, showing no biochemical lesions or clinical symptoms, from whom these bacteria could be isolated by enrichment culture of their feces. *Bacillus thiaminolyticus* (a spore-forming aerobe) and *Clostridium thiaminolyticum* (a sporulating obligate anaerobe) produced thiaminase I, and the third organism *Bacillus aneurinolyticus* (another spore-forming aerobe) was unusual in that it elaborated thiaminase II. These bacteria have since been isolated from the feces of a large variety of animal species, from fodder, and from soils. Kimura (1965) expressed the view that it cannot be considered that thiaminase bacteria are the sole etiological agents of beriberi.

Hamada (1954) studied the effects of oral administration of *Bacillus thiaminolyticus* to various animals, and found that the ease of its establishment in the intestinal tract was in the order: cat, guinea pig, rat, hen, rabbit. Cats developed thiaminase disease (i.e., avitaminosis B_1) easily, but the organism had no effect on sheep. W. C. Evans *et al.* (1958) gave by rumen fistulas, 10-liter cultures of *Bacillus thiaminolyticus* and *Clostridium thiaminolyticum* daily to yearling Welsh Black bullocks for 6 weeks; the animals showed no ill effects whatsoever, either during this period or later. Since then, we have given, intrarumenally, cultures of these three (human) species of bacteria to individual sheep on a normal hay and sheep-pellet diet, for a period of 3 months without producing symptoms of thiamine deficiency. Hamada (1954) observed that the growth of *Bacillus thiaminolyticus* was inhibited by various bile samples; he therefore presumed that the amount of bile and/or bile acids in the intestine were factors determining the ease of establishment of the organism in the alimentary tract of animals. Little is known regarding the relationships and interactions between thiaminase bacteria and their host animals.

b. Cerebrocortical Necrosis (CCN) in Ruminants. In 1956, a disease of sheep and cattle, called polioencephalomalacia, was described by Jensen, Griner, and Adams in the United States; later, Terlecki and Markson (1959) recognized a similar clinicopathological entity in Britain, which they called cerebrocortical necrosis, or CCN. The first symptoms in sheep appeared to be anorexia and aimless wandering, accompanied by amaurosis. Subsequently, ataxia developed and rapidly became worse, exhibiting opisthotonus and nystagmus; coma ensued, and ultimately death. At postmortem, the brain was visibly abnormal, showing a yellowish discoloration and swollen areas in the cerebral gyri. Histopathology revealed a focal necrosis of the cerebral cortex, which has been described in detail by Terlecki and Markson (1961). Later, Pill (1967) showed that these animals were thiamine deficient and, in many cases, responded to vitamin B_1 therapy. It remained unclear how the avitaminosis B_1 was brought about until Edwin *et al.* (1968b; see also Edwin and

Lewis, 1971) observed that rumen liquor from CCN cases possessed thiaminase I activity at higher levels than in healthy ruminants (cf. also Roberts and Boyd, 1974). The source of production of this enzyme is now believed to be of microbial origin (Shreeve and Edwin, 1974). Recently, Edwin and Jackman (1974) reported that, so far, the only thiaminase I-producing isolate from rumen liquor of CCN cases has been *Clostridium sporogenes* (cf. Hayashi *et al.*, 1964, but see Morgan and Lawson, 1974).

The disease has not been experimentally induced by the administration per os of any thiaminase elaborating microorganism or of rumen liquor from CCN cases, to healthy sheep, at least so far as the author is aware. A thiamine antagonist, amprolium [1-(4-amino-2-*n*-propyl-5-pyrimidinylmethyl)-2-picolinum chloride hydrochloride, Merck, Sharp and Dohme Ltd.] in massive doses given orally to preruminant calves (Markson *et al.*, 1966), ruminating calves (Markson *et al.*, 1974), and some adult sheep (Loew and Dunlop, 1972) has produced a condition indistinguishable from CCN. None of the other well-known antagonists, e.g., oxythiamine or pyrithiamine, were effective at the dose level tried (Pill *et al.*, 1966; Markson *et al.*, 1972), and neither was sodium sulfite fed in an attempt to destroy the thiamine (Edwin *et al.*, 1968b).

3. *Thiamine Deficiency Disease Caused by Thiaminases of Plant Origin*

The bracken fern (*Pteridium aquilinum*) is one of the most persistent weeds that the hill farmer has to deal with in the temperate zone. Recent estimates show that a million acres of rough grazings are densely covered by the plant in Britain alone. Reports from the North and South Americas (both the Atlantic and Pacific coasts), Australia, New Zealand, Europe (especially Brittany and Turkey), and Africa (Kenya) indicate its wide distribution and consequent problems. Horsetail (*Equisetum arvense*) is another pteridophyte that infests pastureland, although not so extensively as the bracken fern. W. C. Evans *et al.* (1950) demonstrated biochemically, and by using the rat as a bioassay, that both these plants contain thiaminase I.

a. Horse Bracken Staggers. Bracken staggers in the horse was recorded by Muller in 1897, and since then a similar condition resulting from eating horsetail has been described (Forenbacher, 1950). The visual symptoms are incoordination, the lub-dubb of the heartbeat becomes very pronounced after mild exercise and, as the disease progresses, severe muscular tremors appear; these are followed by convulsive seizures and death. In 1949, W. C. Evans and his collaborators (Roberts *et al.*, 1949; Evans *et al.*, 1951) reproduced this disease experimentally by feeding bracken hay and showed that it was an induced thiamine deficiency;

it responded to thiamine therapy if the vitamin was given at the onset of clinical symptoms. Welsh Mountain ponies grazing bracken-infested hills have been known to develop the condition; they too recover after administration of the vitamin. Bracken that was autoclaved (thus inactivating thiaminase I) was incapable of inducing the disease (Chamberlain, 1959).

Table IV records the sequence of events during the experimental reproduction of horse bracken staggers, and Fig. 4 shows stills from a cine film, taken during a typical stagger, ending in the characteristic stance with the hind legs placed wide apart (E. T. R. Evans et al., 1951). Forenbacher (1950, 1951) investigated the poisoning of horses by *Equisetum* sp. contaminating hay in Yugoslavia and reproduced the condition; its clinical pathology resembled bracken staggers, and the disease responded to thiamine therapy.

b. Bracken Rhizome Poisoning of Pigs. It has been claimed that pigs are useful in clearing bracken-infested land, by virtue of their capacity to root up the rhizomes and trample the fronds. Suspected cases of "bracken poisoning" in pigs had been reported, however, under field conditions, but its nature remained obscure (Blakeway, 1924; Swann and Barrowman, 1959). The animals showed signs of listlessness and partial inappetence, or cases appeared to have succumbed suddenly. The condition was reproduced by I. A. Evans et al. (1963) and W. C. Evans et al. (1972) by feeding a balanced diet mixed with 25% low-temperature-dried ground bracken rhizomes either as a dry or wet wash. The first signs of "poisoning" was a rise in blood pyruvate and a fall in transketolase activity, followed by anorexia; terminal symptoms of recumbency and dyspnea appeared suddenly, and death occurred within about 6 hours

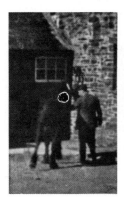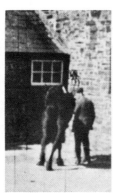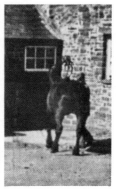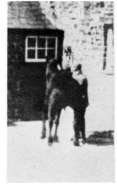

FIG. 4. Bracken staggers in the horse. Stills from a cine-film taken during a typical stagger; note the stance with hind legs well apart, after the stagger is over.

TABLE IV

Observations during the Experimental Reproduction of Bracken Staggers in the Horse

Date, 1949	Days of experiment	Weight (pounds)	Rectal temp. (°F)	Heart rate/minute	Blood pyruvate (mg/100 ml)	Blood thiamine (μg/100 ml)	Thiamine therapy (dose, in mg, subcutaneous injection)
July 8	1	1036	99.4	32	2.2	8.5	—
July 14	7	—	99.5	48	—	—	—
July 22	15	1076	99.8	34	2.6	7.8	—
Aug. 9	33	—	104.5	52	3.5	3.25	—
Aug. 10	34	1018	104	68	—	—	—
Aug. 11	35	—	103.5	68	6.25	2.5	—
Aug. 12	36	—	101.6	Arrhythmia	5.75	3.0	2(100)
Aug. 13	37	—	103	70	3.2	—	100
Aug. 14	38	—	103	66	—	—	100
Aug. 15	39	942	102	40	3.5	—	100
Aug. 16	40	—	100.4	40	—	—	100
Aug. 17	41	989	100	48	3.2	—	100
Aug. 19	43	1030	101.3	35	2.9	11.5	—
Aug. 22	46	—	100.4	48	2.1	7.0	—
Aug. 26	50	—	100.5	32	2.3	—	—
Aug. 31	55	1018	100.8	38	—	—	—
Sept. 7	62	982	98.5	38	—	—	—
Sept. 16	71	968	100	28	4.2	4.0	—
Sept. 21	76	964	101	28	5.8	2.8	—
Sept. 22	77	—	102 (A.M.)	80	8.5	—	4(100)
			104 (P.M.)	80 (app.)			
Sept. 23	78	Dead					

(Fig. 5). Gross postmortem lesions were dominated by an enlarged mottled heart, and evidence in other organs suggestive of acute heart failure. Microscopically, the heart revealed lesions similar to those described in experimental thiamine deficiency in pigs (Fig. 6). The symptoms were all corrected by parenteral injections of thiamine, and, provided these were given periodically, no other effect was observed on prolonged feeding of the rhizome diet.

   c. *Thiamine Deficiency in Sheep, with Lesions Similar to Those of Cerebrocortical Necrosis (CCN).* The naturally occurring disease termed cerebrocortical necrosis of ruminants has been described (Section V, 2, b).

   Acute thiamine deficiency has been produced in lambs and calves by feeding a thiamine-free diet (Draper and Johnson, 1951). Once the rumen flora develops, bacterial synthesis of the B vitamins is able to meet the metabolic requirements of these animals (Kon and Porter, 1954); mature ruminants do not need an exogenous source of these essential nutrients (Virtanen, 1963).

   Homogastric animals, as we have seen, develop avitaminosis B_1 when fed a complete diet mixed with low temperature-dried green bracken frond powder. Ruminating animals do not show clinical thiamine deficiency on such diets. Cattle succumb to the bone-marrow toxin, also present in this plant, to the effects of which this species is particularly sensitive (W. C. Evans *et al.*, 1951, 1954, 1958). Sheep can tolerate higher dosages of this poisonous substance, and simple-stomached animals (e.g., rat pig, and horse) are even more resistant to its action (Humphreys, 1963).

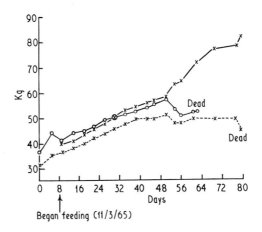

FIG. 5. Bracken rhizome poisoning in the pig. Live weight gains and outcome of the experiment. ×——×, Control pig; ×---×, dry rhizome pig; ○——○, wet rhizome pig.

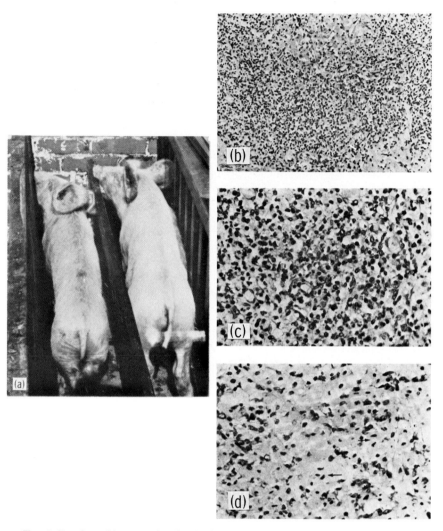

FIG. 6. Bracken rhizome poisoning in the pig. (a) Pig 1 (right) received the basal sow and weaner ration. Pig 2 (left) received the basal ration plus rhizome in a 3:1 mixture. (b–d) The principal histological lesions were in the heart and correspond with those described in experimental thiamine deficiency in the pig (Follis *et al.*, 1943; Miller *et al.*, 1955). (b) Myocardium. Note extensive area of lytic degeneration of muscle fibers with activation and proliferation of endomysium. (c) Detail from (b) showing almost empty network of activated endomysium. (d) Area of more acute necrosis of muscle fibers with eosinophilic, hyaline cytoplasm, and pycnotic nuclei (arrows). (b–d) Hematoxylin and eosin. (b) ×175; (c, d) ×450.

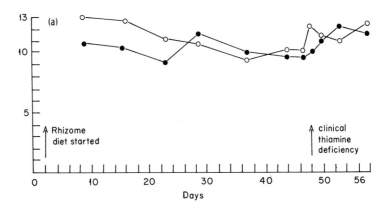

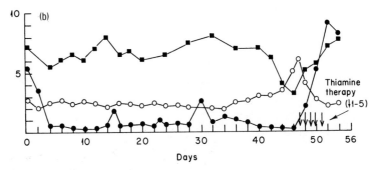

FIG. 7. Hematological and biochemical parameters of a sheep during the induction of acute thiamine deficiency by the bracken rhizome diet. (a) Leukocytes (O——O) $\times 10^3/mm^3$; platelets (●——●) $\times 10^5/mm^3$. Note that these remained within normal limits; sheep are relatively resistant to the cattle bracken poisoning factor (W. C. Evans et al., 1951, 1954). (b) Blood thiamine (■——■), micrograms per 100 ml; blood pyruvic acid (O——O), milligrams per 100 ml; urinary thiamine (●——●), milligrams per 24-hour sample $\times 10$; thiamine therapy (↓, 1–5), 100 mg initially, then 20 mg per day for 4 days, by which time the sheep had recovered.

While investigating the quantitative distribution and seasonal variations of thiaminase I in the bracken plant, it was found that the level of activity of the enzyme in the rhizome is several times higher than in the frond (see Fig. 1). By taking advantage of his fact, W. C. Evans et al. (1975) have now produced acute thiamine deficiency in adult sheep by feeding a well-balanced diet mixed with low temperature-dried rhizome powder. Autoclaving the rhizome powder abolished its capacity to induce avitaminosis B_1, because this procedure inactivated thiaminase I. The rhizome powder used destroyed about 80 μg of thiamine per minute per gram (radiochemical assay), and the minimum quantity required was 15–25% by weight of the pelleted green dried-grass plus cake-concentrate ration. When this plant source of thiaminase I formed 25–35% of the diet, symptoms took from 25 to 40 days to develop—roughly the time required in homogastric animals. Decreasing the concentration to 15% prolonged this time to 3 months, and a 5% level did not produce the disease. Thiaminase I activity was present in the contents from all parts of the alimentary tract and feces of sheep fed the rhizome diets; some particles of rhizome powder escape digestion and can even be seen in the feces. When the concentration of enzyme was insufficient to cause the clinical syndrome, the sheep nevertheless did not thrive as well as animals fed autoclaved rhizome diets.

Sheep made thiamine deficient in this way exhibited all the biochemical and clinical features characteristic of avitaminosis B_1 in simple-stomached animals, and the response to thiamine therapy was dramatic in the early stages of the disease. Figures 7–9 illustrate these findings, in-

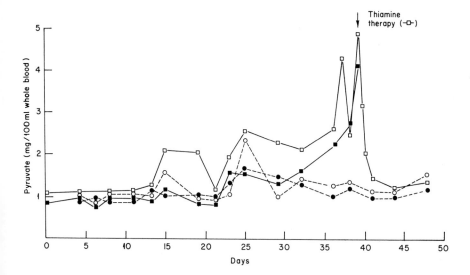

Fig. 8. Blood pyruvic acid of sheep fed rhizome and autoclaved rhizome diets. Sheep 1 (■——■), on active rhizome diet, developed a high blood pyruvic acid and clinical symptoms of acute thiamine deficiency. It was killed on day 40, for biochemical and pathological investigations. Sheep 2 (□——□), on active rhizome diet developed symptoms similar to those of sheep 1; the blood pyruvate returned to within the normal range on thiamine therapy, and the animal recovered. Sheep 3 and 4 (●---●, ○---○), on autoclaved rhizome diets (which inactivate thiaminase), showed blood pyruvates within the normal range, and the animals remained healthy.

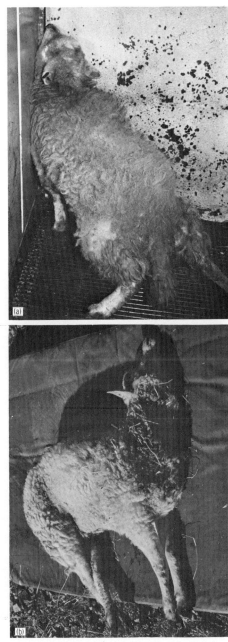

FIG. 9. Stance and opisthotonus exhibited by sheep with acute thiamine deficiency
on the rhizome diet.

cluding the typical opisthotonus exhibited during the acute phase of the clinical syndrome. The gross postmortem appearance was not very informative until the brain was exposed. This was visibly abnormal, with swollen areas in the cerebral gyri, showing a yellowish discoloration; the morbid anatomy appeared identical with field cases of cerebrocortical necrosis (CCN) in sheep. When viewed under UV light, parts of the brain showed a creamy-colored fluorescence, attributed by Ziffo and Inglis (1974) to the necrotic areas. After fixation in 10% neutral formol saline, the brains were sent to the Central Veterinary Laboratory, Weybridge, Surrey, England for histological examination; histopathology confirmed the diagnosis of CCN (Fig. 10).

That thiamine deficiency, accompanied by the histopathological lesions of CCN, can be experimentally induced in sheep by the inclusion of a plant source of thiaminase I at the requisite level in the diet lends credence to the view that CCN is a "thiaminase disease" of ruminants.

There have now been encountered many examples of the consequences to animals of ingesting feedstuffs containing an active source of thiaminase, or those developing a gut microflora that produces this enzyme *in situ* to an excessive degree; these are summarized in Table V.

TABLE V
OCCURRENCE AND EFFECTS OF THIAMINASE IN ANIMALS

Thiaminase (source)	Animal species (avitaminosis B_1)	Authors
Cyprinidae		
Carp viscera	Silver fox (Chastek paralysis)	C. A. Evans *et al.* (1942)
Pteridophytes		
Bracken (fronds)	Rat	Weswig *et al.* (1946)
Bracken (fronds)	Horse (staggers)	Roberts *et al.* (1949)
Bracken (rhizomes)	Pig	I. A. Evans *et al.* (1963)
Bracken (rhizomes)	Sheep	W. C. Evans *et al.* (1975)
Horsetail	Horse (staggers)	Forenbacher (1950)
Microorganisms		
Bacillus thiaminolyticus *Clostridium thiaminolyticum* *Bacillus aneurinolyticus*	Human (a form of beri-beri) (also cats, guinea pigs, rats, hens, and rabbits)	Matsukawa *et al.* (1954), Kimura (1965)
Unidentified	Sheep and cattle (CCN)	Pill (1967)
Clostridium sporogenes?	Sheep and cattle (CCN)	Edwin and Jackman (1974); Morgan and Lawson (1974).

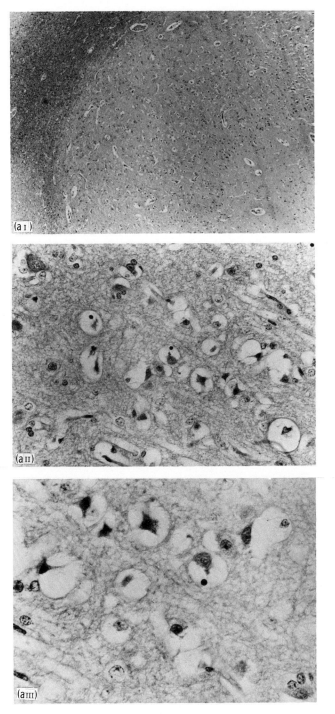

Fig. 10. Thiamine-deficient sheep. (a) Cerebral cortex: (I) ×90, (II) × 387, (III) × 621. (b) Cerebrum of sheep: (I) × 90, (II) × 387, (III) × 621. The sections

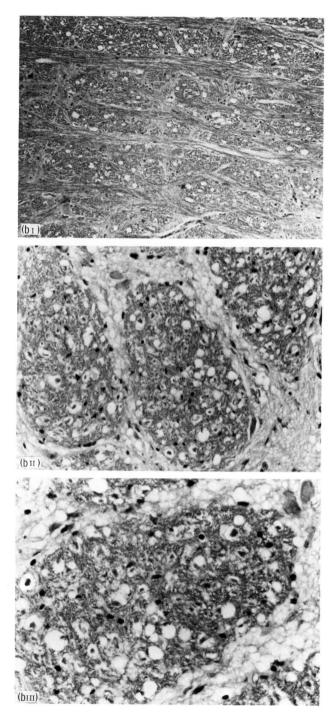

show shrunken and necrotic neurons with perineuronal vacuolation. Hematoxylin and eosin.

VI. PHYSIOLOGICAL SIGNIFICANCE OF THE THIAMINASES

The function of thiaminases in the economy of the cells which contain them is a baffling problem in view of their limited and even bizarre distribution. If the necessary precautions are taken, it can be shown that the thiaminase-containing tissues also yield thiamine (Table VI). This substrate, cosubstrate, and enzyme are therefore either in separate compartments or enzyme action is under the control of some unknown mechanism.

The transfer reaction catalyzed by thiaminase I is reversible with some amines, but *in vitro* the equilibrium is unfavorable for thiamine synthesis (Fujita, 1954); this need not be a stumbling block *in vivo*, since mechanisms may exist for the removal of the thiamine formed from the site of enzyme action. However, the known pathways of thiamine biosynthesis in microbes and plants proceed by other mechanisms (Mitsuda *et al.*, 1969; Nose *et al.*, 1969), and the direct synthesis of thiamine by thiaminase action has never been demonstrated *in vivo*.

Woolley (1951, 1953) suggested that thiamine was not the only substrate of thiaminase within the cell; carp thiaminase I transferred *p*-aminobenzoylglutamate to the pteridine analog of thiamine to produce folic acid, but the yield was extremely small. Fancifully, he visualized a new kind of biosynthetic mechanism in which the driving force resides not in a phosphate bond, but in a quaternary ammonium ion, which is reduced to a tertiary amine during the reaction.

TABLE VI

THIAMINE CONTENTS OF TISSUES CONTAINING THIAMINASE[a]

Species	Thiamine content (μg/gm fresh wt.)
Shellfish	
Meretrix meretrix (clam)	0.50
Paphia philippinarum	0.43
Corbicula laena	0.37
Viviparus mellaetus	0.43
Cristaria plicata	0.50
Plants	
Pteridium aquilinum	0.45
Osmunda japonica	0.65
Equisetum arvense	2.17
Bacteria (peptone broth)	
Bacillus thiaminolyticus	3.20
Bacillus aneurinolyticus	3.0–4.0

[a] Fujita (1954), Murata (1965).

Certain purines and pyrimidines are active as acceptor amines in the thiaminase I reaction; Pirie (1959) found that the infective nucleic acid of tobacco mosaic virus lost its infectivity when treated with a thiaminase preparation from bracken in the presence of thiamine, but not with either alone. It is an assumption, however, that thiaminase was the effective ingredient in the preparation.

Ikehata (1956) made the interesting observation that the production of thiaminase II by *Bacillus aneurinolyticus* was repressed by thiamine in the medium; a specific function for thiaminases of microbial origin has not been discovered.

The elucidation of the role of thiaminases within the cells which contain them remains a task for the future. They may be "fossil" enzymes that once catalyzed an essential reaction since achieved by other mechanisms, but have continued to be coded for, through some quirk of nature, by the genome of a few disparate forms of life.

ACKNOWLEDGMENTS

The author wishes to thank his technical and secretarial staff, research students, colleagues, veterinarians, and farmers for their enthusiastic collaboration and the Agricultural Research Council for their financial support.

REFERENCES

Ågren, G. (1945). *Acta Physiol. Scand.* **10**, 381.
Ågren, G. (1946). *Acta Physiol. Scand.* **12**, 34.
Alexander. L., Green, R. G., Evans, C. A., and Wolf, L. E. (1941). *Trans. Amer. Neurol Ass.* **67**, 119.
Aoki, F. (1955). *Vitamins* **9**, 48.
Asahi, Y. (1960). *Yakugaku Zasshi* **80**, 1093.
Bánhidi, Z. G. (1960). *J. Bacteriol.* **79**, 181.
Barnhurst, J. D., and Hennessy, D. J. (1952). *J. Amer. Chem. Soc.* **74**, 356.
Beruter, J., and Somogyi, J. C. (1967). *Experientia* **23**, 996.
Bhagvat, K., and Devi, P. (1944). *Indian J. Med. Res.* **32**, 131 and 139.
Blakeway, J. (1924). *Vet. J.* **80**, 89.
Brin, M., Tai, M., Ostashever, A. S., and Kalinsky, H. (1960). *J. Nutr.* **71**, 273.
Chamberlain, A. G. (1959). Ph.D. Thesis, University of Wales, Bangor.
Davies, W. E. J., and Evans, W. C. (1974). To be published.
Draper, H. H., and Johnson, B. C. (1951). *J. Nutr.* **43**, 413.
Ebata, J., and Murata, K. (1961). *J. Vitaminol. (Kyoto)* **7**, 115.
Edwin, E. E., and Jackman, R. (1970). *Nature (London)* **228**, 772.
Edwin, E. E., and Jackman, R. (1974). *J. Sci. Food Agr.* **25**, 357.
Edwin, E. E., and Lewis, G. (1971). *J. Dairy Res.* **38**, 79.
Edwin, E. E., Lewis, G., and Allcroft, R. (1968a). *Vet. Rec.* **83**, 176.
Edwin, E. E., Spence, J. B., and Wood, A. J. (1968b). *Vet. Rec.* **83**, 417.
Evans, C. A., Carlson, W. E., and Green, R. G. (1942). *Amer. J. Pathol.* **18**, 79.
Evans, E. T. R., Evans, W. C., and Roberts, H. E. (1951). *Brit. Vet. J.* **107**, 364.
Evans, I. A., Humphreys, D. J., Goulden, L., Thomas, A. J., and Evans, W. C. (1963). *J. Comp. Pathol.* **73**, 229.

Evans, W. C., and Evans, E. T. R. (1949). *Brit. Vet. J.* **105,** 175.

Evans, W. C., and Jones, N. R. (1952). *Biochem. J.* **50,** xxxviii.

Evans, W. C., Jones, N. R., and Evans, R. A. (1950). *Biochem. J.* **46,** xxxviii.

Evans, W. C., Evans, E. T. R., and Hughes, L. E. (1951). *Vet. Rec.* **63,** 444.

Evans, W. C., Evans, E. T. R., and Hughes, L. E. (1954). *Brit. Vet. J.* **110,** 295.

Evans, W. C., Evans, I. A., Thomas, A. J., Watkin, J. E., and Chamberlain, A. J. (1958). *Brit. Vet. J.* **114,** 180.

Evans, W. C., Widdop, B., and Harding, J. D. (1972). *Vet. Rec.* **90,** 471.

Evans, W. C., Evans, I. A., Humphreys, D. J., Lewin, B., Davies, W. E. J., and Axford, R. F. E. (1975). *J. Comp. Pathol.* **85,** 253.

Florkin, M., and Stotz, E. H. eds. (1973). "Comprehensive Biochemistry," Vol. 13. Elsevier, Amsterdam.

Follis, B. H., Miller, M. H., Wintrobe, M. M., and Stein, H. S. (1943). *Amer. J. Pathol.* 19, 341.

Forenbacher, S. (1950). *Vet. Arh.* **20,** 405.

Forenbacher, S. (1951). *Vet. Arh.* **21,** 497.

Fujita, A. (1954). *Advan. Enzymol.* **19,** 389.

Fujita, A. (1972). *J. Vitaminol. (Kyoto)* **18,** 67.

Fujita, A., and Numata, I. (1942). *18th Annu. Meet., Jap. Biochem. Soc.*

Fujita, A., Nose, Y., and Okamoto, T. (1951). *Vitamins* **4,** 138.

Fujita, A., Okamoto, T., and Nose, Y. (1955). *J. Vitaminol.* **1,** 208.

Furness, N. (1962). *Ann. N.Y. Acad. Sci.* **98,** 383.

Green, R. G., Carlson, W. E., and Evans, C. A. (1941). *J. Nutr.* **21,** 243.

Green, R. G., Carlson, W. E., and Evans, C. A. (1942). *J. Nutr.* **23,** 165.

Hamada, K. (1954). *Vitamins* **7,** 65 and 70.

Hamada, K. (1956). *J. Vitaminol. (Kyoto)* **2,** 67.

Harris, L. J., and Wang, Y. L. (1943). *Biochem. J.* **37,** 433.

Hasegawa, E., and Ueda, K. (1953). *Seikagaku* **25,** 81.

Hasegawa, E., Sakamoto, S., Nagayama, K., and Fujita, A. (1956). *J. Vitaminol.* **2,** 31.

Hayashi, R., Yoshii, Z., Harada, T., Nigota, K., Tsubota, Y., Shibutake, M., Sasaki, M., Suzaki, S., and Takagi, T. (1964). *J. Vitaminol. (Kyoto)* **10,** 168.

Humphreys, D. J. (1963). Ph.D. Thesis, University of Wales, Bangor.

Ikehata, H. (1956). *Vitamins* **10,** 233.

Ikehata, H. (1960). *J. Gen. Appl. Microbiol.* **6,** 30.

Jensen, R., Griner, L. A., and Adams, O. R. (1956). *J. Amer. Vet. Med. Ass.* **129,** 311.

Jones, N. R. (1950). M.Sc. Thesis, University of Wales, Bangor.

Jones, N. R. (1952). Ph.D. Thesis, University of Wales, Bangor.

Kenten, R. H. (1957). *Biochem. J.* **67,** 25.

Kenten, R. H. (1958). *Biochem. J.* **69,** 439.

Kimura, R. (1965). In "Beriberi and Thiamin" (N. Shimazoni and E. Katsura, eds.), p. 255. Vitamin B Res. Comm. Japan. "Igaku-Shoin", Tokyo.

Kimura, R., and Aoyama, S. (1951). *Vitamins* **4,** 366.

Kimura, R., Liao, T. H., Hayashi, R., and Nakayama, H. (1952). *Vitamins* **5,** 521.

Kon, S. K., and Porter, J. W. G. (1954). *Vitam. Horm. (New York)* **12,** 53.

Krampitz, L. O. (1969). *J. Vitaminol. (Kyoto)* **15,** 321.

Krampitz, L. O. (1970). "Thiamin Diphosphate and its Catalytic Functions." Dekker, New York.

Krampitz, L. O., and Woolley, D. W. (1944). *J. Biol. Chem.* **152,** 9.

Kupstas, E. E., and Hennessey, D. J. (1957). *J. Amer. Chem. Soc.* **79,** 5217.

Kuratani, K. (1955). *Seikagaku* **27,** 579.

Lieck, H., and Ågren, G. (1944). *Acta Physiol. Scand.* **8,** 203.

Loew, F. M., and Dunlop, R. H. (1972). *Amer. J. Vet. Res.* **33,** 2195.

Makino, K., and Koike, M. (1954). *Nature (London)* **173,** 34.

Makino, K., Kinoshita, T., Aramaki, Y., and Shintani, S. (1954). *Nature (London)* **173,** 275.

Markson, L. M., Terlecki, S., and Lewis, G. (1966). *Vet. Rec.* **79,** 578.

Markson, L. M., Lewis, G., Terlecki, S., Edwin, E. E., and Ford, J. E. (1972). *Brit. Vet. J.* **128,** 488.

Markson, L. M., Edwin, E. E., Lewis, G., and Richardson, C. (1974). *Brit. Vet. J.* **130,** 9.

Matsukawa, D., and Kawakami, T. (1955). *J. Vitaminol.* **1,** 208.

Matsukawa, D., and Misawa, H. (1949). *Proc. Comm. Vitamin B Res.* **31,** 16.

Matsukawa, T., and Yurugi, S. (1952). *J. Pharm. Soc. Jap.* **72,** 33.

Matsukawa, T., and Yurugi, S. (1965). *In* "Beriberi and Thiamin" (N. Shimazono and E. Katsura, eds.), p. 81. Vitamin B Res. Comm. Jap.

Matsukawa, T., Misawa, H., Fujimiya, M., Kobayashi, H., Horikawa, Y., and Takato, T. (1954). *J. Vitaminol. (Kyoto)* **1,** 43.

Matsukawa, T., Hirano, H., Iwatsu, T., and Yurugi, S. (1957). *J. Vitaminol. (Kyoto)* **3,** 218.

Melnick, D., and Field, H., Jr. (1939). *J. Biol. Chem.* **127,** 505.

Miller, E. R., Schmidt, D. A., Hoeffer, J. A., and Luecke, R. W. (1955). *J. Nutr.* **56,** 423.

Mitsuda, H., Tanaka, T., Kawai, F., and Yasumoto, K. (1969). *J. Vitaminol.ʾ (Kyoto)* **15,** 328.

Miura, U., Fujiwara, M., and Watanabe, H. (1950). *Vitamins* **3,** 239.

Morgan, K. T., and Lawson, G. H. K. (1974). *Vet. Rec.* **95,** 361.

Muller, H. (1897). "Landwirthschaftliche Giftlehre" (cited in Lander's "Veterinary Toxicology" Baillière, London, 1926).

Murata, K. (1965). *in* "Beriberi and Thiamin" (N. Shimasono and E. Katsura, eds.), p. 220. Vitam. B Res. Comm. Jap.

Murata, K., and Ebata, J. (1959). *Vitamins* **18,** 497.

Murata, K., Ikehata, H., Koizumi, Y., and Hase, S. (1961a). *Proc. Vitamin Res. Comm. Jap.* No. 124.

Murata, K., Ikehata, H., Koizumi, Y., and Hase, S. (1961b). *Vitamins* **22,** 239.

Murata, K., Ebata, J., Somekawa, M., and Marukawa, S. (1968). *J. Vitaminol. (Kyoto)* **14,** 12.

Murata, K., Tanaka, R., and Yamaoka, M. (1974). *J. Nutr. Sci. Vitaminol* **20,** 351.

Nishio, K. (1957). *Vitamins* **13,** 94.

Nose, Y., Kawasaki, T., and Iwashim, A. (1969). *J. Vitaminol. (Kyoto)* **15,** 329.

Ono, T., and Kawasaki, M. (1968). *J. Vitaminol. (Kyoto)* **14,** 179.

Peters, R. A. (1963). *In* "Biochemical Lesions and Lethal Synthesis" (D. Alexander and Z. N. Bacq, eds.), pp. 6–39. Pergamon, Oxford.

Peters, R. A. (1967). *Ciba Found. Study Group* **28,** pp. 1–8.

Petropulos, S. F. (1960). *J. Cell. Comp. Physiol.* **56,** 7.

Pill, A. H. (1967). *Vet. Rec.* **81,** 178.

Pill, A. H., Davies, E. T., Collings, D. F., and Venn, J. A. J. (1966). *Vet. Rec.* **78,** 737.

Pirie, N. W. (1959). *Proc. Int. Congr. Biochem., 4th, 1958* Vol. 7, p. 45.

Prebluda, H. J., and McCollum, E. V. (1939). *J. Biol. Chem.* **127**, 495.

Roberts, G. W., and Boyd, J. W. (1974). *J. Comp. Pathol.* **84**, 365.

Roberts, H. E., Evans, E. T. R. and Evans, W. C. (1949). *Vet. Rec.* **11**, 549.

Sealock, R. R., and Davies, N. C. (1949). *J. Biol. Chem.* **177**, 987.

Sealock, R. R., and Livermore, A. H. (1944). *J. Biol. Chem.* **156**, 379.

Sealock, R. R., and White, H. S. (1949). *J. Biol. Chem.* **181**, 393.

Sealock, R. R., Livermore, A. H., and Evans, C. A. (1943). *J. Amer. Chem. Soc.* **65**, 935.

Shreeve, J. E., and Edwin, E. E. (1974). *Vet. Rec.* **94**, 330.

Somogyi, J. C. (1949). *Int. Z. Vitaminforsch.* **21**, 341.

Somogyi, J. C. (1952). "Die Antianeurinfaktoren" Huber, Bern.

Somogyi, J. C. (1960). *Bibl. "Nut. Dieta"* **1**, 77.

Somogyi, J. C. (1971). *J. Vitaminol. (Kyoto)* **17**, 165.

Somogyi, J. C., and Bönicke, R. (1969). *Int. Z. Vitaminforsch.* **39**, 65.

Stahl, E. (1969). "Thin-Layer Chromatography" (transl. by M. R. F. Ashworth), 2nd ed. Allen & Unwin, London.

Swann, H. C., and Barrowman, J. C. (1959). *Vet. Rec.* **71**, 493.

Terlecki, S., and Markson, L. M. (1959). *Vet. Rec.* **71**, 508.

Terlecki, S., and Markson, L. M. (1961). *Vet. Rec.* **73**, 23.

Thomas, B., and Walker, H. F. (1949). *J. Soc. Chem. Ind., London* **68**, 6.

Thomas, A. J. (1954). Ph.D. Thesis, University of Wales, Bangor.

Thomas, A. J., Watkin, J. E., Evans, I. A., and Evans, W. C. (1955). *Biochem. J.* **61**, viii.

Virtanen, A. I. (1963). *Biochem. Z.* **338**, 443.

von Muralt, A. (1939). *Naturwissenschaften* **27**, 265.

von Muralt, A. (1958). "Neue Ergebnisse der Nervenphysiologie." Springer-Verlag, Berlin and New York.

von Muralt, A. (1962). *Ann. N.Y. Acad. Sci.* **98**, 383.

Warnock, L. G. (1970). *J. Nutr.* **100**, 1057.

Watkin, J. E. (1955). Ph.D. Thesis, University of Wales, Bangor.

Watkin, J. E., Thomas, A. J., and Evans, W. C. (1953). *Biochem. J.* **54**, xxx.

Weswig, P. H., Freed, A. M., and Haag, J. R. (1946). *J. Biol. Chem.* **165**, 737.

Williams, R. R. (1935). *J. Amer. Chem. Soc.* **57**, 229.

Williams, R. R. (1938). *Ergeb. Vitamin Hormon/forsch.* **1**, 256.

Williams, R. R. (1961). "Towards the Conquest of Beriberi." Harvard Univ. Press, Cambridge, Massachusetts.

Wittcliff, J. L., and Airth, R. L. (1968). *Biochemistry* **7**, 736.

Wittcliff, J. L., and Airth, R. L. (1970). In "Methods in Enzymology" (D. B. McCormick and L. D. Wright, eds.), Vol. 18, p. 229. Academic Press, New York.

Woolley, D. W. (1941). *J. Biol. Chem.* **141**, 997.

Woolley, D. W. (1951). *J. Amer. Chem. Soc.* **73**, 1898.

Woolley, D. W. (1953). *Nature (London)* **171**, 323.

Yasuda, T. (1953). *Vitamins* **6**, 17.

Yoshioka, T. (1958). *Vitamins* **14**, 188.

Yudkin, W. H. (1949). *Physiol. Rev.* **29**, 389.

Ziffo, G. S., and Inglis, D. M. (1974). *Vet. Rec.* **94**, 252.

Zima, O., and Williams, R. R. (1940). *Chem. Ber.* **73**, 941.

Pellagra and Amino Acid Imbalance

C. GOPALAN AND KAMALA S. JAYA RAO

*National Institute of Nutrition, Indian Council of Medical Research,
Hyderabad, India*

I. INTRODUCTION

Pellagra is a classical nutritional deficiency disease which had a world-wide distribution until the beginning of this century. It still continues to be an endemic public health problem in some parts of the technologically developing world. Excellent descriptions of the classical clinical features, which include dermatitis, diarrhea, and dementia, can be found in numerous publications and in standard textbooks of medicine and nutrition. Notwithstanding the statement of Gillman and Gillman (1951) that the typical manifestations of a disease are not the ones to be invariably seen, the dermatitis of pellagra is highly characteristic and diagnostic of the disease. It is bilateral, symmetrical, and seen on those parts of the body that are constantly exposed to sunlight. Thus it is commonly seen on the extensor surfaces of the extremities and on the face and neck. Pigmentation on the face is generally limited to the cheeks and the bridge of the nose, and this characteristic pattern goes by the picturesque name of "butterfly pigmentation." The dermatitis extending over the scapulo-clavicular area is called Casal's necklace or Casal's dermatitis, perpetuating the name of the man who first described this disease in the 18th century.

The remaining two of the classical 3 D's of pellagra, namely, diarrhea and dementia, are not invariable features of the disease. The mental changes, when present, may range from mild symptoms like insomnia and depression to marked emotional instability and mania.

Glossitis and angular stomatitis are seen in most of the cases. Nasolabial dyssebacia is also frequently seen. However, these are generally attributed to associated riboflavin deficiency and are not considered to be a part of the clinical syndrome per se.

II. Etiology

Pellagra has been classically recognized to be a disease of the maize-eating populations. The association was suggested by Casal, Frappoli, and other European physicians in the early 18th century soon after the introduction of the maize crop on the continent. Credit, however, goes to Goldberger, who experimentally confirmed the association between consumption of maize and pellagra, both in humans and in dogs (Goldberger and Wheeler, 1920, 1928). He demonstrated the preventable nature of the disease and, more important, stressed that the disease was attributable to a faulty diet, not to any specific foodstuff. The etiology was suggested to be the deficiency of what Goldberger termed a pellagra-preventive or P-P factor. The beautiful anthology of some of his classical contributions to this field (Terris, 1964) is a testimony to the patience and scientific acumen with which he conducted his studies.

Pellagra was common in the southern states of the United States and in Europe, where maize was commonly consumed by the poorer sections of the community. The disease has now been completely eliminated there. However, it is still encountered among the Bantus of South Africa (Potgeiter et al., 1966), in Egypt, and in the maize-eating populations of India (Shah and Singh, 1967).

In the rice belt of Asia the disease is practically unknown (Aykroyd and Swaminathan, 1940; Gopalan and Srikantia, 1960). However, in the rural areas of the rocky Deccan plateau of India the disease is common among the adult population (Gopalan and Srikantia, 1960). The disease accounts for about 1% of all admissions to general hospitals and for nearly 8–10% of admissions to mental institutions in the city of Hyderabad. The staple diet of these people is a millet, jowar (*Sorghum vulgare*), and the diets are not supplemented by any animal foods. Careful dietary histories of cases admitted to hospitals revealed that in 6% of the cases jowar was the staple food and the diets did not include maize. The rest consumed jowar together with rice whereas in few cases a history of occasional consumption of maize in addition to jowar was obtained.

The disease afflicts both sexes equally. It is usually seen only in adults. Seasonal exacerbations and remissions have been described, the incidence being highest in spring when sunlight is in plenty. In India, where ample sunlight is present all through the year, the seasonal incidence is related to the food consumption pattern. Jowar is eaten during the lean season starting from June–July and the peak incidence of the disease is seen during the months of November to February.

A. Role of Nicotinic Acid Deficiency

Goldberger and Tanner (1925) attributed pellagra to a lack of a pellagra-preventive factor in maize. Elvehjem et al. (1937) identified this factor as nicotonic acid by demonstrating the curative efficacy of this vitamin in canine blacktongue. Soon after, the clinical efficacy of nicotinic acid was also demonstrated in human pellagra (Fouts et al., 1937; Spies et al., 1938). After these conclusive studies, it had come to be generally accepted that pellagra is a disease of nicotinic acid deficiency. Although maize is poor in nicotinic acid, it is no worse in this respect than other cereals (Aykroyd and Swaminathan, 1940). Krehl et al. (1945a) found that the marked growth depressive effect of maize in rats could be counteracted by nicotinic acid or by raising the casein content of the diets to 20%. Rice containing less nicotinic acid produced no such growth depression. The same group of workers (Krehl et al., 1945b) subsequently obtained data attributing the growth-depressive action of maize to its low tryptophan content. Rice is richer in tryptophan than maize. That tryptophan is a precursor of nicotinic acid was subsequently established in experimental animals (Rosen et al., 1946; Singal et al., 1946) and in humans (Perlzweig et al., 1947; Sarett and Goldsmith, 1947). It is generally agreed that approximately 60 mg of tryptophan is equivalent to 1 mg of nicotinic acid (Horwitt et al., 1956; Goldsmith et al., 1961).

From the foregoing observations, it was justifiably assumed that the pellagragenic nature of maize is due to its low content of nicotinic acid and tryptophan. Early workers in Egypt had postulated that pellagra might be due to a lack of tryptophan (Barrett-Connor, 1967). Goldberger was also of the opinion that the disease might be one of amino acid deficiency (Goldberger and Tanner, 1922).

Availability of Nicotinic Acid

Among the poorer sections of the population in Central America, maize forms the staple cereal. Despite providing 80% of the total calories and nearly 70% of the total protein (Bressani et al., 1953), the traditional association between maize consumption and pellagra is belied here, the disease being very rare (Aguirre et al., 1953; Squibb et al., 1959). A possible explanation forwarded for the rarity of pellagra in Central America is that corn is consumed here in the form of tortillas prepared after preliminary lime treatment. Much of the nicotinic acid in maize and other cereals is believed to be present in a bound form (Kodicek, 1940) considered unavailable to animals like chicks (Krehl et al., 1944; Coates et al., 1952), pigs (Kodicek et al., 1956), and rats (Kodicek, 1960). It has been claimed that the bound form is rendered free by alkali hydrolysis (Kodicek, 1940; Kodicek et al., 1959). Thus the rarity of pellagra in Central America has been attributed to the liberation of nicotinic acid consequent on lime treatment (Braude et al., 1955; Kodicek et al., 1956). Goldsmith et al. (1956), however, successfully induced symptoms and signs of nicotinic acid deficiency in human volunteers fed lime-treated maize diets. Another factor mentioned in the context of absence of pellagra in Central America is the high rate of coffee consumption. Roasted coffee contains considerable quantities of nicotinic acid (Teply et al., 1945), and this may make significant contributions to a diet otherwise deficient in tryptophan and nicotinic acid (Teply et al., 1945; Goldsmith et al., 1959).

In view of the reported unavailability of nicotinic acid in maize, the possibility that the vitamin might be present in a bound form in jowar too had to be tested. Although a marked increase in the nicotonic acid content of jowar following alkaline hydrolysis has been reported (Ghosh et al., 1963), Belavady and Gopalan (1966) could not confirm these findings. Nicotinic acid content of jowar was found to range from 2 to 3.5 mg/100 gm. In acid–methanol extracts, 80% of the vitamin was found to be in a free form, and in methanol extracts nearly 60% was found to be in a free form. The growth pattern of rats and pups maintained on diets containing either untreated or lime-treated jowar was found to be similar. These studies supported the data obtained by chemical analysis that much of the nicotinic acid in jowar in its natural state is present in a free and available form. Thus the possibility that pellagra in jowar-eaters may be due to nicotinic acid in the millet being bound and unavailable could be ruled out.

B. Role of Leucine

Analysis of jowar, however, showed that the nicotinic acid and tryptophan content of this millet was similar to that of rice (Gopalan and Srikantia, 1960). Further analysis revealed a high content of leucine, a feature that jowar shares with maize. Leucine constitutes 12–14% of the protein of these foods in contrast to 8% observed in rice (Table I). Excess of certain essential amino acids in the diet has been shown to have a growth-depressive effect in experimental animals (Harper, 1964; Harper et al., 1970). The toxic effect of the excess amino acid was generally found to be more when the diet was inadequate in other respects than when complete. Addition of 1% or more of L-leucine to a 9% casein diet was found to cause growth retardation in rats, but this effect was absent when the animals were fed 18% casein diet (Harper et al., 1955).

Pellagrins subsisting on jowar diets consume daily around 2000 kcal and 45 gm of protein derived almost solely from jowar and sometimes other cereals. Thus they are seen to consume a 9% vegetable protein diet containing 1–1.5% leucine. This observation was the starting point of the investigaton of the possible role of excess leucine in the causation of pellagra. Woolley (1946) and Borrow et al. (1948) questioned the widely accepted theory that pellagra is due to the low tryptophan–nicotinic acid content of maize, and, though they postulated the presence of a toxic pellagragenic agent, they were unable to conclusively demonstrate its presence.

III. Biochemical Changes

A. Urinary Excretion of Tryptophan and Nicotinic Acid Metabolites

Najjar and Wood in 1940 reported the excretion of a whitish blue fluorescent substance in urine following the administration of nicotinic acid. This compound, subsequently demonstrated to be N'-methyl nicotinamide (N'MeN), is one of the major urinary metabolites of nicotinic acid (Huff and Perlzweig, 1943a,b). Search for a second important metabolite (Ellinger and Coulson, 1944; Perlzweig and Huff, 1945) led to the identification of the 6-pyridone of N'MeN (Knox and Grossman, 1946). The principal metabolites of nicotinic acid in urine are now established as N'MeN and N'-methyl 6-pyridone 3-carboxylamide (6-pyridone).

The major pathway of tryptophan metabolism is the kynurenine pathway (Fig. 1). 3-Hydroxyanthranilic acid, a metabolite in this pathway, can either be diverted to the glutarate pathway or be converted to quino-

TABLE I

THE CONTENT[a] OF NICOTINIC ACID AND CERTAIN
AMINO ACIDS IN SOME FOODSTUFFS

Foodstuff	Nicotinic acid	Trypto-phan	Leucine	Iso-leucine
Rice	1.2	1.2	8.0	6.0
Wheat	5.5	1.1	6.5	3.5
Maize	1.4	0.8	14.9	6.4
Jowar	1.8	1.2	12.9	6.1
(Sorghum vulgare)				

[a] Grams per 100 gm of protein.

linic acid (Henderson, 1949; Henderson and Hirsch, 1949; Moline et al.,
1959; Nishizuka and Hayaishi, 1963). Although it was believed that
quinolinic acid could be directly converted to nicotinic acid (Henderson,
1949; Henderson et al., 1949; Sarrett, 1951; Hankes and Segal, 1957),
it has now been conclusively shown that it is an immediate precursor
of nicotinic acid ribonucleotide (Nishizuka and Hayaishi, 1963).

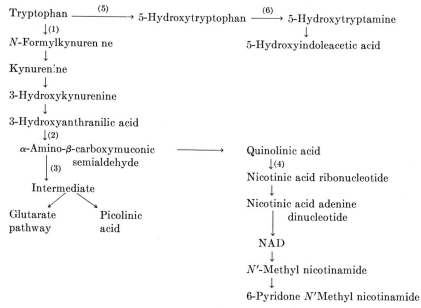

FIG. 1. Pathways of tryptophan catabolism: (1) tryptophan oxygenase, (2) 3-hy-
droxyanthranilate oxygenase, (3) picolinic carboxylase, (4) quinolinate phosphoribosyltransferase, (5) tryptophan hydroxylase, (6) 5-hydroxytryptamine
decarboxylase.

On barely adequate protein diets providing marginal amounts of tryptophan, addition of other amino acids has been shown to cause a disturbance in tryptophan–nicotinic acid metabolism and to result in nicotinic acid deficiency (Rosen and Perlzweig, 1949; Lyman and Elvehjem, 1951; Koeppe and Henderson, 1955). It was inferred that, in a diet providing marginal amounts of all amino acids, tryptophan is spared for conversion to nicotinic acid, whereas when other amino acids are in excess and tryptophan becomes a limiting amino acid, this conversion is impaired (Henderson et al., 1953; Koeppe and Henderson, 1955). Investigations were, therefore, undertaken to see whether excess leucine would also bring about such disturbances in the tryptophan–nicotinic acid interrelationship.

Urinary excretion of N'MeN, 6-pyridone, tryptophan, and quinolinic acid was found to be low in pellagrins (Belavady et al., 1963). Hankes et al. (1971) also observed low levels of N'MeN, nicotinic acid, and kynurenic acid in the urine of pellagrins.

Normal subjects and pellagrins were maintained on diets providing approximately 2300 kcals and 50 gm of protein, derived solely from vegetable sources. The diets provided about 8% protein and were similar to those consumed by the population which suffers from pellagra. Each subject was given in addition every day 10 gm of L-leucine orally. Administration of leucine brought about a marked increase in the excretion of quinolinic acid and a significant decrease in that of 6-pyridone (Belavady et al., 1963). Withdrawal of leucine resulted in a reversal to the basal pattern. Although in a preliminary study there was suggested evidence that leucine administration may increase urinary excretion of N'MeN (Gopalan and Srikantia, 1960), subsequent studies showed that there is no consistent alteration in the excretion of this metabolite (Belavady et al., 1963). The foregoing observations suggested that there might be a block in the further metabolism of quinolinic acid following leucine administration.

More detailed investigations were carried out in experimental rats. Weanling albino rats were fed a basal diet containing 9% casein but adequate in other respects. The animals were also given supplements of either L-leucine or L-tryptophan. Quinolinic acid excretion was markedly increased. Excretion of N'MeN although raised was not significant (Raghuramulu et al., 1965a). Moreover, quinolinic acid excretion was found to increase with increasing doses of leucine. The effect was specific to leucine and was not seen with lysine, glycine, methionine, or threonine. Quinolinic acid excretion was found to be higher in rats fed a jowar diet than in those fed a wheat diet. The excretion of nicotinic acid and N'MeN was also high.

B. PLASMA TRYPTOPHAN LEVELS

Plasma tryptophan levels are in the low range in pellagrins. Truswell *et al.* (1968) were of the opinion that the plasma level of this amino acid may be a good biochemical index of pellagra. However, individual variations in the levels are so wide that it would appear that the plasma tryptophan level may not be of much significance in the pathogenesis of the disease (Ghafoorunissa and Narasinga Rao, 1975). The low plasma tryptophan levels are more likely a reflection of the general undernutrition in the pellagrins, since nonpellagrins from low socioeconomic groups, in which pellagra is common, had levels similar to those in pellagrins. On the other hand, plasma tryptophan levels in well-nourished nonpellagrins were higher than those seen in either of the former two groups. Truswell *et al.* (1968) also observed that plasma tryptophan levels in children suffering from pellagra and kwashiorkor were of similar order.

A decrease in urinary excretion of tryptophan was observed after a leucine load (Belavady *et al.*, 1963). Feeding a high-leucine diet to rats resulted in decreased levels of plasma valine and isoleucine (Rogers *et al.*, 1962), and a similar observation has also been made in human subjects after a leucine load (Swendseid *et al.*, 1965). The studies of Hagihira *et al.* (1960) suggest that these alterations might be due to a competition between the amino acids during intestinal absorption. However, such a mechanism does not appear to operate in the case of leucine and tryptophan. A leucine load did not bring about any alterations in plasma tryptophan levels in normal volunteers (Ghafoorunissa and Narasinga Rao, 1971.) Further, the increase in plasma tryptophan levels following simultaneous administration of tryptophan and leucine was found to be similar to that observed after a tryptophan load alone.

C. NICOTINAMIDE NUCLEOTIDES IN ERYTHROCYTES

The functional forms of nicotinic acid in the body are the two nucleotides nicotinamide adenine dinucleotide (NAD) and nicotinamide adenine dinucleotide phosphate (NADP). In view of the altered nicotinic acid metabolism in pellagra, studies were directed toward investigating the profile of these constituents. The total nucleotide concentration in the erythrocytes of pellagrins was similar to that in normals (Raghuramulu *et al.*, 1965b). This is in line with the observations of Axelrod *et al.* (1941). The rate of nucleotide synthesis was, however, significantly lower in the pellagrins. Supplementation with L-leucine for 5 days did not alter the nucleotide concentration either in pellagrins or in normal subjects, but its rate of synthesis was suppressed in both groups to nearly

60% of the initial values. A rapid reversal to basal conditions occurred following withdrawal of leucine. Leucine added *in vitro* at high concentrations also inhibited the nucleotide synthesis (Belavady *et al.*, 1973). As mentioned earlier, leucine supplementation led to an increased excretion of quinolinic acid and, it may be logically assumed, to an increased concentration in blood. Quinolinic acid was found to inhibit nucleotide synthesis *in vitro*, the inhibition being progressive with increasing concentrations of the compound (Raghuramulu *et al.*, 1965b). A similar mechanism may also be operative *in vivo*. The depressed rate of synthesis may, therefore, be due to a direct action of leucine or of quinolinic acid.

The paradox of a normal concentration of the nucleotide in the face of a depressed synthesizing capacity of the erythrocytes was resolved in subsequent studies. Fractionation of the nucleotides was carried out by paper chromatography using the solvent system 95% ethanol:1 M ammonium acetate, pH 5, in the ratio of 7:3, as described by Preiss and Handler (1958a). Much of the nucleotide in the normal subjects resolved into NAD and NADP. In pellagrins a third spot corresponding to nicotinamide mononucleotide (NMN) was identified. Levels of NAD and NADP were lower than in normals (Srikantia *et al.*, 1968a). Treatment with nicotinic acid brought about a marked reduction in the NMN content of the erythrocytes of pellagrins.

NMN is normally not found in human and dog erythrocytes. However, the monkey, guinea pig, and rat have significant concentrations of NMN in their erythrocytes (Table II). In dogs which developed blacktongue after feeding of jowar or maize diets, the total nucleotide concentration of the erythrocytes was not altered—a finding similar to that observed in pellagrins and in normal volunteers administered L-leucine. Nevertheless, NMN was detected in considerable concentrations. Monkeys fed jowar diets, however, showed a fall in the total concentration of nucleotides in the erythrocytes but no alteration in the NMN concentration (Belavady *et al.*, 1968). Similar observations were also made in monkeys fed leucine (Belavady and Rao, 1973). It appears that there may be species variations in the changes in the nucleotide pattern following consumption of jowar. In species that normally have NMN in erythrocytes, the concentration is not changed, whereas those which normally do not have detectable quantities of the nucleotide show an increase. In the absence of an adequate explanation for the normally observed species variations, it is not wise to speculate further on these divergent observations.

The pathway proposed by Preiss and Handler (1958b) for the biosynthesis of nicotinamide nucleotides from nicotinic acid is depicted in Fig. 2. The incorporation of ^{14}C-labeled nicotinic acid into nicotinic acid ribonucleotide as well as into nicotinic acid adenine dinucleotide

TABLE II

SPECIES DIFFERENCES IN NICOTINAMIDE NUCLEOTIDE[a] CONCENTRATIONS
OF ERYTHROCYTES

Species	Total nucleotides (mg/100 ml of erythrocytes)	NAD (% of total)	NADP (% of total)	NMN (% of total)
Chick (3)[b]	9.5	74	26	Trace
Dog (13)	7.0	74	22	<5
Duckling (7)	13.3	87.5	12.5	Trace
Guinea pig (3)	10.2	64	24.5	10
Monkey (21)	12.4	58	28	14
Rat (6)	12.1	80.5	12	7.5
Man (12)	5.2	65.5	34.5	<5

[a] NAD, nicotinamide adenine dinucleotide; NADP, NAD phosphate; NMN, nicotinamide mononucleotide.

[b] Figures in parenthesis indicate number of observations.

(NAAD) and NAD was found to be lower in the erythrocytes of pellagrins than in those of normal subjects. The activity of the enzyme nicotinate phosphoribosyltransferase, measured according to the method described by Preiss and Handler (1958a), was, however, not altered (Anasuya and Narasinga Rao, 1973). Concentration of ATP in the erythrocytes was found to be low, and the levels increased after treatment. This would indicate that lack of ATP may be an important contributory factor to the reduced synthesis of erythrocyte nicotinamide nucleotide. However, the reason for the reduction in ATP concentration is not clear.

Nicotinic acid + PRPP $\xrightarrow{(1)}$ Nicotinic acid ribonucleotide + PP_i
          (NARN)

NARN + ATP $\xrightarrow{(2)}$ Nicotinic acid adenine dinucleotide + PP_i
          (NAAD)

NAAD + Glutamine + ATP $\xrightarrow{(3)}$ Nicotinamide dinucleotide + Glutamic acid
          + AMP + PP_i
          (NAD)

FIG. 2. Preiss–Handler pathway of nicotinamide nucleotide biosynthesis: (1) nicotinic acid phosphoribosyltransferase, (2) NARN-Adenyltransferase, (3) NAD synthetase.

IV. Effects of Excess Leucine

A. Production of Canine Blacktongue

Belavady and Gopalan (1965) maintained dogs on a modified version of Goldberger's diet (Goldberger and Wheeler, 1928) based on jowar instead of maize. Signs of blacktongue in varying degrees were observed within 30–80 days of starting the experiment. There was a foul odor of the mouth and superficial ulceration of the buccal mucosa followed by profuse salivation and excretion of blood-stained feces. Conclusive evidence of the role of excess leucine in jowar in the development of canine blacktongue was obtained in further experiments.

Pups were maintained on diets providing 20% casein and 3.6% leucine but devoid of nicotinic acid. All the pups developed classical signs of blacktongue within 30–90 days whereas this did not occur when the diet contained only 1.5% leucine (Belavady et al., 1967). Blacktongue could be produced even when the diets provided 300 μg of niacin, but with the level of leucine kept at 2.7% (Belavady et al., 1967). There was degeneration of surface epithelium and inflammatory exudate in the buccal mucosa. Punctate hemorrhages were seen in various parts of the small intestine. Hemorrhagic necrosis and exudation of leukocytes were seen in the duodenum. Villous atrophy was seen in the jejunum and ileum. The large intestine was also the seat of extensive hemorrhagic necrosis. There was atrophy and dilatation of the glands and abnormal regeneration of the crypts. Goblet cells were scarce and periodic acid–Schiff's reagent (PAS) staining showed an absence of secretory activity. Contrary to earlier observations (Chittenden and Underhill, 1917; Goldberger and Wheeler, 1928), neurological changes were relatively minor. Similar histopathological changes were also seen in dogs fed jowar or maize diets (Madhavan et al., 1968).

Signs similar to canine blacktongue could also be induced in monkeys, a species closer to man than dog, by feeding diets based on either jowar or maize (Belavady et al., 1968). As in the dog, the gastrointestinal signs were most dominant and the histopathological picture was somewhat similar. The large intestine was more strikingly involved, with gross attenuation of the transverse folds, hemorrhages, and ulceration. There was large-scale destruction of the epithelium with severe inflammation of the mucosa. Goblet cells were virtually absent, and secretory activity was minimal.

There is a paucity of data regarding the histopathological changes in human pellagra. Salib (1959) on the basis of gastroscopic studies described gastric atrophy. Pellagra in the Middle East, as pointed out by the author, is commonly associated with intestinal parasitism. Since similar studies were not done on suitable control subjects, the contribution of malnutrition, secondary to parasitism, to the gastric atrophy cannot be ruled out. The studies of Hanafy et al. (1968) are similarly handicapped, and more so since their cases were children in whom protein-calorie malnutrition is rampant.

B. Leucine Excess and Maize

Common varieties of maize contain 12–14% leucine. Recently, a hybrid strain, Opaque-2, has been shown to have a protein and amino acid composition markedly different from that of the conventional strains (Mertz et al., 1964). Lysine content of Opaque-2 is much higher and leucine much lower than in the normal maize varieties (Mertz et al., 1965). The availability of this strain afforded an opportunity to test the validity of the postulate that pellagra in maize-eaters may also be due to the high leucine content of this cereal. Dogs were fed diets based on a locally available variety of maize (Deccan Hybrid) or on Opaque-2 maize. Lysine content of the two varieties was 2.5% and 3.5% of the protein, respectively, and the corresponding figures for leucine were 12.3% and 7.8%. The animals were further subdivided and fed either Opaque-2 maize diet whose leucine content was made equal to that of Deccan Hybrid or fed a diet containing the latter with its lysine content equalized to that of Opaque-2. Protein, tryptophan, and nicotinic acid content of all the four diets were similar. All pups fed the Deccan Hybrid maize, whether supplemented or not with lysine, developed classical blacktongue. Treatment with nicotinic acid led to complete remission of the condition. The group receiving Opaque-2 maize alone did not develop the disease, whereas in the group supplemented with leucine classical signs of the disease were observed (Gopalan et al., 1969). Thus evidence was obtained to show that pellagra in maize-eaters may also be due to dietary excess of leucine and that consumption of the cereal with a low content of this aminoacid may not lead to the development of the disease.

C. Effect of Leucine on Enzymes in the Trypotophan-Nicotinic Acid Pathway

Earlier, the effect of leucine on the urinary excretion of quinolinic acid and the 6-pyridone of N′MeN, and also its effect on nicotinamide nucleotide concentration in the tissues, was discussed. Recent studies indicate that the amino acid alters the activity of some enzymes involved in the conversion of tryptophan to nicotinic acid.

Weanling albino rats were fed a basal diet containing 9% protein derived from casein and were supplemented with 1.5% leucine, 3% leucine, or 0.001% nicotinic acid. The activity of quinolinate phosphoribosyltransferase (QPRT), which brings about the conversion of quinolinic acid to nicotinic acid ribonucleotide, was found to be significantly depressed in rats supplemented with 3% leucine. The effect was seen irrespective of the addition or otherwise of nicotinic acid to the diet (Ghafoorunissa and Narasinga Rao, 1973). At this level of leucine the activity of tryptophan oxygenase was markedly increased. A similar effect of leucine was also seen in monkeys fed an 11% protein diet supplemented with 1.5 gm of L-leucine per day.

Picolinic carboxylase activity was not detectable in the livers of either control rats or the leucine-supplemented ones. Lan and Gholson (1965) also reported failure to detect this enzyme in rat livers. However, in the kidney of the leucine-supplemented rats the enzyme activity was high. 3-Hydroxyanthranilate oxygenase was not altered either in rats or monkeys fed leucine.

An increase in tryptophan oxygenase will lead to an increased formation of kynurenine, which in turn will lead to an increased formation of α-amino-β-carboxymuconic semialdehyde, which is a substrate for quinolinic acid synthesis. However, an increased picolinic carboxylase activity would divert this compound toward picolinic acid (see Fig. 1) and make it less available for formation of quinolinic acid. Both these enzymes were elevated in the leucine-supplemented rats. Thus each would tend to cancel the effect of the other and the increased quinolinic acid excretion observed in leucine-supplemented human subjects (Belavady et al., 1963) and animals (Raghuramulu et al., 1965a) could not be due to an elevation of tryptophan oxygenase activity alone. A decrease in QPRT would lead to decreased conversion of quinolinic acid to nicotinic acid ribonucleotide. An inverse relationship between the amount of NAD synthesized from tryptophan and the activity of picolinic carboxylase has been demonstrated (Ikeda et al., 1965). Now a similar relationship has been established between this enzyme and QPRT in leucine-fed animals. Thus the increased quinolinic acid excretion in pellagra may be due to a low QPRT causing an accumulation of quinolinic acid.

V. Mental Changes in Pellagra

A. Clinical Symptoms and Signs

Striking among the protean manifestations of pellagra are the mental changes. In Hyderabad during the peak season nearly 8–10% of the admissions to the mental hospital are cases of pellagra. A majority of the patients exhibit mental changes of a mild nature, which may be so subtle as to be completely missed. These include fatigue, insomnia, and apprehension. Insomnia is in fact a very common complaint. Approximately 1–2% of the cases admitted to the hospital show more severe manifestations, the more noticeable and serious ones being various types of psychoses. Confusion, disorientation, hallucinations, and loss of memory may be encountered. In some others depression, severe paranoid symptoms, and mania may also be present. Acute encephalopathies have also been described (Jolliffe *et al.*, 1940), but these have been notably rare in our series of cases. Paresthesias, burning sensation in hands and feet, and polyneuritis are also quite common, but these are more probably due to the concomitant deficiency of other members of the B-vitamin group. Disturbances in vision have also been reported (Spillane, 1947). In a series of 30 cases studied in our Institute, 25 cases complained of dimness of vision, and 18 of these were found to have a defective vision (Krishnaswamy, 1968). The optical fundus revealed no abnormality. Acuity of vision was found to improve with treatment with nicotinic acid.

In an earlier investigation, where a causal relationship between leucine and pellagra was first suggested, administration of 20–30 gm of the amino acid to two patients was accompanied by a temporary but marked deterioration of their mental condition which could be reversed by leucine withdrawal and treatment with nicotinic acid (Gopalan and Srikantia, 1960). These findings were confirmed in a larger series of patients (Srikantia *et al.*, 1968b). The patients were found to become depressive and emotionally unstable but were not violent. Insomnia, an original complaint, became a distressing symptom. All patients responded to treatment with nicotinic acid within 48 hours of oral administration of the vitamin, but those with severe depression required parenteral therapy. Administration of leucine did not bring about any such mental change in normal subjects.

A study of the electroencephalographic (EEG) pattern showed that in most cases there was either an excess *theta* activity or *delta* activity (Srikantia *et al.*, 1968b). In those who did not initially show such a pattern, administration of 10 gm of L-leucine or 1 gm of quinolinic acid for 10 days revealed considerable *theta* activity. Within 10–40 days of treatment with nicotinic acid, a return to the normal *alpha* rhythm was noted. All the patients who had clinical manifestations of mental changes showed an altered EEG pattern, but the reverse was not necessarily true. Neither leucine nor quinolinic acid brought about similar clinical or EEG alterations in nonpellagrins. Pellagrins are either more sensitive to leucine and respond to it in a short time or, since they are already on a high-leucine diet, administration of extra leucine might have precipitated changes earlier.

B. Biochemical Basis for Altered Mental Function

A quantitatively minor pathway of tryptophan metabolism is the 5-hydroxytryptamine (5-HTP, serotonin) pathway, the existence of which was established by Udenfriend and collaborators (Udenfriend *et al.*, 1956, 1957a). Serotonin is present in appreciable quantities in the brain (Twarog and Page, 1953; Amin *et al.*, 1954) and is mostly localized in the primitive portions of the brain (Bogdanski and Udenfriend, 1956; Udenfriend *et al.*, 1957b). Woolley and Shaw (1954, 1957) put forward the concept and provided evidence that serotonin may be needed for normal functioning of the mental processes.

Pellagrins excrete low amounts of urinary 5-hydroxyindoleacetic acid (5-HIAA), the end product of the serotonin pathway (Belavady *et al.*, 1963). Administration of leucine to normal subjects as well as to pellagrins was found to depress the excretion of this urinary metabolite. Feeding leucine at a level of 5% or 8% of the diet to rats resulted in a significant lowering of brain serotonin content (Yuwiler and Geller, 1965). It may be logically assumed that alterations in the serotonin pathway may play an important role in the alteration of mental status in pellagra. Although Edelstein *et al.* (1962) did not observe lowering of 5-HIAA excretion in urine in canine blacktongue, they attributed this to the fact that the animals died before any mental changes or alteration in EEG pattern had occurred.

Albino rats were fed a basal diet providing 10% protein derived from casein and were supplemented with 1.5%, 3%, or 8% L-leucine. Animals in the last two groups had a significantly low brain serotonin content, thus confirming the observations of Yuwiler and Geller (1965). This reduction was entirely due to a reduction of serotonin content in the synaptosomes. Supplementation with leucine at a level of 1.5% did not alter brain serotonin content. However, when rats were fed a jowar-based diet which provided 10% protein and only 1.6% leucine, the brain amine content was significantly lowered (Ramanamurthy and Srikantia, 1970). The protein in jowar being of a quality inferior to casein, this factor might have potentiated the action of leucine. Pellagrins with mental depression and emotional instability had low levels of serotonin in platelets, the values being invariably less than 0.5 μg per milligram of protein (Krishnaswamy and Ramanamurthy, 1970). Pellagrins without mental changes had levels similar to those of nonpellagrins, the mean value being

0.57 μg per milligram of protein. Nicotinamide and nicotinic acid in small amounts can increase brain serotonin content (Scherer and Kramer, 1972; Krishnaswamy and Raghuram, 1972). However, in pharmacological doses they have been found to lower brain serotonin content further in leucine-fed animals and platelet serotonin in pellagrins (Ramanamurthy and Srikantia, 1970; Krishnaswamy and Ramanamurthy, 1970). It is suggested that serotonin present in a bound form in the storage granules may be released by nicotinic acid and acted upon immediately by mono-amine oxides.

A blood–brain barrier has been demonstrated for serotonin (Udenfriend *et al.*, 1957a; Woolley and Shaw, 1957; Axelrod and Inscoe, 1963). The low levels of serotonin in the brain may, therefore, be due to poor availability of the precursor amino acids, to their impaired uptake by brain, or to a reduced activity of the enzymes involved in their conversion to 5-HTP. When rats fed an 8% leucine diet were given an intraperitoneal injection of 100 mg of 5-HTP per kilogram body weight, the synthesis of serotonin in brain was found to be markedly lowered. However, uptake of ^{14}C-labeled 5-HTP *in vitro* by brain slices of these animals was not depressed (Ramanamurthy and Srikantia, 1970). The uptake of 5-HTP by synaptosomes *in vitro* was also not altered (Kaladhar, 1972). This would suggest that uptake of 5-HTP may not be inhibited by leucine feeding. This is in conflict with earlier observations that leucine added *in vitro*, given as an intraperitoneal injection, or given as a dietary supplement can inhibit 5-HTP uptake by brain (McKean *et al.*, 1962; Schanberg, 1963).

Recent studies have shown that the brain does not depend on a peripheral source of 5-HTP. Tryptophan is actively taken up by the synaptosomes (Grahame-Smith and Parfitt, 1970). Brain serotonin synthesis may, therefore, be limited by the availability of tryptophan (Fernstrom and Wurtman, 1971a). However, neither the uptake of the amino acid nor its concentration in synaptosomes was found to be altered in rats fed 3% leucine (Kaladhar, 1974). Earlier, it was suggested that alterations in plasma tryptophan concentration would be reflected in brain tryptophan content (Fernstrom and Wurtman, 1971b). Recent studies, however, indicate that brain tryptophan concentration is dependent not only on the plasma concentration of this amino acid, but also on the plasma levels of other amino acids, which compete with tryptophan for transport into the brain. Despite an increase in its plasma concentration, if the concentration of tryptophan continues to be low in relation to that of other amino acids, brain tryptophan concentration will not rise (Fernstrom and Wurtman, 1972; Fernstrom *et al.*, 1973). The absence of any significant alteration in plasma amino acid pattern in pellagra (Ghafoorunissa and Narasinga Rao, 1975) could hence explain the nonalteration of brain tryptophan content.

5-Hydroxylation of tryptophan is believed to be the rate-limiting step in the synthesis of serotonin (Green and Sawyer, 1966; Grahame-Smith, 1967). However, the activity of this enzyme was found not to be altered in rats fed 3% leucine (Kaladhar, 1974). The activity of 5-HTP decarboxylase was not altered either, confirming the findings of Geller and Yuwiler (1967). It thus appears that the low serotonin content in the brains of leucine-fed rats may not be due to an impaired uptake of tryptophan nor to its impaired conversion to serotonin. However, the uptake of serotonin by synaptic vesicles, the storage granules within the synaptosomes, was significantly reduced (Kaladhar, 1972), and this probably is the crucial factor in the reduction of brain serotonin. Free serotonin, not taken up by the storage granules is immediately destroyed by monoamine oxidase, the activity of which was not altered in these animals.

VI. The Skin in Pellagra

The symmetrical, photosensitive dermatosis of pellagra is characteristic of the disease. The lesion starts as an intense area of erythema, which later gives place to hyperpigmentation. Desquamation usually follows to expose a smooth, shiny, depigmented but intact epidermis. Hyperkeratinization is also very common, and callus formation may occur on the skeletal pressure parts. A clear-cut demarcation is seen between the normal and affected parts. The symmetrical distribution and this clear-cut distinction are two very striking features of pellagrous dermatitis.

An exhaustive account of the histopathology of the skin in pellagra has been provided by Gillman and Gillman (1951). In a series of cases studied in Hyderabad, hyperkeratosis was commonly seen. There was a severe depletion of melanin in the stratum germinativum while the stratum corneum presented more of the pigmentation than was seen in a normal corneal layer. This redistribution of melanin is the factor underlying the "hyperpigmentation" of pellagra (D. Krishnamurthy, unpublished observations). Neither the total nitrogen content of the skin nor the dermal nitrogen content are altered in pellagra (Vasantha, 1970a). Collagen nitrogen content is low, and understandably the hydroxyproline content of dermis is also low. A marked alteration in the amino acid pattern of the dermis is also found.

The biochemical lesion contributing to the photosensitivity of pellagrous dermatitis has not been investigated. The major ultraviolet-absorbing compound in the skin is urocanic acid (Tabachnick, 1957), which may protect the skin from the erythema-producing effect of sunlight, sunburn (Zenisek *et al.*, 1955). Exposure of guinea pigs to UV light has been shown to decrease the urocanic acid content of their skin (Anglin *et al.*, 1961). A marked reduction in urocanic acid, in its precursor, histidine, and in histidinase, the enzyme which converts histidine to urocanic acid, has been observed in the stratum corneum of pellagrins (Vasantha, 1970b). This suggests that the lowered histidine and urocanic acid content of the skin may play an important role in the photosensitivity of pellagrous dermatitis.

Copper Metabolism

The pathogenesis of the skin lesions has also not been fully worked out. In animals reared on copper-deficient diets, histopathological changes suggestive of a disturbed connective tissue metabolism have been described (O'Dell *et al.*, 1961; Shields *et al.*, 1962). Alterations in elastin, collagen, and hydroxyproline content have been reported in the tissues of such animals (Weissman *et al.*, 1963; O'Dell *et al.*, 1966), and an essential role for copper in maturation of collagen has been suggested (Chou *et al.*, 1968).

In the light of the above observations, investigations of copper metabolism in pellagra acquire significance. Total serum copper levels were raised in this condition, the mean value being 166.6 μg/100 ml as against a value of 91.5 μg/100 ml in nonpellagrins (Krishnamachari, 1974). The serum ceruloplasmin content was not altered, however, indicating that the increase in total copper concentration is due to an increase in the nonceruloplasmin portion of serum copper. Administration of 5 gm of L-leucine orally to normal persons also resulted in a similar increase in serum copper levels. Urinary excretion of copper is high in pellagrins as well as in normal human volunteers fed leucine. Histidine has a very high affinity for copper (Sarkar and Kruck, 1966; Neumann and Sass-Kortsak, 1967), and amino acids are believed to help in the transport of the metal across the cells (Sarkar and Kruck, 1966). In view of Vasantha's observation (Vasantha, 1970b) that the histidine content of skin is low in pellagra, the possibility of a resultant lowering of copper content of the skin contributing to dermatitis needs to be considered. Recent studies have shown that the molybdenum content of some varieties of jowar is high. Normal volunteers fed high-molybdenum diets excrete excess quantities of copper in urine (Deosthale and Gopalan, 1974). A study of the interrelationship between copper and molybdenum may help in the further investigations on pellagra.

VII. Leucine–Isoleucine Imbalance

Leucine content of maize and jowar, the two cereals whose consumption is associated with pellagra, is high. Sauberlich *et al.* (1953) observed that isoleucine was one of the limiting amino acids in low-protein diets based on maize. These findings were subsequently confirmed by Benton *et al.* (1955). Harper *et al.* (1955) also observed that the growth-retarding effect of excess dietary leucine on rats could be counteracted to a large extent by the simultaneous addition of isoleucine to the diet. Harper and co-workers (1970) concluded that excess of any branched-chain amino acid in diet might increase the requirement for other amino acids of the same group. Administration of 5 gm DL-isoleucine for 10–15 days can bring about a remarkable clinical cure of pellagra and can, in a majority of the cases, reverse the abnormal EEG pattern (Krishnaswamy and Gopalan, 1971). The increased excretion of urinary quinolinic acid in rats fed a 1.5% leucine-containing diet could be reversed by the addition of 0.2% DL-isoleucine (Raghuramulu *et al.*, 1965a). It counteracts the suppressive action of leucine on nicotinamide nucleotide synthesis (Belavady and Rao, 1973; Belavady *et al.*, 1973). Similarly, administration of isoleucine was shown to prevent the rise in total serum copper levels and increased urinary copper excretion brought about by leucine feeding to human volunteers (Krishnamachari, 1974). In rats, it can counteract the serotonin-lowering effect of leucine in brain (Krishnaswamy and Raghuram, 1972). These findings strongly point to a leucine-isoleucine imbalance being a possible etiopathogenic factor in the development of pellagra.

VIII. Summary and Concluding Remarks

Pellagra has long been recognized as a disease resulting from nicotinic acid deficiency. It has been classically associated with diets in which the staple is maize and has been attributed to the low tryptophan content and to the poor availability of nicotinic acid in maize. More recently, endemic pellagra has been identified among population groups whose staple food is jowar (sorghum), a millet that is not low in tryptophan and wherein nicotinic acid is freely available.

A common feature of maize and sorghum is their high leucine content. Evidence presented in this review indicates that the etiological factor in the pathogenesis of endemic pellagra could be the high content of leucine in the diet and also probably an imbalance between leucine and isoleucine. Canine blacktongue and signs of nicotinic acid deficiency in monkeys could be produced by feeding the animals high-leucine, marginal-protein diets. While canine blacktongue could be consistently produced by feeding traditional maize varieties, the disease could not be produced by feeding Opaque-2 maize, which contains low amounts of leucine. Biochemical changes seen in pellagra could be produced in experimental animals as well as in normal human volunteers be feeding high doses of leucine. These changes could be prevented by simultaneous administration of isoleucine and cured by nicotinic acid.

These observations provide the first instance of an important nutritional disease mediated through amino acid imbalance and call for a revision of our concept regarding the pathogenesis of pellagra. The significance of these observations lies in the fact that they provide a practical basis for an approach toward prevention and control of a disease, which is still a major public health problem in some parts of the world. Varietal differences in the leucine/isoleucine composition of jowar samples exist, and it may be possible to identify and selectively propagate jowar varieties with relatively low leucine concentration. Recent studies in areas where jowar is grown also indicate good possibilities of intercropping of jowar and red gram (*Cajanus cajan*) with satisfactory amino acid composition. Since it will be clearly impossible to totally replace jowar as the staple in communities where pellagra is endemic, the practical answer must lie in these directions.

REFERENCES

Aguirre, F., Bressani, R., and Scrimshaw, N. S. (1953). *Food Res.* 18, 273.

Amin, A. H., Crawford, T. B. B., and Gaddum, J. H. (1954). *J. Physiol. (London)* 126, 596.

Anasuya, A., and Narasinga Rao, B. S. (1973). Annual Report, p. 47. National Institute of Nutrition, Hyderabad, India.

Anglin, J. H., Bever, A. T., Everett, M. A., and Lamb, J. H. (1961). *Biochim. Biophys. Acta* 53, 409.

Axelrod, A. E., Spies, T. D., and Elvehjem, C. A. (1941). *J. Biol. Chem.* 138, 667.

Axelrod, J., and Inscoe, J. K. (1963). *J. Pharmacol. Exp. Ther.* 141, 161.

Aykroyd, W. R., and Swaminathan, M. (1940). *Indian J. Med. Res.* 27, 667.

Barrett-Connor, E. (1967). *Amer. J. Med.* 42, 859.

Belavady, B., and Gopalan, C. (1965). *Lancet* 2, 1220.

Belavady, B., and Gopalan, C. (1966). *Indian J. Biochem.* 3, 44.

Belavady, B., and Rao, P. U. S. (1973). *Int. J. Vitam. Nutr. Res.* 43, 454.

Belavady, B., Srikantia, S. G., and Gopalan, C. (1963). *Biochem. J.* 87, 652.

Belavady, B., Madhavan, T. V., and Gopalan, C. (1967). *Gastroenterology* 53, 749.

Belavady, B., Madhavan, T. V., and Gopalan, C. (1968). *Lab. Invest.* 18, 94.

Belavady, B., Rao, P. U. S., and Khan, L. (1973). *Int. J. Vitam. Nutr. Res.* 43, 442.

Benton, D. A., Harper, A. E., and Elvehjem, C. A. (1955). *Arch. Biochem. Biophys.* **57**, 13.

Bogdanski, D. F., and Udenfriend, S. (1956). *J. Pharmacol. Exp. Ther.* **116**, 7.

Borrow, A., Fowden, L., Stedman, M. M., Waterlow, J. C., and Webb, R. A. (1948). *Lancet* **1**, 752.

Braude, R., Kon, S. K., Mitchell, K. G., and Kodicek, E. (1955). *Lancet* **1**, 898.

Bressani, R., Arroyave, G., and Scrimshaw, N. S. (1953). *Food Res.* **18**, 261.

Chittenden, R. H., and Underhill, F. P. (1917). *Amer. J. Physiol.* **44**, 13.

Chou, W. S., Savage, J. E., and O'Dell, B. L. (1968). *Proc. Soc. Exp. Biol. Med.* **128**, 948.

Coates, M. E., Ford, J. E., Harrison, G. F., Kon, S. K., Shepheard, E. E., and Wilby, F. W. (1952). *Brit. J. Nutr.* **6**, 75.

Deosthale, Y. G., and Gopalan, C. (1974). *Brit. J. Nutr.* **31**, 351.

Edelstein, E. L., Pfeifer, Y., Steiner, J. E., and Sulman, F. G. (1962). *Proc. Soc. Exp. Biol. Med.* **110**, 13.

Ellinger, P., and Coulson, R. A. (1944). *Biochem. J.* **38**, 265.

Elvehjem, C. A., Madden, R. J., Strong, F. M., and Woolley, D. W. (1937). *J. Amer. Chem. Soc.* **59**, 1767.

Fernstrom, J. D., and Wurtman, R. J. (1971a). *Science* **173**, 149.

Fernstrom, J. D., and Wurtman, R. J. (1971b). *Science* **174**, 1023.

Fernstrom, J. D., and Wurtman, R. J. (1972). *Science* **178**, 414.

Fernstrom, J. D., Larin, F., and Wurtman, R. J. (1973). *Life Sci.* **13**, 517.

Fouts, P. J., Helmer, O. M., Lepkovsky, S., and Jukes, T. H. (1937). *Proc. Soc. Exp Biol. Med.* **37**, 405.

Geller, E., and Yuwiler, A. (1967). *J. Neurochem.* **14**, 725.

Ghafoorunissa and Narasinga Rao, B. S. (1971). *Indian J. Med. Res.* **59**, 1861.

Ghafoorunissa and Narasinga Rao, B. S. (1973). *Biochem. J.* **134**, 425.

Ghafoorunissa and Narasinga Rao, B. S. (1975). *Amer. J. Clin. Nutr.* **28**, 325.

Ghosh, H. P., Sarkar, P. K., and Guha, B. C. (1963). *J. Nutr.* **79**, 451.

Gillman, J., and Gillman, T. (1951). "Perspectives in Human Malnutrition," p. 15. Grune & Stratton, New York.

Goldberger, J., and Tanner, W. F. (1922). *Pub. Health Rep.* **37**, 462.

Goldberger, J., and Tanner, W. F. (1925). *Pub. Health Rep.* **40**, 54.

Goldberger, J., and Wheeler, G. A. (1920). *Hyg. Lab. Bull.* No. 120, p. 7.

Golberger, J., and Wheeler, G. A. (1928). *Pub. Health Rep.* **43**, 172.

Goldsmith, G. A., Gibbens, J., Unglaub, W. G., and Miller, O. N. (1956). *Amer. J. Clin. Nutr.* **4**, 151.

Goldsmith, G. A., Miller, O. N., Unglaub, W. G., and Kercheval, K. (1959). *Proc. Soc. Exp. Biol. Med.* **102**, 579.

Goldsmith, G. A., Miller, O. N., and Unglaub, W. G. (1961). *J. Nutr.* **73**, 172.

Gopalan, C., and Srikantia, S. G. (1960). *Lancet* **1**, 954.

Gopalan, C., Belavady, B., and Krishnamurthy, D. (1969). *Lancet* **2**, 956.

Grahame-Smith, D. G. (1967). *Biochem. J.* **105**, 351.

Grahame-Smith, D. G., and Parfitt, A. G. (1970). *J. Neurochem.* **17**, 1339.

Green, H., and Sawyer, J. L. (1966). *Anal. Biochem.* **15**, 53.

Hagihira, H., Ogata, M., Takedatsu, N., and Suda, M. (1960). *J. Biochem. (Tokyo)* **47**, 139.

Hanafy, M. M., Konbar, A. A., Zeitoun, M. M., and Hassan, A. I. (1968). *J. Trop. Med. Hyg.* **71**, 125.

Hankes, L. V., and Segal, I. H. (1957). *Proc. Soc. Exp. Biol. Med.* **94**, 447.

Hankes, L. V., Leklem, J. E., Brown, R. R., and Mekel, R. C. P. M. (1971). *Amer. J. Clin. Nutr.* **24**, 730.

Harper, A. E. (1964). *Mammalian Protein Metab.* **2**, 115.

Harper, A. E., Benton, D. A., and Elvehjem, C. A. (1955). *Arch. Biochem. Biophys.* **57**, 1.

Harper, A. E., Benevenga, N. J., and Wohlhueter, R. M. (1970). *Physiol. Rev.* **50**, 428.

Henderson, L. M. (1949). *J. Biol. Chem.* **181**, 677.

Henderson, L. M., and Hirsch, H. M. (1949). *J. Biol. Chem.* **181**, 667.

Henderson, L. M., Ramasarma, G. B., and Johnson, B. C. (1949). *J. Biol. Chem.* **181**, 731.

Henderson, L. M., Koeppe, O. J., and Zimmerman, H. H. (1953). *J. Biol. Chem.* **201**, 697.

Horwitt, M. K., Harvey, C. C., Rothwell, W. S., Cutler, J. L., and Haffron, D. (1956). *J. Nutr.* **60**, Suppl. 1.

Huff, J. W., and Perlzweig, W. A. (1943a). *Science* **97**, 538.

Huff, J. W., and Perlzweig, W. A. (1943b). *J. Biol. Chem.* **150**, 395.

Ikeda, M., Tsuji, H., Nakamura, S, Ichiyama, A., Nishizuka, Y., and Hayaishi, O. (1965). *J. Biol. Chem.* **240**, 1395.

Jolliffe, N., Bowman, K. M., Rosenblum, L. A., and Fein, H. D. (1940). *J. Amer. Med. Ass.* **114**, 307.

Kaladhar, M. (1972). Annual Report, p. 90. National Institute of Nutrition, Hyderabad, India.

Kaladhar, M. (1974). Annual Report, p. 70. National Institute of Nutrition, Hyderabad, India.

Knox, W. E., and Grossman, W. I. (1946). *J. Biol. Chem.* **166**, 391.

Kodicek, E. (1940). *Biochem. J.* **34**, 712.

Kodicek, E. (1960). *Brit. J. Nutr.* **14**, 13.

Kodicek, E., Braude, R., Kon, S. K., and Mitchell, K. G. (1956). *Brit. J. Nutr.* **10**, 51.

Kodicek, E., Braude, R., Kon, S. K., and Mitchell, K. G. (1959). *Brit. J. Nutr.* **13**, 363.

Koeppe, O. J., and Henderson, L. M. (1955). *J. Nutr.* **55**, 23.

Krehl, W. A., Elvehjem, C. A., and Strong, F. M. (1944). *J. Biol. Chem.* **156**, 13.

Krehl, W. A., Teply, L. J., and Elvehjem, C. A. (1945a). *Science* **101**, 283.

Krehl, W. A., Teply, L. J., Sarma, P. S., and Elvehjem, C. A. (1945b). *Science* **101**, 489.

Krishnamachari, K. A. V .R. (1974). *Amer. J. Clin. Nutr.* **27**, 108.

Krishnaswamy, K. (1968). M. D. Thesis, Osmania University, Hyderabad, India.

Krishnaswamy, K., and Gopalan, C. (1971). *Lancet* **2**, 1167.

Krishnaswamy, K., and Raghuram, T. C. (1972). *Life Sci., Part II* **11**, 1191.

Krishnaswamy, K., and Ramanamurthy, P. S. V. (1970). *Clin. Chim. Acta* **27**, 301.

Lan, S. J., and Gholson, R. K. (1965). *J. Biol. Chem.* **240**, 3934.

Lyman, R. L., and Elvehjem, C. A. (1951). *J. Nutr.* **45**, 101.

McKean, C. M., Schanberg, S. M., and Giarman, N. J. (1962). *Science* **137**, 604.

Madhavan, T. V., Belavady, B., and Gopalan, C. (1968). *J. Pathol. Bacteriol.* **95**, 259.

Mertz, E. T., Bates, L. S., and Nelson, O. E. (1964). *Science* **145**, 279.

Mertz, E. T., Veron, O. A., Bates, L. S., and Nelson, O. E. (1965). *Science* **148**, 1741.

Moline, S. W., Walker, H. C., and Schweigert, B. S. (1959). *J. Biol. Chem.* **234**, 880.

Najjar, V. A., and Wood, R. W. (1940). *Proc. Soc. Exp. Biol. Med.* **44**, 386.

Neumann, P. Z., and Sass-Kortsak, A. (1967). *J. Clin. Invest.* **46**, 646.

Nishizuka, Y., and Hayaishi, O. (1963). *J. Biol. Chem.* **238**, 3369.

O'Dell, B. L., Hardwick, B. C., Reynolds, G., and Savage, J. E. (1961). *Proc. Soc. Exp. Biol. Med.* **108**, 402.

O'Dell, B. L., Bird, D. W., Ruggles, D. L., and Savage, J. E., (1966). *J. Nutr.* **88**, 9.

Perlzweig, W. A., and Huff, J. W. (1945). *J. Biol. Chem.* **161**, 417.

Perlzweig, W. A., Rosen, F., Levitas, N., and Robinson, J. (1947). *J. Biol. Chem.* **167**, 511.

Potgeiter, J. F., Fellingham, S. A., and Neser, M. L. (1966). *S. Afr. J. Nutr.* 2(2), 22. Supplement to *S. Afr. Med. J.* **40**, 504.

Preiss, J., and Handler, P. (1958a). *J. Biol. Chem.* **233**, 488.

Preiss, J., and Handler, P. (1958b). *J. Biol. Chem.* **233**, 493.

Raghuramulu, N., Narasinga Rao, B. S., and Gopalan, C. (1965a). *J. Nutr.* **86**, 100.

Raghuramulu, N., Srikantia, S. G., Narasinga Rao, B. S., and Gopalan, C. (1965b). *Biochem. J.* **96**, 837.

Ramanamurthy, P. S. V., and Srikantia, S. G. (1970). *J. Neurochem.* **17**, 27.

Rogers, Q. R., Spolter, P. D., and Harper, A. E. (1962). *Arch. Biochem. Biophys.* **97**, 497.

Rosen, F., and Perlzweig, W. A. (1949). *J. Biol. Chem.* **177**, 163.

Rosen, F., Huff, J. W., and Perlzweig, W. A. (1946). *J. Biol. Chem.* **163**, 343.

Salib, M. (1959). *Gastroenterology* **36**, 816.

Sarkar, B., and Kruck, T. P. A. (1966). *In* "Biochemistry of Copper" (J. Peisach, P. Aisen, and W. E. Blumberg, eds.), p. 183. Academic Press, New York.

Sarrett, H. P. (1951). *J. Biol. Chem.* **193**, 627.

Sarrett, H. P., and Goldsmith, G. A. (1947). *J. Biol. Chem.* **167**, 293.

Sauberlich, H. E., Chang, W. Y., and Salmon, W. D. (1953). *J. Nutr.* **51**, 623.

Schanberg, S. M. (1963). *J. Pharmacol. Exp. Ther.* **139**, 191.

Scherer, B., and Kramer, W. (1972). *Life Sci., Part I* **11**, 189.

Shah, D. R., and Singh, S. V. (1967). *J. Ass. Physicians India* **15**, 1.

Shields, G. S., Coulson, W. F., Kimball, D. A., Carnes, W. H., Cartwright, G. E., and Wintrobe, M. M. (1962). *Amer. J. Pathol.* **41**, 603.

Singal, S. A., Briggs, A. P., Sydenstricker, V. P., and Littlejohn, J. M. (1946). *J. Biol. Chem.* **166**, 573.

Spies, T. D., Cooper, C., and Blankenhorn, M. A. (1938). *J. Amer. Med. Ass.* **110**, 622.

Spillane, J. D. (1947). "Nutritional Disorders of the Nervous System," p. 29. Livingstone, Edinburgh.

Squibb, R. L., Braham, J. E., Arroyave, G., and Scrimshaw, N. S. (1959). *J. Nutr.* **67**, 351.

Srikantia, S. G., Narasinga Rao, B. S., Raghuramulu, N., and Gopalan, C. (1968a). *Amer. J. Clin. Nutr.* **21**, 1306.

Srikantia, S. G., Reddy, V., and Krishnaswamy, K. (1968b). *Electroencephalogr. Clin Neurophysiol.* **25**, 386.

Swendseid, M. E., Villalobos, J., Figueroa, W. S., and Drenick, E. J. (1965). *Amer. J. Clin. Nutr.* **17**, 317.

Tabachnick, J. (1957). *Arch. Biochem. Biophys.* **70**, 295.

Teply, L. J., Krehl, W. A., and Elvehjem, C. A. (1945). *Arch. Biochem.* **6**, 139.

Terris, M. (1964). "Goldberger on Pellagra." Louisiana State Univ. Press, Baton Rouge.

Truswell, A. S., Hansen, J. D. L., and Wannenburg, P. (1968). *Amer. J. Clin. Nutr.* **21**, 1314.

Twarog, B. M., and Page, I. H. (1953). *Amer. J. Physiol.* **175**, 157.

Udenfriend, S., Titus, E., Weissbach, H., and Peterson, R. E. (1956). *J. Biol. Chem.* **219**, 335.

Udenfriend, S., Weissbach, H., and Bogdanski, D. F. (1957a). *J. Biol. Chem.* **224**, 803.

Udenfriend, S., Weissbach, H., and Bogdanski, D. F. (1957b). *Ann. N.Y. Acad. Sci.* **66**, 602.

Vasantha, L. (1970a). *Clin. Chim. Acta* **27**, 543.

Vasantha, L. (1970b). *Indian J. Med. Res.* **58**, 1079.

Weissman, N., Shields, G. S., and Carnes, W. H. (1963). *J. Biol. Chem.* **238**, 3115.

Woolley, D. W. (1946). *J. Biol. Chem.* **163**, 773.

Woolley, D. W., and Shaw, E. (1954). *Brit. Med. J.* **2**, 122.

Woolley, D. W., and Shaw, E. N. (1957). *Ann. N.Y. Acad. Sci.* **66**, 649.

Yuwiler, A., and Geller, E. (1965). *Nature (London)* **208**, 83.

Zenisek, A., Kral, J. A., and Hais, I. M. (1955). *Biochim. Biophys. Acta* **18**, 589.

Myo-inositol Lipids

J. N. HAWTHORNE AND D. A. WHITE

*Department of Biochemistry, University Hospital and Medical School,
Nottingham, England*

I. INTRODUCTION

Myo-inositol is generally included among the vitamins, although its status there is not completely secure since it can be synthesized from glucose in various tissues. Its function is still not well understood in molecular terms, but it seems clear that a major role (if not the only one) involves the membrane phospholipids which contain inositol. Several important advances have been made in this area during the last year or two.

This article is intended to supplement an earlier review by one of us (Hawthorne, 1964) and therefore deals briefly with the general metabolism of myo-inositol lipids. Much new information has been published in the last decade and an exhaustive compilation would be merely exhausting, so we have not attempted this.

A few related reviews may be of interest. Hokin (1968) has considered inositol lipid metabolism and zymogen secretion by pancreas. Phosphoinositides in the nervous system have been reviewed by Hawthorne and Kai (1970) and L. E. Hokin (1969), and phospholipid metabolism in relation to transport across cell membranes is the subject of a chapter by Hawthorne (1973). A recent article by Michell (1975) deals with receptor activation and phosphatidylinositol metabolism. A conference of the New York Academy of Sciences in 1968 was devoted to cyclitols and phosphoinositides (Eisenberg, 1969), and the treatise of Posternak (1965) on cyclitols has a great deal of useful information.

II. METABOLISM IN OUTLINE

A. STRUCTURES

This brief account deals only with phosphatidylinositol (PI) (I), phosphatidylinositol 4-phosphate (diphosphoinositide, DPI) (II), and phosphatidylinositol 4,5-bisphosphate (triphosphoinositide, TPI) (III). Nomenclature of compounds II and III is still confused. In the absence

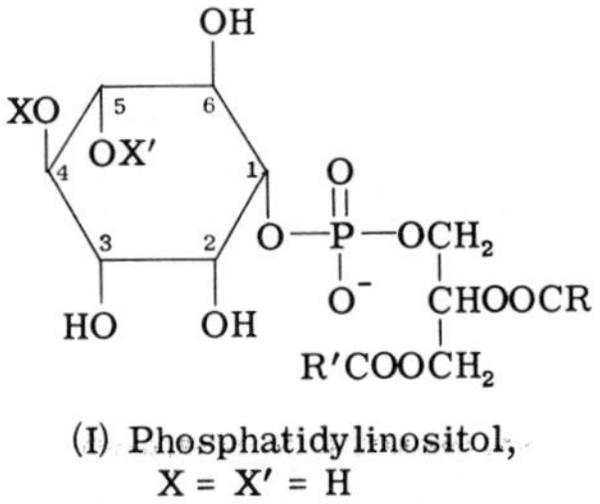

(I) Phosphatidylinositol,
X = X' = H
(II) Diphosphoinositide,
X = PO_3^{2-}, X' = H
(III) Triphosphoinositide,
X = X' = PO_3^{2-}

of an internationally agreed terminology, the shorter names diphospho-inositide and triphosphoinositide are used here. Klyashchitskii *et al.* (1969a) discuss the nomenclature of phosphatidylinositol and derivatives.

B. BIOSYNTHESIS

The major route, in which CDP-diacylglycerol is a key intermediate, is given in Fig. 1. Phosphatidylinositol biosynthesis takes place on the membranes of the endoplasmic reticulum whereas the phosphorylations of the 4- and 5-hydroxyls to give DPI and TPI are associated with plasma membranes and other parts of the cell, which vary from tissue to tissue.

C. CATABOLISM

Enzymes that hydrolyze all three phosphoinositides to diacylglycerol and an inositol phosphate are widely distributed in animal tissues. There are also phosphomonoesterases which convert TPI to DPI and DPI to phosphatidylinositol.

Dawson *et al.* (1971) have shown that D-inositol 1,2-cyclic phosphate (IV) is produced by the enzyme that hydrolyzes phosphatidylinositol in many tissues, rather than the D-inositol 1-phosphate, as was originally thought. A further diesterase converts the cyclic phosphate to D-inositol 1-phosphate (Dawson and Clarke, 1972). This enzyme is particularly active in kidney, where it is located in the brush borders of the proximal tubules (Clarke and Dawson, 1972).

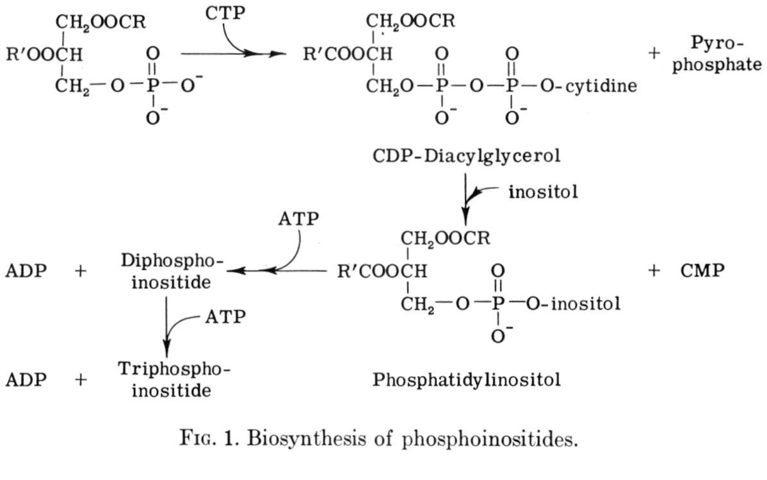

FIG. 1. Biosynthesis of phosphoinositides.

(IV)

Inositol cyclic phosphates may also be produced by enzymic hydrolysis of DPI and TPI, but these reactions have not yet been studied in detail.

III. CHEMICAL SYNTHESIS OF PHOSPHATIDYLINOSITOL

The major problems of chemical synthesis of PI have involved the synthesis of a protected myoinositol with a free hydroxyl at C-1 on the inositol ring and also the isolation of an optically active product. Before the final elucidation of the structure of PI by Brockerhoff and Ballou (1961), Davies and Malkin (1959) condensed sn-1:2-distearoyl-3-iodoglycerol with silver-2(1:3:4:5:6-penta-o-acetyl) myo-inositol phenylphosphate, forming the 2-isomer of PI on removal of the protecting acetyl groups. Early studies on the chemical synthesis of PI have been reviewed by Klyashchitskii et al. (1969b). The group of Preobrazhenski in Russia (Luk'yanov et al. 1965) have synthesized a racemic PI and also claim (Zhelvakova et al., 1970) to have synthesized a PI having the stereo-chemistry of the natural product. However, they failed to give experimental conditions and their method has been criticized by Gent et al. (1970). These latter workers described the synthesis of racemic PI by two methods using the benzyl group to protect the inositol hydroxyls. The first method involves condensation of the silver salt of 2,3,4,5,6-penta-o-benzylmyo-inositol-1-benzylphosphate (I) with 1,2-dipalmitoyl-3-iodoglycerol to produce a fully protected PI. In the second method, they allowed the sodium salt of (I) to react with 1:2-dipalmitoyl-L-glycerol in the presence of triisopropylbenzene sulfonyl chloride in dry pyridine, again producing the fully substituted PI. The products from both methods were converted to the free acid, separated by alumina column chromatography, and treated with hydrogen over palladium on charcoal to remove the protecting benzyl groups. In each case the purified lipid gave elemental analyses in excellent agreement with the theoretical. The disadvantages of the methods are that (1) the product is a racemic mixture and thus further separation of the isomers is required, and (2) the final hydrogenation for removal of the benzyl groups precludes synthesis of unsaturated molecular species of PI.

An alternative synthetic route which overcomes the second disadvantage has been published by Molotkovskii and Bergel'son (1971). These workers synthesized the silver salt of *rac*-1-benzylphosphoryl-(2,3,4,5,6)-penta-*o*-acetyl-myo-inositol and allowed this to react with 1-lauroyl-2-oleoyl-*sn*-glycerol-3-iodohydrin in a reaction similar to the first method of Gent *et al.* (1970). However, the acetyl protecting groups were removed by hydrazinolysis and thus left any unsaturated bonds in the fatty acids of the molecule intact. The PI synthesized in this way was indistinguishable from yeast PI on thin-layer chromatography (TLC) in basic, neutral, and acid solvents and gave a white powder of $[\alpha_D]$ $+2.3°$ and melting point $180°–185°C$ (decomp) on recrystallization from chloroform–acetone. Elemental analysis was in excellent agreement with the theoretical values and the overall yield was about 10%.

Phosphatidylinositol synthesized by these methods has not as yet been used in any biological studies but could prove to be very useful particularly in physical experiments when defined fatty acid composition is required. The problem of separating the isomers from the racemic product has not yet been overcome, but it would be of interest to see whether both isomers or just one of them act as substrates in, for instance, the PI kinase reaction—indeed any specificity might prove useful in the separation of the isomers.

IV. Extraction and Separation Methods

A. Extraction of Inositol Lipids

Bulk preparations of the inositides may be obtained from animal tissues, particularly brain, by methods based on those of Folch (1942, 1949) using a sequential extraction of the tissue with acetone, ethanol, and petroleum ether. Ethanol precipitation of the petroleum ether extract redissolved in diethyl ether gives an inositide-rich fraction. From this fraction, PI may be prepared by repeated methanol precipitation of DPI and TPI from chloroform, leaving PI in solution (Dittmer and Dawson, 1961). The major contaminants, phosphatidylserine and phosphatidylethanolamine, can be separated from the PI by alumina (Long and Owens, 1962; Luthra and Sheltawy, 1972a) and silicic acid chromatography (Spanner, 1973) respectively.

Ansell and Hawthorne (1964) described a method of preparing PI on silicic acid in high yield from a chloroform–methanol (2:1, v/v) extract of frozen peas, and a convenient reproducible method for the preparation of PI from asolectin (a commercially available preparation of soybean phosphatides) has been reported by Colacicco and Rapport (1967). In this method PI was precipitated with methanol from a solution of asolectin in chloroform and further purified on a silicic acid column. Plant PI has also been purified from various commercially available seeds using a countercurrent distribution technique involving hexane–alcohol–water systems to separate the two major inositol-containing fractions (Carter and Kisic, 1969). Phytoglycolipid partitioned in the hexane phases, and PI was found in the alcohol phases. The extraction of inositides from yeast presents problems unless the cell wall is at least partially removed. S. Steiner and Lester (1972) treated *Saccharomyces cerevisiae* with snail juice enzyme to hydrolyze the cell wall prior to extraction with an ethanol–water–ether–pyridine mixture (15:15:5:1, by volume) at 60°C for 15 minutes. Under these conditions PI, DPI, and TPI and an inositol-containing sphingolipid, ceramide-$(inositol)_2$-$(phosphate)_2$-mannose were extracted.

Quantitative extraction of PI, particularly from small quantities of tissue and from tissue homogenates and subcellular fractions, has usually utilized chloroform–methanol mixtures. In the system of Bligh and Dyer (1959) the sample is extracted with chloroform–methanol (1:2, v/v) and further chloroform and water added later to give a final chloroform–methanol–water ratio of 1:1:0.9 (by volume), a two-phase system in which lipid partions in the lower chloroform layer and water-soluble material partitions in the upper phase. Insoluble protein lies at the interphase. Folch *et al.* (1957) used a salt solution instead of the additional water. Such a system has been criticized by Palmer (1971), who showed that not all of the acidic lipids partitioned into the chloroform layer, particularly in the presence of insoluble protein where some of the acidic lipids are adsorbed onto the protein at the interphase. The loss of PI in this way appears to be random, suggesting that complete extraction of the lipid occurs followed by random readsorption on to the protein surface. Addition of small amounts of divalent cation reduced the readsorption. This had previously been demonstrated for TPI by Dawson (1965), who showed that the sodium salt of TPI partitioned in the upper phase of a two-phase chloroform–methanol–water system but partitioned in the lower phase on addition of Ca^{2+} or Mg^{2+}. On further addition of serum albumin some of the Ca^{2+}-TPI bound to the protein at the interphase and was insoluble in chloroform–methanol (2:1, v/v). However, it was soluble in acidified chloroform–methanol.

The extraction of the higher inositides from tissues has received much attention since these are not extracted by the usual neutral chloroform–methanol mixtures. Also, during the acetone extraction of the Folch procedure much of the tissue TPI undergoes autolysis to DPI (Kerr *et al.*, 1964; Wells and Dittmer, 1965; Dawson and Eichberg, 1965), and during prolonged extraction procedures hydrolysis of both DPI and TPI occurs (Hayashi *et al.*, 1966; Eichberg and Hauser, 1967; Dittmer and Douglas, 1969). In addition the petroleum ether extractions of the Folch procedure did not extract all the DPI and TPI from the tissue (rat and ox brain, Wells and Dittmer, 1965; guinea pig and ox brain, Dawson and Eichberg, 1965). Further DPI and TPI were recovered on reextraction with acidified chloroform–methanol. Higher recoveries were obtained by homogenizing fresh frozen tissue in chloroform–methanol (2:1 v/v containing 0.25% HCl) and then separating the phases with 1 M HCl. Since this extracts all the tissue lipids and complicates the separation of DPI and TPI, subsequent procedures involved extraction of the tissue with neutral chloroform–methanol (2:1 v/v) to remove all lipids except DPI and TPI. These higher inositides were then extracted using acidified chloroform–methanol. No further combined inositiol was recovered following such a procedure (Le Baron *et al.*, 1963; Dawson and Eichberg, 1965). A comprehensive review of various extraction methods appears in the paper of Wells and Dittmer (1965).

More recently, the recovery of higher inositides has been investigated by Michell *et al.* (1970), who quantitatively extracted DPI and TPI from guinea pig brain with a chloroform–methanol–2 M KCl mixture after previous extraction of the tissue with neutral chloroform–methanol (2:1, v/v). Such extracts were essentially free of chloroform-insoluble material and inorganic phosphate. Extracts obtained with acidified solvents are often highly colored and yield residues insoluble in chloroform–methanol on drying, although Wells and Dittmer (1963) removed much of the latter by pretreatment of the extract with Sephadex. Michell *et al.* (1970) further showed that less than 5% of the total higher inositides of the tissue was recovered on reextraction with acidified chloroform–methanol. However, the principles governing this salt extraction procedure are unclear, and polyphosphoinositides were not extracted from guinea pig liver or from several other tissues.

Because of the rapid loss of phosphoinositides from brain post mortem due to phosphomonoesterase activity (e.g., 63% of ^{32}P-labeled TPI of guinea pig brain is lost after 10 minutes at 30°C post mortem, Hayashi *et al.*, 1966), Eichberg and Hauser (1973) suggested that satisfactory quantitative extraction of DPI and TPI can be made only from tissue frozen *in situ* immediately after death. Lipids extracted into chloroform–methanol–HCl (200:100:1, by volume) are stable for at least 18 hours at 4°C (Hayashi *et al.*, 1966), and Sheltawy and Dawson (1969) noted that addition of butylated hydroxytoluene to the extract improved recovery and subsequent chromatography. These conditions have been improved recently by Hauser and Eichberg (1973) particularly for extractions from tissue homogenates and subcellular fractions, where some time elapses before extraction. These authors have recommended the addition of calcium chloride (60 μmoles per gram of tissue) to the neutral chloroform–methanol (1:1, v/v) mixture and that the tissue be extracted with at least 15 volumes of this solvent before extracting with acidified chloroform–methanol. Since the TPI phosphomonoesterase of brain has little activity at alkaline pH, higher recoveries of TPI from homogenates and subcellular fractions of immature rat brains were obtained by homogenizing the tissue in sucrose buffered to pH 9.5 with Tris Cl maintained at 0°C, and then extracting with neutral and acidified chloroform–methanol as for the whole tissue. However, the increased recoveries of TPI under these conditions may only reflect the phosphomonoesterase activity and low calcium levels of immature brains, since similar large differences were not seen with adult brain or kidney. The authors suggested that calcium aided retention of polyphosphoinositides in the tissue by formation of a protein–Ca^{2+}–TPI complex (viz. Dawson, 1965). Since the calcium levels in adult brain and kidney were higher than levels in the immature brain, addition of calcium during the extraction had no effect.

Thus, in general, extraction of inositides with acidified chloroform–methanol should be made immediately from fresh tissue or from tissue frozen immediately on death. An initial extraction with neutral chloroform–methanol removes phosphatidylinositiol and all other phospholipids except DPI and TPI. For extraction from tissue homogenates and subcellular fractions, homogenization conditions should be modified to minimize the activity of hydrolytic degradative enzymes during the fractionation procedure. In this respect the hydrolysis of PI should not be ignored, since, during fractionation of pancreas, White *et al.* (1971) and Meldolesi *et al.* (1971) reported hydrolysis of phospholipids, including phosphatidylinositol, during fractionation even though the temperature throughout was kept at 4°C.

B. Chromatographic Separations

The final isolation and separation of inositol lipids has been carried out in a number of ways including column, paper, and thin-layer chromatography.

1. Column Chromatography

Prior to the development of techniques for the separation of intact lipids, ion exchange chromatography was used to separate the water-soluble phosphate esters derived from alkaline hydrolysis. Ellis *et al.* (1963) used mild alkaline conditions to hydrolyze the DPI fraction of ox brain and separated the products on Dowex-1 (formate) by eluting with an ammonium formate–sodium borate–formic acid gradient. Because such hydrolyses incur losses due to further hydrolysis of the phosphodiester linkage, Wells and Dittmer (1965) modified the alkaline methanolysis procedure of Brockerhoff (1963) and separated the products on Bio-Rad AG1-X2 at pH 9.5 with a formate–borate gradient using a method developed by Lester (1963). The extraction, methanolysis, and separation by anion exchange chromatography of inositides of *S. cerevisiae* has been described in detail by Lester and Steiner (1968).

Separation of intact phosphoinositides by ion exchange on DEAE-cellulose acetate was first reported by Hendrickson and Ballou (1964), who eluted the lipids with a gradient of 0–0.5 M ammonium acetate. This is particularly useful for large-scale preparations of the inositides. Cooper and Hawthorne (1973) described a separation of inositides on silicic acid impregnated with potassium oxalate eluting with chloroform–methanol–ammonia, a method based on the TLC method of Gonzalez-Sastre and Folch-Pi (1968).

Little information on the quantitative isolation of phosphatidylmanno-sides from bacterial sources is available but they appear to be extracted by neutral chloroform–methanol (Brennan and Lehane, 1971).

PI may be purified by chromatography on alumina and silicic acid, and a comprehensive monograph on the use of these columns has recently appeared (Kates, 1972).

2. *Paper Chromatography*

Acid and alkaline hydrolysis of inositides and separation of the water-soluble products by two-dimensional paper chromatography ionophoresis was reported by Dawson and Dittmer (1961) and Eichberg and Dawson (1965).

Intact phosphoinositides were separated on formaldehyde-impregnated papers by Wagner *et al.* (1963). Santiago-Calvó *et al.* (1964) separated DPI and TPI from other phospholipids on silicic acid-impregnated papers developed in a phenol–ammonia solvent. These methods give good separations of the inositides, but the former papers are rather tedious to prepare and, although silicic acid-impregnated papers can now be obtained commercially, both have in general been replaced by TLC. However, many systems are available for separation of PI from other phospholipids on silicic acid-impregnated papers (e.g., Wuthier, 1966), and S. Steiner and Lester (1972) have separated DPI and TPI in a two-dimensional system on EDTA-treated, silicic acid-impregnated papers.

3. *Thin-Layer Chromatography*

Numerous solvent systems have been described for the separation of phospholipids on silica gel, but a major problem has been the separation of PS from PI, particularly in one-dimensional systems. Skipski *et al.* (1964) used basic silicic acid (containing 1 mM Na$_2$CO$_3$) developed in chloroform–methanol–acetic acid–water (25:15:4:2, by volume) to separate them, but this has not been very reproducible, and Rouser *et al.* (1969) have developed two-step one-dimensional systems. More consistent separations have been obtained using two-dimensional TLC developing the plate in an acidic solvent in one dimension and then in a basic solvent in the other. Again many systems have been described, and those of Pumphrey (1969) and Rouser *et al.* (1967) have proved useful in the authors' hands. In the former system DPI and TPI remain at the origin whereas the latter system resolves them. A rapid one-dimensional system for separation of PI, DPI, and TPI on silica gel H, impregnated with 1 mM potassium oxalate, was reported by Gonzalez-Sastre and Folch-Pi (1968). Hauser *et al.* (1971a) have recently reported a one-dimensional two-step system for separation of inositides on silicic acid.

4. *Gas–Liquid Chromatography and Mass Spectroscopy*

A novel method of analysis and assay of brain phosphoinositides was reported by Cicero and Sherman (1971). After extraction of the fresh frozen tissue with neutral chloroform–methanol, DPI and TPI were extracted with acidified chloroform–methanol and deacylated with methanolic sodium hydroxide. After conversion to the free acid, the water-soluble GPIP and GPIP$_2$ were further converted to their trimethylsilyl derivatives and separated on a column of 1% SE-30 on Gas Chrom Q using helium as carrier gas. Peaks eluting from the column were analyzed by mass spectroscopy. The authors claim to be able to measure DPI and TPI levels in 1 mg or less of tissue, a sensitivity over 100-fold greater than by other methods (Cicero and Sherman, 1973).

C. ANALYSIS OF MOLECULAR SPECIES OF INOSITOL LIPIDS

The fatty acid composition of inositol lipids has been determined by the usual process of gas–liquid chromatography (GLC) of the methyl esters of fatty acids released on alkaline methanolysis. However, more recently analysis of individual molecular species of the inositides has been obtained, particularly from the laboratories of Holub and Sheltawy.

Holub *et al.* (1970) isolated PI, DPI, and TPI of ox brain and used a specific brain phosphodiesterase to hydrolyze them to diglycerides, which were identified and quantitated as their acetates by argentation chromatography and GLC. Complete positional analysis was obtained by treating the diglycerides with pancreatic lipase and determining the released fatty acid by GLC. Holub and Kuksis (1971a) reported the separation of molecular species of intact unmodified PI, prepared from rat liver, by argentation chromatography. Although mono- and dienoic species cochromatographed, they were well separated from the tri- and tetraenoic species. Good agreement was obtained between the fatty acid composition of the original and reconstituted PI, suggesting that no significant losses of any molecular species had occurred during the argentation chromatography.

Akino and Shimojo (1970) used the procedure of Renkonen (1968) to separate molecular species of PI. After isolation, the lipid was subjected to acetolysis and the resulting diglyceride acetates were separated on silver nitrate-impregnated plates. The recovery of 1:2-diglyceride acetates was greater than 90%, but the method is somewhat limited in that studies of the phosphate and inositol moieties cannot be made.

Luthra and Sheltawy (1972a,b,c) developed two methods of separating molecular species of PI purified from lamb's liver and ox brain. Both involved modification of the inositol ring prior to argentation chromatography. In the first method the inositol ring was oxidized with periodate to yield phosphatidic acid, which was esterified to its dimethyl ester with diazomethane. The molecular species of dimethylphosphatidic acid thus formed were analyzed by argentation chromatography. The method was made quantitative by eluting the dimethylphosphatidic acids from the plates and analyzing the radioactive fatty acid methyl esters released by alkaline methanolysis using ^{3}H-labeled methanol.

In a second method the phosphatidylinositol was acetylated to its tri-O-acetyl derivative and methylated with diazomethane. These dimethyl triacetyl phosphatidylinositols were then separated by argentation chromatography and quantitated by methanolysis in ^{3}H-labeled methanol as before. Both methods gave good separation of mono-, di-, tri-, and tetraenoic species, and results were in good agreement. However, the latter method has an advantage over the former since the inositol ring is retained intact and allows metabolic studies of this part of the molecule.

Thus it is now possible to extract and analyze quantitatively inositides from a range of tissues, and, using the methods of Holub and Sheltawy described above, a complete analysis of each part of the molecule and its metabolism can be made.

V. Analysis and Distribution

The phosphatidylinositol content of some mammalian and plant tissues is given in Tables I and II. More extensive analyses of PI content and fatty acid composition of PI of subfractions of tissues have been compiled by Galliard (1973) and White (1973). The higher inositide content of tissues such as those in Table III will depend very much on the extraction conditions as discussed in Section IV, and thus the values quoted in Table III should be considered minimal. It is not known whether, under various metabolic conditions, all the PI of the tissues can be converted to DPI and TPI as reported for erythrocytes (Buckley and Hawthorne, 1972).

The molecular species of PI from liver of rat and lamb and brain of ox are given in Table IV. In rat liver and bovine brain the arachidonoyl-tetraenoic species are predominant. Holub et al. (1970) detected 27 different molecular species of PI in ox brain but $C_{18:0}$, $C_{20:4}$-tetraene constituted greater than 40% of the total PI. The molecular species of DPI and TPI from ox brain showed a similar distribution pattern to PI

TABLE I

PHOSPHATIDYLINOSITOL AS PERCENTAGE OF TOTAL PHOSPHOLIPID P FROM VARIOUS MAMMALIAN TISSUES

Tissue	Total lipid P (mg P/gm wet wt)	PI (% total lipid P) Human	Rat	Cow	References
Heart	0.66 (human)	6.1	3.7	4.1	Simon and Rouser (1969) Dawson et al. (1962)
Liver	1.32 (human)	8.6	7.2	7.9	Rouser et al. (1969) Wuthier (1966) Dawson et al. (1962)
Kidney	0.58 (human)	5.5	5.9	7.2	Rouser et al. (1969)
Spleen	0.79 (human)	4.4	5.5	4.3	Rouser et al. (1969)
Lung	0.14 (human)	3.2	3.9	3.3	Baxter et al. (1969)
Skeletal muscle	0.53 (human)	6.0	8.9	5.6	Simon and Rouser (1969)
Erythrocytes	—	0	3.5	3.7	Dawson et al. (1962), Nelson (1967)
Pancreas	0.87 (bovine)	—	8.7	8.7	Prottey and Hawthorne (1966) Gurr et al. (1965)
Thyroid	0.24 (bovine)	—	—	11.7	Macchia and Pastan (1968)
Thymus	0.39 (rat)	—	11.9	0.2	Abramson and Blecher (1965) Rose and Frenster (1965)
Pituitary	0.61 (human)	4.2	15.5	6.3	Singh and Carroll (1970) Clement et al. (1963)
Intestinal mucosa	—	—	4.1	—	Gurr et al. (1965)

TABLE II

PHOSPHATIDYLINOSITOL CONTENT OF NONMAMMALIAN TISSUES

Source	PI (as % total phospholipid)	Reference
Yeast: *Saccharomyces cerevisiae*	22.5	S. Steiner and Lester (1972)
S. pombe	17.6	White and Hawthorne (1970)
Protozoan: *Crithidia fasciculata*	16.3	Palmer (1973a)
Insect larvae: *Aedes aegypt*	7.0	Townsend *et al.* (1972)
Leaves: Maize	7	Roughan and Batt (1969)
Lettuce	7	Roughan and Batt (1969)
Tomato	5	Roughan and Batt (1969)
Tobacco	22	Benson and Maruo (1958)
Pumpkin	13	Roughan (1970)
Lucerne alfalfa	63	Kuiper (1970)
Sweet clover	18	Benson and Maruo (1958)
Runner bean	9	Sastry and Kates (1964)
Pine	16	Roughan and Batt (1969)
Cotyledon: Pea	18	Quarles and Dawson (1969)
Root: Parsnip	13	Roughan and Batt (1969)
Tuber: Potato	26	Lepage (1968)
Fruit: Apple	13	Galliard (1968)
Bud: Cotton	26	Thompson *et al.* (1968)
Seed: Soybean	25	Paulose *et al.* (1966)
Cotton	37	Vijayalakshmi *et al.* (1969)
Cocoa	25–29	Parsons *et al.* (1969)
Green algae: *Chlorella vulgaris*	14	Sastry and Kates (1965)
Euglena gracilis	9	Calvayrac and Douce (1970)

TABLE III

PHOSPHOINOSITIDE CONTENT[a] OF SOME MAMMALIAN TISSUES

Tissue	PI	DPI	TPI	Reference
Rat brain (7 day)	—	164	86	Eichberg and Hauser (1973)
Adult (34 day)	—	279	300	Eichberg and Hauser (1973)
Adult	—	160	440	Baker and Thompson 1972)
Guinea pig brain				
Gray matter	—	41.9	287	Sheltawy and Dawson (1969)
White matter	—	403.3	677	Sheltawy and Dawson (1969)
Rat kidney	—	67	130	Sheltawy and Dawson (1969)
Rat kidney	1348	306	503	Tou *et al.* (1972)
Erythrocytes, pig	—	16.8	43.7	Schneider and Kirschner (1970)

[a] All values are expressed as nanomoles per gram wet weight of tissue except for erythrocytes, which are expressed in nanomoles per milliliter of cells.

TABLE IV

MOLECULAR SPECIES OF PHOSPHATIDYLINOSITOL FROM SOME MAMMALIAN TISSUES

Tissue	Molecular species	% total PI	Fatty acids as % total						Reference
			16:0	18:0	18:1	18:2	20:3	20:4	
Liver, rat	Monoenes	2.1	—	—	—	—	—	—	Akino and Shimojo (1970)
	Dienes	8.0	9.7	50.4	—	37.8	—	—	
	Trienes	3.2	—	—	—	—	—	—	
	Tetraenes	86.8	3.3	52.4	—	—	—	41.4	
Liver, lamb	Monoenes	60	6.1	38.8	51.8	—	—	—	Luthra and Sheltawy (1972b)
	Dienes	6	—	39.1	—	59.0	—	—	
	Trienes	11	—	59.0	—	—	36.0	—	
	Tetraenes	17	—	56.6	—	—	—	41.8	
	Pentaenes	3	—	47.9	—	—	—	19.0	
	Hexaenes	4	—	27.0	—	—	42.6	—	
Brain, ox	Monoenes	9.6	27.5	22.0	44.0	—	—	—	Holub et al. (1970)
	Dienes	6.1	19.0	15.5	24.0	15.0	—	—	
	Trienes	9.2	4.5	45.5	—	—	50.0	45.5	
	Tetraenes	71.9	—	41.5	4.5	16.5	0.5	33.5	
	Pentaenes	2.5	—	—	33.5	—	—	—	

(Holub *et al.*, 1970). In lamb liver, however, the $C_{18:0}$, $C_{18:1}$-monoene is the major molecular species (Luthra and Sheltawy, 1972b), and the fully saturated species of PI predominate in lung surfactant of rabbit, sheep, and cow (J. L. Harwood and R. Richards, personal communication).

The final molecular species pattern says little about the biosynthesis and metabolism of PI in the tissue. As discussed in Section VII, the dienoic species of PI appear to be the major species synthesized *de novo* by rat liver *in vivo*, and this later undergoes deacylation and reacylation to give the tetraenoic species, which predominate in the tissue. Also, Luthra and Sheltawy (1976) have studied the metabolism of different molecular species of phosphatidic acid and PI after intracranial injection of ^{32}P and [^{14}C]glucose. Acylation of glycerophosphate gave predominantly a monoenoic phosphatidate while the tetraenoic compound was least readily formed. The diacylglycerol kinase route, on the contrary, accepted the tetraenoic compound most avidly and the monoenoic or saturated diacylglycerols least. This supports the scheme of Fig. 2 (p. 562), in which tetraenoic diacylglycerol arises from PI. Formation of phosphatidylinositol *de novo* made use of various CPD-diacylglycerols, but arachidonate was incorporated largely by transacylation.

VI. Physical Properties of Phosphoinositides

A. Micelles and Smectic Mesophases

The highly acidic polyphosphoinositides disperse readily in water, forming much smaller micelles than phosphatidylcholine, for instance. Hendrickson (1969) quotes a micellar weight of 78,100 for TPI, determined from sedimentation data. The corresponding figure for phosphatidylcholine is well over a million, and this lipid is likely to form extended lamellar structures whereas TPI micelles are probably spherical. Hendrickson made his measurements in a buffer of N-ethylmorpholine, pH 8. Sodium or potassium salts of all the phosphoinositides are readily dispersed in water, but salts with divalent cations such as Mg^{2+} or Ca^{2+} are insoluble, although they readily dissolve in chloroform.

Bangham (1968) has shown that many phospholipids, when sonicated in aqueous media, form smectic mesophases ("liposomes") in which an aqueous compartment is surrounded by one or more concentric bimolecular membranes. The polyphosphoinositides do not seem to form such structures, but ox brain phosphatidylinositol formed very regular liposomes after sonication for 45 minutes (Papahadjopoulos and Miller, 1967). Electron microscopy, using negative staining, showed that they consisted of one or two lamellae only and most were 300–400 Å in diameter. Phosphatidylcholine liposomes were multilamellar in structure and generally about ten times larger. Litman (1973) has prepared mixed vesicles of phosphatidylinositol and phosphatidylcholine. As the proportion of the inositol lipid increased, the trapped volume of aqueous phase decreased until the mole fraction reached 0.5. After that the volume remained constant.

B. Monolayers

Hauser and Dawson (1968) measured the binding of radioactive calcium ions to a phosphatidylinositol monolayer at an air–water interface. A surface concentration of one Ca^{2+} to 3.7 phospholipid molecules was reached surface at pressures between 20 and 30 dyne/cm. At higher or lower pressures, less calcium was bound. Certain narcotic or excitatory drugs displaced calcium ions in proportion to their ability to penetrate the lipid film. There was little adsorption of calcium at pH below 3 (Quinn and Dawson, 1972). Between pH 3 and pH 6.5 initial adsorption was followed by loss, while at pHs higher than 6.5 there was permanent adsorption, affinity increasing up to pH 11. The binding of calcium ions to cell membranes containing phosphatidylinositol could thus vary considerably as pH shifted slightly either side of the physiological value. Papahadjopoulos (1968) also studied binding of calcium and magnesium to phospholipid monolayers. The acidic lipids had a high affinity for these ions in the presence of physiological concentrations of univalent salts. Adsorption increased the surface potential and condensed the film.

DPI and TPI also have a high affinity for divalent ions, and TPI can form insoluble complexes with the basic protein of myelin (Palmer and Dawson, 1969). Complexes of this type and of basic protein with cerebroside sulfate could be important in the structure of myelin.

C. Clustering of Lipid Species in Membranes

Electron spin resonance (ESR) spectroscopy has recently been used to study the motion of phospholipids in model and natural membranes, making use of nitroxide derivatives. The nitroxide group can be attached to the polar head group of a phospholipid or to one of the fatty acid chains. In some experiments spin-labeled fatty acids are simply allowed to dissolve in the membrane, though here the results may be less definitive. Schnepel et al. (1974) used spin-labeled stearic acid to investigate the mobility of plant phosphatidylinositol dispersions. Addition of calcium ions reduced the mobility of the head groups, but not of the fatty acid chains.

Several theories about the function of phosphoinositides in natural membranes depend on the formation of clusters of, for example, phosphatidylinositol in the membrane. ESR spectroscopy can provide evidence of this, as shown by Ito and Ohnishi (1974) using spin-labeled phospholipids. Addition of calcium ions caused clustering of phosphatidic acid in phosphatidic acid–phosphatidylcholine membranes as judged by exchange-broadening of the spectra. Ohnishi and Ito (1974) detected similar clustering of phosphatidylserine in phosphatidylcholine membranes. The aggregating effect of Ca^{2+} was inhibited by tetracaine. No clustering of phosphatidylinositol was seen under these conditions. The authors considered that for clustering each phospholipid head group required two anionic sites. The polyphosphoinositides have not been studied, but by this criterion they would readily form clusters. How far such studies are applicable to natural membranes, where acidic phospholipids may be bound to proteins, remains to be seen.

VII. Metabolism in Various Tissues and Organisms

This section surveys those tissues for which enzymes involved in the metabolism of inositides have been reported. The presence of DPI and TPI in many tissues (Hawthorne and Michell, 1966) implies the presence of PI and DPI kinases, but these are included here only where the particular kinase has been described. Quantitative results on PI, DPI, and TPI from various sources are given in Table III. The route of synthesis of PI in many of the tissues exhibiting stimulated turnover of PI (Section VIII), has not yet been reported, but it seems likely that the major pathway is via CDP-diglyceride (Section II).

A. Nervous Tissue

1. *Phosphatidylinositol*

Much of the work on phosphatidylinositol metabolism in nervous tissue is covered in Section V, since it related to changes on stimulation. Some recent biosynthetic studies are outlined here.

Hokin and Brown (1969) studied the effects of various isomers of hexachlorocyclohexane on phosphatidylinositol biosynthesis. The γ-isomer (Gammexane), related to mucoinositol in configuration, inhibited the stimulation of labeling caused by acetylcholine in brain slices. Control phosphatidylinositol labeling was unaffected. The microsomal synthesis of phosphatidylinositol from CDP-diacylglycerol was strongly inhibited by S-hexachlorocyclohexane, the isomer with the myo-inositol conformation. The biosynthesis of other phospholipids was also inhibited.

Baker and Thompson (1972) showed that [³H]arachidonic acid was rapidly incorporated into phosphatidylinositol after intracerebral injection. Comparison with [¹⁴C]glycerol labeling of the lipid indicated an acyl exchange mechanism rather than synthesis *de novo* for the incorporation of the arachidonate. Labeling of DPI and TPI was less rapid, suggesting that much of the highly labeled phosphatidylinositol was not in metabolic equilibrium with the polyphosphoinositides. The same authors (1973) reported that 1-acylglycerophosphorylinositol was acylated in the 2-position by acyl-CoA in the presence of microsomal fraction from rat brain. Arachidonoyl-CoA was much the most effective acylating agent, suggesting that incorporation of this fatty acid into the phosphoinositides depended on the Lands type of acyl exchange. The work with labeled arachidonate *in vivo* supports this, but the necessary phospholipase A has not yet been characterized in brain.

Eliasson *et al.* (1972) studied the biosynthesis of phosphatidylinositol in brain from rabbits suffering from hereditary ataxia. In this defect, brain stem and cerebellar areas are deficient in all three phosphoinositides and there are deposits of glycogen. Biosynthesis of phosphatidylinositol from CDP-diacylglycerol was not inhibited by the glycogen, but the reaction rate was low in the affected areas of brain. This seemed to be due to hydrolysis of CDP-diacylglycerol. The kinases responsible for DPI and TPI synthesis seemed normal, as was TPI phosphodiesterase.

Keough *et al.* (1972) showed that 60% of the diacylglycerol of rat brain was the 1-stearoyl, 2-arachidonoyl compound, suggesting that it had been produced by hydrolysis of phosphoinositides, in which this species predominates. This is relevant to the cycle of reactions discussed in Section V.

2. Diphosphoinositide and Triphosphoinositide

a. Occurrence in Myelin and Other Structures. Iacobelli (1969) found appreciable DPI kinase activity in myelin purified from sciatic nerve, but earlier work suggested that central myelin was not very active (see Hawthorne and Kai, 1970). There is a good deal of evidence that PI kinase is a plasma membrane enzyme in many tissues, and this may relate to the presence of the polyphosphoinositides in myelin, which is produced from plasma membranes of glial or Schwann cells (Hawthorne and Kai, 1970).

Hauser *et al.* (1971a) found the lowest concentrations of DPI and

TPI (112.9 and 103.2 nmoles per gram wet weight, respectively) in cortical gray matter of rat brain, and the highest (235.5 and 549.5) in brain
stem, with intermediate concentrations in whole brain, forebrain, thala-
mus–hypothalamus, and cerebellum. The rats were 34 days old. There
was relatively more DPI in gray matter than in white. The loss of both
DPI and TPI post mortem was greatest in gray matter. Regional distribution of the stable polyphosphoinositide pool resembled that of galacto-
lipid, suggesting a location in myelin. The labile DPI and TPI were presumably in other structures. These concepts were confirmed by studies
of ^{32}P incorporation *in vivo* (Gonzalez-Sastre *et al.*, 1971). Specific activities of DPI and TPI from different regions of brain were compared in
tissue rapidly frozen in liquid N_2 and in tissue analyzed after 10 minutes
at room temperature. In brain stem, where myelin predominates, the
delay of 10 minutes did not affect specific radioactivities, but the rapidly
frozen sample of cortical gray matter, forebrain, or cerebellum had TPI
of considerably higher activity than the 10-minute postmortem sample.
It can be concluded that a labile fraction of polyphosphoinositides is associated with gray matter and nonmyelin structures and that the myelin
DPI and TPI are relatively inert.

Hauser *et al.* (1971b) also studied DPI and TPI levels in brains of
"quaking" mutant mice, where myelination is inadequate. Such brains
had 20% of the normal cerebroside, 27% TPI, and 61% DPI, suggesting
that some TPI and much DPI were present in other structures than
myelin. Eichberg and Hauser (1973) have compared the subcellular distribution of DPI and TPI in brains of 7-day (unmyelinated) and 34-day
(myelinated) rats. In the unmyelinated brains, distribution somewhat
resembled that of 5′-nucleotidase and acetylcholinesterase, indicating the
presence of polyphosphoinositides in neuronal and glial plasma membranes. In myelinated brains over half the DPI and 75% of the TPI
were in myelin-rich fractions. The ratio DPI/TPI was 0.47 for the main
myelin fraction and 1.96 for synaptosomes.

Keough and Thompson (1970, 1972) characterized the brain phospho-
diesterase(s) attacking PI, DPI, and TPI with the release of diacylglycerol. Both particulate and soluble forms of the enzyme were found, and
the subcellular distribution with TPI as substrate resembled that of
5′-nucleotidase. Levels of the enzyme rose during myelination. A limited
purification was achieved.

b. Possible Functions of Polyphosphoinositides. Changes in DPI or TPI
labeling in response to stimulation at synapses have sometimes been described, but PI seems to be more important in synaptic transmission.
Yagihara *et al.* (1969) incubated rat vagus and sciatic nerves and sympathetic ganglia for 3 hours in a medium containing ^{32}P. The most highly

labeled phosphoinositide in the ganglia was PI, but TPI was most active in vagus and sciatic.

One of us has argued elsewhere (Hawthorne and Kai, 1970) that poly-phosphoinositides may be important in calcium binding and permeability changes related to axonal conduction. Hendrickson and Reinertsen (1971) used metal complex stability constants and acid association constants of deacylated DPI and TPI to calculate that conversion of TPI to DPI would release 70% of bound Ca^{2+} and decrease ligand charge by 25%. They concluded that such changes would affect Na^+ and K^+ permeability.

Various attempts have been made to relate changes in brain activity and particularly axonal conduction with the metabolism of polyphospho-inositides. Schacht and Agranoff (1972) found increased incorporation of ^{32}P and [^3H]inositol into TPI and PI of goldfish brain a few minutes after convulsions induced electrically or with a drug. Birnberger et al. (1971) prelabeled lobster claw and leg nerve phospholipids with ^{32}P and then stimulated the nerves electrically for 5 minutes in a medium with only nonradioactive phosphate. Increased loss of label from TPI indi-cated increased turnover as a result of nerve stimulation. Salway and Hughes (1972) stimulated rabbit vagus for 2 minutes in the presence of ^{32}P and found increases of DPI and TPI labeling that were not statisti-cally significant. Tetrodotoxin had no effect. Using a more refined incuba-tion system, White and Larrabee (1973) found a 25% decrease in labeling of rat vagus TPI by ^{32}P as a result of stimulation for 3 hours. With a similar system but only a 30-minute period of stimulation, White et al. (1974) observed increases in labeling of most phospholipids, though nucleotides were unaffected. The only statistically significant increases ($P = 0.02$) were in TPI (181%) and DPI (192%). Again, tetrodotoxin had no effect.

Although more sophisticated experiments are needed, it seems likely that short periods of electrical stimulation of vagus nerve cause increased turnover of the monoester phosphates of TPI. Whether this is related to permeability changes remains to be seen.

The polyphosphoinositides do not show consistent metabolic changes that can be related to synaptic transmission, although some changes have been reported. Torda (1972) provided evidence that cyclic AMP (cAMP) activates DPI kinase and suggests that this may be by interaction with a regulatory subunit of the enzyme. The process is considered to be part of the mechanism by which cAMP hyperpolarizes postsynaptic mem-branes. Torda (1973) also claimed that depolarization of such membranes is caused when acetylcholine binds to nicotinic receptors which are regula-tory subunits of TPI phosphatase. Acetylcholine binding releases inhibition by the subunit and the resulting hydrolysis of TPI leads to release of membrane-bound Ca^{2+} with increased membrane permeability which causes depolarization. On the whole, the experimental support for these ideas is not yet adequate. In particular, the enzymes and supposed regulatory subunits are by no means pure.

B. LIVER

The major molecular species of PI of rat liver are the stearoyl-arachidonoyl tetraenes (Holub and Kuksis, 1971a). However, Akino and Shimojo (1970) and Holub and Kuksis (1971b) have presented evidence that the polyunsaturated species are not synthesized *de novo* via phosphatidate but are derived from the mono- and dienoic species. Holub and Kuksis (1972) measured the specific radioactivity of individual molecular species of PI of rat liver following injection *in vivo* of [^{32}P]orthophosphate or [^{14}C]glycerol and found with either isotope that up to 3 hours post injection the specific activity of linoleoyl dienes was 17-fold greater than that of the arachidonoyl tetraenes and 8-fold greater than the tri- and polyenes. Thus after 5 minutes the mono- + dienes (7% total PI) contained 65% of the total PI radioactivity whereas the tetraenes (77% total PI) contained only 17% of the PI radioactivity. Over a 9-hour period the radioactivity recovered in the mono- + dienes decreased to 17% of the total radioactivity while there was a concomitant rise to about 70% in the recovery of radioactivity from the tetraenes suggesting that polyunsaturates, the major species of PI in the tissue, are formed from mono- and dienoic species by a deacylation–reacylation at C_2 of the glycerol moiety involving arachidonic acid.

Holub (1974) compared the distribution of [^{3}H]inositol in molecular species of PI of rat liver *in vivo* with its distribution *in vitro* following the Mn^{2+} stimulated incorporation of [^{3}H]inositol into rat liver microsomal fraction (exchange pathway) and showed that initial entry of free inositol into PI *in vivo* occurs via *de novo* synthesis of the lipid from CDP-diglyceride, not by the Mn^{2+} stimulated exchange of inositol.

The occurrence of a PI kinase in liver was suggested by the appearance of radioactive DPI in rat liver following injection *in vivo* of [^{32}P]orthophosphate (Hölzl and Wagner, 1964). Hawthorne and Michell (1966) described a PI kinase in the nuclear fraction of liver and further subfractionation by Michell *et al.* (1967) localized the enzyme in a plasma membrane-enriched fraction. Harwood and Hawthorne (1969) presented evidence for a second PI kinase in the endoplasmic reticulum which differed from the plasma membrane enzyme in its pH optimum and response to the nonionic detergent Cutscum. It is probable that earlier reports of a

PI kinase of rat liver mitochondria (reviewed by Hawthorne and Michell, 1966) are due to contamination of mitochondria by microsomal and/or plasma membranes.

C. KIDNEY

The synthesis and degradation of DPI and TPI in rat kidney has been extensively studied by Huggins and co-workers, who reported a microsomal PI kinase which had an absolute requirement for Mn^{2+} or Mg^{2+} and was inhibited by Ca^{2+} (Tou et al., 1968, 1969). Harwood and Hawthorne (1969) presented evidence of two PI kinases in rat kidney which, like the liver enzymes, differed in pH optimum and response to Cutscum. The Cutscum-stimulated PI kinase was associated with the endoplasmic reticulum while a second kinase unaffected by Cutscum was present in a plasma membrane-enriched fraction. Tou et al. (1970) found that the DPI kinase of rat kidney was also predominantly localized in the plasma membrane and exhibited properties similar to those of the PI kinase. An in vivo study using [^{32}P]orthophosphate showed that the phosphomonoester groups of DPI and TPI underwent rapid turnover which was unaffected by starvation (Tou et al., 1972). The phosphodiester phosphorus did not exhibit this rapid metabolism.

The catabolism of DPI and TPI by phosphomonoesterase activity was reported by Lee and Huggins (1968a,b). This enzyme, which appeared to be microsomal, was activated by Mg^{2+} and inhibited by Ca^{2+}. TPI was hydrolyzed to PI + inorganic phosphate with DPI as a transient intermediate. A partially purified enzyme preparation hydrolyzed both monophosphates from TPI, although Cooper and Hawthorne (1975) suggested from subfractionation studies that the TPI and DPI phosphomonoesterases are separate enzymes exhibiting a dual distribution, partly soluble and partly membrane bound. Recently Tou et al. (1973) reported a TPI phosphodiesterase activity in the supernatant fraction of rat kidney cortex. This activity, which cleaved TPI and DPI, but not PI, to 1,2-diglyceride was freed from monoesterase activity by acid precipitation and ammonium sulfate fractionation. An active phosphodiesterase specific for PI has been reported by Dawson et al. (1971). The products of this activity were 1,2-diglyceride and inositol-1,2-cyclic diphosphate (see Section II, B).

D. THYROID

Jungalwala et al. (1971) reported that all the enzymes required for PI synthesis in pig thyroid are microsomal and demonstrated the incorporation of [^{3}H]inositol into PI in the presence of CDP-diglyceride or CTP + ATP. Incubation of a microsomal fraction, prelabeled with ^{32}P and [³H]inositol, with unlabeled inositol in the presence of nucleotide co-enzymes resulted in loss of tritium, but not ³²P, from PI. Such a phospho-lipase D activity, which would leave membrane-bound phosphatidic acid for recycling, has not been demonstrated in mammalian tissues, and the authors suggest that the appearance of [³H]inositol might be due to a reversal of the CDP-diglyceride–inositol phosphoryltransferase activity. These workers also described a soluble, Ca^{2+}-dependent PI phosphodies-terase which gave inositol 1:2-cyclic diphosphate as its major water-soluble product (65%). Synthesis and degradation of PI were inhibited by 1 mM chlorpromazine, which also suppresses thyrotropin-induced stimulated activity of thyroid slices. It was suggested that chlorpro-mazine enters the plasma membrane and displaces calcium required for the phosphodiesterase. Such an enzyme is very active on stimulation of thyroid with TSH (Scott et al., 1968). Macchia and Pastan (1968) reported that sphingomyelinase (like TSH) rapidly increases the turn-over of PI in dog and bovine thyroid, as measured by the incorporation of [³²P]orthophosphate.

E. LYMPHOCYTES

The treatment of small lymphocytes with a variety of agents, including phytohemagglutinin, causes the cells to develop into lymphoblasts and to divide. A rapid turnover of phosphatidylinositol occurs in the early stages of these processes (Fisher and Mueller, 1968). Allan and Michell (1974a,b) have postulated that the hydrolysis of PI to diglyceride and inositol 1:2-cyclic phosphate is regulated by extracellular external stim-uli. These workers have reported two PI hydrolase activities of a soluble fraction derived from pig lymphocytes. The activity at pH 5.5 required 50 μM Ca^{2+} for optimal activity while that at pH 7.0 required 0.7 μM Ca^{2+}, a calcium concentration near the free calcium level of the cell (1 μM). Allan and Michell (1974b) suggested that the pH 5.5 activity which has been detected in several other tissues [e.g., intestinal mucosa, Ather-ton and Hawthorne (1968); thyroid, Jungalwala et al. (1971)] is not the physiological activity and that the pH 7.0 activity operates in vivo. Previous reports on the high concentrations of calcium required for PI hydrolase activity possibly reflect the calcium buffering capacity of PI and that when the PI substrate concentration is high, much calcium is bound to the substrate and lowers the effective free calcium concentra-tion. This implies that calcium is required for binding to the enzyme rather than for modifying the form of the substrate PI (Jungalwala et al., 1971) and this is supported by the fact that cations, such as chlorpro-mazine and cinchocaine, which displace calcium from PI enhance the hydrolase activity at low calcium concentrations. These results suggest that PI breakdown in intact cells is controlled in part by changes in intracellular calcium concentration.

F. ERYTHROCYTES

Sloviter and Tanaka (1967) showed that intact immature erythrocytes (reticulocytes), obtained from rabbits, incorporated [^{3}H]inositol into PI; Percy et al. (1973) later demonstrated the synthesis of PI from CDP-diglyceride and inositol in membranes derived from rabbit reticulocytes. Maximal synthesis of PI was achieved on addition of CDP-diglyceride, but there was no absolute requirement for the liponucleotide, suggesting that the membranes were rich in CDP-diglyceride, contaminated with an intracellular component rich in CDP-diglyceride, or that a separate enzyme not requiring CDP-diglyceride, possibly an exchange enzyme, was present. This ability to synthesize PI *de novo* is lost on maturation, but the mature erythrocyte can still incorporate ^{32}P from [^{32}P]ATP into the monoesterified phosphates of phosphatidic acid (PA), DPI, and TPI (L. E. Hokin and Hokin, 1964; Redman, 1971), and Harwood and Hawthorne (1969) described a PI kinase of human erythrocyte membranes. The synthesis and turnover of DPI and TPI in intact pig erythrocytes (Peterson and Kirschner, 1970) and in pig erythrocyte ghosts (Schneider and Kirschner, 1970) was too slow for these lipids to be intermediates in the magnesium-dependent Na$^+$-K$^+$ stimulated ATPase. Neither synthesis nor turnover required sodium or potassium ions, and neither was affected by ouabain. Buckley and Hawthorne (1972) suggested that the higher inositide levels produced by PI kinase activity may regulate intracellular calcium levels since, as the membrane DPI level rose, so the Ca^{2+} bound to the erythrocyte membrane rose concomitantly in the ratio 2 PO$_4{}^{2-}$ (from 2 molecules of DPI) per Ca^{2+}, and in this state the membranes exhibited increased Ca^{2+}-ATPase activity. However, polyphosphoinositide metabolism does not change during Ca^{2+} transport (Buckley, 1974).

G. PLATELETS

Lucas et al. (1970) reported the properties of a CDP-diglyceride-inositol phosphatidate transferase of human platelet membranes. Its activity from patients with diseases interfering with the clot-promoting function of platelets was similar to the normal. The further phosphorylation of PI is regulated by environmental factors. Thus, Cohen et al. (1971) showed that ^{32}P incorporation into phosphoinositides of human platelets was dependent on the ionic environment of the cells. In changing the incubation medium from 150 mOsm, where all phospholipids are highly labeled, to 300 mOsm, only DPI and TPI become labeled to any extent. Stimulated labeling also occurred on raising Na^+ and lowering K^+ concentrations in 300 mOsm media. The significance of this is not known, but it did not appear to be due to thrombocytolysis since freezing and thawing abolished the stimulated ^{32}P incorporation. Addition of ADP to a suspension of rabbit platelets caused aggregation of the platelets and an immediate (within 30 seconds) increase in incorporation of ^{32}P into PA, DPI, and TPI but not into PI or other phospholipids. Increased incorporation into PI was seen after 3 minutes, probably as a result of metabolism of PA (Lloyd et al., 1972a,b).

H. ADRENALS

Trifaró (1969a) reported that PA was an intermediate in phosphatidyl-inositol synthesis in bovine adrenal medulla, suggesting that the CDP-diglyceride pathway was operative in this tissue. The same author (Trifaró and Dworkind, 1971) described the phosphorylation of the chromaffin granule membranes of the tissue on incubation of the isolated granules with $[\gamma\text{-}^{32}P]$-ATP. Two components of the membrane were phosphorylated, a membrane protein and a lipid that was isolated and identified as DPI by Buckley et al. (1971). TPI may also be formed by varying the incubation conditions (Lefebvre, 1974). The properties of the granule membrane PI kinase have been described by Phillips (1973) and Lefebvre (1974). The latter author compared the granular PI kinase with the PI kinase activity of the microsomal (plasma?) membrane and found them to be identical under many conditions. They had the same pH optimum, were inhibited by Cutscum and Ca^{2+}, and were stimulated by Mg^{2+}. In contrast to the phosphorylated erythrocyte membranes, the phosphorylated granules did not exhibit enhanced calcium binding. The catabolism of granule-membrane DPI occurred by phosphomonoesterase and phosphodiesterase activities of the supernatant and microsomal fractions. There was no catabolic activity associated with the granule itself, and ^{32}P-phosphorylated granules lost radioactivity only very slowly. The function of DPI of the granules is not known, but it may be related to the high concentrations of ATP in the granule. Similar experiments designed to demonstrate PI kinase in vesicle membranes of other secretory tissues indicated that the synaptic vesicles of guinea pig brain may contain a PI kinase although elimination of plasma membrane and microsomal activity is difficult (Bleasdale, 1974). However, isolated zymogen granules of bovine pancreas failed to elicit any PI kinase activity, although this may be a reflection of the high catabolic activities of this tissue (Lefebvre, 1974).

I. PANCREAS

Prottey and Hawthorne (1967) reported the incorporation *in vivo* of [^{32}P]orthophosphate into PI of guinea pig pancreas. Biosynthesis appeared to follow the CDP-diglyceride pathway, and the authors characterized the final enzyme of the pathway, CDP-diglyceride-inositol phosphoryltransferase. White *et al.* (1971) reported a phospholipase A$_1$ activity of guinea pig pancreas which was capable of hydrolyzing endogenous PI during fractionation procedures even at 4°C. Keenan and Hokin (1964) had earlier described the acylation of lyso-PI in a variety of pigeon tissues including pancreas, but this was not part of a *de novo* synthetic route. However, in view of the results on the biosynthesis of molecular species of PI in rat liver (Holub and Kuksis, 1972), such an enzyme might well play an important role in the conversion of one species to another. PI kinase activity was found in bovine pancreas homogenates, but no further localization of the enzyme was reported (Lefebvre, 1974).

J. MUSCLE

The incorporation of ^{32}P into rat hemidiaphragm PI *in vivo* was selectively inhibited by denervation (Steinberg and Durell, 1971), and the authors suggested that this is related to the change in Ca^{2+} levels of the muscle. Further evidence for this was reported by Lennon and Steinberg (1973), who found that ethyleneglycoltetraacetate (EGTA) caused a concentration-dependent inhibition of ^{32}P incorporation into PI of rat diaphragm incubated in calcium-free media. There was no effect on the labeling of other phospholipids. The inhibition was reversed by addition of calcium. EGTA also enhanced [^{3}H]inositol incorporation into PI, probably via the calcium-independent exchange reaction, but this was not due to any direct effect on the enzyme, since EGTA treatment increased [^{3}H]inositol uptake into the tissue. It was suggested that EGTA binds membrane calcium, thus inhibiting a Ca^{2+}-dependent PI hydrolase in the membrane and preventing PI turnover.

The turnover of PI in rat skeletal muscle membranes was used to monitor the state of membranes *in vitro* following *in vivo* denervation (Appel *et al.*, 1974). All the enzymes of PI synthesis and degradation occurred in the membrane. PI turnover was enhanced in membrane subfractions derived from denervated muscle, and this appeared to be a general response since both sarcoplasmic reticulum and surface membranes exhibited the effect. This enhanced turnover was not stimulated by exogenous diglyceride or PA and did not increase the size of the PI pool. It was also independent of neurotransmitter addition. The significance of such observations is as yet unclear, but Appel *et al.* suggest that the observed changes could have significant effects on the structure and function of membrane proteins, particularly if PI was intimately associated with such proteins, and it is of interest that Levey (1971) has shown that PI restores the responsiveness of solubilized adenyl cyclase (a plasma membrane-associated enzyme) of cat heart to norepinephrine.

Harwood and Hawthorne (1969) demonstrated the occurrence of a PI kinase in rat heart.

K. Other Tissues

1. *Polymorphonuclear Leukocytes*

The rapid labeling of PI of polymorphonuclear leukocytes during phagocytosis was reported by Karnovsky and Wallach (1961). The total amount of PI in the cells was unaffected during the process, suggesting increased turnover of the lipid. This was confirmed by Sastry and Hokin (1966), who showed that labeling of PI was independent of the increased turnover of PA. Tou and Stjernholm (1974) measured the effect of phagocytosis on incorporation of $^{32}P_i$ and [^{3}H]inositol into PI, DPI, and TPI of guinea pig polymorphonuclear leukocytes and showed enhanced incorporation of both precursors into all three inositides. Phagocytosis did not stimulate loss of label from cells that had been prelabeled with $^{32}P_i$ and [^{3}H]inositol, indicating that increased radioactivity in the inositides was due to a greater rate of synthesis of these lipids rather than increased rate of turnover. This is at variance with the results of Karnovsky and Wallach (1961) and does not agree with results found for some other tissues undergoing stimulated turnover of PI in response to external stimuli discussed in Section V. Harwood and Hawthorne (1969) reported a PI kinase activity in a plasma membrane fraction from polymorphonuclear leukocytes.

2. *Embryonic Fibroblasts*

During exponential growth the ^{3}H/^{32}P ratio of PI of embryonic mouse fibroblasts, which had been prelabeled with [^{3}H]inositol and ^{32}P, increases; this increase suggests that, during this phase of growth, hydrolysis to diglyceride and possibly inositol cyclic phosphate occurs and that the diglyceride is specifically recycled (Diringer and Koch, 1973). At

confluency the ^{3}H/^{32}P ratio for PI remained constant, indicating a
blocked turnover of PI under conditions of high cell density. The authors
suggested that cleavage of PI was linked to regulation of cell growth.
This inhibition of PI turnover was not evident in SV40-transformed fibroblasts at confluency (Koch and Diringer, 1973).

L. PHOSPHATIDYLINOSITOL EXCHANGE BETWEEN MEMBRANES

When ^{32}P-labeled rat liver microsomal fraction was incubated with unlabeled mitochondria, in the presence of supernatant fraction, exchange
of radioactive phosphatidylcholine (PC) and phosphatidylethanolamine
(PE), but not cardiolipin, occurred, and radioactivity was found in the
mitochondria on subsequent fractionation. The radioactivity in the mitochondria could not be accounted for by cross contamination of fractions
(Wirtz and Zilversmit, 1968; Akiyama and Sakagami, 1969). A similar
rapid exchange of PI between membranes of rat liver was reported by
McMurray and Dawson (1969). The rate of exchange of PI was comparable to PC whereas PE and PA exchanged only slowly. Exchange was
dependent on a heat-labile component of the supernatant fraction but
did not require energy in the form of ATP + Mg^{2+}. Miller and Dawson
(1972) demonstrated a similar exchange *in vitro* of phospholipids, including PI, between membranes prepared from guinea pig brain, where the
rates of exchange were similar. The rapid transfer of PI from pig thyroid
microsomal membranes to mitochondria in the presence of a supernatant
fraction has also been reported by Jungalwala *et al.* (1971).
    Specific proteins responsible for the transfer of PI between membranes
have been purified from bovine liver and brain (Harvey *et al.*, 1973;
Helmkamp *et al.*, 1974; Possmayer, 1974). Two acidic proteins (MW
29,000 and 30,000) were isolated from bovine brain cortical tissue supernatant fraction. Both of these were able to catalyze the transfer of
[^{3}H]inositol-PI from rat liver microsomes to liposomes. Although there
was a marked preference for the transfer of PI they also transferred PC
to a lesser degree, but not PE, and in this respect differed from the supernatant preparation of guinea pig brain described above, which transferred
all three phospholipids at the same rate (Miller and Dawson, 1972).
Under normal assay conditions, both donor and acceptor membranes contained PI, and thus exchange of PI probably occurs (Demel *et al.*, 1973),
but Helmkamp *et al.* (1974) have reported net transfer of PI from labeled
microsomal fraction to liposomes containing no PI.
    Brammer and Sheltawy (1975) reported the purification from bovine
brain of two proteins, each MW 22,000, which exchange PI and PC between mitochondria of bovine brain and PI/PC liposomes. Although the
proteins exhibit the same isoelectric point on isoelectric focusing, the ex-

change of PC was inhibited by increasing the PI content of the liposomes and was abolished when PI constituted 40% of the liposomes. The pH optimum of the exchange protein was rather broad and was unaffected by calcium.

The role (if any) of such specific exchange (transfer?) proteins *in vivo* is not yet known but may be related to the redistribution of newly synthesized phospholipids (Miller and Dawson, 1972). Synthesis of the major phospholipids occurs only in the endoplasmic reticulum, and thus these proteins may constitute part of a membrane-repair or renewal mechanism in membranes, such as those of mitochondria, which are incapable of synthesizing phospholipids.

M. YEAST

The major pathway for PI synthesis in *S. cerevisiae* appears to be via CDP-diglyceride (M. R. Steiner and Lester, 1972). This was not the sole route, however, since under acidic growth conditions or increased calcium, ^{32}P and ^{14}C from doubly labeled sn-$[^{14}C]$glycero-3-$[^{32}P]$phosphate were not incorporated into PI at the same rate. The authors suggested that this might be explained by a phosphodiesterase (phospholipase C) activity operating in reverse and catalyzing the reaction of 1,2-$[^{14}C]$diglyceride with inositol 1,2-cyclic phosphate derived from endogenous PI, thus accounting for the observed increase in $^{14}C/^{32}P$ ratio in PI. An alternative route for PI synthesis in *S. pombe* was also suggested by the results of White and Hawthorne (1970). PI was synthesized *in vitro*, by an apparently energy-independent route, in the absence of endogenous CDP-diglyceride and was interpreted as an exchange reaction mediated through a phospholipase D activity. However, CMP stimulated incorporation of $[^3H]$inositol into PI, and the observation might be due to a reversal of the terminal step of PI synthesis forming CDP-diglyceride at an appropriate site in the membrane for reaction with $[^3H]$inositol and thus not requiring exogenous CDP-diglyceride.

Saccharomyces cerevisiae cells which had been uniformly prelabeled with ^{32}P and $[2-^3H]$inositol lost both labels from PI at the same rate (half-life of two generations) on transfer to unlabeled medium (Angus and Lester, 1972). At the same time, both labels were incorporated into the major phosphosphingolipid, ceramide-(inositol)$_2$-(phosphate)$_2$-mannose (Steiner *et al.*, 1969) in a ratio the same as that of the original PI, suggesting a phosphodiesterase activity releasing inositol-phosphate (cyclic?), which is incorporated intact into the sphingolipid. During logarithmic growth glycerylphosphorylinositol (GPI) was released into the extracellular medium in an amount proportional to the cell density and equivalent to about one-fourth of the cellular PI. The $^3H/^{32}P$ ratio of the released GPI was the same as the original PI and is presumably derived from a specific phospholipase A activity toward PI, since only small amounts of GPC and GPE appeared in the medium. This is a major fate of the PI in a growing culture, accounting for about one-half of the labeled [³H]inositol and ³²P disappearing from the PI pool; the GPI is not reutilized.

The presence of DPI and TPI in yeast (S. cerevisiae) was first reported by Lester and Steiner (1968). S. Steiner and Lester (1972) described the rapid metabolism of the phosphomonoester groups during growth, and Talwalkar and Lester (1973) suggested, from studies with a respiratory-deficient mutant of S. cerevisiae, that absolute cellular concentrations of the higher inosetides in vivo were rapidly and reversibly altered by changes in ATP concentration or adenylate charge. Such a regulation during growth would help to conserve ATP.

PI kinase activity was detected in a plasma membrane fraction of S. cerevisiae prepared on a discontinuous sucrose density gradient (Wheeler et al., 1972). Talwalkar and Lester (1974), however, described a PI kinase of the soluble fraction of a yeast cell homogenate and found little kinase activity in the sedimentable fraction. Possibly the enzyme was solubilized during preparation of the homogenate. It could be precipitated with ammonium sulfate and redissolved into a fully soluble form on dilution. Such a preparation may prove to be very useful in determining factors regulating PI kinase activity and perhaps helping to find a biological role for the higher inositides.

Detailed studies by Lester's group have resulted in chemical characterization of all the major inositol-containing lipids of S. cerevisiae (i.e., containing $>1\%$ total inositol). Thus, besides PI (60%; Lester and Steiner, 1968) and DPI + TPI (1%: Talwalkar and Lester, 1973), Steiner et al. (1969) isolated a novel sphingolipid of composition mannose-(inositol-P)$_2$-ceramide, and Smith and Lester (1974) have recently characterized a group of sphingolipids containing a single phosphorylinositol moiety. The major lipid of this latter group was characterized as inositol phosphorylceramide containing hydroxysphinganine and a hydroxy C_{26} fatty acid. Two other inositol phosphorylceramides differing in their ceramide moieties were also identified. Evidence was also presented for the existence of two other glycolipids, one of which had the composition mannosylinositol phosphorylceramide.

N. Microorganisms

Phosphatidylinositol is found both free and covalently bound to mannose in certain classes of microorganisms, and much of our knowledge of the structure and biosynthesis of these mannophosphoinositides has come from the laboratories of Lederer and Ballou. The occurrence, structure, and biosynthesis of these glycolipids have been comprehensively reviewed by Ambron and Pieringer (1973). A family of mannophosphoinositides containing one to five mannose units is present in mycobacteria (Vilkas and Lederer, 1960; Nojima, 1959a,b; Vilkas, 1960; Lederer, 1961; Lee and Ballou, 1965). Mannose is linked via a glycosidic bond to the hydroxyl at C-2 on the inositol ring in the monomannoside. A second mannose in the dimannophosphoinositide is linked glycosidically to the hydroxyl at C-6 of the inositol ring. Subsequent mannose residues in the tri and tetra homologs are linked 1:6 to the mannose at C-6 on the inositol ring. In the PI pentamannoside, the terminal mannose is covalently linked to the oligosaccharide chain in an $\alpha1:2$ bond. Pangborn and McKinney (1966) showed that acylation of the hydroxyls of mannose occurred in *Mycobacterium tuberculosis* and separated two dimannosides containing (per phosphate) two fatty acids, two dimannosides containing three or four fatty acids, and two pentamannosides containing three or four fatty acids, respectively. Similar results were found in *M. phlei* (Brennan and Ballou, 1967). The biosynthesis of these mannophosphoinositides is catalyzed by one or more particulate mannosyltransferases which transfer mannose from GDP-mannose to phosphatidylinositol (Hill and Ballou, 1966; Brennan and Ballou, 1967, 1968a). Acylation requires fatty acyl-CoA or a fatty acyl-CoA synthesizing system and occurs at the level of the mono- or dimannoside prior to further mannosylation to the higher mannosides.

A diacyl myoinositol monomannoside in which D-mannose is glycosidically linked to C_2 of inositol was described in propionibacteria by Prottey and Ballou (1968) and Shaw and Dinglinger (1968). Two fatty acids were esterified at C-6 of mannose and C-1 of inositol, respectively. Because of its structural resemblance to the deacylated PI-mannosides, Shaw and Dinglinger (1969) proposed an alternative route for PI-mannoside biosynthesis whereby myo-inositol is mannosylated with GDP-mannose to 2-O-α-D-mannopyranosyl-myo-inositol, which is acylated to its 2,6'-diacyl derivative and reacted with CDP-diglyceride to form diacyl PI monomannoside.

The metabolism of these PI-mannosides is somewhat obscure and Akamatsu et al. (1967) showed from ^{32}P-labeling studies with *M. phlei* that they turn over only slowly. Apart from the mycobacteria, they have also been detected in propionibacteria (e.g., Brennan and Ballou, 1968b), corynebacteria (e.g., Brennan, 1968), and actinomycetes (Kataoka and Nojima, 1967).

The occurrence of phosphoinositides in a protist *Crithidia fasciculata* was reported by Palmer (1973a). Turnover of polyphosphoinositides was very rapid and was quantitatively increased in cells at the end of the logarithmic growth phase. Palmer (1973b) has also reported a phosphodiesterase specific for TPI in homogenates prepared from the organism. The enzyme activity was associated with both particulate and supernatant fractions and did not hydrolyze PI.

Lester *et al.* (1974) extracted and separated six [^{3}H]inositol-containing lipids from *Neurospora crassa* grown on [^{3}H]inositol and ^{32}P$_i$. The major inositol lipid was PI while 40–60% of the ^{3}H-labeled lipid appeared to be sphingolipid. The major sphingolipid was similar in structure to that of *S. cerevisiae* (Steiner *et al.*, 1969), having a composition mannose (inositol-P)$_2$-ceramide. Three other monophosphorylinositol sphingolipids similar to those characterized in yeast (Smith and Lester, 1974) were also identified. It seems possible that PI serves as a phosphorylinositol donor to the phosphorylinositol sphingolipid, as in the yeast system. A [^{3}H]inositol pulse-chase experiment using an inositol-requiring mutant showed that during exponential growth ^{3}H was lost from PI concomitant with an increase in incorporation of [^{3}H] inositol into the sphingolipid. Such changes also occur during inositol starvation, demonstrating that PI degradation and sphingolipid synthesis continue even when growth of the organism ceases.

VIII. Phosphatidylinositol Turnover and Plasma Membrane Activation

Activation of a wide variety of cells with secretory functions of one sort or another is accompanied by increased turnover of phosphatidylinositol and phosphatidic acid, but not of the other phospholipids. Much of the work has been done with ^{32}P as tracer and most workers agree that the effect is not simply a reflection of increased ATP labeling of activated cells (see, for example, Yagihara and Hawthorne, 1972). The subject was recently reviewed by one of us (Hawthorne, 1973), but a good deal of information has appeared since then and we can now understand at least the initial biochemical changes much better, though the physiological function remains somewhat obscure. This section attempts a critical review of the field, therefore, with emphasis on very recent data.

A. Tissues Showing the Phosphatidylinositol Effect

Table V gives a representative selection of tissues that respond to stimulation by increased labeling of PI and (usually) phosphatidic acid.

TABLE V

TISSUES SHOWING A PHOSPHATIDYLINOSITOL EFFECT

Tissue	Stimulus	Response	Increase in labeling[a]		Reference
			PI	PA	
Nervous					
Whole brain	Carbamylcholine	?	1.8	2.0	Friedel and Schanberg (1972)
Whole brain	α-Adrenergic	?	2	3	Friedel et al. (1973)
Rat superior cervical ganglion	Electrical	Impulse transmission	1.8	1.1	Larrabee et al. (1963)
Vagus nerve	Cinchocaine	?	4.1	—	Salway and Hughes (1972)
Eel electroplax	Acetylcholine	?	3.8	1.6[b]	Rosenberg (1973)
Endocrine					
Adrenal medulla	Acetylcholine	Epinephrine secretion	2.7	3.4	Trifaró (1969a)
Pineal	Norepinephrine	?	2.6	1.5	Eichberg et al. (1973)
Thyroid	Thyroid-stimulating hormone	Thyroxine secretion	3.6	1.8	Freinkel (1957)
Exocrine					
Pancreas	Acetylcholine	Enzyme secretion	19.3	3.1	Hokin and Hokin (1958)
Parotid gland	Acetylcholine	Amylase secretion	5.2	4.8	Eggman and Hokin (1960)
Peptic mucosa	Acetylcholine	Pepsin secretion	2.1	2.4	Eggman and Hokin (1960)
Avian salt gland	Acetylcholine	NaCl secretion	3.2	13.3	Hokin and Hokin (1960)
Sweat gland	Acetylcholine	NaCl and mucus secretion	2.1	2.2	Hokin et al. (1963)
Other tissues					
Adipose	Insulin	?	1.9	1.8	De Torrontegui and Berthet (1966)
Fibroblasts	Serum	Relief of contact inhibition	4.5	—	Pasternak (1972)
Lymphocytes	Phytohemagglutinin	Activation, mitosis	17.6	3.5	Fisher and Mueller (1971)
Platelets	ADP (etc.)	Shape change	1.2	1.7	Lloyd et al. (1972a)
Polymorphonuclear leukocytes	Starch granules (etc.)	Phagocytosis	3.2	5.5	Karnovsky and Wallach (1961)
Heart	Epinephrine	?	2.1	—	Gaut and Huggins (1966)

[a] PI, phosphatidylinositol; PA, phosphatidic acid.
[b] Not statistically significant.

1. *Are the Phospholipid Changes Merely Side Effects?*

Since phosphatidic acid can be formed directly from ATP by diacylglycerol kinase, both this lipid and PI have ready access to the nucleotide pool in tissues containing this enzyme. Changes in the labeling of this pool, however, do not account for the phospholipid effect, as already pointed out.

In several tissues, the response to the stimulus e.g., secretion of zymogens by slices of pancreas (Hokin, 1966) requires calcium ions in the medium, but the enhanced labeling of PI is calcium-independent. The same applies to secretion of catecholamines by adrenal medulla (Trifaró, 1969b). At first sight this seems to suggest that there is no connection between the phospholipid labeling and the tissue's secretory response. The same is implied by the fact that secretion often precedes the lipid labeling, as in the adrenal medulla (Trifaró, 1969a).

These objections lose their force if, as seems likely, the initial stimulus leads to phosphatidylinositol hydrolysis and the labeling is associated with resynthesis. A cycle of reactions can be considered, as in Fig. 2. This cycle was suggested by M. R. Hokin and Hokin (1964) for salt gland and later by Durell *et al.* (1969) for brain, and the four enzymes involved have been found in many tissues.

2. *Is Phosphatidylinositol Hydrolysis the Key Response?*

Enzymes hydrolyzing PI to diacylglycerol and an inositol phosphate are widely distributed. The enzymes are soluble, have an acid pH optimum, and require Ca^{2+} for activity (Kemp *et al.*, 1961; Atherton and Hawthorne, 1968; Thompson, 1967). More recent work indicates that the product is an inositol cyclic phosphate (Dawson *et al.*, 1971). Allan and

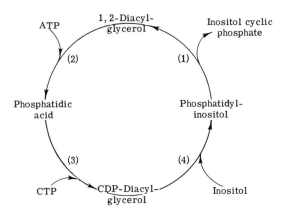

Fig. 2. Phosphatidylinositol cycle.

Michell (1974b) pointed out that an enzyme with a pH optimum near 5.5 and a calcium requirement around 5 mM is unlikely to be physiologically effective. In lymphocytes, they found a soluble enzyme that degrades PI at pH 7.0, maximum activity being obtained with 0.7 μM Ca^{2+} (free), a concentration likely to be found within many cells. Activity at pH 7.0 was also found in subcellular fractions of rat cerebral cortex (Lapetina and Michell, 1973), although the calcium requirement was 2 mM. About half the activity was particle-bound, much of it associated with plasma membranes, to judge from acetylcholinesterase distribution. Stimulation of such a plasma membrane enzyme would provide the first step in the cycle of reactions outlined in Fig. 2, and it is of interest that Canessa de Scarnati and Rodriguez de Lores Arnaiz (1972) have claimed that acetylcholine stimulates a similar enzyme. Other workers failed to confirm this effect (Lapetina and Michell, 1973; Yagihara and Hawthorne, 1972).

In tissue slices, however, there is now clear evidence that acetylcholine causes hydrolysis of PI. Jones and Michell (1974) showed that 10 μM acetylcholine/100 μM eserine caused the loss of 32% of tissue PI from rat parotid gland fragments incubated for 1 hour. With 2 mM acetylcholine, a similar loss took place in 5 minutes. The effect was blocked by atropine and seemed to be associated with muscarinic cholinergic receptors. Hokin-Neaverson (1974) obtained similar results with pancreas. In this case the loss of PI was accompanied by an equivalent rise in phosphatidic acid concentration. Atropine reversed these changes.

It is no longer foolhardy therefore, to conclude that, in these tissues at least, the PI cycle is stimulated at reaction (1) of Fig. 2. If this is the case, loss of this lipid from the plasma membrane should be detectable. Evidence on this important point is not yet available. The subcellular localization of the phospholipid effect has only been sought so far in terms of PI labeling, which is a measure of resynthesis rather than breakdown. Both in rat brain (Lapetina and Michell, 1972) and guinea pig pancreas (De Camilli and Meldolesi, 1974) labeling of PI was stimulated in most subcellular membranes. Biosynthesis of this phospholipid takes place in the endoplasmic reticulum, whence it may be transferred to other membranes by specific exchange proteins (Helmkamp et al., 1974; Possmayer, 1974). The newly formed PI is thus likely to be widely distributed in the cell, and its location will provide little information about the site of the original breakdown.

B. THE PHOSPHATIDYLINOSITOL EFFECT IN BRAIN

This subject has been reviewed previously (L. E. Hokin, 1969; Hawthorne and Kai, 1970; Hawthorne, 1973), and so the emphasis here will be on recent work using synaptosomes. This work suggests that phospholipid changes are associated with presynaptic events, probably release of transmitters, as well as with the depolarization of the postsynaptic neuron. Increased turnover of phospholipid in response to a stimulus is seen only in whole cells generally, but Durell and Sodd (1966) were able to detect an increased labeling of phosphatidic acid by ^{32}P when a brain subcellular fraction rich in nerve endings was incubated with acetylcholine. In this respect then, the synaptosome (nerve-ending particle) is behaving like an intact cell. This is not surprising since it has a plasma membrane capable of maintaining ionic gradients and a cytoplasm containing mitochondria as well as transmitter vesicles. A section of the postsynaptic membrane is also usually attached to the synaptosome.

In synaptosomes incubated with acetylcholine and eserine, the increased labeling of phosphatidic acid was chiefly due to changes in the transmitter vesicle fraction according to Yagihara et al. (1973). Schacht et al. (1974), however, found no vesicle effect and considered that the increased labeling was associated with membranes containing acetylcholinesterase, probably plasma membranes. These differences have not yet been resolved, although Lunt and Pickard (1975) found loss of PI from a synaptic vesicle fraction after prelabeling in vivo with ^{32}P and intraventricular injection of carbamylcholine with eserine.

The experiments with synaptosomes in vitro are artificial in the sense that nerve endings are concerned more with release of transmitters such as acetylcholine than with response to them, although there are probably presynaptic membrane receptors that mediate feedback inhibition of transmitter release. Bleasdale and Hawthorne (1975) argued that the phosphatidic acid changes are not part of this system. Widlund and Heilbronn (1974) consider that carrier-mediated uptake of acetylcholine is not involved either.

Electrical stimulation of synaptosomes in suspension causes release of transmitter. In the presence of ^{32}P$_i$, increased labeling of phosphatidate, synchronous with transmitter release, was seen in the synaptic vesicle fraction (Bleasdale and Hawthorne, 1975). Unlike the phospholipid changes provoked by acetylcholine, this effect depended on the presence of calcium ions in the medium (Hawthorne and Bleasdale, 1975).

Although PI labeling with ^{32}P is also increased by stimulation of synaptosomes, the effect seems more variable and less marked than with phosphatidate. It is still too soon to say whether the initial change at the plasma membrane is hydrolysis of PI, although the experiments in vivo of Lunt and Pickard (1975) suggest this. With cholinergic agonists, hydrolysis of phosphatidate occurs in vitro (Yagihara et al., 1973; Schacht and Agranoff, 1974), but effects of such agents on synaptosomes are difficult to relate to synaptic transmission. M. R. Hokin (1969 ,1970) has studied effects of adrenergic and other neurotransmitters on ^{32}P incorporation into phospholipids of slices from various areas of guinea pig brain. Norepinephrine (10^{-4} M) increased incorporation into phosphatidic acid of cerebellar cortex, cerebral cortex, and hypothalamus, other areas being unaffected. All areas studied responded to 10^{-2} M 5-hydroxytryptamine by increased labeling of this lipid. γ-Aminobutyric acid (10^{-3} M) reduced labeling of both phosphatidic acid and PI in cerebral cortex, but other regions were not affected. With 10^{-4} M dopamine only hypothalamus showed an increase, which was limited to phosphatidic acid. Hokin suggested that decreased labeling might be associated with inhibitory effects of a neurotransmitter. Woelk et al. (1974) have shown that norepinephrine increased the incorporation of phosphate into PI of both neurons and glial cells of rabbit cerebral cortex in vivo. Using cerebral cortex slices, Abdel-Latif et al. (1974) found increased labeling of PI, phosphatidate, and phosphatidylcholine by acetylcholine, norepinephrine, and other transmitters to be widely distributed among subcellular fractions. Synaptosomes showed a marked effect, but stimulation was also seen in microsomal, mitochondrial, and nuclear fractions. Glial cells, as well as neurons, exhibited increases. Results from whole brain or brain slices are almost impossible to interpret, but it can no longer be stated that the phospholipid effect is limited to the cell body of the postsynaptic neuron.

Quinn (1973) subjected the PI phosphodiesterase from rat brain supernatant to chromatography on columns of DEAE-Sephadex and considered that a subunit of microtubular protein interacted with it. The interaction was promoted by the effect of cAMP on microtubular protein, and Quinn suggested that if the activity of the phosphodiesterase was affected by the association this might provide a link between PI hydrolysis and membrane activation. A more rigorous purification of the proteins concerned will be required before this interesting suggestion can be evaluated.

Eichberg et al. (1973) have made an interesting study of ^{32}P$_i$ incorporation into phospholipids of rat pineal glands in organ culture. Both norepinephrine and β-adrenergic blocking agents markedly stimulated labeling of PI and even more markedly of phosphatidylglycerol. This latter compound had not previously been implicated in responses to neurotransmitters. Further work from this laboratory (Hauser et al., 1974) suggests that the norepinephrine was acting through α-adrenergic receptors. This is consistent with the adipose tissue results outlined below.

C. Adipose Tissue

De Torrontegui and Barthet (1966) showed that insulin increased the incorporation of ^{32}P into PI of rat epididymal fat pads incubated in vitro.

Increased labeling of other phospholipids also occurred, but was less reproducible. The effects could be due to the increased availability of glycerophosphate as a result of insulin action, but a genuine phospholipid effect is also possible. Stein and Hales (1972) studied the actions of epinephrine and α- and β-adrenergic blocking agents on the same system. Epinephrine caused lipolysis and increased ^{32}P labeling of only phosphatidylcholine. In the presence of the β-blocking agent propanolol, epinephrine no longer caused lipolysis, and in this case labeling of phosphatidylcholine was reduced while there was a marked increase in labeling of phosphatidic acid and PI compared with cells incubated with only epinephrine. Similar experiments with epinephrine and phenoxybenzamine, an α-blocking drug, showed stimulation of lipolysis and decreased labeling of all the phospholipids compared with epinephrine alone. Stein and Hales pointed out that interpretation of the phospholipid changes is difficult when the specific activity and concentration of ATP are not known under the various conditions. It is possible, however, that increased turnover of PI is a response to α-receptors in fat cells. More light is thrown on this possibility by the studies of Hayashi et al. (1974) on inositol-deficient rats. Such rats developed fatty livers, and this was apparently due to increased mobilization of fatty acid from adipose tissue. If this lipolysis was due to ineffective α-receptor activity, a possible explanation would be lack of PI, which is involved somehow in the response to these receptors.

The α-adrenergic stimulus usually counteracts the activation of adenyl cyclase by β-adrenergic agents. Levey (1971) has shown that heart adenyl cyclase sensitivity to the β-adrenergic stimulus required the presence of PI. If α- and β-receptors occupied adjacent sites on the plasma membrane, α stimulation leading to hydrolysis of PI might at the same time uncouple the β-receptor regulation of adenyl cyclase (Michell, 1975), thus reinforcing the α effect. These speculations are not easy to reconcile with those in the preceding paragraph for adipose tissue, but the two regulatory systems could be quite different. It seems likely that both α-adrenergic and muscarinic cholinergic activities involve PI breakdown. Further work will show whether this lipid plays a part in other related regulatory systems.

ACKNOWLEDGMENT

We are indebted to Mrs. D. Paxton for her patience and care in preparing the manuscript.

REFERENCES

Abdel-Latif, A. A., Yan, S.-J., and Smith, J. P. (1974). J. Neurochem. 22, 383–393.
Abramson, D., and Blecher, M. (1965). Biochim. Biophys. Acta 98, 117–127.

Akamatsu, Y., Ono, Y., and Nojima, S. (1967). *J. Biochem. (Tokyo)* **59**, 176–182.

Akino, T., and Shimojo. T. (1970). *Biochim. Biophys. Acta* **210**, 343–346.

Akiyama, M., and Sakagami, T. (1969). *Biochim. Biophys. Acta* **187**, 105–112.

Allan, D., and Michell, R. H. (1974a). *Biochem. J.* **142**, 591–598.

Allan, D., and Michell, R. H. (1974b). *Biochem. J.* **142**, 599–604.

Ambron, R. T., and Pieringer, R. A. (1973). *In* "Form and Function of Phospholipids" (G. B. Ansell, R. M. C. Dawson, and J. N. Hawthorne, eds.), pp. 289–331. Elsevier, Amsterdam.

Angus, W. W., and Lester, R. L. (1972). *Arch. Biochem. Biophys.* **151**, 483–495.

Ansell, G. B., and Hawthorne, J. N. (1964). "The Phospholipids." Elsevier, Amsterdam.

Appel, S. H., Andrew, C. G., and Almon, R. R. (1974). *J. Neurochem.* **23**, 1077–1080.

Atherton, R. S., and Hawthorne, J. N. (1968). *Eur. J. Biochem.* **4**, 68–75.

Baker, R. R., and Thompson, W. (1972). *Biochim. Biophys. Acta* **270**, 489–503.

Baker, R. R., and Thompson, W. (1973). *J. Biol. Chem.* **248**, 7060–7065.

Bangham, A. D. (1968). *Progr. Biophys. Mol. Biol.* **18**, 29–95.

Baxter, C. F., Rouser, G., and Simon, G. (1969). *Lipids* **4**, 243–244.

Benson, A. A., and Maruo, B. (1958). *Biochim. Biophys. Acta* **27**, 189–195.

Birnberger, A. C., Birnberger, K. L., Eliasson, S. G., and Simpson, P. C. (1971). *J. Neurochem.* **18**, 1291–1298.

Bleasdale, J. E. (1974). Ph.D. Thesis, University of Nottingham, England.

Bleasdale, J. E., and Hawthorne, J. N. (1975). *J. Neurochem.* **24**, 373–379.

Bligh, E. G., and Dyer, W. J. (1959). *Can. J. Biochem. Physiol.* **37**, 911–917.

Brammer, M. J., and Sheltawy, A. (1975). *J. Neurochem.* **25**, 699–705.

Brennan, P. J. (1968). *Biochem. J.* **109**, 158–160.

Brennan, P. J., and Ballou, C. E. (1967). *J. Biol. Chem.* **242**, 3046–3056.

Brennan, P. J., and Ballou, C. E. (1968a). *J. Biol. Chem.* **243**, 2975–2984.

Brennan, P. J., and Ballou, C. E. (1968b). *Biochem. Biophys. Res. Commun.* **30**, 69–75.

Brennan, P. J., and Lehane, D. P. (1971). *Lipids* **6**, 401–409.

Brockerhoff, H. (1963). *J. Lipid Res.* **4**, 96–99.

Brockerhoff, H., and Ballou, C. E. (1961). *J. Biol. Chem.* **236**, 1907–1911.

Buckley, J. T. (1974). *Biochem. J.* **142**, 521–526.

Buckley, J. T., and Hawthorne, J. N. (1972). *J. Biol. Chem.* **247**, 7218–7223.

Buckley, J. T., Lefebvre, Y. A., and Hawthorne, J. N. (1971). *Biochim. Biophys. Acta* **239**, 517–519.

Calvayrac, R., and Douce, R. (1970). *FEBS (Fed. Eur. Biochem. Soc.) Lett.* **7**, 259.

Canessa de Scarnatti, O., and Rodriguez de Lores Arnaiz, G. (1972). *Biochim. Biophys. Acta* **270**, 218–225.

Carter, H. E., and Kisic, A. (1969). *J. Lipid Res.* **10**, 356–362.

Cicero, T. J., and Sherman, W. R. (1971). *Biochem. Biophys. Res. Commun.* **42**, 428–433.

Cicero, T. J., and Sherman, W. R. (1973). *Anal. Biochem.* **54**, 32–39.

Clarke, N., and Dawson, R. M. C. (1972). *Biochem. J.* **130**, 229–238.

Clement, J., Clement, G., and Fontaine, H. (1963). *C. R. Soc. Biol.* **157**, 1716–1721.

Cohen, P., Broekman, M. J., Verkley, A., Lisman, J. W. W., and Derksen, A. (1971). *J. Clin. Invest.* **50**, 763–772.

Colacicco, G., and Rapport, M. M. (1967). *J. Lipid Res.* **8**, 513–515.

Cooper, P. H., and Hawthorne, J. N. (1973). *J. Chromatogr.* **87**, 267–268.

Cooper, P. H., and Hawthorne, J. N. (1975). *Biochem. J.* **150**, 537–551.

Davies, J. H., and Malkin, T. (1959). *Chem. Ind. (London)* **37**, 1155–1156.

Dawson, R. M. C. (1965). *Biochem. J.* **97**, 134–138.

Dawson, R. M. C., and Clarke, N. (1972). *Biochem. J.* **127**, 113–118.

Dawson, R. M. C., and Dittmer, J. C. (1961). *Biochem. J.* **81**, 540–545.

Dawson, R. M. C., and Eichberg, J. (1965). *Biochem. J.* **96**, 634–643.

Dawson, R. M. C., Hemington, N., and Davenport, J. B. (1962). *Biochem. J.* **84**, 497–501.

Dawson, R. M. C., Freinkel, N., Jungalwala, F. B., and Clarke, N. (1971). *Biochem. J.* **122**, 605–607.

De Camilli, P., and Meldolesi, J. (1974). *Life Sci.* **15**, 711–721.

Demel, R., Wirtz, K. W. A., Kamp, H. H., Geurts van Kessel, W. S. H., and Van Deenen, L. L. M. (1973). *Nature (London) New Biol.* **246**, 102–105.

De Torrontegui, G., and Berthet, J. (1966). *Biochim. Biophys. Acta* **116**, 477–481.

Diringer, H., and Koch, M. A. (1973). *Biochem. Biophys. Res. Commun.* **51**, 967–971.

Dittmer, J. C., and Dawson, R. M. C. (1961). *Biochem. J.* **81**, 535–540.

Dittmer, J. C., and Douglas, M. G. (1969). *Ann. N.Y. Acad. Sci.* **165**, 515–525.

Durell, J., and Sodd, M. A. (1966). *J. Neurochem.* **13**, 487–491.

Durell, J., Garland, J. T., and Friedel, R. O. (1969). *Science* **165**, 862–866.

Eggman, L. D., and Hokin, L. E. (1960). *J. Biol. Chem.* **235**, 2569–2572.

Eichberg, J., and Dawson, R. M. C. (1965). *Biochem. J.* **96**, 644–658.

Eichberg, J., and Hauser, G. (1967). *Biochim. Biophys. Acta* **144**, 415–422.

Eichberg, J., and Hauser, G. (1973). *Biochim. Biophys. Acta* **326**, 210–223.

Eichberg, J., Shein, H. M., Schwartz, M., and Hauser, G. (1973). *J. Biol. Chem.* **248**, 3615–3622.

Eisenberg, F., Jr. (1969). *Ann. N.Y. Acad. Sci.* **165**, 509–819.

Eliasson, S. G., Scarpellini, J. D., and Fox, R. R. (1972). *Arch. Neurol (Chicago)* **27**, 535–539.

Ellis, R. B., Galliard, T., and Hawthorne, J. N. (1963). *Biochem. J.* **88**, 125–131.

Fisher, D. B., and Mueller, G. C. (1968). *Proc. Nat. Acad. Sci. U.S.* **60**, 1396–1402.

Fisher, D. B., and Mueller, G. C. (1971). *Biochim. Biophys. Acta* **248**, 434–448.

Folch, J. (1942). *J. Biol. Chem.* **146**, 35–44.

Folch, J. (1949). *J. Biol. Chem.* **177**, 505–519.

Folch, J., Lees, M., and Sloane-Stanley, G. H. (1957). *J. Biol. Chem.* **226**, 497–509.

Freinkel, N. (1957). *Endocrinology* **61**, 448–460.

Friedel, R. O., and Schanberg, S. M. (1972). *J. Pharmacol. Exp. Ther.* **183**, 326–332.

Friedel, R. O., Johnson, J. R., and Schanberg, S. M. (1973). *J. Pharmacol. Exp. Ther.* **184**, 583–589.

Galliard, T. (1968). *Phytochemistry* **7**, 1915–1922.

Galliard, T. (1973). *In* "Form and Function of Phospholipids" (G. B. Ansell, R. M. C. Dawson, and J. N. Hawthorne, eds.), pp. 253–288. Elsevier, Amsterdam.

Gaut, Z. N., and Huggins, C. G. (1966). *Nature (London)* **212**, 612–613.

Gent, P. A., Gigg, R., and Warren, C. D. (1970). *Tetrahedron Lett.* **30**, 2575–2578.

Gonzalez-Sastre, F., and Folch-Pi, J. (1968). *J. Lipid Res.* **9**, 532–533.

Gonzalez-Sastre, F., Eichberg, J., and Hauser, G. (1971). *Biochim. Biophys. Acta* **248**, 96–104.

Gurr, M. I., Prottey, C., and Hawthorne, J. N. (1965). *Biochim. Biophys. Acta* **106**, 357–370.

Harvey, M. S., Wirtz, K. W. A., Kamp, H. H., Zegers, B. J. M., and Van Deenen, L. L. M. (1973). *Biochim. Biophys. Acta* **323**, 234–239.

Harwood, J. L., and Hawthorne, J. N. (1969). *Biochim. Biophys. Acta* **171**, 75–88.

Hauser, G., and Eichberg, J. (1973). *Biochim. Biophys. Acta* **306**, 201–209.

Hauser, G., Eichberg, J., and Gonzalez-Sastre, F. (1971a). *Biochim. Biophys. Acta* **248**, 87–95.

Hauser, G., Eichberg, J., and Jacobs, S. (1971b). *Biochem. Biophys. Res. Commun.* **43**, 1072–1080.

Hauser, G., Shein, H. M., and Eichberg, J. (1974). *Nature (London)* **252**, 482–483.

Hauser, H., and Dawson, R. M. C. (1968). *Biochem. J.* **109**, 909–916.

Hawthorne, J. N. (1964). *Vitam. Horm. (New York)* **22**, 57–79.

Hawthorne, J. N. (1973). *In* "Form and Function of Phospholipids" (G. B. Ansell, R. M. C. Dawson, and J. N. Hawthorne, eds.), pp. 423–440. Elsevier, Amsterdam.

Hawthorne, J. N., and Bleasdale, J. E. (1975). *Mol. Cell. Biochem.* **8**, 83–87.

Hawthorne, J. N., and Kai, M. (1970). *In* "Handbook of Neurochemistry" (A. Lajtha, ed.), Vol. 3, pp. 491–508. Plenum, New York.

Hawthorne, J. N., and Michell, R. H. (1966). *In* "Cyclitols and Phosphoinositides" (H. Kindl, ed.), pp. 49–55. Pergamon, Oxford.

Hayashi, E., Maeda, T., and Tomita, T. (1974). *Biochim. Biophys. Acta* **360**, 134–145 and 146–155.

Hayashi, K., Yagihara, Y., Nakamura, I., and Yamazoe, S. (1966). *J. Biochem. (Tokyo)* **60**, 42–51.

Helmkamp, G. M., Harvey, M. S., Wirtz, K. W. A., and Van Deenen, L. L. M. (1974). *J. Biol. Chem.* **249**, 6382–6389.

Hendrickson, H. S. (1969). *Ann. N.Y. Acad. Sci.* **165**, 668–676.

Hendrickson, H. S., and Ballou, C. E. (1964). *J. Biol. Chem.* **239**, 1369–1373.

Hendrickson, H. S., and Reinertsen, J. L. (1971). *Biochem. Biophys. Res. Commun.* **44**, 1258–1274.

Hill, D. L., and Ballou, C. E. (1966). *J. Biol. Chem.* **241**, 895–902.

Hokin, L. E. (1966). *Biochim. Biophys. Acta* **115**, 219–221.

Hokin, L. E. (1968). *Int. Rev. Cytol.* **23**, 187–208.

Hokin, L. E. (1969). *In* "The Structure and Function of Nervous Tissue" (G. H. Bourne, ed.), Vol. 3, pp. 161–184. Academic Press, New York.

Hokin, L. E., and Hokin, M. R. (1958). *J. Biol. Chem.* **233**, 805–826.

Hokin, L. E., and Hokin, M. R. (1960). *J. Gen. Physiol.* **44**, 61–85.

Hokin, L. E., and Hokin, M. R. (1964). *Biochim. Biophys. Acta* **84**, 563–575.

Hokin, L. E., Hokin, M. R., and Lobeck, C. C. (1963). *J. Clin. Invest.* **42**, 1232–1237.

Hokin, M. R. (1969). *J. Neurochem.* **16**, 127–134.

Hokin, M. R. (1970). *J. Neurochem.* **17**, 357–364.

Hokin, M. R., and Brown, D. F. (1969). *J. Neurochem.* **16**, 475–483.

Hokin, M. R., and Hokin, L. E. (1964). *In* "Metabolism and Physiological Significance of Lipids" (R. M. C. Dawson and D. N. Rhodes, eds.). pp. 423–434. Wiley, New York.

Hokin-Neaverson, M. R. (1974). *Biochem. Biophys. Res. Commun.* **58**, 763–768.

Holub, B. J. (1974). *Biochim. Biophys. Acta* **369**, 111–122.

Holub, B. J., and Kuksis, A. (1971a). *J. Lipid Res.* **12**, 510–512.

Holub, B. J., and Kuksis, A. (1971b). *J. Lipid Res.* **12**, 699–705.

Holub, B. J., and Kuksis, A. (1972). *Lipids* **7**, 78–80.

Holub, B. J., Kuksis, A., and Thompson, W. (1970). *J. Lipid Res.* **11**, 558–564.

Hölzl, J., and Wagner, H. (1964). *Biochem. Z.* **339**, 327–330.

Iacobelli, S. (1969). *J. Neurochem.* **16**, 909–911.

Ito, T., and Ohnishi, S. (1974). *Biochim. Biophys. Acta* **352**, 29–37.

Jones, L. M., and Michell, R. H. (1974). *Biochem. J.* **142**, 583–590.

Jungalwala, F. B., Freinkel, N., and Dawson, R. M. C. (1971). *Biochem. J.* **123**, 19–33.

Karnovsky, M. L., and Wallach, D. F. H. (1961). *J. Biol. Chem.* **236**, 1895–1901.

Kataoka, T., and Nojima, S. (1967). *Biochim. Biophys. Acta* **144**, 681–683.

Kates, M. (1972). "Techniques of Lipidology." North-Holland Publ., Amsterdam.

Keenan, R. N., and Hokin, L. E. (1964). *Biochim. Biophys. Acta* **84**, 458–460.

Kemp, P., Hübscher, G., and Hawthorne, J. N. (1961). *Biochem. J.* **79**, 193–200.

Keough, K. M. W., and Thompson, W. (1970). *J. Neurochem.* **17**, 1–11.

Keough, K. M. W., and Thompson, W. (1972). *Biochim. Biophys. Acta* **270**, 324–336.

Keough, K. M. W., Macdonald, G., and Thompson, W. (1972). *Biochim. Biophys. Acta* **270**, 337–347.

Kerr, S. E., Kfoury, G. A., and Djibelian, L. G. (1964). *J. Lipid Res.* **5**, 481–483.

Klyashchitskii, B. A., Shvets, V. I., and Preobrazhenskii, U. A. (1969a). *Chem. Phys. Lipids* **3**, 393–400.

Klyashchitskii, B. A., Sokolov, S. D., and Shvets, V. I. (1969b). *Russ. Chem. Rev.* **38**, 345–353.

Koch, M. A., and Diringer, H. (1973). *Biochem. Biophys. Res. Commun.* **55**, 305–311.

Kuiper, P. J. C. (1970). *Plant Physiol.* **45**, 684–686.

Lapetina, E. G., and Michell, R. H. (1972). *Biochem. J.* **126**, 1141–1147.

Lapetina, E. G., and Michell, R. H. (1973). *Biochem. J.* **131**, 433–442.

Larrabee, M. G., Klingman, J. D., and Leicht, W. S. (1963). *J. Neurochem.* **10**, 549–570.

Le Baron, F. N., McDonald, C. P., and Sridhara Ramarao, B. S. (1963). *J. Neurochem.* **10**, 677–683.

Lee, T.-C., and Huggins, C. G. (1968a). *Arch. Biochem. Biophys.* **126**, 206–213.

Lee, T.-C., and Huggins, C. G. (1968b). *Arch. Biochem. Biophys.* **126**, 214–220.

Lee, Y. C., and Ballou, C. E. (1965). *Biochemistry* **4**, 1395–1404.

Lederer, E. (1961). *Biochem. J.* **81**, 31P-32P.

Lefebvre, Y. A. (1974). Ph.D. Thesis, University of Nottingham, England.

Lennon, A. M., and Steinberg, H. R. (1973). *J. Neurochem.* **20**, 337–345.

Lepage, M. (1968). *Lipids* **3**, 477–481.

Lester, R. L. (1963). *Fed. Proc., Fed. Amer. Soc. Exp. Biol.* **22**, 415.

Lester, R. L., and Steiner, M. R. (1968). *J. Biol. Chem.* **243**, 4889–4893.

Lester, R. L., Smith, S. W., Wells, G. B., Rees, D. C., and Angus, W. A. (1974). *J. Biol. Chem.* **249**, 3383–3387.

Levey, G. S. (1971). *J. Biol. Chem.* **246**, 7405–7407.

Litman, B. J. (1973). *Biochemistry* **12**, 2545–2554.

Lloyd, J. V., Nishizawa, E. E., Halder, J., and Mustard, J. F. (1972a). *Brit. J. Haematol.* **23**, 571–585.

Lloyd, J. V., Nishizawa, E. E., Joist, J. H., and Mustard, J. F. (1972b). *Brit. J. Haematol.* **24**, 589–604.

Long, C., and Owens, K. (1962). *Biochem. J.* **85**, 34P.

Lucas, C. T., Call, F. L., and Williams, W. J. (1970). *J. Clin. Invest.* **49**, 1949–1955.

Luk'yanov, A. V., Lyutik, A. I., Shvets, V. I., and Preobrazhenskii, N. A. (1965). *Dokl. Chem.* **165**, 1079–1082.

Lunt, G. G., and Pickard, M. R. (1975). *J. Neurochem.* **24**, 1203–1208.

Luthra, M. G., and Sheltawy, A. (1972a). *Biochem. J.* **126**, 251–253.

Luthra, M. G., and Sheltawy, A. (1972b). *Biochem. J.* **126**, 1231–1239.
Luthra, M. G., and Sheltawy, A. (1972c). *Biochem. J.* **128**, 587–595.
Luthra, M. G., and Sheltawy, A. (1976). *J. Neurochem.* (in press).
Macchia, V., and Pastan, I. (1968). *Biochim. Biophys. Acta* **152**, 704–712.
McMurray, W. C., and Dawson, R. M. C. (1969). *Biochem. J.* **112**, 91–108.
Meldolesi, J., Jamieson, J. D., and Palade, G. E. (1971). *J. Cell Biol.* **49**, 130–149.
Michell, R. H. (1975). *Biochim. Biophys. Acta* **415**, 81–147.
Michell, R. H., Harwood, J. L., Coleman, R., and Hawthorne, J. N. (1967). *Biochim. Biophys. Acta* **144**, 649–658.
Michell, R. H., Hawthorne, J. N., Coleman, R., and Karnovsky, M. L. (1970). *Biochim. Biophys. Acta* **210**, 86–91.
Miller, E. K., and Dawson, R. M. C. (1972). *Biochem. J.* **126**, 823–835.
Molotkovskii, Y. G., and Bergel'son, L. D. (1971). *Dokl. Adad. Nauk SSSR* **198**, 461–464.
Nelson, G. J. (1967). *Biochim. Biophys. Acta* **144**, 221–232.
Nojima, S. (1959a). *J. Biochem.* (*Tokyo*) **46**, 499–506.
Nojima, S. (1959b). *J. Biochem.* (*Tokyo*) **46**, 607–620.
Ohnishi, S., and Ito, T. (1974). *Biochemistry* **13**, 881–887.
Palmer, F. B. St. C. (1971). *Biochim. Biophys. Acta* **231**, 134–144.
Palmer, F. B. St. C. (1973a). *Biochim. Biophys. Acta* **316**, 296–304.
Palmer, F. B. St. C. (1973b). *Biochim. Biophys. Acta* **326**, 194–200.
Palmer, F. B. St. C., and Dawson, R. M. C. (1969). *Biochem. J.* **111**, 637–646.
Pangborn, M. C., and McKinney, J. A. (1966). *J. Lipid Res.* **7**, 627–633.
Papahadjopoulos, D. (1968). *Biochim. Biophys. Acta* **163**, 240–254.
Papahadjopoulos, D., and Miller, N. (1967). *Biochim. Biophys. Acta* **135**, 624–638.
Parsons, J. G., Keeney, P. G., and Patton, S. (1969). *J. Food Sci.* **34**, 497–499.
Pasternak, C. A. (1972). *J. Cell Biol.* **53**, 231–234.
Paulose, M. M., Venkob Rao, S., and Achaya, K. T. (1966). *Indian J. Chem.* **4**, 529–532.
Percy, A. K., Schmell, E., Earles, B. J., and Lennarz, W. J. (1973). *Biochemistry* **12**, 2456–2461.
Peterson, S. C., and Kirschner, L. B. (1970). *Biochim. Biophys. Acta* **202**, 295–304.
Phillips, J. H. (1973). *Biochem. J.* **136**, 579–587.
Possmayer, F. (1974). *Brain Res.* **74**, 167–174.
Posternak, T. (1965). "The Cyclitols." Holden-Day, San Francisco, California.
Prottey, C., and Ballou, C. E. (1968). *J. Biol. Chem.* **243**, 6196–6201.
Prottey, C., and Hawthorne, J. N. (1966). *Biochem. J.* **101**, 191–196.
Prottey, C., and Hawthorne, J. N. (1967). *Biochem. J.* **105**, 379–392.
Pumphrey, A. M. (1969). *Biochem. J.* **112**, 61–70.
Quarles, R. H., and Dawson, R. M. C. (1969). *Biochem. J.* **112**, 787–794.
Quinn, P. J. (1973). *Biochem. J.* **133**, 273–281.
Quinn, P. J., and Dawson, R. M. C. (1972). *Chem. Phys. Lipids* **8**, 1–9.
Redman, C. M. (1971). *J. Cell Biol.* **49**, 35–49.
Renkonen, O. (1968). *Biochim. Biophys. Acta* **152**, 114–135.
Rose, H. G., and Frenster, J. H. (1965). *Biochim. Biophys. Acta* **106**, 577–591.
Rosenberg, P. (1973). *J. Pharm. Sci.* **62**, 1552–1554.
Roughan, P. G. (1970). *Biochem. J.* **117**, 1–8.
Roughan, P. G., and Batt, R. D. (1969). *Phytochemistry* **8**, 363–369.
Rouser, G., Kritchevsky, G., and Yamamoto, A. (1967). "Lipid Chromatographic Analysis," Vol. 1, pp. 99–162. Dekker, New York.

Rouser, G., Simon, G., and Kritchevsky, G. (1969). *Lipids* **4**, 599–606.

Salway, J. G., and Hughes, I. E. (1972). *J. Neurochem.* **19**, 1233–1240.

Santiago-Calvó, E., Mulé, S., Redman, C. M., Hokin, M. R., and Hokin, L. E. (1964). *Biochim. Biophys. Acta* **84**, 550–562.

Sastry, P. S., and Hokin, L. E. (1966). *J. Biol. Chem.* **241**, 3354–3361.

Sastry, P. S., and Kates, M. (1964). *Biochemistry* **3**, 1271–1280.

Sastry, P. S., and Kates, M. (1965). *Can. J. Biochem.* **43**, 1445–1454.

Schacht, J., and Agranoff, B. W. (1972). *J. Neurochem.* **19**, 1417–1421.

Schacht, J., and Agranoff, B. W. (1974). *J. Biol. Chem.* **249**, 1551–1557.

Schacht, J., Neale, E. A., and Agranoff, B. W. (1974). *J. Neurochem.* **23**, 211–218.

Schneider, R. P., and Kirschner, L. B. (1970). *Biochim. Biophys. Acta* **202**, 283–294.

Schnepel, G. H., Hegner, D., and Schummer, U. (1974). *Biochim. Biophys. Acta* **367**, 67–74.

Scott, T. W., Mills, S. C., and Freinkel, N. (1968). *Biochem. J.* **109**, 325–332.

Shaw, N., and Dinglinger, F. (1968). *Biochem. J.* **109**, 700–701.

Shaw, N., and Dinglinger, F. (1969). *Biochem. J.* **112**, 769–775.

Sheltawy, A., and Dawson, R. M. C. (1969). *Biochem. J.* **111**, 147–155.

Simon, G., and Rouser, G. (1969). *Lipids* **4**, 607–614.

Singh, H., and Carroll, K. K. (1970). *Lipids* **5**, 121–127.

Skipski, V. P., Peterson, R. F., and Barclay, M. (1964). *Biochem. J.* **90**, 374–378.

Sloviter, H. A., and Tanaka, S. (1967). *Biochim. Biophys. Acta* **137**, 70–79.

Smith, S. W., and Lester, R. L. (1974). *J. Biol. Chem.* **249**, 3388–3394.

Spanner, S. (1973). *In* "Form and Function of Phospholipids" (G. B. Ansell, R. M. C. Dawson, and J. N. Hawthorne, eds.), pp. 43–65. Elsevier, Amsterdam.

Stein, J. M., and Hales, C. N. (1972). *Biochem. J.* **128**, 531–541.

Steinberg, H. R., and Durell, J. (1971). *J. Neurochem.* **18**, 277–286.

Steiner, M. R., and Lester, R. L. (1972). *Biochim. Biophys. Acta* **260**, 222–243.

Steiner, S., and Lester, R. L. (1972). *Biochim. Biophys. Acta* **260**, 82–87.

Steiner, S., Smith, S., Waechter, C. J., and Lester, R. L. (1969). *Proc. Nat. Acad. Sci. U.S.* **64**, 1042–1048.

Talwalkar, R. T., and Lester, R. L. (1973). *Biochim. Biophys. Acta* **306**, 412–421.

Talwalkar, R. T., and Lester, R. L. (1974). *Biochim. Biophys. Acta* **360**, 306–311.

Thompson, A. C., Henson, R. D., Minyard, J. P., and Hedin, P. A. (1968). *Lipids* **3**, 373–374.

Thompson, W. (1967). *Can. J. Biochem.* **45**, 853–861.

Torda, C. (1972). *Biochim. Biophys. Acta* **286**, 389–395.

Torda, C. (1973). *Naturwissenschaften* **60**, 436.

Tou, J.-S, and Stjernholm, R. L. (1974). *Arch. Biochem. Biophys.* **160**, 487–494.

Tou, J.-S., Hurst, M. W., and Huggins, C. G. (1968). *Arch. Biochem. Biophys.* **127**, 54–58.

Tou, J.-S., Hurst, M. W., and Huggins, C. G. (1969). *Arch. Biochem. Biophys.* **131**, 596–602.

Tou, J.-S., Hurst, M. W., Huggins, C. G., and Foor, W. E. (1970). *Arch. Biochem. Biophys.* **140**, 492–502.

Tou, J.-S., Hurst, M. W., Baricos, W. H., and Huggins, C. G. (1972). *Arch. Biochem. Biophys.* **149**, 146–152.

Tou, J.-S., Hurst, M. W., Baricos, W. H., and Huggins, C. G. (1973). *Arch. Biochem. Biophys.* **154**, 593–600.

Townsend, D., Jenkin, H. M., and Yang, T.-K. (1972). *Biochim. Biophys. Acta* **260**, 20–25.

Trifaró, J. M. (1969a). *Mol. Pharmacol.* **5**, 382–393.
Trifaró, J. M. (1969b). *Mol. Pharmacol.* **5**, 424–427.
Trifaró, J. M., and Dworkind, J. (1971). *Mol. Pharmacol.* **7**, 52–65.
Vijayalakshmi, B., Venkob Rao, S., and Achaya, K. T. (1969). *Fette, Seifen, Anstrich.* **71**, 757.
Vilkas, E. (1960). *Bull. Soc. Chim. Biol.* **42**, 1005–1011.
Vilkas, E., and Lederer, E. (1960). *Bull. Soc. Chim. Biol.* **42**, 1013–1022.
Wagner, H., Hölzl, J., Lissau, A., and Hörhammer, I. (1963). *Biochem. Z.* **339**, 34.
Wells, M. A., and Dittmer, J. C. (1963). *Biochemistry* **2**, 1259–1263.
Wells, M. A., and Dittmer, J. C. (1965). *Biochemistry* **4**, 2459–2468.
Wheeler, G. E., Michell, R. H., and Rose, A. H. (1972). *Biochem. J.* **127**, 64P.
White, D. A. (1973). *In* "Form and Function of Phospholipids" (G. B. Ansell, R. M. C. Dawson, and J. N. Hawthorne, eds.), pp. 441–482. Elsevier, Amsterdam.
White, D. A., Pounder, D. J., and Hawthorne, J. N. (1971). *Biochim. Biophys. Acta* **242**, 99–107.
White, G. L., and Hawthorne, J. N. (1970). *Biochem. J.* **117**, 203–213.
White, G. L., and Larrabee, M. G. (1973). *J. Neurochem.* **20**, 783–798.
White, G. L. Schellhase, H. U., and Hawthorne, J. N. (1974). *J. Neurochem.* **22**, 149–158.
Widlund, L., and Heilbronn, E. (1974). *J. Neurochem.* **22**, 991–998.
Wirtz, K. W. A., and Zilversmit, D. B. (1968). *J. Biol. Chem.* **243**, 3596–3602.
Woelk, H., Kanig, K., and Peiler-Ichikawa, K. (1974). *J. Neurochem.* **23**, 1057–1063.
Wuthier, R. E. (1966). *J. Lipid Res.* **7**, 544–550.
Yagihara, Y., and Hawthorne, J. N. (1972). *J. Neurochem.* **19**, 355–367.
Yagihara, Y., Salway, J. G., and Hawthorne, J. N. (1969). *J. Neurochem.* **16**, 1133–1139.
Yagihara, Y., Bleasdale, J. E., and Hawthorne, J. N. (1973). *J. Neurochem.* **21**, 173–190.
Zhelvakova, E. G., Klyashchitskii, B. A., Shvets, V. I., Evstigneeva, R. P., and Preobrazhenskii, N. A. (1970). *J. Gen. Chem. U.S.S.R.* **40**, 227.

Hormonal Regulation of Cartilage Growth and Metabolism*

HAROLD E. LEBOVITZ AND GEORGE S. EISENBARTH

*Departments of Medicine and Physiology, Duke University Medical Center,
Durham, North Carolina*

I. INTRODUCTION

The central role of cartilage in linear growth has been appreciated since the process of endochondral ossification was recognized (see review by Sissons, 1972). Many hormone excesses and deficiencies are associated with aberrations of statural growth, and it is therefore not surprising that a number of investigators turned their attention to questions relating to hormonal control of epiphyseal cartliage growth. The observations made indicate that a number of hormones affect epiphyseal cartilage growth and/or maturation. Evidence for regulation of nonossifying cartilage (nasal, laryngeal, articular) by hormones portends that all cartilage may be under some degree of hormonal control.

Certain aspects of the biochemistry and physiology of cartilage appear

* The authors' studies have been supported by grants from the National Institute of Arthritis, Metabolic, and Digestive Diseases (AM 01324 and 5 T1 AM 5074).

to be unique. In spite of the great increase in knowledge about basic cartilage metabolism, relatively little is known concerning its hormonal regulation. The scope of this contribution is to focus on the current status of our knowledge of hormone regulation of cartilage growth and metabolism; to reflect on the significance of this knowledge, and to project, on the basis of recent knowledge about basic cartilage metabolism, future directions for research in this area.

Cartilage is a specialized connective tissue whose primary function is to make a matrix that is resilient and resists deformation and compression. Several different types of cartilage exist in animals, and each appears to be adapted to its own specific function by the chemical composition of its matrix. The matrix compositions of the three major types of cartilage, elastic, fibrous, and hyaline, are given in Table I. All cartilage matrix consists of varying proportions of glycosaminoglycans, collagen, elastin, and noncollagenous protein. Fibrous cartilage, such as occurs in the intervertebral discs, contains virtually only collagen and has therefore a very fibrillar matrix with limited resilience. Elastic cartilage, such as in the auricle of the ear, contains much elastin and has elastic properties.

TABLE I

CHEMICAL COMPOSITION OF VARIOUS CARTILAGES

Type of cartilage	Source	Glycos-amino-glycans[a]	Colla-gen[a]	Elastin[a]	Non-col-lage-nous pro-tein[a]
Elastic	Bovine auricle[b]	12	53	19	16
Fibrocartilage	Human meniscus[b]	2.4	78	0.6	19
	Bovine meniscus[b]	2	82	0	16
Hyaline	Bovine nasal[b]	43	35	0	22
	Bovine epiphyseal[b]	22	51	0	27
	Bovine articular[b]	14	72	0	14
	Calf articular[d]	29	64	0	20
	Fetal ox articular[d]	41	46	0	32
	Rat epiphyseal[c]	20	30	0	50
	Rachitic chick[e] epiphyseal	31	22	0	47
	Calf epiphyseal[d]	38	56	0	6

[a] Percent dry weight.
[b] Peters and Smille (1971).
[c] Guri and Bernstein (1965).
[d] Campo and Tourtellotte (1967).
[e] Cipera (1962).

Hyaline cartilage has a smooth granular matrix, which contains large quantities of both glycosaminoglycans and collagen. Glycosaminoglycans are polysaccharide macromolecules that usually contain free carboxyl and sulfate groups. Their chemical characteristics are such that they avidly bind large quantities of water and, additionally, act as cation exchangers (Schubert, 1964, 1966; Gerber and Schubert, 1964; reviewed by Barrett, 1968; Serafini-Fracassini and Smith, 1974). Hyaline cartilage, therefore, is smooth and markedly resilient. Most cartilages that function to provide weight bearing or protection (immature skeleton, epiphyses, costal, laryngeal, tracheal, and nasal cartilages) or smooth resilient gliding surfaces (articular cartilage) are hyaline.

Hyaline cartilage is especially essential in the development and function of the skeletal system. Epiphyseal cartilage plates in the bones of immature animals control the rate of linear growth of the skeleton through the process of endochondral ossification (Sissons, 1972; Vaughan, 1970). Articular cartilage covering the surfaces of the bones in a movable joint allow the smooth and frictionless movement of the skeletal system.

Endochondral ossification is an effective way to promote the growth of bones of the skeleton (Vaughan, 1970; Sissons, 1972). Cartilage increases in size by appositional and interstitial growth in contrast to bone, which can enlarge only by appositional growth. Growth at the epiphyseal cartilage plate occurs by cell division of the chondroblasts in the area most remote from the surface of vascularization. The chondroblasts migrate toward the diaphysis and become columns of mature chondrocytes producing matrix. Upon continued migration, the cells become hypertrophied, the lacunae swell, and matrix production lessens. As they approach the diaphysis, the matrix becomes calcified, the chondrocytes die, and the spongiosa of the diaphysis with its blood vessels grows into the region. The growth and maturation of the epiphyseal cartilage of immature animals is a complex process, which appears to be regulated by several hormones.

Articular cartilage is composed of three ill-defined layers (Vaughan, 1970): (1) a superficial layer in which the cells are small, flat, and lie with their long axes parallel to the joint surface; (2) an intermediate layer of cells that are larger and round and make most of the matrix; (3) a deep layer adjacent to the bone with large cells whose matrix calcify and which is replaced by bone during periods of growth.

II. Chemistry and Physiology of Hyaline Cartilage

Cartilage is an avascular tissue and consists of cells (chondroblasts and chondrocytes) separated by an extensive matrix. The matrix, which is a product of the cells, consists primarily of proteoglycans (glycosaminoglycans covalently linked to proteins) and collagen. The cartilage matrix is divided into that immediately adjacent to chondrocytes (territorial matrix) and surrounded by the territorial capsule and that which occupies the interstices between territorial capsules (interterritorial matrix). Hyaline cartilages from different sites show marked variation in glycosaminoglycan and collagen content (Table I).

The chemistry of cartilage proteoglycans is extremely complex and is discussed in detail in several reviews (Barrett, 1968; Rodén, 1970; Rosenberg, 1973; Serafini-Fracassini and Smith, 1974). Proteoglycans are macromolecules consisting of many glycosaminoglycan chains covalently linked to a protein core (Schatton and Schubert, 1954). The basic proteoglycan unit is the smallest species that is not dissociable without breaking covalent bonds (Rosenberg, 1973). Glycosaminoglycans are polysaccharides consisting of repeating disaccharide units linked together to yield an unbranched macromolecule (Barrett, 1968; Campo, 1970; Rodén, 1970). In each repeating dissacharide unit one member is invariably a hexosamine and the other is usually a hexuronic acid, but may be a hexose. Usually the amino group of the hexosamine is acetylated, and one of the members of the unit is ordinarily sulfated. There are many types of glycosaminoglycans depending on the nature of the repeating dissaccharide unit. The major glycosaminoglycans present in cartilage are chondroitin 4-sulfate, chondroitin 6-sulfate, and keratin sulfate (Table II). In addition, hyaluronic acid has been detected as a very minor component in some cartilages (Seno and Anno, 1961; Szirmai et al., 1967). The concentration and distribution of the glycosaminoglycans vary according to age, type of cartilage, and morphological areas within the tissue (Conklin, 1963; Szirmai, 1963; Loewi, 1965; Schubert and Hammerman, 1965; Stockwell and Scott, 1965; Quintarelli and Dellovo, 1966; Szirmai, 1966; Scott and Stockwell, 1967; Szirmai et al., 1967).

TABLE II
GLYCOSAMINOGLYCANS OF CARTILAGE

Type	Repeating subunit	Location of sulfate
Chondroitin 4-sulfate	D-N-Acetylgalactosamine D-Glucuronic acid	Position 4 of N-acetylgalactosamine
Chondroitin 6-sulfate	D-N-Acetylgalactosamine D-Glucuronic acid	Position 6 of N-acetylgalactosamine
Keratin sulfate	D-N-Acetylglucosamine D-Galactose	Position 6 of either N-acetylglucosamine or galactose
Hyaluronic acid	D-N-Acetylglucosamine D-Glucuronic acid	None

Fibrous cartilage of the intervertebral disc has a high content of keratin sulfate, which increases with age (Gardell, 1955; Hallén, 1958, 1962; Davidson and Woodhall, 1959; Davidson and Small, 1963; Buddecke and Sziegoleit, 1964). In the newborn human, the chondroitin 4-sulfate to chondroitin 6-sulfate ratio in costal cartilage is 0.7. With increasing age chondroitin 4-sulfate steadily decreases with no change in chondroitin 6-sulfate, so that after three decades the ratio falls to 0.25 or less. Keratin sulfate, which is absent in the embryo and during early life, rises progressively from the first to fourth decade, when the value reaches 55% of the total glycosaminoglycan concentration (Meyer et al., 1958; Kaplan and Meyer, 1959; Rosenberg et al., 1965; Stidworthy et al., 1958; Mathews and Glagov, 1966). Similar changes in keratin sulfate occur in articular and bovine nasal cartilage (Kühn and Leppelman, 1958; Goh and Lowther, 1966).

Mathews (1971) has proposed that the proteoglycan unit is a single peptide of 2000 amino acids which contain repeating regions of 45 amino acid residues: 10 amino acids in a doublet to each end of which polysaccharide chains are attached and 35 amino acids separating the doublets from each other. Most cartilage proteoglycans exist as proteoglycan aggregates formed by the noncovalent association of proteoglycan units with each other and with another protein species called the glycoprotein link (Rosenberg, 1973). Proteoglycans aggregate with cartilage collagen through noncovalent links.

The biosynthesis of chondroitin sulfate is schematically depicted in Fig. 1 (see reviews of Barrett, 1968; Rodén, 1970; Serafini-Fracassini and Smith, 1974). Initiation begins with the synthesis of the core protein in the rough endoplasmic reticulum of the chondrocyte. The monosaccharides are individually attached to the chain through their UDP derivatives under the control of the specific transferases. The xylose-O-linkage to serine is specific to some unique aspect of the amino acid sequence of the core protein (perhaps the doublet), as free serine is not a suitable acceptor for the xylosyltransferase (Baker et al., 1971; Stoolmiller et al., 1972). The two galactoses of the trisaccharide linkage require separate enzymes for their transfer from UDP-galactose (Helting and Rodén, 1968, 1969). The synthesis of the linkage region seems to occur in the rough endoplasmic reticulum. The addition of the glucuronic acid and the subsequent repeating subunit occurs primarily in the Golgi region. The monosaccharides of the repeating subunits are added individually, not as a completed subunit (Tesler et al., 1966). Incorporation of sulfate into chondroitin sulfate occurs intracellularly in the Golgi region (Goodman and Lane, 1966) through a sulfate transfer system. The sulfate is first activated and then transferred to the acceptor. The activated deriva-

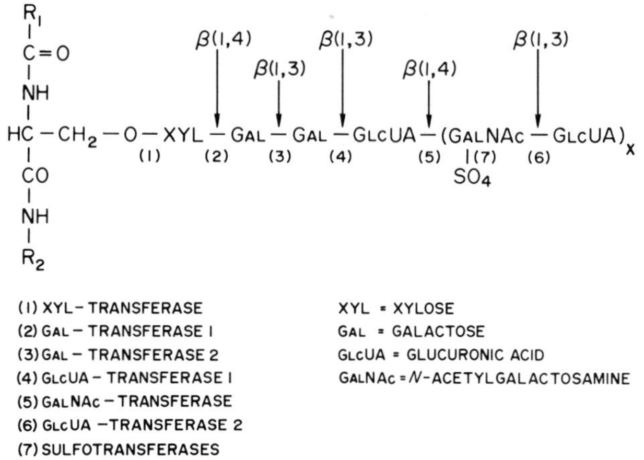

$$
\begin{array}{c}
R_1 \\
| \\
C=O \\
| \\
NH \\
| \\
HC - CH_2 - O - XYL - GAL - GAL - GLcUA - (GALNAc - GLcUA)_x \\
\end{array}
$$

(1) XYL – TRANSFERASE   XYL = XYLOSE
(2) GAL – TRANSFERASE I   GAL = GALACTOSE
(3) GAL – TRANSFERASE 2   GLcUA = GLUCURONIC ACID
(4) GLcUA – TRANSFERASE I   GALNAc = N-ACETYLGALACTOSAMINE
(5) GALNAc – TRANSFERASE
(6) GLcUA – TRANSFERASE 2
(7) SULFOTRANSFERASES

FIG. 1. Schematic representation of the biosynthesis of proteoglycans. The type of glycosidic linkage is given by the arrows. The numbers 1 to 7 in parentheses refer to the specific enzymes.

tive 3′-phosphoadenosine 5′-phosphosulfate (PAPS) is formed from inorganic sulfate in a two-step process (Robbins and Lipman, 1956, 1957; Adams, 1960; Suzuki and Strominger, 1960a,b,c).

$$SO_4^{2-} + ATP \rightarrow \text{adenosine 5′-phosphosulfate (APS)} + PP_i$$

$$APS + ATP \rightarrow \text{3′-phosphoadenosine 5′-phosphosulfate (PAPS)} + ADP$$

The two enzymes involved in these sulfate-activating reactions are ATP:sulfate adenyltransferase (EC 2.7.7.4) and ATP:adenylsulfate 3′-phosphotransferase (EC 2.7.1.25). Specific sulfotransferases (EC 2.8.2) are present in cartilage and probably determine the specific sites that are sulfated (D'Abramo and Lipmann, 1957; Adams and Rienitz, 1961; Hasegawa et al., 1961; Silbert, 1964; Perlman et al., 1964). Formation of the disaccharide units and sulfation probably occur simultaneously (Silbert et al., 1970). The newly synthesized proteoglycans are secreted rapidly into the territorial matrix, and as they migrate into the interterritorial matrix they polymerize with other simple proteoglycan units and with collagen (Serafini-Fracassini and Smith, 1974). Colchicine and vinblastine, compounds known to disrupt microtubules and interfere with microtubule-mediated cell function, inhibit the secretion and synthesis of glycosaminoglycans by chondrocytes in culture, and it seems likely that the secretion of proteoglycans is mediated by the microtubular system (Jansen and Bornstein, 1974). The factors that control the length of the polysaccharide chains and the extent and position of sulfation are not known.

Keratin sulfate is composed of repeating units of galactose and

N-acetylglucosamine linked by alternating $\beta1,4$ and $\beta1,3$ linkages (Barrett, 1968). The sulfate group may be located in position 6 of either galactose or N-acetylglucosamine. Keratin sulfate is linked to serine or threonine of the peptide chains. The exact nature of the linkage is unknown.

The formation and interconversion of the UDP-monosaccharides involved in the synthesis of cartilage glycosaminoglycans are shown in Fig. 2. Two major sites for the enzymic regulation of glycosaminoglycan synthesis are known; they are depicted by the heavy arrows. Neufeld and Hall (1965) reported that UDP-xylose specifically inhibits UDP-glucose:NAD oxidoreductase, thereby interfering with the conversion of UDP-glucose to UDP-glucuronate. This has been confirmed in cornea (Balduini *et al.*, 1970) and cartilage (Aureli *et al.*, 1969). Any accumulation of UDP-xylose due to a reduced rate of protein synthesis might be expected to cause immediate reduction of one of the activated intermediates for chondroitin sulfate synthesis.

The pool of UDP-N-acetylhexosamine is regulated by a feedback

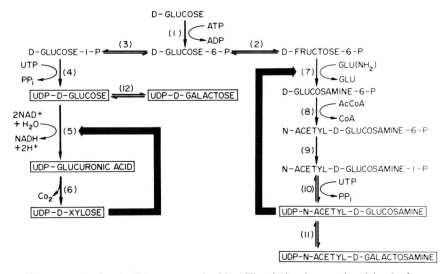

Fig. 2. Synthesis of UDP monosaccharides. The derivatives enclosed in the boxes are the intermediates involved in glycosaminoglycan synthesis. The heavy solid arrows refer to the two known sites of feedback regulation. The numbers in parentheses refer to the following specific enzymes: (1) hexokinase, EC 2.7.1.1; (2) glucose phosphate isomerase, EC 5.3.1.9; (3) phosphoglucomutase, EC 2.7.5.1; (4) glucose-1-phosphate uridylyltransferase, EC 2.7.7.9; (5) UDP-glucose:NAD oxidoreductase, EC 1.1.1.22; (6) UDP-glucuronic acid carboxy-lyase, EC 4.1.1.35; (7) L-glutamine-D-fructose-6-phosphate aminotransferase, EC 5.3.1.19; (8) phosphoglucosamine transacetylase, EC 2.3.1.4; (9) acetylglucosamine phosphomutase, EC 2.7.5.2; (10) UDP-glucosamine pyrophosphorylase, EC 2.7.7.23; (11) UDP-N-acetylglucosamine-4-epimerase, EC 5.1.3.7; (12) UDP-glucose 4-epimerase, EC 5.1.3.2.

mechanism since UDP-N-acetylglucosamine inhibits the L-glutamine:D-fructose-6-phosphate aminotransferase that catalyzes the conversion of fructose 6-phosphate to D-glucosamine 6-phosphate, the first step in UDP-N-acetylglucosamine synthesis (Kornfeld et al., 1964). Winterburn and Phelps (1971) showed that this inhibition could be relieved by UTP.

Collagen is the other major matrix protein in hyaline cartilage. Its chemistry is also quite complex and has been reviewed recently (Bornstein, 1974; Serafini-Fracassini and Smith, 1974). Several features of cartilage collagen are unique and need to be reviewed here. Cartilage collagen has a structure that is remarkably different from that of bone, skin, tendon, and other tissue collagen (Miller and Matukas, 1969). All collagens have a coiled three-chain structure, and in most vertebrae collagens the amino acid composition of one of the chains ($\alpha2$) is quite different from the other two, which are identical ($\alpha1$). Cartilage collagen is composed of three identical $\alpha1$ subunits. Structural studies of the $\alpha1$ subunit of cartilage collagen show that it is distinctly different from $\alpha1$ subunits of other collagens. It has been designated $\alpha1$ (II) in contradistinction to $\alpha1$ (I) ($\alpha1$ subunit of other collagens) (Miller and Matukas, 1969; Miller, 1971a,b, 1972; Miller and Lunde, 1973; Miller et al., 1971).

The $\alpha1$ (II) subunit amino acid composition is similar in cartilage from different species and in different sites within the same species. Table III gives the amino acid composition of $\alpha1$ (II) chains from chick and ox cartilage and compares them to $\alpha1$ (I) chains from other collagen in the same species. As can be noted from Table III, there are significant differences in the amino acid composition of $\alpha1$ (II) from $\alpha1$ (I). The majority (approximately two-thirds) of the lysyl residues of $\alpha1$ (II) are hydroxylated. In this regard $\alpha1$ (II) is similar to collagen obtained from glomerular basement membranes (Spiro, 1967a,b,c; Kefalides and Denduchis, 1969) and lens capsule (Fukushi and Spiro, 1969; Denduchis et al., 1970). In addition, similarly to glomerular basement membrane collagen (Spiro, 1967a,b) and lens capsule, $\alpha1$ (II) exhibits a high degree of glycosylation of the hydroxylysine residues. However, the extent of glycosylation of hydroxylysine residues observed for $\alpha1$ (II) is 40%, which is approximately one-half that observed for basement membrane and lens capsule collagens, and the carbohydrate appears to be almost equally distributed between disaccharide glucosylgalactose and monosaccharide galactose in $\alpha1$ (II) whereas essentially all the hydroxylysine-linked carbohydrate is in the disaccharide form in basement membrane collagens. $\alpha1$ (II) from chick cartilage contains nine times as much hydroxylysine-linked carbohydrates as $\alpha1$ (I) from bone and skin.

Hydroxylation of proline and lysine in collagen occur after the synthesis of protocollagen and are regulated by the enzymes protocollagen pro-

TABLE III

AMINO ACID COMPOSITION OF α1 (I) AND α1 (II) CHAINS OF COLLAGEN[a]

Component	Chick[b]		Ox[c]	
	Bone α1 (I)	Cartilage α1 (II)	Bone α1 (I)	Cartilage α1 (II)
3-Hydroxyproline	1.0	2.2		
4-Hydroxyproline	102	103	84	95
Aspartic acid	42	42	47	49
Threonine	19	26	22	21
Serine	29	26	40	27
Glutamic acid	78	87	80	80
Proline	118	115	135	114
Glycine	330	329	329	329
Alanine	129	104	108	103
Valine	14	16	12	20
Methionine	8.2	11	7	10
Isoleucine	6.1	7.8	11	12
Leucine	20	26	22	26
Tyrosine	2.0	2.2	2	2
Phenylalanine	14	15	14	15
Hydroxylysine	5.1	23	8	28
Lysine	30	13	26	15
Histadine	2.0	2.0	5	6
Arginine	51	50	50	46
Amide nitrogen	(39)	(50)		

[a] Amino acids are calculated as residues per 1000 amino acid residues.
[b] Miller (1971b,c).
[c] Strawich and Nimni (1971).

line hydroxylase, and protocollagen lysine hydroxylase, respectively (see reviews by Bornstein, 1974; Serafini-Fracessini and Smith, 1974). Both enzymes are oxygenases and require molecular oxygen, ferrous ions, α ketoglutarate, and a reducing agent.

Glycosylation occurs at the time of or immediately after hydroxylation. It involves the addition of galactose O-glycosidically linked to hydroxylysines. Glucose is subsequently added to the galactose so that disaccharide units are attached to the hydroxylysines. In order to add the monosaccharides they must first be activated to their UDP derivatives. The enzymes UDP-galactose:hydroxylysine-collagen galactosyltransferase and UDP-glucose:galactosylhydroxylysine-collagen glucosyltransferase have been shown to be present with high levels of activity in cartilage (Blumenkrantz and Prockop, 1970; Spiro and Spiro, 1971).

An additional aspect of cartilage metabolism that needs to be emphasized is its low oxygen consumption and heavy dependence on anaerobic glycolysis for energy (Kuwabara, 1932; Bywaters, 1936, 1937; Dickens and Weil-Malherbe, 1936; Hills, 1940; Laskin et al., 1952; Eeg-Larsen, 1956). This probably arises from the avascular nature of the tissue so that nutrients including oxygen must diffuse from the periphery of the cartilage through the matrix to the chondrocytes. Oxygen consumption for cartilage has been reported to range from 0.005 to 2.2 ml per gram dry weight per hour (see review by Delbrück, 1970). Growing and ossifying cartilage consumes more oxygen than resting cartilage (Whitehead and Weidmann, 1959). Anaerobic glycolysis is still the predominant source of energy in growing and epiphyseal cartilage. Glycolytic enzyme activities have been measured in epiphyseal and articular cartilage (Delbrück, 1970) and shown to change in response to cortisone treatment in vivo (Meyer and Kunin, 1969) or low oxygen tension in a cell culture system (Marcus and Srivastava, 1973). The respiratory chain enzymes and mitochondria are present in cartilage and are probably more active in epiphyseal plate chondrocytes at specific stages of their life cycle (Martin and Matthews, 1969; Fine and Person, 1970). The dependence of cartilage on glucose for anaerobic glycolysis serves to intensify the essential role of glucose in cartilage metabolism since it is utilized in the structure of the matrix proteins as well as for energy.

III. Effects of Hormones on Cartilage Growth and Metabolism

A. Growth Hormone

Cessation of growth following hypophysectomy and its restoration by treatment with growth hormone were studied extensively in the 1940s (see review by Simpson et al., 1950). Histological changes in epiphyseal cartilage following hypophysectomy are those of decreased activity and include a decrease in chondrocyte size, a marked diminution in the width of the epiphyseal cartilage growth plate and the development of a lamina of bone which seals the growth plate from the marrow. Growth hormone treatment of hypophysectomized animals causes the cartilage to become more cellular, the epiphyseal cartilage growth plate to increase in width in proportion to the dose of growth hormone given, and the sealing lamina of bone to be removed (Simpson et al., 1950). The ability of growth hormone to increase the size of the epiphyseal cartilage plates of hypophysectomized rats was specifically applied to the rat tibia and adapted as an in vivo bioassay for growth hormone activity (Greenspan et al., 1949; Geschwind and Li, 1955). This effect is not absolutely specific for growth hormone as thyroxine administration will cause a small increase in the tibial epiphyseal cartilage width of hypophysectomized rats (mean maximal increase 31 μm compared to growth hormone effects of 200 μm) (Marx *et al.*, 1944; Greenspan *et al.*, 1949). More recently, it has been shown that various derivatives of aniline, *N*-acetyl-*p*-aminophenol, and methyl thiocyanate can cause small increases in the tibial cartilage epiphyseal width in hypophysectomized rats, and this may lead to some confusion in assaying for growth hormone biological activity (Pena *et al.*, 1972).

After the demonstration that $^{35}SO_4$ is taken up by cartilage and incorporated into chondroitin sulfate (Dziewiatkowski *et al.*, 1949; Boström and Mansson, 1952), a number of investigators determined the effects of growth hormone on radiolabeled sulfate incorporation into cartilage *in vivo*. Ellis *et al.* (1953) administered $^{35}SO_4$ to normal, hypophysectomized, and growth hormone-treated hypophysectomized immature rats; sacrificed them 13, 19, and 25 hours later, and measured plasma and rib cartilage sulfate specific activity. Hypophysectomy reduced cartilage sulfate uptake to less than 11% that of normal rats. Growth hormone (25 μg daily for 3 days) increased the cartilage sulfate uptake to 33% of normal. Denko and Bergenstal (1955) found that $^{35}SO_4$ incorporation into costal cartilage *in vivo* was markedly reduced in young hypophysectomized rats and administration of 100 μg of growth hormone daily for 8 days increased $^{35}SO_4$ incorporation 3- to 4-fold. The sulfate incorporation in the treated hypophysectomized rats was higher than that in normal animals. Although hypophysectomy did not decrease $^{35}SO_4$ incorporation into tibial caps and xiphoid cartilage, growth hormone treatment of hypophysectomized rats increased $^{35}SO_4$ incorporation into these cartilages. Administration of growth hormone to normal rats did not increase $^{35}SO_4$ incorporation into costal, tibial, or xiphoid cartilage. Similar results were obtained by Murphy *et al.* (1956), who showed that *in vivo* $^{35}SO_4$ uptake by the proximal tibial epiphysis declined progressively for 20 days after hypophysectomy of young rats and then stabilized. Growth hormone treatment of hypophysectomized rats increased *in vivo* sulfate uptake of tibial and nasal cartilage. Administration of growth hormone (10–250 μg) to normal rats had no effect on cartilage $^{35}SO_4$ uptake *in vivo*.

Herbai (1971a,c), utilizing a method that measures the size of the total body sulfate pool and allows calculation of the cartilage sulfate uptake from measurement of $^{35}SO_4$ incorporation, has made a number of observations concerning *in vivo* cartilage sulfate uptake in normal, hypophysectomized, and dwarfed mice. Immature male mice (3–8 weeks of age) have significantly greater costal cartilage sulfate uptake than age-matched female mice. Older mice have very low costal cartilage sulfate uptake, and no sex difference is present. By 6–12 days after hypophysectomy, costal cartilage sulfate incorporation is reduced to 30 or 40% of normal. Starvation of normal mice for 24 hours similarly reduced costal cartilage sulfate incorporation. Sulfate incorporation of genetically dwarfed mice is 37% that of controls. Treatment of hypophysectomized mice with porcine and ovine growth hormone, but not bovine or human growth hormone, restored costal cartilage sulfate incorporation to normal and promoted significant weight gain. Ovine growth hormone treatment to normal mice had no effect on sulfate incorporation into cartilage. Hypophysectomy in mice reduced sulfate uptake in ear (13%), tracheal (37%), and xiphoid (24%) cartilage, as well as costal cartilage. However, growth hormone treatment, which restored costal cartilage sulfate incorporation to normal, had no effect on sulfate incorporation into ear, tracheal, or xiphoid cartilage. Growth hormone stimulation of costal cartilage sulfate uptake in hypophysectomized mice occurs only after a latent period of 8–17 hours. Measurement of radiosulfate incorporation in costal cartilage of hypophysectomized rats has been reported to be a better *in vivo* assay of growth hormone activity than the increase in tibial width (Collins *et al.*, 1961).

Histological studies of the effect of growth hormone treatment of animals on cartilage have been somewhat conflicting. Rigal (1964) administered growth hormone to normal rabbits, then removed explants from the proximal tibial epiphyses and incubated them *in vitro* with tritiated thymidine. Growth hormone treatment *in vivo* had no detectable effect on the cartilage either macroscopically or by conventional histological methods. In contrast, autoradiographs showed a marked change from controls. Whereas only 5% of the cells in the germinal zone of the epiphyseal cartilage of control animals took up thymidine, 25–50% of all the germinal zone cells took up tritiated thymidine in the growth hormone-treated animals. Kember (1971) studied the effects of growth hormone treatment on cell division in the growth cartilage of normal and hypophysectomized rats by autoradiographic studies with tritiated thymidine. In normal rats (up to 42 days of age) sacrificed 1 hour after injection of tritiated thymidine, 8–10% of the nuclei in the tibial epiphyses were labeled. After hypophysectomy the percentage of labeled nuclei fell, by 4 days, to 1.5–2.0%. Growth hormone treatment (100–1600 μg of bovine growth hormone) of the hypophysectomized rats restored the percentage of nuclei labeled but only after a delay of 8–16 hours. The percentage of labeled nuclei did not increase in normal rats treated with growth hormone. Yablon *et al.* (1974) treated dogs that had articular cartilage transplants with growth hormone (0.5 mg/kg per day for 3 weeks) and showed that [³H]proline incorporation as [³H]hydroxyproline, and ³⁵SO₄ incorporation into proteoglycans of the transplanted cartilages were 10-fold greater than those of transplanted cartilages in control (nontreated) animals.

The above *in vivo* data indicate that growth hormone exerts a key role in the regulation of cartilage metabolism. Attempts to demonstrate a direct effect of growth hormone on cartilage metabolism in an *in vitro* system have not been successful. *In vitro* incubation of costal cartilage from young, hypophysectomized rats with bovine growth hormone is not accompanied by a significant increase in $^{35}SO_4$ incorporation (Salmon and Daughaday, 1957), conversion of [U-^{14}C]proline to labeled hydroxyproline (Daughaday and Mariz, 1962), or increase in [^{3}H]methylthymidine incorporation into DNA (Daughaday and Reeder, 1966). Rigal (1964) was unable to show any effect of growth hormone *in vitro* in increasing tritiated thymidine uptake into rabbit chondrocyte nuclei. Studies with embryonic chicken cartilage incubated *in vitro* likewise have failed to show significant growth hormone stimulation of $^{35}SO_4$ incorporation into proteoglycan (Adamson and Anast, 1966; Hall, 1970; Beuttel et al., 1975), [^{3}H]leucine incorporation into cartilage proteins (Beuttel et al., 1975), [^{3}H]uridine incorporation into RNA (Beuttel et al., 1975), α-aminoisobutyrate transport (Drezner et al., 1975), or cyclic AMP (cAMP) generation (Drezner et al., 1975). Meier and Solursh (1972a) have reported that ovine growth hormone *in vitro* stimulates the incorporation of $^{35}SO_4$ by cultured chick embryo chondrocytes. Subsequent studies (Meier and Solursh, 1972b) indicated that bovine growth hormone would also stimulate, but rat and procine growth hormone inhibit, $^{35}SO_4$ incorporation while human growth hormone had no effect. The culture system used for these studies was a complicated one that included 10% fetal calf serum. Heat inactivation of the fetal calf serum abolished the effect of growth hormone in their system. More recently they have shown that ovine growth hormone stimulation of $^{35}SO_4$ incorporation is not accompanied by proteoglycan synthesis and does not occur if the medium amino acids (particularly valine) are increased (Meier and Solursh, 1973). The most probable explanation for their effect is that the ovine growth hormone alters some artifact of the *in vitro* tissue culture system. From the available data it is thus reasonable to conclude that growth hormone does not exert direct effects on cartilage metabolism. The effects observed *in vivo* are secondary, as described in the next section (III, B).

B. Somatomedins

Salmon and Daughaday (1957) were the first to describe the mechanism by which growth hormone regulates cartilage metabolism. They demonstrated that normal rat serum contains a nondialyzable component which stimulates $^{35}SO_4$ incorporation into cartilage chondroitin sulfate *in vitro*. This material is not present in serum of hypophysectomized rats but appears in the serum after treatment with growth hormone. The substance is not growth hormone, since growth hormone itself has no effects on cartilage metabolism *in vitro*. Salmon and Daughaday initially called this material sulfation factor. Subsequent studies have shown that the serum sulfation factor may be a family of growth hormone-dependent circulating peptides, mediates all the action of growth hormone on cartilage, exerts effects on many tissues other than cartilage, and has insulin-like activities. For these reasons the name sulfation factor was thought to be inappropriate and has been replaced by the term somatomedin (Daughaday *et al.*, 1972). Many comprehensive reviews concerning somatomedin are available (Daughaday, 1971; Daughaday and Garland, 1972; Grant, 1972; Hall and VanWyk, 1974; Hall and Luft, 1974).

The sites of sulfation factor production and the mechanisms by which it is generated by growth hormone are unknown. Salmon and Daughaday (1957) initially showed that high concentrations of insulin could mimic the effects of serum sulfation factor on cartilage (see Section III, C). This led Salmon (1960b) to explore the relationship between serum sulfation factor and insulin. He measured *in vivo* $^{35}SO_4$ incorporation into cartilage (costal, nasal, and xiphoid) of hypophysectomized and alloxan-diabetic hypophysectomized rats (blood glucose greater than 300 mg/dl) treated with saline or growth hormone. Sulfate incorporation was significantly reduced in alloxan-diabetic hypophysectomized and hypophysectomized rats. Growth hormone treatment markedly stimulated $^{35}SO_4$ incorporation into cartilage in both groups. The serum from alloxan-diabetic hypophysectomized rats had low or absent sulfation factor activity, which was restored to normal by growth hormone treatment. Salmon concluded from his studies that serum sulfation factor was not related to insulin or any product of insulin action or degradation. However, Yde (1969a,b) has claimed that serum sulfation factor activity in patients with diabetes mellitus is significantly reduced and the reduction is inversely related to the blood glucose level. The reasons for suppression of serum sulfation factor activity in the intact animal or man are many (see Section IV, C), and such data are not useful in determining the direct relationship between serum sulfation factor and insulin.

Since growth hormone stimulates nucleic acid and protein synthesis *in vitro* in muscle (Kostyo, 1968), liver (Jefferson and Korner, 1967), and adipose tissue (Goodman, 1963), these might be reasonable sites for somatomedin generation. Growth hormone generation of somatomedin probably requires protein synthesis since administration of cycloheximide before hypophysectomized rats were treated with growth hormone prevented the expected rise in serum somatomedin activity (Uthne and Uthne, 1972).

Hall and Bozovic (1969) extracted pieces of various tissues with Tyrode's medium and measured the ability of the extracts to stimulate $^{35}SO_4$ incorporation into embryonic chick cartilage in vitro. Brain, skeletal muscle, and heart muscle contained the greatest activity. Liver, spleen, and placenta contained significant but lesser quantities, and lung and kidney had no activity. The somatomedin assays were done in medium without amino acids and are of questionable validity since amino acids themselves stimulate $^{35}SO_4$ incorporation into cartilage in vitro (Salmon and Daughaday, 1957, 1958; Salmon, 1960a). Muscle extract did increase $^{35}SO_4$ uptake in medium containing amino acids. The muscle factor was not precipitated by 80% ethanol and on Sephadex G-25 chromatography it eluted with very low molecular weight substances (Hall et al., 1970). Growth hormone incubation with pieces of muscle increased extractable sulfation activity (Hall and Bozovic, 1969). Saline extracts of pituitary, liver, spleen, and kidney from normal rats did not stimulate in vitro $^{35}SO_4$ uptake by cartilage from hypophysectomized rats and removal of spleen, kidney, and intestine from normal rats did not result in a decrease of sulfation factor activity in serum (Daughaday, 1971). Salmon (1972), using a similar assay technique, found very small amounts of sulfation activity in pancreas, heart, kidney, and pituitary. Liver showed no activity and muscle was not tested. In totally eviscerated hypophysectomized rats, human growth hormone treatment did not induce any detectable somatomedin activity in serum (Hall and Luft, 1974).

Evidence that the liver is the site of somatomedin production has been presented in several studies. Perfusion of the in situ liver with Weymouth's medium containing bovine growth hormone (10 μg/ml) caused a significant increase in sulfation factor activity in the medium by the third recirculation (McConaghey and Sledge, 1970). Liver slices in vitro release somatomedin activity into the medium and the activity is greatly increased if bovine growth hormone (10 μg/ml) is added (McConaghey, 1972). Serum somatomedin levels in normal rats fall (75% decrease) 4–6 hours after partial hepatectomy and return to normal at the same rate as the liver regenerates to normal (Uthne and Uthne, 1972). Growth hormone treatment of hypophysectomized rats results in 40% less serum somatomedin activity if they had undergone partial hepatectomy (Uthne and Uthne, 1972). Similarly, Sledge (1973) showed that hypophysectomized-hepatectomized rats are unresponsive to growth hormone both in incorporation of [^{3}H]thymidine into their costal cartilage and in generation of serum somatomedin. Serum somatomedin levels are reduced in many patients with chronic liver disease in spite of their having normal or elevated plasma growth hormone levels (Wu *et al.*, 1974).

Somatomedin production by perfused kidneys and kidney slices from normal and hypophysectomized rats has been demonstrated (McConaghey and Dehnel, 1972). Bovine growth hormone (10 μg/ml) added to the medium perfusing normal and hypophysectomized rat kidneys stimulated the production of sulfation factor. Similarly, bovine growth hormone addition to kidney slices from normal rats caused the appearance of significant somatomedin activity in the medium. Medium from kidney slices from hypophysectomized rats unexpectedly contained very high basal levels of somatomedin, and this was not increased by addition of bovine growth hormone.

The studies reviewed do not give any unequivocal answers to the site of origin of serum somatomedin activity. Sulfation activity is measured in extracts from several tissues. Perfusion and incubation of slices of liver and kidney with growth hormone give rise to sulfation activity. The identity and characteristics of these various materials have not been determined. Further studies are necessary to clarify the significance of the various observations and which, if any, are related to the growth hormone-dependent serum somatomedins.

Little is known concerning the mechanism by which growth hormone causes the generation of serum sulfation factor activity. There is no evidence that this activity results from a chemical alteration in the growth hormone molecule itself or an active fragment released from the metabolism of growth hormone (Kostyo and Nutting, 1973; Nutting *et al.*, 1972; Mills *et al.*, 1973; Holladay *et al.*, 1975).

Two sets of observations suggest that growth hormone is not the only factor that can stimulate the generation of serum sulfation factor activity. Hypophysectomized rats infected with *Spirometra mansonoides* spargana grow rapidly for 4–6 weeks and then plateau (Mueller, 1963; Steelman *et al.*, 1970, 1971). When actively growing their serum contains a very potent growth factor (spargana growth factor), which is produced and secreted by the plerocercoid. This factor can stimulate growth in noninfected hypophysectomized rats. It is immunologically distinct from growth hormone, has characteristics that indicate that it is not serum sulfation factor, and does not have any *in vitro* effects on cartilage metabolism (Steelman *et al.*, 1971; Daughaday and Garland, 1972). It exerts its effects *in vivo* by generating serum sulfation factor activity (Garland *et al.*, 1971; Daughaday and Garland, 1972). The resistance to the spargana growth factor which develops appears to be the result of the development of neutralizing antibodies.

The second set of observations demonstrate that patients (with hypothalamic tumors or following resection of a craniopharyngioma) who have no measurable serum growth hormone (either random measurements or after provocative stimulatory tests) can have normal serum somatomedin levels with normal growth rates (Finkelstein et al., 1972; Kenny et al., 1973). What these other factors are that can stimulate somatomedin generation and the mechanisms by which they cause their effects remain questions for further investigations.

Many schemes have been proposed for the isolation and purification of somatomedins from serum (Liberti, 1970, 1973; VanWyk et al., 1969, 1971, 1972, 1973, 1974; Van den Brande et al., 1971; Hall, 1972; Uthne, 1973; Hall and Luft, 1974; Salmon and Duvall, 1970a,b). Somatomedin in plasma exists as a high molecular weight material that is retained on a Millipore filter with a pore size of 50,000 daltons (VanWyk et al., 1971, 1972) and elutes from Sephadex with a higher molecular weight than growth hormone (Daughaday and Kipnis, 1966; VanWyk et al., 1969, 1971, 1972; Bala et al., 1970). After acid–ethanol extraction, somatomedin has a much lower molecular weight (Van Wyk et al., 1969, 1971, 1972; Hall, 1972; Uthne, 1973). After acid–ethanol extractions from serum Cohn fraction IV, human somatomedin has been purified by gel filtration, ion exchange chromatography, electrofocusing, and high voltage electrophoresis (Uthne, 1973; VanWyk et al., 1973, 1974; Hall and Luft, 1974). Using these techniques, three somatomedins have so far been isolated: somatomedin A, a neutral peptide of about 7000 daltons which stimulates $^{35}SO_4$ incorporation into embryonic chick cartilage; somatomedin B, an acidic peptide of about 5000 daltons, which stimulates thymidine incorporation into glial cells in tissue culture; somatomedin C, a basic peptide which stimulates $^{35}SO_4$ and [^{3}H]thymidine incorporation into costal cartilage from hypophysectomized rats. Some preliminary data suggest that somatomedin C does not stimulate $^{35}SO_4$ incorporation into embryonic chick cartilage; that somatomedin A will not support growth in hypophysectomized rats, nor stimulate $^{35}SO_4$ and [^{3}H]thymidine incorporation in costal cartilage from hypophysectomized rats; that somatomedin B does not stimulate $^{35}SO_4$ incorporation into any cartilage (Van Wyk et al., 1973, 1974; Uthne, 1973). Radioreceptor assays, using placental membrane fractions, for human somatomedin A (Hall et al., 1974) and human somatomedin C (Marshall et al., 1974) and a radioimmunoassay for human somatomedin B (Yalow et al., 1975) have been described recently. Human somatomedin B is immunologically detected in human and monkey serum but not in nonprimate serum. Somatomedins A and C and NSILA-S do not cross react with the somatomedin B antibody. Somatomedin B levels are higher (19.3 $\pm$ 2.3 μg/ml) in acromegalic

than in hypopituitary patients (6.6 ± 0.5 μg/ml). Serum somatomedin
A and C levels are similarly reported to be higher in acromegalic than
in hypopituitary patients (Hall et al., 1974; Marshall et al., 1974). The
somatomedin C receptor assay does cross react with a number of other
hormones (bovine TSH, human menopausal gonadotropin, nerve growth
factor, epidermal growth factor, and glucagon). It is not known whether
somatomedins A and C displace each other from their respective placental
receptors. The difference in serum levels of the three somatomedins in
acromegalic patients as compared to hypopituitary patients has been used
as evidence that these these factors are growth hormone dependent.

Biological work with these three separate factors has not been sufficient
to characterize their specific effects on cartilage metabolism. It is not
possible to determine which of these factors, if any, is responsible for
the various biological effects of crude or partially purified serum sulfation
factors that have been reported previously. VanWyk et al. (1973, 1974)
have proposed that the definition of a somatomedin be changed and that
it include any substance that (1) is under growth hormone control (at
least partially), (2) is insulinlike in its action, and (3) stimulates cell
growth in one or more tissues. Whether this expanded definition, which
excludes specificity on the skeletal system and makes growth-hormone
dependence less rigorous, will serve to be more useful or more confusing
remains to be determined.

Most of the studies of the effect of serum sulfation factor on cartilage
metabolism in vitro have been conducted using serum containing sulfation
factor activity or a partially purified fraction of serum containing such
activity. For these studies the ultimate proof that the effect was due to
serum sulfation factor required the following criteria: (1) growth hormone itself had very little or no effect; (2) serum from hypophysectomized animals had little or no activity; (3) normal serum had activity;
(4) activity could be restored to the serum of hypophysectomized animals
if they were treated with growth hormone. These studies employed costal
cartilage (nasal and xiphoid cartilage were occasionally used) from hypophysectomized rats or cartilage from 10- to 13-day chick embryos.

Table IV summarizes the metabolic effects of serum sulfation factor
in vitro on hypophysectomized rat costal cartilage. Similar effects are
not obtained with costal cartilage removed from normal rats, but this
is attributed to the finding that cartilage binds serum sulfation factor
(Daughaday et al., 1968) and cartilage from normal rats still has significant sulfation factor bound to it. Incubation of cartilage from normal
animals for 24 hours reduces sulfate uptake to that observed in tissue
from hypophysectomized rats and causes the tissue to become responsive
to in vitro addition of sulfation factor (Yde, 1968). Costal cartilage from

TABLE IV

METABOLIC EFFECTS OF SERUM SULFATION FACTOR *in Vitro* ON COSTAL
CARTILAGE FROM HYPOPHYSECTOMIZED RATS

1. Increase incorporation of $^{35}SO_4$ into chondroitin sulfate (Salmon and Daughaday, 1957)
2. Increase L-[U-^{14}C]leucine incorporation into polysaccharide–protein complex (proteoglycan) (Salmon and Duvall, 1970a)
3. Increase conversion of [U-^{14}C]proline into free and collagen [^{14}C]hydroxyproline (Daughaday and Mariz, 1962)
4. Increase [^{3}H]uridine incorporation into RNA (Salmon and Duvall, 1970a)
5. Increase [^{3}H]thymidine incorporation into DNA (Daughaday and Reeder, 1966)

fetal rats or older rats (greater than 190 gm) is unresponsive to serum sulfation factor *in vitro* (Heins *et al.*, 1970). Amino acids in the incubation medium increase basal and sulfation factor-stimulated metabolic activity (Salmon and Daughaday, 1958; Salmon, 1960a). Sulfation of rat cartilage macromolecules is inhibited *in vitro* by puromycin or actinomycin D, and both inhibit serum sulfation factor stimulation of cartilage metabolic processes (Salmon *et al.*, 1967). Salmon has hypothesized that the earliest event in sulfation factor action on cartilage is an increase in protein synthesis (Salmon and Duvall, 1970a).

Studies with embryonic chick cartilage *in vitro* have yielded results quite similar to those with rat costal cartilage (Table V). Adamson has carried out a series of studies on the transport of metabolizable and nonmetabolizable amino acids in embryonic chick cartilage *in vitro*. She has shown that sulfate incorporation is dependent on the presence in the medium of Na$^+$ and K$^+$ and is inhibited by ouabain (Adamson *et al.*, 1964). Subsequently, she showed that embryonic chick cartilage *in vitro* actively transports amino acids and that transport is inhibited by ouabain, fluoride, N-ethylmaleamide, or incubation at 4°C and is stimulated by serum

TABLE V

METABOLIC EFFECTS OF SERUM SULFATION FACTOR *in Vitro* ON EMBRYONIC
CHICK CARTILAGE

1. Increase amino acid transport (both nonmetabolizable, such as α-aminoisobutyrate and cycloleucine, and metabolizable) (Adamson and Anast, 1966; Drezner *et al.*, 1975)
2. Increase cartilage cyclic AMP (Drezner *et al.*, 1975)
3. Increase $^{35}SO_4$ incorporation into chondroitin sulfate (Adamson and Anast, 1966; Hall, 1970; Delcher *et al.*, 1973)
4. Increase radiolabeled amino acid incorporation into proteins (Herington *et al.*, 1972; Eisenbarth *et al.*, 1973)
5. Increase incorporation of [^{3}H]uridine into RNA (Eisenbarth *et al.*, 1973)

sulfation factor (Adamson *et al.*, 1966a; Adamson and Anast, 1966). Active transport of sulfate, glucose, and 3-*O*-methylglucose could not be demonstrated. Puromycin added to the incubation medium blocked protein synthesis and amino acid transport (Adamson *et al.*, 1966b). Adamson interprets her studies to mean that the primary action of serum sulfation factor is to increase amino acid transport (Adamson, 1970; Herington *et al.*, 1972; Adamson *et al.*, 1972). Drezner *et al.* (1975) have shown that serum sulfation factor probably stimulates cartilage amino acid transport through a cAMP-dependent mechanism. They demonstrated that serum sulfation factor increases cartilage cAMP content as well as α-aminoisobutyrate transport and that the correlation between the two effects is striking (Fig. 3). Exogenous cAMP, butyrylated cAMP derivatives, and theophylline were shown to stimulate cartilage amino acid transport (Drezner *et al.*, 1975). It is unlikely that all the effects of serum sulfation factor on cartilage can be attributed to its effects on amino acid transport.

Serum sulfation factor and somatomedins cause effects on tissues other than cartilage (Table VI). The most prominent action of the partially purified somatomedins is insulinlike action on adipose tissue and skeletal

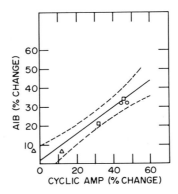

FIG. 3. Correlation between percentage of stimulation of cartilage α-aminoisobutyrate transport and percentage of increase in cartilage cyclic AMP (cAMP) in response to incubation in medium containing 5% serum from normal (○), hypophysectomized (△), and growth hormone-treated hypophysectomized (□) rats. In each experiment paired groups of cartilages [one for α-aminoisobutyrate (AIB) uptake and one for cAMP content] were incubated in medium with the appropriate serum added and compared to paired groups of control cartilages incubated in medium without any serum added. The data are expressed as the percentage of change from the mean values of the control cartilages. Each point is the mean of five observations of cAMP and α-aminoisobutyrate uptake in the paired cartilage groups. The dashed lines represent the 95% confidence limits of the calculated line. α-Aminoisobutyrate uptake and cAMP concentration are highly correlated ($r = 0.977$; $P < 0.001$). Reprinted from Drezner *et al.*, *Biochim. Biophys. Acta* **381**, 384 (1975).

TABLE VI

EFFECTS OF SERUM SULFATION FACTOR OR PARTIALLY PURIFIED SOMATOMEDINS ON
TISSUES OTHER THAN CARTILAGE

A. Serum fraction with sulfation factor activity
   1. Stimulates growth of HeLa cells in tissue culture (Salmon and Hosse, 1971)
   2. Increases [³H]leucine incorporation into muscle protein (Salmon and Duvall, 1970b)
B. Partially purified somatomedin
   1. Increases oxidation of [1-¹⁴C]glucose to ¹⁴CO₂ by rat epididymal adipose tissue and isolated fat cells *in vitro* (Hall and Uthne, 1971; VanWyk *et al.*, 1973, 1974)
   2. Inhibits *in vitro* glycerol release in epinephrine-stimulated rat epididymal fat pad segments (Underwood *et al.*, 1972)
   3. Increases α-aminoisobutyrate and 3-O-methylglucose transport in skeletal muscle (Hall and Uthne, 1972; Uthne *et al.*, 1974)
   4. Increases [³H]leucine incorporation into skeletal muscle protein (Hall and Uthne, 1972; Uthne *et al.*, 1974)
   5. Increases [³H]thymidine incorporation into human glialike cells in tissue culture (Uthne, 1973)
   6. Inhibits adenylate cyclase activity in crude membrane homogenates from fat cells, liver, and spleen lymphocytes of the rat and chondrocytes from chick embryonic cartilage (Tell *et al.*, 1973)

muscle. There is also promotion of growth of various cell lines in tissue culture. The effects of somatomedins on adipose tissue are identical to those reported for nonsuppressible insulinlike activity (NSILA). The *in vitro* actions on skeletal muscle are insulinlike (very rapid and not inhibited by puromycin or theophylline) rather than like those of growth hormone (Kostyo *et al.*, 1973). The inhibition of adenylate cyclase occurs with concentrations markedly in excess of those that circulate and is probably an artifact, especially since serum sulfation factor increases cartilage cAMP content.

The insulinlike activities of partially purified somatomedins suggested that they are related to insulin and may be the nonsuppressible insulinlike materials in the serum. Hintz *et al.* (1972) showed that somatomedin and insulin compete for insulin receptors of adipocytes, chondrocytes, and liver membranes. Somatomedin displaced labeled insulin as well as unlabeled insulin from the liver membranes and adipocytes. Their data were compatible with somatomedin and insulin competing for the same receptor. In contrast, somatomedin displaced labeled insulin very poorly from chondrocytes. Subsequent studies with receptors in human placental membranes indicate distinct insulin and somatomedin receptors. The insulin receptor interacts with insulin, somatomedin, and a number of other, as yet unidentified, molecules. The somatomedin receptor is more specific for somatomedin and reacts with insulin rather poorly (Marshall *et al.*, 1974).

Several important questions are raised by the biological data: (1) What is the relationship of serum sulfation factor to insulin, nonsuppressible insulinlike activity of serum, and other growth factors? (2) What are the metabolic effects of the different somatomedins and which control the various aspects of cartilage metabolism? (3) Do somatomedins mediate all the effects of growth hormone?

VanWyk *et al.* (1973, 1974) and Hall and Luft (1974) have reviewed the relationship between somatomedins and other growth factors such as insulin, NSILA, Temin's multiplication-stimulating activity, erythropoietin, epidermal growth factor, and nerve growth factor. All these hormones stimulate cell growth in their target tissues. Whether their formation is regulated by physiological alterations in growth hormone secretion is not known. The extent to which they all have insulinlike activity has still to be tested. The hypothesis that they and the somatomedins are growth hormone-dependent, insulinlike factors which control cell growth through similar mechanisms is intriguing and amenable to experimental validation. The specific effects of some of these factors on cartilage metabolism are discussed in subsequent sections.

The question of whether somatomedins mediate all the effects of growth hormone is a difficult one. Since liver, muscle, and adipose tissue incubated *in vitro* with growth hormone synthesize nucleic acids and proteins, it is possible that the primary effect of growth hormone is to generate somatomedin, which then exerts the biological effects. Those tissues that cannot generate somatomedin in response to growth hormone would be expected not to respond to growth hormone *in vitro*. Kostyo and Nutting (1973) showed that acute *in vivo* administration of growth hormone to hypophysectomized rats caused an increase in L-[^{14}C]leucine incorporation into skeletal muscle and liver proteins within 30 minutes, which was hours before serum insulin or thymidine factor increased. Although they concluded that the acute effects of growth hormone treatment could not be due to circulating insulin or somatomedin, they did not exclude somatomedin production in the tissues as the primary action. Somewhat more convincing evidence of independent actions of growth hormone is the demonstration that cyanogen bromide fragments A of human and porcine growth hormone stimulate amino acid transport and protein synthesis in liver and muscle of hypophysectomized rats both *in vivo* and *in vitro*, but fail to stimulate the production of serum sulfation factor or cause linear growth (Nutting *et al.*, 1972). These fragments did stimulate *in vitro* glucose oxidation by adipose tissue from hypophysectomized rats. This dissociation of effects on muscle and adipose tissue metabolism from cartilage metabolism does suggest that growth hormone might have direct metabolic effects. Comparison of growth hormone and somatomedin action on skeletal muscle *in vitro* is compatible with the concept that growth hormone acts by generating somatomedins. Growth hormone action occurs only after a latent period of 30 minutes, and its action is blocked by puromycin and theophylline. Somatomedin action occurs very rapidly and is not blocked by puromycin or theophylline (Kostyo *et al.*, 1973; Uthne *et al.*, 1974). Additional studies are necessary to resolve this question.

The methods of assay for serum somatomedin activity and the clinical relevance of these measurements are outside the scope of this review and may be found in several excellent published reviews (Hall and Luft, 1974; Hall and VanWyk, 1974; Grant, 1972; Daughaday, 1971).

C. Insulin

Since 1953 an increasing number of observations have been made which suggest that insulin could play a role in the growth and metabolism of developing cartilage and bone. Most of the studies required large pharmacological doses of insulin to demonstrate effects in unphysiological systems; it is difficult, therefore, to determine whether the effects reported are meaningful in terms of physiological regulation. The recent studies of the relationship of soluble NSILA of serum to serum somatomedins, reviewed in the previous section, lends more credence to the possibility that some of these effects of insulin may be physiologically meaningful.

The first series of observations to suggest that insulin might function as a growth hormone were made by Salter and Best (1953), who showed that the administration of increasing doses of protamine zinc insulin (to a maximum of 3 U/day for 15 days) to hypophysectomized rats on an unrestricted diet resulted in a 38-gm increase in body weight, a 2.5-gm increase in body protein, and a 65% increase in the width of the tibial epiphyseal growth plate. Histological examination of the tibial epiphyseal cartilage plates of the insulin-treated hypophysectomized rats showed them to be the same as those of normal rats, indicating that insulin had corrected the defect caused by hypophysectomy. The insulin treatment caused a marked increase in the rats' food consumption. The effects of insulin on nitrogen retention and cartilage growth were not as dramatic (50% as great) as those occurring with growth hormone treatment that caused an equivalent body weight gain. In subsequent studies the same investigators (Lawrence *et al.*, 1954) noted a linear relationship between the percentage of ingested nitrogen retained in body protein and the amount of insulin given the hypophysectomized rats. Wagner and Scow (1957) controlled the food intake of hypophysectomized rats by tube feeding and found that a food intake of 9–11 gm/day caused them to gain 32 gm in 22 days, and, though two-thirds of the weight gain was fat, there was a 2.7-gm gain in the protein content of the animals. Administration of 2–3 U of regular insulin per day (divided in equal doses and administered immediately after each meal) had no effect on body weight or composition of tube-fed hypophysectomized rats. Wagner and Scow concluded that insulin had no growth effect other than through increasing caloric consumption.

Electron microscopic studies of the effect of insulin treatment on the articular cartilage of dwarf mice have been conducted and compared with similar studies of the effect of growth hormone treatment (Silberberg et al., 1966). Mice were given either 0.003 U of insulin and intraperitoneal glucose or intraperitoneal glucose alone. Insulin treatment caused an increased prominence of the Golgi apparatus and of multivesicular bodies and a coarsening of mitochondria; enlargement of the cytoplasm with formation of many cytoplasmic footlets and increased endoplasmic reticulum; accelerated glycogen deposition in the chondrocytes of the midzone and deep layers. Treatment with glucose alone caused similar changes, but much less marked than those seen following insulin and glucose. However, there was a degree of dilatation of the Golgi vacuoles seen after glucose that was not seen after insulin. The action of insulin was not identical with that of growth hormone. Growth hormone caused proliferation of chondrocytes and it enhanced cell size far more than did insulin. Growth hormone more markedly stimulated the endoplasmic reticulum and the appearance of free ribosomes than did insulin. The effects of the two hormones on the Golgi structures, the mitochondria, and glycogen deposition were similar. The data available do not allow us to determine whether the histological differences reflect differences in quantitative or qualitative action of the two hormones.

A number of in vitro studies have shown direct effects of insulin on cartilage metabolism. Salmon and Daughaday (1957) observed that insulin (0.1–1.0 U/ml) stimulated radiolabeled sulfate incorporation into costal cartilage pieces from hypophysectomized rats (62% increase at 1.0 U/ml) or normal fasted rats in vitro. It is of particular interest that insulin stimulated $^{35}SO_4$ incorporation into cartilage pieces occurred in medium which contained no glucose or amino acids. Addition of amino acids to the medium increased insulin-mediated $^{35}SO_4$ incorporation, but glucose addition had no effect (Salmon, 1960a). An unexplained observation is that insulin did not stimulate $^{35}SO_4$ incorporation into cartilage incubated in medium containing amino acids, except for valine, when it did so in cartilages incubated in medium containing no amino acids (Salmon, 1960a). Insulin stimulated $^{35}SO_4$ incorporation into nonossifying cartilage like nasal and xiphoid, as well as costal cartilage. Later studies by Salmon *et al.* (1968) extended the original observations by demonstrating that 0.1 U of insulin per milliliter stimulated $^{35}SO_4$ and [^3H]leucine incorporation *in vitro* into the protein–polysaccharide complexes of cartilage, as well as [^3H]uridine into cartilage RNA and [^3H]thymidine into cartilage DNA. Both inhibition of RNA synthesis by actinomycin D and of protein synthesis by puromycin blocked the incorporation of $^{35}SO_4$ and [^3H]leucine into cartilage protein polysaccharides in the presence or absence of insulin. The conclusions drawn from the experiments measuring the *in vitro* effects of insulin on costal cartilage pieces from hypophysectomized rats were that pharmacological doses of insulin could simulate the effects of serum sulfation factor on cartilage, and that is was unlikely that physiological concentrations of insulin affected cartilage metabolism *in vivo*.

Further studies of the *in vitro* actions of insulin on cartilage have been conducted utilizing pelvic leaflets from 10–12-day chick embryos. Hall and Uthne (1971), employing insulin concentrations from 62.5 to 4000 μU/ml, showed a slight, and not always significant, stimulation of the uptake of radiolabeled sulfate. However, recent studies from our laboratory have shown that insulin, 200–10,000 μU/ml, consistently and significantly stimulates cartilage proteoglycan, general protein, RNA and DNA synthesis (Beuttel *et al.*, 1975). Additionally, insulin stimulates glucose and amino acid transport and glucose oxidation by embryonic chick cartilage *in vitro*.

Several effects of insulin on bone and cartilage growth *in vitro* have been proposed, but the experimental designs and lack of consistent results make them difficult to interpret. Prasad and Rajan (1970) claimed that insulin facilitates the repair of cultured bone. In their *in vitro* culture system, which employs tibia from 14-day chick embryos, insulin has no effect on bone length, hexosamine or collagen content. However, in bone damaged by fracture or proteolytic digestion, insulin (0.01 U/ml) significantly increased bone repair as measured by bone length and weight, and bone hexosamine content. An effect of insulin (0.001 U/ml) but not of growth hormone in stimulating collagen synthesis by newborn rat bone *in vitro* has been reported (Wettenhall *et al.*, 1969; Schwartz *et al.*, 1970). The effect has been demonstrated in a steady-state culture system, but only after 42 hours of incubation. In contrast, Perlish *et al.* (1973) found a slight increase in collagen synthesis by 10-day embryonic chick tibia incubated *in vitro* with 154 μg of insulin per milliliter for 2–4 hours. More prolonged incubation failed to show any effect of insulin on collagen synthesis.

Insulin action on isolated bone cells *in vitro* has been demonstrated, and similar actions probably occur with chondrocytes. Peck and Messinger (1970) showed that insulin (4.6–460 ng/ml) stimulates uridine uptake or phosphorylation by isolated fetal rat bone cells in culture. This effect results in increased radioactivity in uridine nucleotide pools with a consequent increase in radioactive uridine incorporated into RNA. A similar effect of insulin on cytidine, but not adenosine or guanosine, suggests that insulin regulates pyrimidine, but not purine, ribonucleoside incorporation into isolated bone cells. The effect of insulin can be mimicked by dithiothreitol (Peck et al., 1971). Insulin stimulation of α-aminoisobutyrate and L-proline transport in fetal rat calvaria in vitro has been shown by Hahn et al. (1969, 1972). The transport is time dependent, can be blocked by inhibitors of protein synthesis, and involves an increase in V_{max} with no change in K_m. Insulin stimulation of amino acid transport is sodium dependent. In preliminary studies in our laboratory, insulin stimulates α-aminoisobutyrate transport and either uridine transport or phosphorylation in embryonic chick cartilage in vitro (Beuttel et al., 1975).

Very large pharmacological doses of insulin administered either in vitro or in vivo to very young chick embryos are teratogenic and cause cartilage necrosis, calcification, and decreased sulfation of matrix proteins in the regions of necrosis (Rabinovitch and Gibson, 1972; Hickey and Klein, 1971). It is very unlikely that these studies have any physiological meaning.

Whether insulin has any physiological effect on the regulation of cartilage metabolism and growth is still an unanswered question. Most of the studies that have been reviewed suggest that it does not. A few, such as our own in vitro studies and the in vivo studies of Salter and Best, suggest that it might. More data on the nature of the effect of NSILA-S on cartilage metabolism and the relationship between receptors for NSILA-S and insulin would be helpful in resolving the question. Laron et al. (1972) recently reviewed the clinical evidence which suggests that insulin, indeed, may be a growth-promoting hormone. The data are circumstantial and by no means conclusive, but they call attention to certain clinical situations in which normal growth occurs in the absence of growth hormone secretion but in the presence of normal, or exaggerated, insulin secretion.

D. Nonsuppressible Insulinlike Activity

Serum from normal individuals or animals contains substances that cause insulinlike effects in vitro on adipose tissue and diaphragm muscle (see review by Oelz et al., 1972). Some of the insulinlike activity of serum can be blocked by the addition of excess guinea pig anti-insulin serum.

This component is termed suppressible insulinlike activity, comprises 7% of the total insulinlike activity in serum from normal fasting individuals, and is probably identical to immunoreactive insulin (Froesch et al., 1963; Oelz et al., 1972). The remaining 93% of insulinlike activity in the serum of normal fasted individuals is not altered by guinea pig anti-insulin serum and is called nonsuppressible insulinlike activity (NSILA). NSILA levels in normal subjects (determined by in vitro adipose tissue assays) range between 100 and 200 μU per milliliter of serum (Froesch et al., 1963). Human serum NSILA does not increase after glucose administration and is not altered in juvenile diabetes mellitus, adult-onset diabetes mellitus, or organic hyperinsulinism. The only consistent change observed in NSILA levels is an increase noted after prolonged fasting in obese individuals (see review by Oelz et al., 1972). The relationship of NSILA to the pancreas and insulin is not resolved. Some reports indicate that pancreatectomy has no effect on serum NSILA (Leonards et al., 1962; Steinke et al., 1962; Schoeffling et al., 1965; Froesch et al., 1967; Kajinuma et al., 1969; Ide et al., 1969), whereas others indicate that it causes a total disappearance of activity in the plasma (Slater et al., 1961; Samaan et al., 1963; Gjedde, 1964, 1968). Administration of alloxan to rats, as well as prolonged fasting and pancreatectomy, have been reported to result in the disappearance of NSILA activity from their plasma (Foresch, 1963; Antoniades, 1969; Samaan et al., 1965; Rasio et al., 1965).

Isolation and purification studies have identified two separate and non-interchangeable forms of NSILA in human serum (Jakob et al., 1968). NSILA-S, a small molecule (7500 daltons), is soluble in acid–ethanol, is heat stable, and comprises 10–20% of the total NSILA activity of serum. NSILA-P, a large molecule (about 100,000–150,000 daltons), is insoluble in acid–ethanol, is heat labile, and comprises 80–90% of the total serum NSILA activity.

NSILA-S has been extensively purified (activity 450 mU per milligram of protein), and the amino acid composition reported (Table VII) shows no similarity to that of insulin or proinsulin (Labhart et al., 1972). Reduction of the disulfide bridges and aminoethylation does not alter the molecular weight, indicating that it is a single chain. Reduction and alkylation abolish biological activity. The effects of NSILA-S on in vitro carbohydrate and lipid metabolism of adipose tissue and diaphragm muscle are similar to insulin both qualitatively and quantitatively (see reviews by Oelz et al., 1972; Renner et al., 1973). NSILA-S is more resistant to degradation by the isolated perfused rat liver than is insulin (Solomon et al., 1967; Oelz et al., 1970). Partially purified NSILA-S administered in vivo to normal or diabetic animals causes the same quali-

602   HAROLD E. LEBOVITZ AND GEORGE S. EISENBARTH

TABLE VII
AMINO ACID COMPOSITION OF PURIFIED NSILA-S AFTER REDUCTION
AND AMINOETHYLATION[a]

Amino acid residue	Moles/mole	Nearest integer
Lys	3.4	3–4
AE-Cys	7.0	7
His	0	0
Arg	6.6	6–7
Asp	5.2	5
Thr	2.8	3
Ser	4.0	4
Glu	6.0	6
Pro	5.5	5–6
Gy	7.3	7
Ala	6.0	6
Val	2.9	3
Met	0.9	1
Ile	0.8	1
Leu	6.0	6
Tyr	2.0	2
Phe	4.0	4

[a] Labhart et al. (1972).

tative effects as insulin, but they are more prolonged, probably because of its resistance to destruction (Oelz et al., 1972). NSILA-P in vitro influences all indices of adipose tissue metabolism, save glycogen synthesis, in a similar manner to insulin (Oelz et al., 1972). Administration of NSILA-P intraperitoneally to rats increases glycogen formation in diaphragm muscle. It is unlikely that serum NSILA is ordinarily involved in the regulation of glucose homeostasis in vivo. The serum concentrations do not change in patients suffering from hyperinsulinism or diabetic ketosis. Pancreatectomized dogs develop ketoacidosis and die although the levels of NSILA remain unchanged (Froesch et al., 1967). Acute diabetes induced by injection of anti-insulin serum does not reduce NSILA levels (Oelz et al., 1972). Thus, circulating NSILA appears to be inactive. This is in contrast to its marked in vitro and in vivo effects after extraction and purification.

Recently a radioreceptor assay has been developed for NSILA-S (Megyesi et al., 1974). In five normal adults, plasma NSILA-S was 1200–2200 ng/ml. Elevated plasma NSILA-S (2400–16,000 ng/ml) was found in five of seven patients with hypoglycemia associated with extrapancreatic tumors. A few patients with acromegaly and insulin-producing tumors had NSILA-S levels in the same range as the normals. Two of three patients with pituitary insufficiency had low plasma NSILA-S levels. The authors estimated that by their radioreceptor assay, normal individuals have about 100 μU of insulinlike activity due to NSILA-per milliliter of plasma. They speculated that the failure of this concentration of NSILA-S to produce hypoglycemia in normals or prevent ketoacidosis in diabetics may be due to most of the plasma NSILA-S being bound to a large molecule which keeps it inactive.

Since partially purified preparations of sulfation factor had been shown to have nonsuppressible insulinlike activity (see Section III, B), the effects of NSILA-S on fibroblasts and cartilage *in vitro* were studied. Morell and Froesch (1973a,b) compared the effects of insulin and NSILA-S on fibroblasts in tissue culture. Both agents stimulated growth (but not nearly as well as 5% fetal calf serum), [³H]thymidine incorporation into DNA, and glucose consumption and lactate production. NSILA-S was about 1000 times more potent than insulin per microunit of insulinlike activity on adipose tissue and about 20 times more potent on a molar basis. Zingg and Froesch (1973) tested the effect of three partially purified NSILA-S preparations (0.8 mU/mg, 17 mU/mg, 61 mU/mg) on sulfate incorporation *in vitro* into costal cartilage from 3-day starved rats and showed that all three increased $^{35}SO_4$ incorporation in the dose range from 0.1 to 10 μU of NSILA activity per milliliter of medium. Comparable stimulation with insulin occurred from 1 to 10 mU/ml. The slope of the dose-response curve and the maximal stimulation of $^{35}SO_4$ incorporation was greater with serum than with NSILA-S or insulin, suggesting that NSILA-S is not the only substance in serum that stimulates sulfate incorporation into cartilage. They were also able to demonstrate stimulation of $^{35}SO_4$ incorporation into embryonic chick cartilage *in vitro* with 5 μU of NSILA-S or 100 mU of insulin per milliliter.

The relationship of NSILA-S to the various somatomedins is unclear. Zingg and Froesch (1973) estimated that 1 sulfation unit of NSILA-S is equivalent to 10–20 μU of NSILA-S. Hall and Uthne (1972) calculated 1 sulfation unit of their somatomedin preparation to be 200 μU of NSILA. Froesch (1974) has chromatographed serum from normal subjects and patients with pituitary dwarfism and acromegaly and bioassayed it for NSILA-S and sulfation activity. Serum from hypopituitary dwarfs had less, and serum from acromegalic patients more, NSILA-S and sulfation activity than serum from normals. NSILA-S and sulfation activity were frequently comparable in the same serum pool but not always, so that the correlation between activities was statistically significant but not extremely impressive. Hall and Luft (1974), in a review, state that their preliminary amino acid analysis of somatomedin A differs from that reported for NSILA-S (Table VII). NSILA-S is immunologically quite distinct from somatomedin B (Yalow *et al.*, 1975). Similarities of somatomedin C and NSILA-S exist, and future studies will determine whether they are the same or different substances.

E. MULTIPLICATION-STIMULATING ACTIVITY

The multiplication of chicken embryo fibroblasts under standard cell culture conditions is completely dependent on the amount of serum in the medium (Temin, 1966). High concentrations of insulin partially substitute for serum in promoting DNA synthesis and cell replication in cultures of chicken embryo fibroblasts (Temin, 1967). On the basis of that information, Pierson and Temin (1972) hypothesized that the factor or factors in serum responsible for stimulating cell multiplication might be one of the various insulinlike activities present in serum. Utilizing isolation and purification techniques devised for obtaining the insulinlike factors from serum, they were able to purify 6000-fold from calf serum an activity that stimulated DNA synthesis and cell multiplication. They called this partially purified material multiplication-stimulating activity (MSA). It is heat stable and treatment with chymotrypsin, periodate, or dithiothreitol, but not with DNase or RNase, inactivates it. MSA has an approximate molecular weight of 4000–5000 daltons. It has nonsuppressible insulinlike activity on rat epididymal fat pad cells *in vitro* (5 mU per milligram of protein).

A line of buffalo rat liver cells cloned by Coon can multiply in cell culture in the absence of serum. On the assumption that the rat liver cells might be independent of MSA, because they produced it, Dulak and Temin (1973a) assayed serum-free medium conditioned by the growth of Coon's buffalo rat liver cells (CRL) and found that it contained as much or more MSA than calf serum. Purification of CRL MSA was accomplished, and its biological activities were tested. A preparation that had 35,000 U of MSA activity per milligram of protein had 200 μU of NSILA activity per milligram on rat epididymal fat pad and 5000 U of sulfation factor activity per milligram on costal cartilage from hypophysectomized rats (Temin *et al.*, 1974). Additionally, it competed with labeled insulin for binding to receptors of rat liver cell membranes. The CRL MSA differs from MSA in calf serum in that it stimulates only half as many cultured chick embryo fibroblasts to incorporate [^{3}H]thymidine into DNA, and its kinetics of activity are also different (Temin *et al.*, 1974). The preparation of CRL MSA can be separated into at least four rapidly migrating polypeptides by polyacrylamide gel electrophoresis in sodium dodecyl sulfate (Dulak and Temin, 1973b).

Temin's MSA appears to be another family of peptides that stimulate cell growth, have NSILA activity, and stimulate sulfate uptake in cartilage. Whether these factors are the same or uniquely different from the previously recognized somatomedins and NSILA-S remains to be determined.

F. THYROID HORMONES

Thyroid hormone insufficiency in man and other mammals leads to impaired linear growth and delayed ossification of the skeleton (Wilkins, 1957; Simpson et al., 1950). Thyroid hormone excess causes accelerated ossification of the skeleton and in some instances can result in short-term increases in linear growth rates (Schlesinger and Fisher, 1951; Farrehi, 1968). These observations indicate that thyroid hormone in vivo has at least two major actions on epiphyseal cartilage: growth and maturation.

The role of thyroid hormones in cartilage growth and osseous maturation and its relationship to growth hormone have been extensively studied in the rat (Simpson et al., 1950; Ray et al., 1954; Riekstniece and Asling, 1966; Asling et al., 1968). Hypophysectomy of immature rats (6–28 days of age) results in a cessation of linear growth when the rats reach 30 days of age. Osseous maturation, as determined by X-ray identification of epiphyseal ossification centers and closure of epiphyseal cartilage plates, continues to a maturational age 18–21 days in excess of the chronological age at the time of hypophysectomy and then ceases. Histological examination shows narrowing of the width of the epiphyseal cartilage plates and sealing of the growth plates from marrow by a lamina of bone. Thyroidectomy of rats at 1 day of age causes a marked decrease in subsequent linear growth and failure to increase bone age beyond 20–24 days, even if the animals live to 140 days. Histological studies show that the epiphyseal cartilage plate width is not different from that of normal animals of comparable age. Some minimal proliferation of chondrocytes and erosion of the cartilage plate adjacent to the marrow continue.

Treatment of hypophysectomized, thyroidectomized, and thyroidectomized-hypophysectomized immature rats with growth hormone, thyroxine, or a combination of both, provide significant insight into the effects of these hormones on cartilage metabolism (Simpson et al., 1950; Ray et al., 1950, 1954; Asling et al., 1949; Scow et al., 1949). Table VIII summarizes the salient points from such studies. Growth hormone stimulates chondrocyte proliferation and matrix production, but has no effect on the maturation process that causes cartilage to be replaced by bone. Although growth hormone can stimulate cartilage growth in thyroidec-

TABLE VIII

EFFECTS OF GROWTH HORMONE AND THYROXINE ON OSSEOUS MATURATION IN NORMAL, HYPOPHYSECTOMIZED (HYPX), THYROIDECTOMIZED (THX), AND THYROIDECTOMIZED-HYPOPHYSECTOMIZED (THX-HYPX) RATS

Rats	Growth hormone	Thyroxine	Growth hormone + thyroxine
Normal	1. Increases linear growth; causes gigantism 2. No effect on osseous maturation	1. No effect on linear growth 2. Increases osseous maturation. Causes premature skeletal aging	— —
Hypx	1. Restores linear growth 2. Causes dose-related increase in epiphyseal cartilage width 3. Resorbs bone lamina sealing cartilage plate 4. No effect on osseous maturation 5. Prolonged treatment results in gigantism	1. Barely detectable increase in linear growth 2. Reduces width of epiphyseal cartilage 3. Resorbs bone lamina sealing cartilage plate; causes cartilage plate erosion 4. Restores osseous maturation to normal	1. Normal or increased growth rate — — 4. Normal or increased osseous maturation rate
Thx	1. Restores linear growth but requires 25 × dose for Hypx rats 2. No effect on osseous maturation	1. Restores linear growth to normal 2. Restores osseous maturation to normal	— —
Thx-Hypx	1. Significant increase in body length 2. Increases tibial length 3. No effect on osseous maturation	1. Significant increase in body length 2. Increases tibial length 3. Osseous maturation normal or increased	1. Normal or increased growth rate 2. Marked increase in tibial length 3. Normal or increased osseous maturation rate

tomized rats, it cannot cause gigantism as it does in hypophysectomized rats. Riekstniece and Asling (1966) and Asling *et al.*, (1968) have shown that thyroxine augments growth hormone effects on chondrogenesis in epiphyseal cartilage plates and they have postulated that tiny amounts of thyroxine are necessary to augment full growth hormone action on cartilage. Thyroxine can cause some increase in bone length and body length in the absence of growth hormone. This was disputed by Goodall and Gavin (1966). However, more recent studies by Thorngren and Hansson (1973) using tetracycline labeling have confirmed that thyroxine does indeed increase longitudinal bone growth in hypophysectomized rats. The most dramatic effects of thyroxine are on osseous maturation. It causes the appearance and enlargement of ossification centers, and in the epiphyseal plate it causes calcification and erosion of the cartilage plate adjacent to the marrow, chondrogenesis in the proliferative zone, and enlargement of the chondrocytes near the diaphysis. Thus, thyroxine causes proliferative changes in chrondrocytes and destruction of the ends of the epiphyseal plates with replacement by endochondral bone.

The failure of thyroidectomized animals to grow is due as much to a deficiency of growth hormone secretion from the anterior pituitary as to lack of thyroid hormone action on cartilage. Anterior pituitaries of thyroidectomized rats contain significantly fewer acidiophiles than those of normal controls of the same chronological age. Treatment with growth hormone further depresses the number of acidiophiles, and thyroxine treatment restores the number and size of pituitary acidiophiles to normal (Koneff *et al.*, 1949; Evans *et al.*, 1964). Growth hormone content of anterior pituitary glands from hypothyroid animals is markedly reduced and is restored to normal by thyroxine treatment (Contopoulos *et al.*, 1958; Solomon and Green, 1959; Schooley *et al.*, 1966; Peake *et al.*, 1973). Growth hormone synthesis and secretion may be so reduced in hypothyroid humans that their circulating plasma growth hormones are unmeasurable, and they may show no rise in response to stimuli (insulin-induced hypoglycemia or intravenous arginine) (Sheikholislam *et al.*, 1966; Katz *et al.*, 1969).

Effects of thyroid hormone on cartilage proteoglycan have been suggested by a number of *in vivo* studies, but the data are somewhat confusing. Dziewiatkowski (1951) administered $^{35}SO_4$ to suckling rats that had been treated with thiouracil, thyroxine, or a combination of both. He found that thiouracil treatment reduced $^{35}SO_4$ uptake in both the blood and knee articular cartilage. Concurrent treatment with thyroxine abolished the effects of thiourea, but thyroxine treatment alone had no effect or depressed $^{35}SO_4$ uptake by articular cartilage. Thiourea treatment decreased and thyroxine treatment increased the rate of degradation of previously radiolabeled articular cartilage chondroitin sulfate. Confirmation that hypothyroidism depresses $^{35}SO_4$ incorporation into cartilage chondroitin sulfate was obtained in studies with epiphyseal cartilage from rats made hypothyroid by thyroidectomy (at 28 days of age) or ^{131}I ablation of the thyroid gland (at birth) (Dziewiatkowski, 1957, 1964). The depressed specific activity of chondroitin sulfate $^{35}SO_4$ was even more impressive since the specific activity of $^{35}SO_4$ in the serum of the hypothyroid animals was greater than in the control or thyroxine-replaced animals. Thyroxine replacement for 14 days increased $^{35}SO_4$ incorporation into cartilage chondroitin sulfate almost to normal. Murphy et al. (1956) found that L-thyroxine, 5 μg/day for 3 days, increased in vivo $^{35}SO_4$ incorporation into the proximal tibial epiphysis of hypophysectomized immature rats Herbai (1971a) measured the body total sulfate pool and costal cartilage sulfate uptake in growing mice given L-thyroxine (0.01–10 μg per mouse). Thyroxine increased the total sulfate pool about 30–70%, and low doses of thyroxine (0.01–1.0 μg) inhibited costal cartilage sulfate uptake 30–40%, while the high dose (10 μg) increased it 23%. Radio-iodine-induced hypothyroidism in rats changes the distribution of acidic glycosaminoglycans in tracheal cartilage with a decrease in dermatan sulfate, an increase in hyaluronic acid and no change in heparin sulfate chondroitin 4-sulfate, or chondroitin 6-sulfate (Kofoed et al., 1969). Replacement with L-thyroxine restores the distribution to normal. It is difficult from the reported studies to get a clear understanding of what specific effects thyroid hormones play in vivo in regulating cartilage proteoglycan metabolism. The difficulty is 2-fold: thyroid hormone promotes both the formation and destruction of cartilage and sulfate incorporation, at any particular instant, will depend on the balance of these actions; and, thyroid hormone may affect qualitative as well as quantitative changes in proteoglycans.

In addition to their effects on cartilage growth and maturation in immature animals, thyroid hormones are thought to be significant in embryonic chondrogenesis. Treatment of embryonic chickens from 8 days to 18 days with sufficient thiourea to cause hypothyroidism results in a 62% retardation in weight and a 24% reduction in length of the tibia (at 18 days) compared to control embryos (Hall, 1973). While total embryo weight is also depressed, the depression of tibial growth is more marked and occurs with a shorter duration of treatment. The decreased tibial growth is attributable to decreased rate of maturation of chondroblasts into chondrocytes, reduction of chondrocyte hypertrophy and defective deposition of matrix proteoglycans. The tibial articular cartilages in treated animals were eroded and fragile, indicating a dependence of articular cartilage on thyroid hormones for normal development and maintenance of integrity. In this series of experiments, thyroxine (100 pg to 1 μg) also impaired the growth of the tibia. Hall interprets his data as showing that thyroxine has a physiological role in chondrocyte maturation and matrix production during normal development. The failure to attempt to reverse the effects of thiourea with thyroxine, and indeed the suppressive effects of thyroxine itself on tibial growth, fail to support his thesis.

Pawelek (1969) measured the effects of thyroxine and low oxygen tension on embryonic chick sternal chondrocytes in cell culture and made the following observations: thyroxine (10^{-6} M) markedly stimulated chondrogenic expression as assessed by both morphology and chondroitin sulfate synthesis in monolayers and clones of the cultured cells. Low oxygen tension, in the presence of thyroxine, stimulated monolayers to increase chondroitin sulfate synthesis even more. In the absence of thyroxine, low oxygen tension had no effects on chondroitin sulfate synthesis. The data imply that thyroxine and low oxygen tension promote chondrogenesis. Marcus (1973) in studies with cultured articular chondrocytes from 6- to 8-week rabbits found that thyroxine (3×10^{-7} M) had no effect on cell growth or radiosulfate incorporation, and low oxygen tension inhibited radiosulfate incorporation. He concluded that neither is important in controlling chondrogenesis, but his studies were not conducted with fetal tissue or epiphyseal cartilage. Nevo et $al.$ (1972) confirmed the chondrogenic effects of low oxygen tension but not thyroxine. Other evidence suggestive of a role of thyroxine in promoting chondrogenesis is that derived from experiments which indicate that thyroxine (0.01 μM) blocks the hyaluronate inhibition of chondrogenesis in stationary cultures of trypsinized 5-day chick embryo somites (Toole, 1973). As is obvious, the nature and significance of thyroid hormone action in promoting chondrogenesis is not well defined, but this is true of most control mechanisms for cartilage differentiation. These are discussed in some detail in a recent review by Levitt and Dorfman (1974).

The few studies of the effect of thyroid hormones on cartilage metabolism in $vitro$ that have been carried out have failed to define the mechanisms by which thyroid hormones influence cartilage growth and maturation. Salmon and Daughaday (1957) were unable to show any in $vitro$ effect of L-thyroxine or L-triiodotyronine on the incorporation of radiolabeled sulfate in costal cartilage from immature hypophysectomized rats. Adamson, in a series of studies, failed to demonstrate any effects of triiodothyronine or thyroxine on the synthesis of macromolecules in embryonic chick cartilage in $vitro$. However, she did find that triiodothyronine and thyroxine increase the transport of some neutral amino acids (tryosine, phenylalanine, tryptophan, cycloleucine histidine, leucine, and methionine), decrease the transport of others (glycine, valine, and isoleucine), and have no effect on the transport of acidic or basic amino acids (Adamson and Ingbar, 1967a,b,c). She concluded that thyroid hormones interact specifically with the L transport site, causing changes in the affinities of affected amino acids for that site. The effect of thyroid hormones was thought not to be mediated by cAMP (Adamson, 1970). Utilizing the *in vitro* incorporation of [^{14}C]hydroxyproline in ulnas from 16-day mouse embryos, Halme *et al.* (1972) showed that triiodothyronine inhibits the synthesis of cartilage collagen and promotes its degradation. Blumenkrantz and Prockop (1970) showed that thyroid hormones decrease the proportion of glycosylgalactosylhydroxylysine to galactosylhydroxylysine in collagen in embryonic chick cartilage incubated *in vitro*, suggesting that thyroid hormones may alter cartilage collagen structure in addition to altering its rate of synthesis or degradation.

It seems reasonable to conclude that the studies which have been conducted fail to provide an understanding of how thyroid hormones affect cartilage growth and maturation.

G. ESTROGENS

Estrogen effects on cartilage were initially recognized in the 1930s. Zondek (1936) observed that natural estrogen (5000 MU) administered parenterally twice a week to 30–50-gm rats (4–6 weeks old) for 3–4 months, inhibited weight gain 45% and body length 13% as compared to control animals. Similar impairment of weight gain and body length were noted when White Leghorn chickens were treated with estrogen for 16 weeks. Histological examination of the chicken bones showed that the bones were small and shortened, the medullary cavity was filled with loose osseous tissue, and the epiphyseal centers showed delayed closure. Estrogen effects on chicken growth were shown to persist even after hormone administration was discontinued, but the changes were reversed if the chickens were subsequently treated with pituitary extract containing growth hormone activity. These observations led Zondek to propose that estrogens exert their effects on the skeletal system by blocking the release of growth hormone from the anterior pituitary gland. Noble (1938) confirmed that estrogens inhibit growth in rats, but he made two additional observations which suggested to him that estrogens inhibited growth by a direct action on cartilage: stilbestrol (a synthetic estrogen) inhibited growth in very young rats whose growth is maintained even in the absence of growth hormone; and stilbestrol partially blocked the growth of growth hormone-treated hypophysectomized rats. Gaarenstroom and

Levie (1939) showed that stilbestrol inhibited growth in mature rats and administration of growth hormone containing extracts could not reverse the effects. In contrast, Richards and Kueter (1941) reported that the effects of stilbestrol in inhibiting growth in young rats could be reversed by treatment of the animals with growth hormone. In these early experiments little attention was given to the effect of estrogen administration on appetitie and food intake. Meites (1949) examined this question and found that administration of diethylstilbestrol (DES) (0.001, 0.01, or 0.1 mg daily) markedly inhibited food and water intake in rats. The growth rate of control rats pair-fed with the DES-treated groups paralleled that of the DES-treated animals. These observations suggested that the growth inhibition of estrogens was related to decreased food intake. However, in the same study, natural estrogens were shown to decrease growth rate, but their effects could not be correlated with reduced food intake. Thus, the early studies (1930s and 1940s) indicated that *in vivo* administration of estrogens is accompanied by reduction in linear growth, but the mechanisms by which this occurs were obscure.

Extensive studies of the histological response of mouse articular and rat eiphyseal cartilage to estrogen treatment have been carried out. Silberberg *et al.* (1965) administered 60 μg of α-estradiol benzoate or placebo to 4-week-old male mice and, after sacrifice at 2, 4, 8 or 24 hours or 2, 3, or 7 days, examined sections of the femoral heads by light and electron microscopy. The single injection of estradiol caused a profound alteration in the structure of the articular chondrocytes. Within a few hours the Golgi apparatus was markedly hypertrophied and the granular endoplasmic reticulum became abundant, with the formation of large cisterns. Multivesicular bodies containing vesicles, delicate electron dense granules, or filaments were increased in size and number. Mitochondria were increased in number and enlarged in size and some were vacuolated or distorted. Intracellular glycogen deposits increased, particularly in surface chondrocytes. Mature chondrocytes had densely packed intracellular banded fibrils similar to those noted pericellulary. The matrix showed increased numbers of relatively thick collagen fibrils with little intervening ground substance. Advanced calcification of the midzone and deep zone matrix was present. Most of the changes were maximal 16–24 hours after the estrogen administration and had not regressed at 1 week. More chronic treatment of mice with α-estradiol benzoate (8 μg once a week for 4 weeks) did not cause any greater change in the chondrocytes of the femoral articular cartilage, but the matrix accretion of collagen to form thick, densely packed fibrils was increased (Silberberg and Silberberg, 1965).

Fahmy *et al.* (1971b) studied the ultrastructure of upper tibial epiphy-

seal cartilage plates from male weanling rats given 1 μg of aqueous estradiol per gram body weight per day. Observations (light and electron
microscopic) were made from 3 hours to 6 days. Their findings were quite
similar to those that Silberberg et al. found in articular cartilage.

Relatively little is known about the specific biochemical alterations
induced in cartilage by estrogen treatment of animals. Estradiol benzoate
(0.33 mg/day) administered for 3 weeks to adult rats markedly inhibits
the incorporation of $^{35}SO_4$ into costal cartilage. This was demonstrated
by injecting $^{35}SO_4$ into the rats 24 hours prior to sacrifice and subsequently determining the uptake; or sacrificing the animals and incubating
pieces of costal cartilage with $^{35}SO_4$ in vitro for 4 hours with subsequent
determination of the uptake (Priest et al, 1960). Time courses indicated
that at least 3 days of estradiol treatment were necessary for the effect
to occur. In the same series of experiments, testosterone propionate (0.25
mg/day) treatment had no effect on $^{35}SO_4$ incorporation into costal cartilage. Estradiol treatment had the same inhibitory effect on $^{35}SO_4$ incorporation into costal cartilage from hypophysectomized rats as in normal
rats, indicating that the estrogen effect was not dependent on the presence
of the pituitary gland. The decreased $^{35}SO_4$ incorporation into cartilage
of estradiol-treated rats is due to decreased synthesis of acid mucopolysaccharides (Priest and Koplitz, 1962). They demonstrated that $^{35}SO_4$
incorporation into isolated acid mucopolysaccharides accounted for all
the measurable inhibition of sulfate uptake and that inhibition of
[^{14}C]glucose incorporation into the acid mucopolysaccharide paralleled
the inhibition of $^{35}SO_4$.

Lack of estrogen, as induced by ovariectomy in weanling rats, causes
an increase in body weight gain as compared to controls. Chemical
changes noted in proximal tibial epiphyseal growth plates (2–4 weeks
after ovariectomy) were increased water content and decreased percentage of calcium. Significant increases occurred in the hexosamine/collagen
ratio, owing mainly to an increase in hexosamine with no significant
change in collagen (Minot and Hillman, 1967). In contrast, estradiol
treatment (0.1 mg/day for 5–15 days) in weanling rats resulted in retardation of body growth and in the following chemical changes in the
epiphyseal cartilage: decrease in water content, increase in calcium concentration, and a decrease in the hexosamine/collagen ratio caused primarily by a reduced hexosamine content (Minot and Hillman, 1967).
Similar changes are found in body growth and chemical composition of
epiphyseal cartilage plates of rabbits treated with estradiolbenzoate 2.5
mg every other day for 30 days (Berntsen, 1968). All the chemical
changes in epiphyseal growth plates that occur in estrogen-treated animals are those normally seen in cartilage plates from older animals. This

suggests that the administration of estrogen hastens the aging process in epiphyseal cartilage.

The question of the mechanism of the *in vivo* effect of estrogen in inhibiting growth has been examined by several more recent studies. Estrogens in pharmacologic doses inhibit growth (as measured by tibial epiphyseal cartilage plate thickness) in hypophysectomized rats (Strickland and Sprinz, 1973). Estrogen administration is able partially (Josimovich *et al.*, 1967) or completely (Strickland and Sprinz, 1973) to block the effect of growth hormone treatment in increasing the width of the tibial epiphyseal cartilage plate in hypophysectomized rats. Similarly, estrogen therapy completely blocks the effect of growth hormone in increasing $^{35}SO_4$ incorporation into costal cartilage from growing male mice (Herbai, 1971b). That the inhibitory effect of estrogen on growth processes is not due to decreased food consumption was shown by studies using pair-fed (Josimovich *et al.*, 1967; Priest *et al.*, 1960) or starved (Herbai, 1971b) animals. The effects of estrogens of different potency in inhibiting body growth in mice are highly correlated with their ability to inhibit $^{35}SO_4$ incorporation into costal cartilage but are not strictly related to their classic estrogen effects, as measured by uterotropic action (Herbai, 1971d). Inhibition of $^{35}SO_4$ incorporation into cartilage that does not ossify (aural, xiphoid, tracheal) occurs in growing female mice given stilbestrol (10–100 μg/day) (Herbai, 1971b). The above data plus studies which indicate that estrogen administration increases plasma growth hormone (Dickerman *et al.*, 1971; Frantz and Rabkin, 1965), rather than lowering it, preclude estrogens inhibiting growth by altering the secretion of growth hormone from the anterior pituitary.

Studies on the *in vitro* effects of estrogens on fragments of cartilage or chondrocyte cultures have not yielded uniform results. Table IX summarizes these data. Most investigators have been unable to demonstrate *in vitro* effects of estrogens. Whether these data indicate that estrogens exert their effects on cartilage secondarily, or whether the *in vitro* systems are deficient, cannot be presently answered.

The possibility that estrogens exert their *in vivo* effects by altering the formation of serum somatomedins has been suggested. Almqvist *et al.* (1961) measured the effect of ethynylestradiol (1 mg/day) treatment on the clinical course and serum somatomedin levels of eight acromegalic patients. In four, serum somatomedin activity was significantly reduced, and this was accompanied by a decrease in the clinical activity of the disease. In the other four, serum somatomedin activity did not change and little or no clinical improvement was noted. Most of the patients had also been treated with X-ray to the pituitary, and it is difficult to determine whether this complicated the results. Confirmation of the suppres-

TABLE IX

In Vitro Effects of Estrogens on Cartilage Metabolism

Author	Cartilage	Animal	Incubation medium	Estrogen	Sulfate incorporation	Acetate incorporation
Priest et al. (1960), Priest and Koplitz (1962)	Costal	Rat	Tyrode's	Estradiol	No effect	—
Endo et al. (1969)	Femur	Chick embryo, 9 days	Chick embryo extract:horse serum:Gey's saline solution (1:5:4)	Estradiol (10^{-6} to 10^{-4} M)	Decreased 10–20%	—
Herbai (1971b)	Costal	Mouse	Krebs–Ringer phosphate with glucose (0.25%) and albumin (2%)	17 β-Estradiol 10 μg/ml or methallenstril-OH 25 μg/ml	Decreased 51%	Decreased 48%
	Costal	Hypox mouse	Same	Methallenstril-OH 25 μg/ml	No effect	—
Wiedemann and Schwartz (1972)	Costal	Hypox rat	Phosphosaline with added essential amino acids	Ethynylestradiol or estradiol-17-β 0.1 and 100 μg/ml added to reference serum	No effect	—
Phillips et al. (1973)	Costal	Pig	Phosphosaline with added essential amino acids	Estradiol 0.2 ng/ml added to reference serum	No effect	—
	Pelvic rudiment	Chick embryo, 10 days	Same	Same	No effect	—

sion of serum somatomedin activity by estrogens was shown by Wiede-mann and Schwartz (1972). In four acromegalic patients, ethynylestra-diol, 0.5–1.0 mg/day for 7–18 days, reduced elevated serum somatomedin levels, hypercalciuria and hydroxyprolinuria without affecting basal plasma growth hormone levels or plasma growth hormone responses to suppression or stimulation. In three growth hormone-treated hypopitu-itary patients, ethynylestradiol prevented the rise in serum somatomedin activity. The data are too scanty to allow evaluation of the metabolic effects of the estrogen alterations in serum somatomedin activity, but the findings did suggest that anabolic effects of growth hormone were not blocked in the estrogen growth hormone-treated hypopituitary pa-tients, while they may have been in the estrogen-treated acromegalic patients. Additional studies will be needed to clarify this very important point. Phillips et al. (1973) have shown that treatment of young male hypophysectomized rats with estradiol, 20 ng/day for several days, blocks the rise in serum somatomedin activity that occurs with bovine growth hormone treatment (200 μg, every 12 hours for 2 doses). Addition-ally, they demonstrated that $^{35}SO_4$ incorporation in the costal cartilage of the treated animals was reduced by the estradiol. They concluded from their study that the primary effect of estrogens is to inhibit the generation of serum somatomedins.

The information currently available on the effects of estrogens on carti-lage metabolism cannot be synthesized into a simple scheme. Estrogen deficiency (ovariectomy) causes the epiphyseal growth zone to close later than ordinarily and the centers of ossification to be delayed in appear-ance. Body size or the length of certain tubular bones or of tails may be temporarily or permanently increased (Silberberg and Silberberg, 1972). Histological and chemical studies of both immature epiphyseal and articular cartilage are compatible with the concept that ovariectomy delays the normal physiological effects of aging in cartilage (Silberberg and Silberberg, 1972; Minot and Hillman, 1967). In contrast, estrogen excess stunts body growth, causes earlier closure of epiphyseal growth zones and earlier appearance of ossification centers, and inhibits proteo-glycan synthesis (Silberberg and Silberberg, 1972; Frasier and Smith, 1968). Minot and Hillman (1967) have suggested that estrogens increase physiological aging in epiphyseal cartilage. The electron microscopic studies of articular and epiphyseal cartilage indicate that pharmacologi-cal doses of estrogens cause profound and unique ultrastructure changes (Silberberg et al., 1965; Fahmy et al., 1971b). All the above observations would seem to indicate that estrogens exert a direct effect on cartilage metabolism. In vitro studies, for the most part, have failed to show such effects.

Other evidence supports the concept that the effects of administered estrogens on cartilage metabolism may be secondary to some other *in vivo* effect. Estrogens seem to inhibit the generation of somatomedin, but this is an untenable explanation for the mechanism of estrogen action on cartilage since the physiological, chemical, and histological changes ensuing from estrogen therapy are quite different from those observed in cartilage from hypophysectomized animals. The observation that a time lag exists between estrogen administration and the inhibition of cartilage proteoglycan synthesis (Priest *et al.*, 1960) is compatible with the concept that estrogen action on cartilage *in vivo* is a secondary effect. Future studies directed toward defining physiological versus pharmacological effects of estrogen *in vivo* and more fruitful *in vitro* studies of the effects of estrogens on cartilage metabolism are necessary to answer some of these unresolved questions.

H. ANDROGENS

Androgens significantly influence statural growth through their general anabolic actions and their specific effects on cartilage metabolism. Most of our information relative to androgen effects is derived from studies involving spontaneous or acquired androgen deficiency or administration of exogenous androgens.

Testicular deficiency in immature animals or man occurring either spontaneously or following orchiectomy results in marked retardation of the development of the skeletal system (Wilkins, 1957; see review by Silberberg and Silberberg, 1972). Epiphyseal ossification centers and epiphyseal closure that occur prior to puberty are unaffected by testicular insufficiency. However, epiphyseal closures that ordinarily occur at puberty are significantly retarded, and those that ordinarily occur after puberty may remain open indefinitely. The delay in epiphyseal closure leads to a more prolonged period of growth, however, usually at a normal or delayed rate, but excessive growth leading to gigantism is not seen (Clark and Gavin, 1962; Wilkins, 1957; Silberberg and Silberberg, 1972). The differential effects of androgen deficiency on the various parts of the skeleton result in a disproportionate growth of the long bones of the extremities (since epiphyseal closure occurs after puberty) and eunuchoidal proportions ensue. The entire skeleton is delicate and occasionally osteoporotic, and the shape of the pelvis remains infantile. Orchiectomy in large animals results in increased standing height while in small animals it frequently leads to stunted growth even though the tubular bones are still increased in length relative to the body size.

By histological examination the epiphyseal cartilage plates of androgen-deficient animals show increased numbers of chondrocytes in the maturing columnar zone and a delay in the hypertrophy of the chondrocytes. The replacement of the provisional zone of calcified cartilage by bone is delayed. In some strains of mice which develop spontaneous osteoarthritis, orchiectomy delays the development, suggesting that articular cartilage aging is also delayed in testicular insufficiency.

Testosterone administration to normal or orchiectomized animals causes growth, presumably through its anabolic actions, and cartilage maturation through its androgenic effects. Small doses of testosterone stimulate the rate of linear growth, but do not lead to increased final length (Rubinstein and Solomon, 1941b; Joss et al., 1963; Foss, 1965). Large doses of testosterone accelerate osseous maturation in excess of any stimulatory effects on chondrocyte proliferation and growth, with the result that the final body length is stunted (Rubinstein and Solomon, 1941a; Howard, 1962, 1963; Joss et al., 1963; Silberberg and Silberberg, 1971). Studies with immature female mice suggest that testosterone stimulates proliferation of chondrocytes and the growth of the epiphyseal plate until 40 days of age, after which it depresses growth (Puche and Romano, 1971). The depression of growth caused by testosterone is not mediated through any hypophyseal hormones, as testosterone depresses endochondral growth produced by growth hormone treatment of hypophysectomized rats (Reiss et al., 1946).

The effects of a single, large dose of testosterone (50 μg/gm) on the ultrastructure of the epiphyseal cartilages of mature rats has been examined by electron microscopy (Fahmy et al., 1971a). While significant changes were noted by 24 hours, the most striking findings occurred after 3 or 4 days. Cell division appeared to be stimulated as the number of clones of dividing cells in the columnar region were increased. The chondrocytes showed evidence of increased secretory activity particularly in the earlier stages of development, giving the impression of acceleration of mature chondrocytes into hypertrophied chondrocytes. Unusually large accumulations of lipids and glycogen were present in early mature chondrocytes. In the zone of prehypertrophy, the interterritorial matrix contained foci of early and premature calcification and thicker and longer collagen fibers than in controls. The results of this acute study indicate that large doses of testosterone probably accelerate chondrocyte proliferation, development and maturation in the growth zones of epiphyseal cartilage.

Similar studies of the effect of acute and subacute administration of testosterone on the ultrastructure of articular cartilage of the femoral heads of growing male mice were carried out by Silberberg and Hasler (1972). Starting within a few hours after testosterone administration and persisting for several days, the hormone caused hypertrophy of the nuclei and cytoplasm, accentuated development of organelles (endoplasmic reticulum, polysomes, Golgi apparatus) and increased glycogen deposition. Chondrocyte proliferation was stimulated. A somewhat later manifestation of hormone action was an increase in matrix fibrillarity. The changes in articular cartilage are similar to those in epiphyseal cartilage with evidence of both growth-promoting and age-accelerating actions.

The effects of androgens on sulfate incorporation into cartilage glycosaminoglycans has been studied both *in vivo* and *in vitro*. Testosterone given to rats or cockerels failed to increase *in vivo* sulfate incorporation by cartilage (Priest *et al.*, 1960; Kowalewski, 1958). Salmon *et al.* (1963) showed that neither castration nor testosterone administration to normal immature rats has any effect on *in vitro* sulfate uptake by cartilage (costal, nasal, or xiphoid). However, hypophysectomized rats treated with testosterone or similar androgens had a consistent increase in costal cartilage sulfate uptake *in vitro*. Direct effects of testosterone added *in vitro* to costal cartilage from hypophysectomized rats could not be demonstrated. Testosterone treatment of hypophysectomized rats did not restore sulfation factor activity to their plasma. Collins and Anilane (1959) have reported similar findings in that testosterone propionate increased sulfate uptake *in vivo* by costal cartilage of hypophysectomized, but not of normal, rats. Herbai (1971e) found that orchiectomy in male mice reduced *in vivo* sulfate uptake by costal cartilage. Testosterone treatment of immature female mice had no effect on sulfate incorporation into costal cartilage except for very large doses (1 mg/day for 6 days) which caused suppression. In contrast, Endo *et al.* (1969) reported that testosterone (10^{-6} to 10^{-4} M) stimulated $^{35}SO_4$ incorporation into 9-day chick embryo femora *in vitro*. Synthetic steroids with primarily anabolic activities, such as methandrosternolone or 17-ethyl-19-nortestosterone, have been reported to increase the growth of embryonic tibia cultivated *in vitro* and increase *in vivo* sulfate incorporation into cartilage of growing cockerels (Prévot and Schneider, 1966; Kowalewski, 1958).

The failure of testosterone *in vivo* and *in vitro* to alter sulfate incorporation into cartilage from normal or gonadectomized animals suggest that either testosterone action *in vivo* is mediated by some other as yet unidentified factor or that the effects of testosterone are other than influencing the rate of synthesis of sulfated glycosaminoglycans. The stimulatory effect of testosterone on cartilage sulfate uptake in hypophysectomized rats might be construed to suggest that testosterone increases sulfation factor production. Salmon *et al.* (1963) were unable to demonstrate this, and Phillips *et al.* (1973) recently showed that testosterone administration to suboptimally growth hormone-treated hypophysectomized rats has no effect on the quantity of sulfation factor generated. Kofoed *et al.* (1970) measured the effects of both orchidectomy and testosterone treatment on the concentration and synthesis of the glycosaminoglycans of rat tracheal cartilage. Testosterone increased hyaluronic acid concentration greater than 2-fold, probably by increasing synthesis. No effect of testosterone was found on any of the sulfated proteoglycans (heparin sulfate, chondroitin 4-sulfate, chondroitin 6-sulfate, or dermatan sulfate). It is clear that the mechanisms of androgen action on the growth and maturation of cartilage have yet to be elucidated.

I. Glucocorticoids

Glucocorticoids have been known to affect growth since the demonstrations that either pituitary extracts rich in ACTH (Moon, 1937) or purified adrenal cortical hormones (Ingle *et al.*, 1938) given to normal rats inhibited somatic growth. Marx *et al.* (1943) suggested that ACTH antagonized the peripheral actions of growth hormone as they demonstrated that ACTH inhibited growth hormone-induced body weight gain and tibial epiphyseal plate enlargement in hypophysectomized rats without causing alterations in food intake. Soyka and Crawford (1965) showed that cortisone (0.1–1.0 mg/day) antagonized the growth-promoting effect of growth hormone in hypophysectomized rats.

Experiences with cortisone treatment in children indicate that the rates of statural growth and osseous maturation in humans are slowed after several weeks or more of therapy (Blodgett *et al.*, 1956). The dose required to produce these effects varies with the specific physiological or pathological state being treated. Effects are noted in hypopituitary patients with as little as 4–20 mg per square meter of body surface per day; in patients with congenital adrenal hyperplasia, with 35–50 mg/m^2 per day; and in normal children, with greater than 45 mg/m^2 per day. The antagonism between growth hormone and glucocorticoid actions on linear growth occur with physiological doses of glucocorticoids, as replacement therapy with cortisone markedly impairs the growth response to growth hormone treatment in hypopituitary patients (Soyka and Crawford, 1965). Administration of human growth hormone to dwarfed prepubertal children who were on chronic corticosteroid therapy caused only a minimal increase in nitrogen and had no effect on retention of phosphorus (Morris *et al.*, 1968b). More prolonged treatment with large doses of human growth hormone (40–120 mg/week for 4–8 months) failed to improve their growth rate. These data clearly demonstrated that glucocorticoids antagonize the effects of growth hormone on peripheral tissues.

Because studies in adult humans had indicated that chronic high-dosage glucocorticoid therapy inhibits growth hormone secretion (Hartog *et al.* 1964; Frantz and Rabkin, 1964), it was initially thought that inhibition of growth hormone release might contribute to the growth-retarding effects of glucocorticoids. However, studies with growth-retarded children on glucorticoid therapy usually show normal basal and stimulated levels of plasma growth hormone (Morris *et al.*, 1968a; Root *et al.*, 1969). Long-acting intramuscular glucocorticoids, such as 6α-methylprednisolone, may significantly inhibit growth hormone secretion (Stempfel *et al.*, 1968). It seems most reasonable to conclude that the inhibition of linear growth and osseous maturation that occur in children on glucocorticoid therapy result from peripheral antagonism of growth hormone and perhaps other hormone actions. The peripheral effects of growth hormone, that are blocked, could be the generation of serum sulfation factor activity or the actions of serum sulfation factor on cartilage metabolism.

Histological changes in epiphyseal cartilage following administration of glucocorticoid are those of decreased growth and maturation. The cartilage plate is markedly thinner than normal, and fewer chondrocytes are present. The matrix is decreased in quantity. Hypertrophy of the chondrocytes and ossification are retarded (Silberberg and Silberberg, 1971). The effects of cortisone acetate (5 mg/day for 5 days) on the ultrastructure of tibial epiphyseal plates of immature rats has been studied by Dearden and Mosier (1972). The chondrocytes are smaller and more spindle-shaped than normal. The rough endoplasmic reticulum and free ribosomes are much reduced. The Golgi apparatus shows evidence of hypertrophy with an increase in vesicles and vacuoles. The mitochondria are bizarre in shape and vacuolated. Cytoplasmic dense bodies and vacuoles are increased. Cellular glycogen is increased. Similar ultrastructural changes have been noted in articular chondrocytes from cortisone-treated rats (Silberberg and Silberberg, 1971).

Because of the known antianabolic actions of glucocorticoids, Layton (1951) investigated the effects of cortisone on chondroitin sulfate synthesis *in vitro* and showed that it inhibited radiolabeled sulfate uptake. Many studies of the effects of glucocorticoids on the synthesis of cartilage macromolecules both *in vivo* and *in vitro* have followed. The results of the studies are not uniform and are probably influenced by the use of different cartilage preparations, experiment designs, incubation medium, etc. While a general overall view can be abstracted from the data, one must nevertheless be concerned about the discrepancies. Clark and Umbreit (1954), using an *in vitro* system with xiphoid cartilage from adult rats, found that cortisone inhibited and hydrocortisone stimulated $^{35}SO_4$ incorporation into macromolecules. Cartilage from adrenalectomized rats incorporated the same amount of $^{35}SO_4$ as that from normal rats. There was no obvious reason for the different effects of cortisone and hydrocortisone (cortisol). Murphy et al. (1956) gave either hydrocortisone or cortisone (1 mg/day for 4 days) to normal rats, and following administration of $^{35}SO_4$ the proximal tibial epiphyses took up significantly less radiolabeled sulfate into chondroitin sulfate than did epiphyses from control animals. In a subsequent study, Daughaday and Mariz (1962) treated normal rats with cortisol (2 mg/100 gm body weight for 4 days) and then removed the costal cartilages and incubated them in vitro with $^{35}SO_4$ and [^{3}H]proline for 6 or 24 hours. No effect on [^{3}H]hydroxyproline incorporation in cartilage collagen and an increase in $^{35}SO_4$ incorporation into chondroitin sulfate were found. If the cortisol (0.9 μg/ml) was added directly to normal rat costal cartilage in vitro, it inhibited [^{3}H]hydroxyproline incorporation into cartilage collagen, and somewhat higher concentrations (5 μg/ml) inhibited $^{35}SO_4$ incorporation.

Addition of glucocorticoids to 3-day-old chick embryo somites in tissue culture decreases growth and reduces $^{35}SO_4$ incorporation into chondroitin sulfate (Whitehouse and Lash, 1961; Lash and Whitehouse, 1961). Total uronic acid content was unchanged, and chromatography of the isolated polysaccharides showed an increase in unsulfated chondroitin. On the basis of these data it was proposed that glucocorticoids interfere with either the sulfate-activating or transfer systems, not with the synthesis of the peptide or carbohydrate unit of the proteoglycan. Similar results were obtained using beef costal cartilage in vitro and measuring $^{35}SO_4$ incorporation and total cartilage sulfate and polysaccharide ($^{35}SO_4$ incorporation was depressed and total sulfate and polysaccharide were unchanged).

Subsequent studies have indicated that glucocorticoids do inhibit the synthesis of the proteoglycan subunit. Whitehouse and Boström (1962) studied the in vitro effect of cortisol and a number of its analogs on the metabolism of beef costal cartilage in vitro. Cortisol (2.5×10^{-4} M) inhibited $^{35}SO_4$, [^{14}C]glucose, and [^{14}C]acetate incorporation into cartilage glycosaminoglycans. It also inhibited cartilage glucose and fatty acid oxidation. Cortisol had a 2-hour delay before its effects on glycosaminoglycan synthesis began, and its effects were reversible. From the many analogs studied, no good correlation could be found between the known glucocorticoid activity and the in vitro effects on cartilage. Barrett et al. (1966) incubated tibias and femurs from 7-day chick embryos in vitro with cortisol (2.1×10^{-9} M to 2.1×10^{-7} M) and showed that $^{35}SO_4$ incorporation into proteoglycans was reduced with a proportionate decrease in uronic acid content indicating that the synthesis of glycosaminoglycans was blocked. No qualitative change in the nature of the carbohydrate subunit occurred, as the glucosamine to galactosamine ratio was unchanged. Reynolds (1966) incubated femurs and humeri from 7-day chick embryos in tissue culture for 6 days and found that cortisol (0.01–10 μg/ml) inhibited growth, reduced water content, decreased DNA and matrix polysaccharide synthesis, and increased collagen synthesis. Ebert and Prockop (1967) injected cortisol (0.05 to 0.15 mg) into chick embryos and, after administering the appropriate radiolabeled precursor, homogenized the embryo and measured incorporation into products. Sulfate incorporation into mucopolysaccharides, proline incorporation into hydroxyproline of collagen, and tryptophan incorporation into noncollagen proteins were inhibited. No effect on orotic acid incorporation into RNA could be demonstrated. These data suggest that glucocorticoids inhibit the synthesis of collagen and other proteins, as well as proteoglycans. In the same series of studies, tibias from 10-day chick embryos were incubated in vitro with hydrocortisone. High concentrations (100 μg/ml) significantly inhibited sulfate, proline, and hydroxyproline incorporation, but only after a latent period of at least 30 minutes. If the cortisol was given in vivo and the tibias were removed and incubated in vitro, collagen synthesis was inhibited but sulfate incorporation into chondromucoprotein was increased. Thus the majority of studies suggest that glucocorticoids inhibit cartilage proteoglycan and collagen synthesis. The reasons for some of the disparate results are unknown.

Several studies have reported observations that are difficult to understand but could perhaps bear on the question of disparate results. Murota et al. (1967, 1969) have shown that femurs from 9-day chick embryos can metabolize cortisol in vitro to dihydrocortisol and tetrahydrocortisol, and, while cortisol inhibits sulfate uptake by cartilage incubated in synthetic medium, it stimulates uptake in natural medium (Containing chick embryo extract and horse serum). Kaplan and Fisher (1964) gave methylprednisolone (3 mg/day for 3 days) to rabbits and isolated the mucopolysaccharide from rib cartilage. They found no reduction in total mucopolysaccharides, but the ratio of glucosamine to galactosamine was significantly increased, suggesting the possibility that more keratin sulfate was being synthesized. These findings are the exact opposite to those found by Barrett et al. (1966) with embryonic chick cartilage.

Many mechanisms have been proposed to explain how glucocorticoids inhibit the synthesis of cartilage macromolecules. Whitehouse and Boström (1961) proposed that the steroids and other anti-inflammatory agents that inhibit cartilage metabolism do so by decreasing ATP production. Kunin and his collaborators have proposed that the primary action of glucocorticoids is to inhibit glycolysis and thereby decrease energy production. Kunin and Meyer (1969) treated rats with cortisone (5 mg/day for 3 days), sacrificed the animals, isolated the tibial epiphyseal cartilages, and either measured metabolites or incubated them *in vitro* with various substrates. Cortisone treatment caused a significant weight loss and reduction in food intake by the animals. The tibial epiphyseal width was reduced 50%; DNA content per epiphyseal plate was unchanged; water content was reduced; and total glucose (glycogen plus free glucose) was 50% of that in cartilage from control animals. Cortisone treatment reduced cartilage lactate production *in vitro* from endogenous substrates to zero, and from exogenous glucose to 30% of normal. It also reduced glucose oxidation by the pentose phosphate shunt 50%, but it had no effect on oxidation of glucose via the tricarboxylic acid cycle. Accompanying the inhibition of anaerobic glycolysis by cortisone was a decrease in epiphyseal cartilage phosphofructokinase, aldolase, pyruvate kinase, and lactate dehydrogenase (Meyer and Kunin, 1969). Other enzymes (hexokinase and glucose-6-phosphate dehydrogenase) were also reduced, but in proportion to the decrease of all proteins that was seen. Starvation resulted in similar changes in intermediary metabolism and glycolytic enzyme activities; and since the glucocorticoid-treated rats lose weight it is difficult to be sure if the changes ascribed to glucocorticoid therapy are really such. No effects of cortisone or starvation were found on oxidative enzyme activities of rat epiphyseal cartilage (Meyer and Kunin, 1973). Histochemical studies of the epiphyseal cartilage of the cortisone-treated rats showed that the most dramatic effects on glycolysis occurred in the maturing columnar and early hypertrophy regions. These areas ordinarily show the greatest content of glycogen, phosphorylase, glyceraldehyde-3-phosphate dehydrogenase, and lactate dehydrogenase, and cortisone treatment markedly decreases them (Balogh and Kunin, 1971). These studies provide the basis for Kunin's proposal that a primary action of glucocorticoid is to decrease energy production by interfering with anaerobic glycosis.

Peck and his collaborators (1967, 1969) have studied the effects of glucocorticoids on isolated bone cells from fetal rat calvaria in cell culture. Hydrocortisone ($10^{-5} M$ to $10^{-4} M$) was found to inhibit the incorporation of [^{14}C]proline into collagen and noncollagen proteins. No effect on protein degradation was found, and it was felt that these findings were indicative of inhibition of synthesis. Hydrocortisone also inhibited the uptake of [2-^{14}C]uridine into the tissue pool of free uridine and uridine nucleotides as well as its incorporation into RNA. Total RNA content was reduced (5–10% in 5 hours, 20–30% in 15 hours). No effects on DNA or thymidine incorporation were noted. The primary effects of glucocorticoids seemed to be an impaired transport or phosphorylation of free nucleosides and an increased rate of degradation of preformed RNA. The inhibition of free nucleoside uptake by cortisol requires protein synthesis as its effects were blocked by inhibitors of protein synthesis. These data raise the possibility that deprivation of key metabolites and a gradual depletion of total cell RNA may represent additional explanations for glucocorticoid inhibitory effects. Eisenbarth and Lebovitz (1974b) have shown that the glucocorticoid content of normal serum is sufficient to inhibit $^{35}SO_4$ incorporation into cartilage proteoglycans and [^{3}H]uridine incorporation into acid-soluble free uridine and uridine nucleosides and into RNA.

In contrast to direct effects of glucocorticoids in inhibiting cartilage growth and metabolism, Phillips et al. (1973) have shown that cortisol administration to growth hormone-treated hypophysectomized rats inhibits $^{35}SO_4$ incorporation into their cartilage and markedly impairs serum somatomedin generation. They found relatively little effect of glucocorticoids on $^{35}SO_4$ uptake by rat or chick cartilage in vitro (pig cartilage uptake was inhibited at 100–1000 μg of cortisol per deciliter). They concluded that the primary effect of glucocorticoids in interfering with cartilage growth and metabolism was to block somatomedin generation.

The inhibitory effects of glucocorticoids on cartilage growth and metabolism have been reported to occur in fetal rat cartilage if the mothers are treated with glucocorticoids (Ornoy, 1971). The effects of cortisol and glucocorticoids on articular cartilage are similar to those occurring in epiphyseal cartilage (Mankin, 1974). Administration of cortisol into rabbit knee joints produces a substantial decrease in the rates of incorporation of $^{35}SO_4$ and [^{3}H]glycine (Mankin and Conger, 1966; Mankin, 1974). Repeated administration may lead to focal chondromalacia. Chronic treatment of rabbits with cortisone 4.5 mg/kg per day for 9 weeks has no effect on the DNA content of articular cartilage but depresses hexosamine concentration (Mankin et al., 1972). In vitro incorporation of $^{35}SO_4$ and [^{3}H]glycine by removed articular cartilage was markedly inhibited. During the study the animals lost 25% of their body weight and a control starved group of rabbits showed similar changes in the articular cartilages, though not as marked.

Glucocorticoids inhibit cartilage growth and maturation in vivo. These effects are dramatic, particularly when pharmacological doses are given. Many questions remain to be answered. Of fundamental importance is the question of the physiological role of glucocorticoids in controlling growth and cartilage function. The pharmacological effects of glucocorticoids on cartilage metabolism are still confusing. In interpreting the results of studies that have been reported it is important to recognize that factors such as specific steroid, dose, animal species, physiological state of the animal, and side effects of the steroid may influence the in vivo results; while type of cartilage, incubation conditions, and incubation medium may influence *in vitro* results. With the new advances in defining mechanisms of steroid hormone actions on other tissues it is reasonable to expect that some of these techniques will be useful in elucidating the mechanisms of glucocorticoid action on cartilage.

J. Nerve Growth Factor

As discussed in Section III, B, the proposal has been made that many of the growth factors that exist may be related and have common modes of action. They are characterized by having insulinlike actions on their respective target tissues (Hershko *et al.*, 1971). Nerve growth factor (NGF) is such a growth factor. It is found in male mouse submaxillary glands, snake venoms, mesenchymal tumors, glial cells, and many other tissues (see review by Levi-Montalcini and Angeletti, 1968; Varon *et al.*, 1972). NGF from male mouse submaxillary glands has been isolated, and structural studies indicate that it has some homology with proinsulin (Frasier *et al.*, 1972). NGF exerts effects on sympathetic and spinal ganglion cells (increased RNA, protein, and lipid synthesis and increased uptake and utilization of glucose) that are similar to the effects that insulin exerts on its target cells (Levi-Montalcini and Angeletti, 1968; Pearce *et al.*, 1972).

The effects of NGF on embryonic chicken cartilage metabolism *in vitro* have been examined and compared to the effects of insulin and serum sulfation factor (Eisenbarth *et al.*, 1975). Figure 4 shows that NGF has no effect on the incorporation of [^{3}H]thymidine into DNA or [^{3}H]uridine into RNA. It significantly inhibits $^{35}SO_4$ incorporation into proteoglycans and causes a small but significant inhibition of [^{3}H]leucine incorporation into total proteins. Fractionation and isolation studies show that [^{3}H]leucine incorporation is inhibited only into proteoglycans and not into any other cartilage proteins. Thus the data indicate that NGF causes a selective and unique inhibition of cartilate proteoglycan synthesis. Its action on cartilage metabolism is therefore quite different from that of serum sulfation factor or insulin.

K. Parathyroid Hormone and Thyrocalcitonin

Relatively few observations have been made concerning the effects of parathyroid hormone and thyrocalcitonin on cartilage metabolism. Guri and Bernstein (1964) incubated femoral and tibial epiphyses from rachitic rats *in vitro* with both crude parathyroid extract and purified parathyroid hormone. Both preparations increased the uptake of $^{35}SO_4$ and [U-^{14}C]glucose into isolated mucopolysaccharide (glycosaminogly-

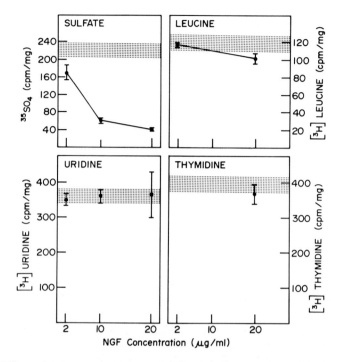

FIG. 4. Effect of nerve growth factor (NGF) on the synthesis of cartilage macromolecules. Cartilages were incubated in medium containing the appropriate radioactive precursor [^{35}SO$_4$ (0.25 mCi/mmole); L-[4,5-^{3}H]leucine (0.6 mCi/mmole; [5-^{3}H]uridine (24.4 Ci/mmole) or [*methyl*-^{3}H]thymidine (96 Ci/mmole)], and incorporation into the specific macromolecule (chondromucoprotein, protein, RNA, or DNA) was determined. The circles are the means and the brackets the standard errors (SE) of five observations. The stippled horizontal region of each panel is the mean ± 1 SE (five observations) of incorporation in medium without added NGF (controls). Incorporation is given as counts per minute per milligram wet weight and is plotted against the NGF concentration. Reprinted from Eisenbarth *et al.*, *J. Pharmacol. Exp. Ther.* **192**, 630 (1975).

can). The peak effect was noted with parathyroid hormone concentrations of 16 μU per flask (2.5–3 ml of medium were in each flask), and at concentrations above 64 μU per flask there was a tendency to depress ^{35}SO$_4$ incorporation. Hjertquist and Vejlens (1968) measured the effect of treatment of dogs with 20–30 USP units of parathyroid extract for 3–5 days on the glycosaminoglycans of epiphyseal cartilage. No effect was noted on the molecular weight of the chondroitin sulfate or in the total hexosamine content of cartilage glycosaminoglycans. Gaillard and co-workers (1968) incubated isolated chondrocytes from epiphyseal cartilages of 16-day-old Swiss albino mice embryos in tissue culture with parathyroid extract (2 U/ml) added. After 4–5 hours there were fewer aggregates of cells than normal, and those that were present were less stable. After 6–9 days in culture, histochemical analysis of the cells suggested that the parathyroid extract caused the chondrocytes to secrete an intracellular substance containing acid mucopolysaccharide with fewer sulfate groups. These data were not confirmed by chemical or isotope incorporation studies. Cipera and Cherian (1969) were unable to show any effects of injected parathyroid hormone on either collagen or glycosaminoglycan synthesis in epiphyseal cartilage of 3-week-old chicks. However, parathyroidectomy in immature chicks resulted, within 24 hours, in a rise in collagen (determined as hydroxyproline) with no change in glycosaminoglycans (determined as hexosamine) in tibial epiphyseal cartilage. Treatment of the parathyroidectomized chicks with bovine parathyroid extract decreased the elevated hydroxyproline content toward normal and had no effect on hexosamine content. Neither parathyroidectomy nor treatment with parathyroid extract altered the epiphyseal cartilage content of glucosamine or galactosamine. As a whole, the reported studies do not present data that are consistent with any specific actions of parathyroid hormone on cartilage metabolism. Recent data from our laboratory (Machledt and Lebovitz, 1975) indicate that parathyroid hormone stimulates the synthesis of macromolecules in embryonic chicken cartilage *in vitro*. Whether this is related to the action of cAMP is not clear (see Section IV, A).

Calcitonin effects on cartilage are equally confusing. Bélanger *et al.* (1973) administered salmon calcitonin to hatchling turtles which had been fed a calcium-deficient diet for 11–19 weeks and then examined bone and epiphyseal cartilage. Calcitonin caused a striking enlargement of the epiphyseal cartilage, and it contained mostly mature chondrocytes. The cartilage was well calcified, as demonstrated in microradiographs. The data suggest that calcitonin inhibits chondrolysis as well as osteocytic osteolysis in young turtles. Thompson and Urist (1973) studied the effects of calcitonin and cortisone upon osteogenesis in a heterotopic muscle site in adult rabbits. Exogenous calcitonin increased cartilage maturation and promoted osteogenesis in such a site. *In vitro* studies of calcitonin action on cartilage are necessary if further information is to be added to our understanding of this hormone's effects on cartilage metabolism.

L. OTHER HORMONES

Studies with various types of cartilage preparations have indicated that many other hormones may influence cartilage metabolism either *in vivo* or *in vitro*. Human placental lactogen (HPL) injected into hypophysectomized rats stimulates costal cartilage such that it increases radiolabeled thymidine incorporation into DNA in subsequent *in vitro* incubations (Murakawa and Raban, 1968; Breuer, 1969). The HPL effect is quite weak compared to human growth hormone, and the dose response curve is rather flat. These observations are in keeping with the low level of growth hormone activity that HPL has been shown to have. Corvol *et al.* (1972) have reported that pituitary glycoprotein hormones, such as TSH, LH, and FSH, contain a contaminant that stimulates the growth of articular chondrocytes in monolayer culture. This material, which they call chondrocyte growth factor, is heat labile, stimulates DNA synthesis, and inhibits $^{35}SO_4$ incorporation into glycosaminoglycans in cultured lapine articular chondrocytes. The material has not been purified, but its effects have been partially characterized (Malemud and Sokoloff, 1974). It increases radiolabeled thymidine incorporation into DNA only for the first 72 hours after it is added to the culture whereas total DNA continues to increase for at least 120 hours. It suppresses the incorporation of $^{35}SO_4$ to the same extent in all the glycosaminoglycans. The nature of the factor and its significance are not at all clear. Reichlin and Haddad (1963) have reported that administration of crude thyroid-stimulating hormone to guinea pigs increases radiosulfate uptake in xiphoid cartilage, certain orbital structures, thyroid, fat, and even the plasma. Again, the meaning of the study, if any, is obscure.

IV. METABOLIC REGULATION

A. CYCLIC AMP

The role of cyclic AMP (cAMP) in regulating cartilage metabolism has only recently received significant attention. Adamson (1970) showed that incubation of embryonic chick cartilage with dibutyryl cAMP caused an increase in amino acid transport and $^{35}SO_4$ incorporation into macromolecules. Theophylline stimulated transport of amino acids and inhibited sulfate incorporation whereas cAMP had no effect on either parameter. Tell *et al.* (1973) found that very high concentrations of a partially purified somatomedin preparation inhibited adenylate cyclase from cartilage and several other tissues and proposed that somatomedin might stimulate cartilage growth and metabolism by lowering cartilage cAMP levels.

Studies from our laboratory have focused on several aspects of the role of cAMP in regulating cartilage metabolism. Exogenous cAMP added to embryonic chick cartilage *in vitro* inhibits the incorporation of $^{35}SO_4$, [^{3}H]leucine, and [^{3}H]uridine into proteoglycans, total protein, and RNA, respectively (Rendall *et al.*, 1972; Drezner and Lebovitz, 1975). Butyrylated cAMP derivatives stimulate the *in vitro* incorporation of the appropriate radiolabeled precursors into embryonic chick cartilage proteoglycans, total proteins, and RNA (Drezner and Lebovitz, 1975). Theophylline in low concentrations (0.1–0.5 mM stimulates *in vitro* incorporation into macromolecules whereas high concentrations (1.0–5.0 mM) inhibit (Rendall *et al.*, 1972; Drezner and Lebovitz, 1975). The reason for the paradoxical effects of exogenous cAMP and the butyrylated cAMP derivatives on the incorporation of precursors into cartilage macromolecules has recently been elucidated (Drezner *et al.*, 1976). Embryonic chick cartilage *in vitro* releases adenosine-3′,5′-monophosphate diesterase and a phosphomonoesterase into the medium. These enzymes break down exogenous cAMP to AMP and adenosine. Adenosine, through some as yet unidentified mechanism(s), inhibits the synthesis of cartilage macromolecules (Drezner *et al.*, 1976). Thus the measured effect of exogenous cAMP on embryonic chick cartilage *in vitro* is an artifact of the system and does not reflect the action of endogenous intracellular cAMP. The low concentrations of theophylline that stimulate labeled precursor incorporation into macromolecules raise cartilage cAMP content significantly (Birch *et al.*, 1973). Thus, the effects of low concentrations of theophylline are probably due to increased tissue cAMP content, and, since they are identical to those caused by butyrylated cAMP derivatives, it seems reasonable to conclude that endogenous cAMP increases the incorporation of labeled precursors into cartilage macromolecules.

Exogenous cAMP, butyrylated cAMP derivatives, and theophylline incubated *in vitro* with embryonic chick cartilage stimulate α-aminoisobutyrate and cycloleucine uptake (Drezner *et al.*, 1975), indicating that cartilage cAMP modulates transport of some amino acids. It is not clear to what extent cartilage cAMP stimulates leucine and uridine transport. Until the specific effects of cartilage cAMP on transport processes are completely defined, it will not be possible to determine whether the effects of cartilage cAMP in increasing radiolabeled precursor incorporation into cartilage macromolecules represents synthesis or changes in the specific activity of the intracellular precursor pools.

Studies of the effect of hormones on cartilage cAMP content indicate that several are capable of elevating it. Serum contains a growth hormone-dependent factor which increases embryonic chicken cartilage cAMP *in vitro* (Drezner *et al.*, 1975). By definition this factor is a serum sulfation factor, but no information is available about its relationship to the various somatomedins or NSILA-S. Parathyroid hormone elevates embryonic chicken cartilage cAMP *in vitro* while other hormones, such as insulin and glucagon, have no effect (Machledt and Lebovitz, 1975).

One can summarize the data as follows: (1) cartilage contains cAMP; (2) cartilage cAMP is under some hormonal control; (3) increases in cartilage cAMP content increase transport of some amino acids and increase incorporation of radiolabeled precursors into macromolecules. Many unresolved questions remain, such as: (1) Is serum sulfation factor action on cartilage mediated solely through cAMP? (2) What is the mechanism of cAMP action on amino acid transport? (3) Does cAMP stimulate the synthesis of cartilage macromolecules and, if so, by what mechanism (gene activation, protein kinase, etc.)? (4) What additional hormones and factors control tissue cAMP concentrations? (5) Are there other second messengers to mediate the actions of protein and peptide hormones that do not alter cAMP levels?

B. Prostaglandins

Prostaglandins appear to have at least two distinct actions on cartilage growth and metabolism. All prostaglandins (A, B, E, and F) increase the cAMP content of pelvic leaflets from 10- to 12-day chick embryos *in vitro* (Eisenbarth *et al.*, 1974a; Eisenbarth and Lebovitz, 1974a). The modest increases in cAMP are capable of increasing amino acid transport (Drezner *et al.*, 1975). In contrast, prostaglandin A (PGA) and, to a lesser extent, prostaglandin B (PGB) cause a marked disruption of embryonic chick cartilage metabolism *in vitro* (Eisenbarth *et al.*, 1974a; Eisenbarth and Lebovitz, 1974a). The synthesis of cartilage DNA, RNA, total proteins, and proteoglycans are remarkably inhibited as estimated by incorporation of radiolabeled precursors. The effects of PGA require a latent period of 1 or 2 hours, but after its effect has started it is irreversible. PGA inhibition of cartilage macromolecule synthesis is dose-related over a concentration range of 1–25 μg/ml. PGB appears to compete equally well with PGA for binding to the site of action that causes inhibition of the synthesis of macromolecules, but its intrinsic activity is about 50% that if PGA (Eisenbarth and Lebovitz, 1974a). Prostaglandins E and F have no effect on cartilage macromolecule synthesis. PGA inhibits *in vitro* macromolecule synthesis in malignant chondrocytes as well as embryonic chondrocytes (Eisenbarth *et al.*, 1974b). Figure 5 schematically represents the two sites of action of prostaglandins on cartilage and indicates the chemical structures that differentiate A and B from E and F classes of prostaglandins.

The mechanism and significance of PGA effects on cartilage are obscure. Tatum and Lebovitz (1975) have shown that PGA inhibits deoxyglucose uptake and lactate production by embryonic chick cartilage *in vitro*. These data do not indicate whether the inhibition of glycolysis is related to the inhibition of macromolecule synthesis. Wong *et al.* (1975)

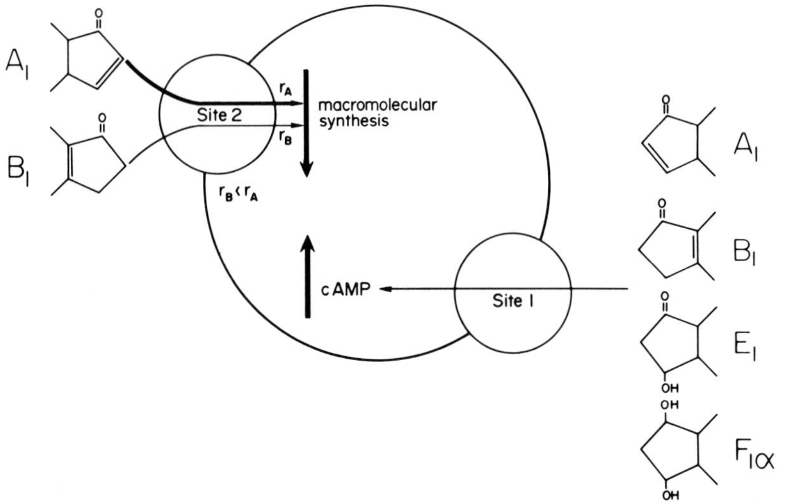

FIGURE 5. Schematic representation of the two sites of prostaglandin action on cartilage. A_1, B_1, E_1, and F_1 refer to prostaglandins A_1, B_1, E_1, and F_1, respectively; $r_B < r_A$ signifies that prostaglandin B has less inhibitory activity on cartilage macromolecule synthesis than does prostaglandin A.

have dissected chick epiphyseal cartilages and measured the prostaglandin synthetic and degradative enzyme activity in each zone. Synthetase activity was highest in the zone of cartilage hypertrophy and degradative enzymes were highest in the zone of cartilage proliferation. These observations raise the interesting possibility that endogenous PGA might play a regulatory role in controlling cartilage growth and maturation with low levels in proliferating chondrocytes and high levels in hypertrophied chondrocytes leading to death and replacement by osseous tissue.

C. FATTY ACIDS

The possibility that circulating fatty acids may play a regulatory role in cartilage growth and metabolism has been raised by several recent studies (Delcher *et al.*, 1973; Eisenbarth *et al.*, 1973). Fatty acids (0.1–1.0 mM) cause a relatively small and frequently statistically insignificant inhibition of $^{35}SO_4$ incorporation into proteoglycans, [^{3}H]leucine incorporation into total proteins and [^{3}H]uridine incorporation into RNA in embryonic chick cartilage *in vitro* under unstimulated (basal) conditions. Striking inhibition of the incorporation of these radiolabeled precursors into macromolecules *in vitro* is found under conditions of serum sulfation factor stimulation. These effects are seen with short (butyrate), medium (octanoate) and long (palmitate and oleate) chain fatty acids

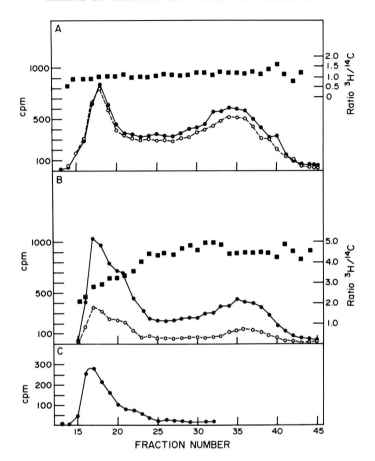

FIGURE 6. (A) The effect of serum stimulation on leucine incorporation *in vitro* into the chondromucoprotein-rich fraction. [^{14}C]Leucine (0.12 μCi) was incubated with four cartilages in the presence of serum; [^{3}H]leucine (0.25 μCi) was incubated with four other cartilages in the absence of serum. The cartilages in each group were pooled and fractionated into chondromucoprotein-rich fractions. The fractions were dissolved in dodecyl sulfate buffer and cochromatographed. The ratio (■) of [^{3}H]leucine (●——●) to [^{14}C]leucine (○- - -○) incorporation is identical throughout the chromatogram, indicating that serum stimulates leucine incorporation into all proteins of the B fraction to the same extent. (B) The effect of 1 mM butyrate on stimulated leucine incorporation into the chondromucoprotein-rich fraction. [^{14}C]Leucine (0.05 μCi) was incubated *in vitro* with four cartilages in the presence of serum, and [^{3}H]leucine (0.25 μCi) was incubated with another four cartilages in the presence of serum plus 1 mM butyrate. The cartilages in each group were pooled and fractioned into chondromucoprotein-rich fractions which were cochromatographed. The ratio (■) of [^{3}H]leucine (●——●) to [^{14}C]leucine (○- - -○) was depressed in the first 25 fractions. This indicates that butyrate inhibits [^{3}H]leucine incorporation to a greater extent in the early protein fractions, as compared to its

but not with ketones (β-hydroxybutyrate and acetoacetate) or acetate. The actions of fatty acids are reversible and are not seen in cartilages incubated in medium containing serum from hypophysectomized rats, suggesting that the effects are somewhat specific for growth hormone-dependent serum factors.

Employing fractionation techniques and specific radiolabeled precursors, it was possible to show that fatty acids inhibit serum sulfation factor stimulation of proteoglycan, collagen, and some other cartilage proteins (Eisenbarth et al., 1973). However, as shown in Fig. 6, fatty acids do not inhibit radiolabeled leucine incorporation into all proteins stimulated by serum sulfation factor. In this particular experiment the cartilage proteins were fractionated into a relatively insoluble collagen-rich fraction and a soluble chondromucoprotein-rich fraction. The data show that serum sulfation factor stimulates radiolabeled leucine incorporation equally into all the proteins of the chondromucoprotein-rich fraction, but that fatty acids primarily inhibit the stimulation of the chondromucoproteins (proteoglycans).

The mechanisms by which fatty acids inhibit the major actions of serum sulfation factor on cartilage metabolism are unknown. Preliminary studies indicate that the effects are uncompetitive with serum sulfation factor, that they occur in costal cartilage from hypophysectomized rats, and that they probably do not result from fatty acid oxidation (Eisenbarth and Lebovitz, 1975).

The data suggest a possible mechanism for dissociating the effects of growth hormone on the skeletal system from its other metabolic actions. Figure 7 depicts such a scheme. Growth hormone secretion results in relatively fixed levels of circulating serum sulfation factor. The actions of the sulfation factor on cartilage would be controlled by the metabolic state of the animal. Conditions leading to decreased fatty acids (food ingestion, insulin, etc.) would facilitate sulfation factor action on cartilage anabolic processes. Conditions leading to increased fatty acids (starvation, stress, illness) would block sulfation factor mediated anabolic activity in cartilage. The other actions of growth hormone would be mediated by the levels of growth hormone and independent of the effects on

effect on smaller proteins that elute later. (C) The chromatography on agarose 4B of $^{35}SO_4$-labeled proteins of the chondromucoprotein-rich fraction. In the presence of 5% serum, $^{35}SO_4$ (0.4 μCi) was incubated in vitro with four cartilages. The cartilages were pooled, the chondromucoprotein-rich fraction was isolated and chromatographed. The elution pattern indicates that the $^{35}SO_4$ is incorporated into large molecules which appear with the exclusion volume of the column. ●——●, $^{35}SO_4$ counts. Reprinted from Eisenbarth et al., Biochem. Biophys. Acta 331, (1973).

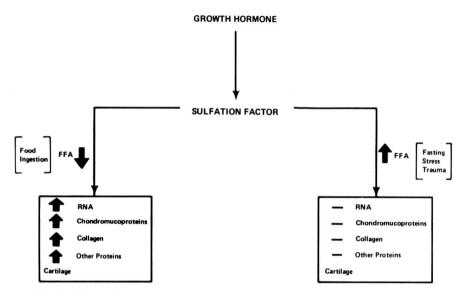

Fig. 7. Schematic representation of fatty acid modulation of growth hormone action on cartilage growth and metabolism. FFA, free fatty acids. See text for further details.

the skeleton. Many additional studies are necessary to test the validity of this hypothesis.

D. Inhibitors

Serum contains one or more factors that are able to interfere with bioassay determinations of serum sulfation factor activity. Relatively little is known about the nature or significance of these factors. Salmon (1973) has reported that serum from hypophysectomized rats contains a non-dialyzable factor, probably a peptide, which inhibits somatomedin action. Eisenbarth and Lebovitz (1974b) showed that circulating glucocorticoids constitute another group of serum factors that inhibit cartilage metabolism. Additional investigations of serum inhibitors of cartilage metabolism need to be made to determine their importance in regulating cartilage metabolism.

V. Summary and Conclusions

While many advances have been made in understanding the basic biochemistry and physiology of cartilage and its matrix proteins, present knowledge about the hormonal and metabolic regulation of these processes is still fragmentary. *In vivo* studies indicate that hormones, such as growth hormone, thyroid hormones, glucocorticoids, estrogens, and androgens, exert profound effects on epiphyseal cartilage in immature animals. Growth hormone and, to a lesser degree, thyroid hormones and androgens, stimulate epiphyseal cartilage anabolic processes and facilitate cartilage growth. Thyroid hormones, estrogens, and androgens stimulate the process of epiphyseal cartilage maturation wherein the epiphyseal cartilage plate becomes less active, narrows and finally is replaced by osseous tissue. Glucocorticoids inhibit both epiphyseal cartilage growth and maturation.

In order to define the mechanisms by which these hormones affect cartilage metabolism many *in vitro* systems have been developed and applied to the study of hormone actions. With the exception of defining the sulfation factor mechanism of growth hormone action, these systems have generally not succeeded in elucidating the mechanisms of hormone actions on cartilage. For example, thyroid hormones, estrogens, and androgens have not consistently influenced *in vitro* cartilage metabolism. Glucocorticoid effects on cartilage metabolism *in vitro* have generally required large concentrations of hormones and the effects vary rather remarkably. These data are consistent with one of the following hypotheses: (1) thyroid and steroid hormones stimulate the production of *in vivo* factors that mediate their actions on cartilage; (2) the *in vitro* systems are incomplete, and, as such, they are unable to support the hormones' actions; or (3) the hormones are affecting processes that have not been measured in the *in vitro* systems.

It has not been feasible to describe the incubation conditions for each *in vitro* study that has been reviewed, but it is noteworthy that many, perhaps most, of the studies have been carried out in incubation media that are either totally deficient in amino acids or contain suboptimal amounts of some amino acids. The importance of the amino acid composition of the medium has been emphasized in the studies of Salmon (1960a), which showed the essential nature of valine for insulin effects on costal cartilage from hypophysectomized rats; and in our own studies (Beuttel *et al.*, 1975), which indicate that deletion of any essential amino acid from the incubation medium markedly alters the effects of hormones, such as insulin, or metabolic regulators, such as butyrylated cAMP derivatives, on embryonic chick cartilage metabolism. The importance of other components of incubation medium on hormone responsiveness of cartilage has received scant attention.

The type of cartilage employed in a study and the nature of the particular *in vitro* system may also influence the observed action of a specific hormone. Cartilage is a complex tissue. Its characteristics change during differentiation and growth of the animal. Hormone responsiveness may be different during each stage of differentiation and growth. The initial phase of cartilage regulation occurs in the embryo, where stem cells differentiate into chondroblasts. The nature of the differentiation process (reviewed by Levitt and Dorfman, 1974) is still poorly understood. The only hormones implicated as possibly playing any role in early chondrogenesis are thyroxine and triiodothyronine (see Section III, F) and glucocorticoids (see Section III, I). After differentiation, cartilage is either replaced by bone or further differentiated into specialized cartilage, such as epiphyseal, articular, intervertebral, or structural (nasal, auricular, rib, laryngeal, and tracheal). Most *in vivo* studies of hormone actions on cartilage metabolism have focused on epiphyseal cartilage. It is not known whether all cartilages respond to the same hormones and, if they do, whether the effects are the same. Since the function of epiphyseal cartilage is so different from that of other types of cartilage, one might presume that some of its responses to hormones would be unique. However, most studies indicate that all types of cartilage respond to somatomedin stimulation with an increase in macromolecule synthesis and growth. Additionally, where appropriate studies have been done, costal cartilage, articular cartilage, and embryonic chick cartilage appear to respond to hormones and metabolic factors similarly to epiphyseal cartilage. Sufficient data are not available to indicate whether any differences in hormone actions occur in different types of cartilage. Therefore, although it seems unlikely, some of the differences in hormone actions noted in various studies could be due to the origin of the particular chondrocytes. Significant differences do exist between results obtained with cartilage incubated *in vitro* in organ culture and chondrocytes grown in tissue culture.

From the data reviewed, it is clear that immature cartilage must be considered a major target organ for hormone actions in much the same manner as liver, muscle, and adipose tissue. Most hormones appear to affect cartilage metabolism. It is of interest that each hormone seems to have a specific and possibly unique spectrum of biological actions on cartilage. Whether these hormone actions are of importance only in the growth and metabolism of immature cartilage, or play key roles in the maintenance and repair of adult cartilage needs to be investigated. There are data to suggest that the development of osteoarthritis and the maintenance of articular cartilage involve the actions of one or more hormones (Mankin, 1974).

Most studies of the action of hormones on cartilage metabolism have limited themselves to quantitative measurement of macromolecule synthesis. Little is known about specific mechanisms of hormone actions;

and the functions of metabolic regulators, such as intracellular cAMP and prostaglandins, and extracellular fatty acids, are just beginning to be explored. As noted in Section II, there are many sites in cartilage metabolic pathways that could be amenable to regulation by hormones and related substances. Alterations of these pathways could lead to qualitative and quantitative changes in cartilage growth, matrix proteins, and cartilage function.

Interference with glycolysis could lead to disruption of energy production and a decrease in chondrocyte synthetic activity and perhaps even loss of viability. This is one of the mechanisms that has been proposed for glucocorticoid action on cartilage. Prostaglandin A interferes with glycolysis. The mechanism of this inhibition of glycolysis and its relationship to inhibition of macromolecule synthesis are currently being investigated. Some authors have suggested that achondroplasia may be associated with a metabolic defect in cartilage glucose utilization (Shephard, 1971).

Regulation might occur in the UDP-monosaccharide synthetic pathway. Figure 2 depicts the sites at which control of this pathway are known to occur. Arrambide et al. (1968) claim that 5'-adenylate inhibits L-glutamine D-fructose-6-phosphate aminotransferase activity in chick cartilage and decreases glucosamine 6-phosphate formation. Direct or indirect effects of hormones or metabolic regulators on the synthesis of UDP-monosaccharides could alter the quantity and nature of glycosaminoglycans being synthesized by cartilage.

Little is known concerning possible effects of hormones in altering the structure of the cartilage proteoglycans or collagen. Kofoed et al. (1969, 1970) have described changes in the proportions of different glycosaminoglycans in tracheal cartilage in thyroid-insufficient rats and in testosterone-treated rats. Lash and Whitehouse (1961) observed results in studies with embryonic chick somites which suggested that glucocorticoids interfere with the sulfation of glycosaminoglycans in developing cartilage. Collagen structure can be modified by incubating chick embryo cartilage with 2-deoxy-D-glucose which inhibits glycosylation and leads to the synthesis of fully hydroxylated but not glycosylated collagen (Blumenkrantz et al., 1969). It therefore seems likely that hormones may regulate the structure of cartilage matrix proteins, as well as the quantity synthesized.

The secretion of cartilage matrix proteins from the chondrocyte into the matrix involves an intracellular microtubular system (Jansen and Bornstein, 1974). No information is available concerning hormone effects on this microtubule system, but in light of other information on the regulation of microtubular function this would be a likely site for hormone control.

Investigations of hormonal and metabolic regulation of cartilage metabolism are in their infancy and knowledge today might be compared to that which existed in the field of hormonal regulation of adipose tissue 15 years ago. Many unresolved questions concerning the specific effects that hormones have on cartilage remain. Little is known about the mechanisms of hormone actions. The regulation of the specialized metabolic pathways in cartilage are yet to be elucidated. The relationships of disease of cartilage to abnormal hormonal or metabolic regulation need to be thoroughly explored. The present review has attempted to summarize our current knowledge of hormone actions on cartilage in light of the present understanding of cartilage biochemistry and physiology. Salient problems for future investigations have been discussed.

REFERENCES

Adams, J. B. (1960). *Biochem. J.* **76**, 520.
Adams, J. B., and Rienitz, K. G. (1961). *Biochim. Biophys. Acta* **51**, 567.
Adamson, L. F. (1970). *Biochim. Biophys. Acta* **201**, 446.
Adamson, L. F., and Anast, C. S. (1966). *Biochim. Biophys. Acta* **121**, 10.
Adamson, L. F., and Ingbar, S. H. (1967a). *J. Biol. Chem.* **242**, 2646.
Adamson, L. F., and Ingbar, S. H. (1967b). *Endocrinology* **81**, 1362.
Adamson, L. F., and Ingbar, S. H. (1967c). *Endocrinology* **81**, 1372.
Adamson, L. F., Gleason, S., and Anast, C. (1964). *Biochim. Biophys. Acta* **83**, 262.
Adamson, L. F., Langeluttig, S. G., and Anast, C. S. (1966a). *Biochim. Biophys. Acta* **115**, 345.
Adamson, L. F., Langeluttig, S. G., and Anast, C. S. (1966b). *Biochim. Biophys. Acta* **115**, 355.
Adamson, L. F., Herington, A. C., and Bornstein, J. (1972). *Biochim. Biophys. Acta* **282**, 352.
Almqvist, S., Ikkos, D., and Luft, R. (1961). *Acta Endocrinol. (Copenhagen)* **37**, 138.
Antoniades, H. N. (1969). *Proc. Congr. Int. Diabetes Fed., 6th, 1967* pp. 171–192.
Arrambide, E., Patrone, M. G., and Calcagno, M. (1968). *Experientia* **24**, 896.
Asling, C. W., Becks, H., Simpson, M. E., and Evans, H. M. (1949). *Anat. Rec.* **104**, 255.
Asling, C. W., Tse, F., and Rosenberg, L. L. (1968). *Proc. Int. Symp. Growth Hor., 1967* Int. Cong. Ser. No. 158, pp. 319–331.
Aureli, G., Rizzotti, M., Balduini, C., and Castellani, A. A. (1969). *Riv. Istochim. Norm. Patol.* **15**, 9.
Baker, J. F., Rodén, L., and Yamagata, S. (1971). *Biochem. J.* **125**, 93P.
Bala, R. M., Ferguson, K. A., and Beck, J. C. (1970). *Endocrinology* **87**, 506.
Balduini, C., Brovelli, A., and Castellani, A. A. (1970). *Biochem. J.* **120**, 719.
Balogh, K., and Kunin, A. S. (1971). *Clin. Orthop. Relat. Res.* **80**, 208.
Barrett, A. J. (1968). *Compr. Biochem.* **26**, Part B, 425–471.
Barrett, A. J., Sledge, C. B., and Dingle, J. T. (1966). *Nature (London)* **211**, 83.
Bélanger, L. F., Dimond, M. T., and Copp, D. H. (1973). *Gen. Comp. Endocrinol.* **20**, 297.
Berntsen, E. (1968). *Acta Endocrinol. (Copenhagen)* **57**, 69.

Beuttel, S. B., Eisenbarth, G. S., and Lebovitz, H. E. (1975). In preparation.
Birch, B. M., Delcher, H. K., Rendall, J. L., Eisenbarth, G. S., and Lebovitz, H. E. (1973). *Biochem. Biophys. Res. Commun.* **52**, 1184.
Blodgett, F. M., Burgin, L., Lezzoni, D., Gribetz, D., and Talbott, N. B. (1956). *N. Engl. J. Med.* **254**, 636.
Blumenkrantz, N., and Prockop, D. J. (1970). *Biochim. Biophys. Acta* **208**, 461.
Blumenkrantz, N., Rosenbloom, J., and Prockop, D. J. (1969). *Biochim. Biophys. Acta* **192**, 81.
Bornstein, P. (1974). *Annu. Rev. Biochem.* **43**, 567.
Boström, H., and Mansson, B. (1952). *J. Biol. Chem.* **196**, 483.
Breuer, C. B. (1969). *Endocrinology* **85**, 989.
Buddecke, E., and Sziegoleit, M. (1964). *Hoppe-Seyler's Z. Physiol. Chem.* **337**, 66.
Bywaters, E. G. L. (1936). *Nature (London)* **138**, 30.
Bywaters, E. G. L. (1937). *J. Pathol. Bacteriol.* **44**, 247.
Campo, R. D. (1970). *Clin. Orthop. Relat. Res.* **68**, 182.
Campo, R. D., and Tourtellotte, C. D. (1967). *Biochim. Biophys. Acta* **141**, 615.
Cipera, J. D. (1962). *Can. J. Biochem. Physiol.* **40**, 65.
Cipera, J. D., and Cherian, A. G. (1969). *Calcif. Tissue Res.* 3, 30.
Clark, G., and Gavin, J. A. (1962). *Anat. Rec.* **143**, 179.
Clark, I., and Umbreit, W. W. (1954). *Proc. Soc. Exp. Biol. Med.* **86**, 558.
Collins, E. J., and Anilane, J. (1959). *Experientia* **15**, 116.
Collins, E. J., Lyster, S. C., and Carpenter, O. S. (1961). *Acta Endocrinol. (Copenhagen)* **36**, 51.
Conklin, J. L. (1963). *Amer. J. Anat.* **112**, 259.
Contopoulos, A. N., Simpson, M. E., and Koneff, A. A. (1958). *Endocrinology* **63**, 642.
Corvol, M. T., Malemud, C. J., and Sokoloff, L. (1972). *Endocrinology* **90**, 262.
D'Abramo, F., and Lipmann, F. (1957). *Biochim. Biophys. Acta* **25**, 211.
Daughaday, W. H. (1971). *Advan. Intern. Med.* **17**, 237.
Daughaday, W. H., and Garland, J. T. (1972). In "Growth and Growth Hormones" (A. Pecile and E. E. Müller, eds.), Int. Congr. Ser. No. 244, pp. 168–179. Excerpta Med. Found., Amsterdam.
Daughaday, W. H., and Kipnis, D. M. (1966). *Recent Progr. Horm. Res.* **22**, 49.
Daughaday, W. H., and Mariz, I. (1962). *J. Lab. Clin. Med.* **59**, 741.
Daughaday, W. H., and Reeder, C. (1966). *J. Lab. Clin. Med.* **68**, 357.
Daughaday, W. H., Heins, J. N., Srivastava, L., and Hammer, C. (1968). *J. Lab. Clin. Med.* **72**, 803.
Daughaday, W. H., Hall, K., Raben, M. S., Salmon, W. D., Van den Brande, J. L., and VanWyk, J. J. (1972). *Nature (London)* **235**, 107.
Davidson, E. A., and Small, W. (1963). *Biochim. Biophys. Acta* **69**, 445.
Davidson, E. A., and Woodhall, B. (1959). *J. Biol. Chem.* **234**, 2951.
Dearden, L. C., and Mosier, H. D. (1972). *Clin. Orthop. Relat. Res.* **87**, 322.
Delbrück, A. (1970). *Enzymol. Biol. Clin.* **11**, 130.
Delcher, H. K., Eisenbarth, G. S., and Lebovitz, H. E. (1973). *J. Biol. Chem.* **248**, 1901.
Denduchis, B., Kefalides, N. A., and Bezkorovainy, A. (1970). *Arch. Biochem. Biophys.* **138**, 582.
Denko, C. W., and Bergenstal, D. M. (1955). *Endocrinology* **57**, 76.
Dickens, F., and Weil-Malherbe, H. (1936). *Nature (London)* **138**, 125.
Dickerman, E., Dickerman, S., and Meites, J. (1972). In "Growth and Growth Hor-

mones" (A. Pecile and E. E. Müller, eds.), Int. Congr. No. 244, pp. 252–260. Excerpta Med. Found., Amsterdam.

Drezner, M. K., and Lebovitz, H. E. (1975). In preparation.

Drezner, M. K., Eisenbarth, G. S., Neelon, F. A., and Lebovitz, H. E. (1975). *Biochim. Biophys. Acta* **381**, 384.

Drezner, M. K., Neelon, F. A., Delcher, H. K., and Lebovitz, H. E. (1976). In preparation.

Dulak, N. C., and Temin, H. M. (1973a). *J. Cell. Physiol.* **81**, 153.

Dulak, N. C., and Temin, H. M. (1973b). *J. Cell. Physiol.* **81**, 161.

Dziewiatkowski, D. D. (1951). *J. Biol. Chem.* **189**, 717.

Dziewiatkowski, D. D. (1957). *J. Exp. Med.* **105**, 81.

Dziewiatkowski, D. D. (1964). *Biophys. J., Suppl.* **4**, 215.

Dziewiatkowski, D. D., Benesch, R. E., and Benesch, R. (1949). *J. Biol. Chem.* **178**, 931.

Ebert, P. S., and Prockop, D. J. (1967). *Biochim. Biophys. Acta* **136**, 45.

Eeg-Larsen, N. (1956). *Acta Physiol. Scand.* **38**, Suppl., 128.

Eisenbarth, G. S., and Lebovitz, H. E. (1974a). *Prostaglandins* **7**, 11.

Eisenbarth, G. S., and Lebovitz, H. E. (1974b). *Endocrinology* **95**, 1600.

Eisenbarth, G. S., and Lebovitz, H. E. (1975). In preparation.

Eisenbarth, G. S., Beuttel, S. C., and Lebovitz, H. E. (1973). *Biochim. Biophys. Acta* **331**, 397.

Eisenbarth, G. S., Beuttel, S. C., and Lebovitz, H. E. (1974a). *J. Pharmacol. Exp. Ther.* **189**, 213.

Eisenbarth, G. S., Wellman, D. K., and Lebovitz, H. E. (1974b). *Biochem. Biophys. Res. Commun.* **60**, 1302.

Eisenbarth, G. S., Drezner, M. K., and Lebovitz, H. E. (1975). *J. Pharmacol. Exp. Ther.* **192**, 630.

Ellis, S., Huble, J., and Simpson, M. E. (1953). *Proc. Soc. Exp. Biol. Med.* **84**, 603.

Endo, H., Murota, S. I., and Enomoto, H. (1969). *Endocrinol. Jap.* **16**, 115.

Evans, E. S., Rosenberg, L. L., Evans, A. B., and Koneff, A. A. (1964). *Endocrinology* **74**, 770.

Fahmy, A., Lee, S., and Johnson, P. (1971a). *Calcif. Tissue Res.* **7**, 12.

Fahmy, A., Talley, P., Frazier, H. M., and Hillman, J. W. (1971b). *Calcif. Tissue Res.* **7**, 139.

Farrehi, C. (1968). *Clin. Pediat.* **7**, 134.

Fine, A. S., and Person, P. (1970). *Calif. Tissue Res.* **5**, 85.

Finkelstein, J. W., Kream, J., Ludan, A., and Hellman, L. (1972). *J. Clin. Endocrinol. Metab.* **35**, 13.

Foss, G. L. (1965). *Arch. Dis. Childhood* **40**, 66.

Frantz, A. G., and Rabkin, M. T. (1964). *N. Engl. J. Med.* **271**, 1375.

Frantz, A. G., and Rabkin, M. T. (1965). *J. Clin. Endocrinol. Metab.* **25**, 1470.

Frasier, S. D., and Smith, F. G. (1968). *J. Clin. Endocrinol. Metab.* **28**, 416.

Frazier, W. A., Angeletti, R. H., and Bradshaw, R. A. (1972). *Science* **176**, 482.

Froesch, E. R. (1963). In "Fortschritte Der Diabetes Forschung" (K. Oberdisse, ed.), pp. 30–36. Thieme, Stuttgart.

Froesch, E. R. (1974). *Recent Progr. Horm. Res.* **30**, 295.

Froesch, E. R., Bürgi, H., Ramseier, E. B., Bally, P., and Labhart, A. (1963). *J. Clin. Invest.* **42**, 1816.

Froesch, E. R., Bürgi, H., Müller, W. A., Humbel, R. E., Jakob, A., and Labhart, A. (1967). *Recent Progr. Horm. Res.* **23**, 565.

Fukushi, S., and Spiro, R. G. (1969). *J. Biol. Chem.* **244**, 2041.

Gaarenstroom, J. H., and Levie, L. H. (1939). *J. Endocrinol.* **1**, 420.

Gaillard, P. J., Moskalewski, S., Verhoog, M. J., and Wassenaar, A. M. (1968). *Calcif. Tisue Res., Suppl.* **49**.

Gardell, S. (1955). *Acta Chem. Scand.* **9**, 1035.

Garland, J. T., Ruegamer, W. R., and Daughaday, W. H. (1971). *Endocrinology* **88**, 924.

Gerber, B. R., and Schubert, M. (1964). *Biopolymers* **2**, 259.

Geschwind, I. I., and Li, C. H. (1955). *In* "The Hypophyseal Growth Hormone: Nature and Actions" (R. W. Smith, Jr., O. H. Gaebler, and C. N. H. Long, eds.), pp. 28–53. McGraw-Hill, New York.

Gjedde, F. (1964). *In* "Structure and Metabolism of Pancreatic Islets" (S. E. Brolin, B. Hellman, and H. Knutson, eds.), pp. 469–476. Permagon, Oxford.

Gjedde, F. (1968). *Acta Endocrinol. (Copenhagen)* **57**, 505.

Goh, A. T.-W., and Lowther, D. A. (1966). *Nature (London)* **210**, 1270.

Goodall, C. M., and Gavin, J. B. (1966). *Acta Endocrinol. (Copenhagen)* **51**, 315.

Goodman, G. C., and Lane, N. (1966). *J. Cell Biol.* **21**, 353.

Goodman, H. M. (1963). *Endocrinology* **73**, 421.

Grant, D. B. (1972). *Clin. Endocrinol. (Oxford)* **1**, 387.

Greenspan, F. S., Li, C. H., Simpson, M. E., and Evans, H. M. (1949). *Endocrinology* **45**, 455.

Guri, C. D., and Bernstein, D. S. (1964). *Proc. Soc. Exp. Biol. Med.* **116**, 702.

Guri, C. D., and Bernstein, D. S. (1965). *Proc. Soc. Exp. Biol. Med.* **118**, 650.

Hahn, T. J., Downing, S. J., and Phang, J. M. (1969). *Biochim. Biophys. Acta* **184**, 675.

Hahn, T. J., Downing, S. J., and Phang, J. M. (1971). *Amer. J. Physiol.* **220**, 1717.

Hall, B. K. (1973). *Anat. Rec.* **176**, 49.

Hall, K. (1970). *Acta Endocrinol. (Copenhagen)* **63**, 338.

Hall, K. (1972). *Acta Endocrinol. (Copenhagen) Suppl.* **163**, 3.

Hall, K., and Božović, M. (1969). *Horm. Metab. Res., Suppl.* **1**, 235.

Hall, K., and Luft, R. (1974). *Advan. Metab. Disord.* **7**, 1.

Hall, K., and Uthne, K. (1971). *Acta Med. Scand.* **190**, 137.

Hall, K., and Uthne, K. (1972). *In* "Growth and Growth Hormones" (A. Pecile and E. E. Müller, eds.) Int. Congr. Ser. No. 244, pp. 192–198. Excerpta Med. Found., Amsterdam.

Hall, K., and Van Wyk, J. J. (1974). *Curr. Top. Exp. Endocrinol.* **2**, 155.

Hall, K., Holmbren, A., and Lindahl, U. (1970). *Biochim. Biophys. Acta* **201**, 398.

Hall, K., Takano, K., and Fryklund, L. (1974). *J. Clin. Endocrinol. Metab.* **39**, 973.

Hallén, A. (1958). *Acta Chem. Scand.* **12**, 1869.

Hallén, A. (1962). *Acta Chem. Scand.* **16**, 705.

Halme, J., Uitto, J., and Kivirikko, K. I. (1972). *Endocrinology* **90**, 1476.

Hartog, M., Gaafar, M. A., and Fraser, R. (1964). *Lancet* **2**, 376.

Hasegawa, E., Delbrück, A., and Lipman, F. (1961). *Fed. Proc., Fed. Amer. Soc. Exp. Biol.* **20**, 86.

Heins, J. N., Garland, J. T., and Daughaday, W. H. (1970). *Endocrinology* **87**, 688.

Helting, T., and Rodén, L. (1968). *Biochem. Biophys. Res. Commun.* **31**, 786.

Helting, T., and Rodén, L. (1969). *J. Biol. Chem.* **244**, 2790.

Herbai, G. (1971a). *Acta Pharmacol. Toxicol.* **29**, 164.

Herbai, G. (1971b). *Acta Physiol. Scand.* **83**, 77.

Herbai, G. (1971c). *Acta Endocrinol. (Copenhagen)* **66**, 333.

Herbai, G. (1971d). *Acta Endocrinol. (Copenhagen)* **68**, 249.

Herbai, G. (1971e). *Acta Pharmacol. Toxicol.* **29**, 177.

Herington, A., Adamson, L. F., and Bornstein, J. (1972). *Biochim. Biophys. Acta* **286**, 164.

Hershko, A., Mamont, P., Shields, R., and Tompkins, G. M. (1971). *Nature (London), New Biol.* **232**, 206.

Hickey, E. D., and Klein, N. W. (1971). *Teratology* **4**, 453.

Hills, G. M. (1940). *Biochem. J.* **34**, 1070.

Hintz, R. L., Clemmons, D. R., Underwood, L. E., and VanWyk, J. J. (1972). *Proc. Nat. Acad. Sci. U.S.* **69**, 2351.

Hjertquist, S.-O., and Vejlens, L. (1968). *Calcif. Tissue Res.* **2**, 314.

Holladay, L. A., Levine, J. H., Nicholson, W. E., Orth, D. N., Salmon, W. D., Jr., and Puett, D. (1975). *Biochim. Biophys. Acta* **381**, 47.

Howard, E. (1962). *Endocrinology* **70**, 131.

Howard, E. (1963). *Endocrinology* **72**, 11.

Ide, T., Kuzuya, T., Kajinuma, H., Kanazawa, Y., and Kosaka, K. (1969). *Diabetes* **18**, 65.

Ingle, D. J., Higgins, S. M., and Kendall, E. C. (1938). *Anat. Rec.* **71**, 363.

Jakob, A., Hauri, C., and Froesch, E. R. (1968). *J. Clin. Invest.* **47**, 2678.

Jansen, H. W., and Bornstein, P. (1974). *Biochim. Biophys. Acta* **362**, 150.

Jefferson, L. S., and Korner, A. (1967). *Biochem. J.* **104**, 826.

Josimovich, J. B., Mintz, D. H., and Finster, J. L. (1967). *Endocrinology* **81**, 1428.

Joss, E. C., Zuppinger, N. A., and Sobel, E. H. (1963). *Endocrinology* **72**, 123.

Kajinuma, H., Ide, T., Kuzuya, T., and Kosaka, K. (1969). *Diabetes* **18**, 75.

Kaplan, D., and Fisher, B. (1964). *Biochim. Biophys. Acta* **83**, 102.

Kaplan, D., and Meyer, K. (1959). *Nature (London)* **183**, 1267.

Katz, H. P., Youlton, R., Kaplan, S. L., and Grumbach, M. M. (1969). *J. Clin. Endocrinol. Metab.* **29**, 346.

Kefalides, N. A., and Denduchis, B. (1969). *Biochemistry* **8**, 4613.

Kember, N. F. (1971). *Cell Tissue Kinet.* **4**, 193.

Kenny, F. M., Guyda, J. H., Wright, J. C., and Friesen, H. G. (1973). *J. Clin. Endocrinol. Metab.* **36**, 378.

Kofoed, J. A., Bozzini, C. E., and Tocci, A. A. (1969). *Endocrinology* **45**, 609.

Kofoed, J. A., Bozzini, C. E., and Tocci, A. A. (1970). *Acta Endocrinol. (Copenhagen)* **63**, 193.

Koneff, A. A., Scow, R. O., Simpson, M. E., Li, C. H., and Evans, H. M. (1949). *Anat. Rec.* **104**, 465.

Kornfeld, S., Kornfeld, R., Neufeld, E. F., and O'Brien, P. J. (1964). *Proc. Nat. Acad. Sci. U.S.* **52**, 371.

Kostyo, J. L. (1968). *Ann. N.Y. Acad. Sci.* **148**, 389.

Kostyo, J. L., and Nutting, D. F. (1973). *Horm. Metab. Res.* **5**, 167.

Kostyo, J. L., Uthne, K., Reagan, C. R., and Gimpel, L. P. (1973). *In* "Advances in Human Growth Hormone Research" (S. Raiti, ed.), DHEW Publ. No. (NIH) 74-612, pp. 127–135. US Govt. Printing Office, Washington, D.C.

Kowalewski, K. (1958). *Endocrinology* **63**, 759.

Kühn, R., and Keppelman, H. J. (1958). *Justus Liebigs Ann. Chem.* **611**, 254.

Kunin, A. S., and Meyer, W. L. (1969). *Arch. Biochem. Biophys.* **129**, 421.

Kuwabara, G. (1932). *J. Biochem. (Tokyo)* **16**, 389.

Labhart, A., Oelz, O, Bünzli, H. F., Humbel, R. E., Ritschard, W. J., and Froesch, E. R. (1972). *Isr. J. Med. Sci.* **8**, 901.

Laron, Z., Karp, M., Pertzelan, A., and Kauli, R. (1972). *Isr. J. Med. Sci.* **8**, 440.

Lash, J. W., and Whitehouse, M. W. (1961). *Lab. Invest.* **10**, 388.

Laskin, D. M., Sarnat, B. G., and Bain, J. A. (1952). *Proc. Soc. Exp. Biol. Med.* **79**, 474.

Lawrence, R. T. B., Salter, J. M., and Best, C. H. (1954). *Brit. Med. J.* **2**, 437.

Layton, L. L. (1951). *Proc. Soc. Exp. Biol. Med.* **76**, 596.

Leonards, J. R., Landau, B. R., and Bartsch, G. (1962). *J. Lab. Clin. Med.* **60**, 552.

Levi-Montalcini, R., and Angeletti, P. U. (1968). *Physiol. Rev.* **48**, 534.

Levitt, D., and Dorfman, A. (1974). *Curr. Top. Develop. Biol.* **8**, 103.

Liberti, J. P. (1970). *Biochem. Biophys. Res. Commun.* **39**, 356.

Liberti, J. P. (1973). *Can. J. Biochem.* **51**, 1113.

Loewi, G. (1965). *Ann. Rheum. Dis.* **24**, 528.

McConaghey, P. (1972). *J. Endocrinol.* **52**, 1.

McConaghey, P., and Dehnel, J. (1972). *J. Endocrinol.* **52**, 587.

McConaghey, P., and Sledge C. B. (1970). *Nature (London)* **225**, 1249.

Machledt, J., and Lebovitz, H. E. (1975). In preparation.

Malemud, C. J., and Sokoloff, L. (1974). *J. Cell. Physiol.* **82**, 171.

Mankin, H. J. (1974). *N. Engl. J. Med.* **291**, 1285 and 1335.

Mankin, H. J., and Conger, K. A. (1966). *Lab. Invest.* **15**, 794.

Mankin, H. J., Zarins, A., and Jaffe, W. L. (1972). *Arthritis Rheum.* **15**, 593.

Marcus, R. E. (1973). *Arthritis Rheum.* **16**, 646.

Marcus, R. E., and Srivastava, V. M. L. (1973). *Proc. Soc. Exp. Biol. Med.* **143**, 488.

Marshall, R. N., Underwood, L. E., Voina, S. J., Foushee, D. B., and VanWyk, J. J. (1974). *J. Clin. Endocrinol. Metab.* **39**, 283.

Martin, H. J., and Matthews, J. L. (1969). *Calcif. Tissue Res.* **4**, 184.

Marx, W., Simpson, M. E., Li, C. H., and Evans, H. M. (1943). *Endocrinology* **33**, 102.

Marx, W., Simpson, M. E., and Evans, H. M. (1944). *Proc. Soc. Exp. Biol. Med.* **55**, 250.

Mathews, M. B. (1971). *Biochem. J.* **125**, 37.

Mathews, M. B., and Glagov, S. (1966). *J. Clin. Invest.* **45**, 1103.

Megyesi, K., Kahn, C. R., Roth, J., and Gorden, P. (1974). *J. Clin. Endocrinol. Metab.* **38**, 931.

Meier, S., and Solursh, M. (1972a). *Gen. Comp. Endocrinol.* **18**, 89.

Meier, S., and Solursh, M. (1972b). *Endocrinology* **90**, 1447.

Meier, S., and Solursh, M. (1973). *Develop. Biol.* **30**, 290.

Meites, J. (1949). *Amer. J. Physiol.* **159**, 281.

Meyer, K., Hoffman, P., and Linker, A. (1958). *Science* **128**, 896.

Meyer, W. L., and Kunin, A. S. (1969). *Arch. Biochem. Biophys.* **129**, 431.

Meyer, W. L., and Kunin, A. S. (1973). *Arch. Biochem. Biophys.* **156**, 122.

Miller, E. J. (1971a). *Biochem. Biophys. Res. Commun.* **42**, 1024.

Miller, E. J. (1971b). *Biochemistry* **10**, 1652.

Miller, E. J. (1971c). *Biochemistry* **10**, 3030.

Miller, E. J. (1972). *Biochemistry* **11**, 4903.

Miller, E. J., and Lunde, L. G. (1973). *Biochemistry* **12**, 3153.

Miller, E. J., and Matukas, V. J. (1969). *Proc. Nat. Acad. Sci. U.S.* **64**, 1264.

Mills, J. B., Regan, C. R., Rudman, D., Kostyo, J. L., Zachariah, P., and Wilhelmi, A. E. (1973). *J. Clin. Invest.* **52**, 2941.

Minot, A. S., and Hillman, J. W. (1967). *Proc. Soc. Exp. Biol. Med.* **126**, 60.

Moon, H. D. (1937). *Proc. Soc. Exp. Biol. Med.* **37**, 34.

Morell, B., and Froesch, E. R. (1973a). *Eur. J. Clin. Invest.* **3**, 112.

Morrell, B., and Froesch, E. R. (1973b). *Eur. J. Clin. Invest.* **3**, 119.

Morris, H. G., Jorgensen, J. R., and Jenkins, S. A. (1968a). *J. Clin. Invest.* **47**, 427.

Morris, H. G., Jorgensen, J. R., Elrick, H., and Goldsmith, R. E. (1968b). *J. Clin. Invest.* **47**, 436.

Mueller, J. F. (1963). *Ann. N.Y. Acad. Sci.* **113**, 217.

Murakawa, S., and Raben, M. S. (1968). *Endocrinology* **83**, 645.

Murota, S., Endo, M., and Tamaoki, B. (1967). *Biochim. Biophys. Acta* **136**, 379.

Murota, S., Kawashima, K., and Endo, H. (1969). *Endocrinol. Jap.* **16**, 109.

Murphy, W. R., Daughaday, W. H., and Hartnett, C. (1956). *J. Lab. Clin. Med.* **47**, 715.

Neufeld, E. F., and Hall, C. W. (1965). *Biochem. Biophys. Res. Commun.* **19**, 456.

Nevo, Z., Horwitz, A. L., and Dorfman, A. (1972). *Develop. Biol.* **28**, 219.

Noble, R. L. (1938). *Lancet* **2**, 192.

Nutting, D. F., Kostyo, J. L., Miller, J. B., and Wilhelmi, A. E. (1972). *Endocrinology* **90**, 1202.

Oelz, O., Jakob, A., and Froesch, E. R. (1970). *Eur. J. Clin. Invest.* **1**, 48.

Oelz, O., Froesch, E. R., Bünzli, H. F., Humbel, R. E., and Ritschard, W. J. (1972). *In* "Handbook of Physiology" (Amer. Physiol. Soc., J. Field, ed.), Sect. 7, Vol. I, pp. 685–702. Williams & Wilkins, Baltimore, Maryland.

Ornoy, A. (1971). *Teratology* **4**, 383.

Pawelek, J. M. (1969). *Develop. Biol.* **19**, 52.

Peake, G. T., Birge, C. A., and Daughaday, W. H. (1973). *Endocrinology* **92**, 487.

Pearce, F. L., Banks, B. E. C., Banthorpe, D. V., Berry, H., Davies, H. S., and Vernon, C. A. (1972). *In* "Nerve Growth Factor and its Antiserum (E. Zamis and J. Knight, eds.), pp. 3–18. Oxford Univ. Press (Athlone), London and New York.

Peck, W. A., and Messinger, K. (1970). *J. Biol. Chem.* **245**, 2722.

Peck, W. A., Brandt, J., and Miller, I. (1967). *Proc. Nat. Acad. Sci. U.S.* **57**, 1599.

Peck, W. A., Messinger, K., Brandt, J., and Carpenter, J. (1969). *J. Biol. Chem.* **244**, 4174.

Peck, W. A., Messinger, K., and Carpenter, J. (1971). *J. Biol. Chem.* **246**, 4439.

Pena, C., Hecht, J. P., Santome, J. A., Dellacha, J. M., and Palladini, A. C. (1972). *FEBS (Fed. Eur. Biochem. Soc.) Lett.* **27**, 338.

Perlish, J. S., Bashey, R. I., and Fleischmajer, R. (1973). *Proc. Soc. Exp. Biol. Med.* **142**, 1152.

Perlman, R. L., Tesler, A., and Dorfman, A. (1964). *J. Biol. Chem.* **239**, 3623.

Peters, T. J., and Smillie, I. S. (1971). *Proc. Roy. Soc. Med.* **64**, 261.

Phillips, L. S., Herington, A. C., and Daughaday, W. H. (1973). *In* "Advances in Human Growth Hormone Research" (S. Raiti, ed.), DHEW Publication No. (NIH) 74-612, pp. 50–67. US Govt. Printing Office, Washington, D.C.

Pierson, R. W., and Temin, H. M. (1972). *J. Cell. Physiol.* **79**, 319.

Prasad, G. C., and Rajan, K. T. (1970). *Acta Orthop. Scand.* **41**, 44.

Prévôt, H., and Schneider, C. (1966). *Acta Endocrinol. (Copenhagen)* **51**, 49.

Priest, R. E., and Koplitz, R. M. (1962). *J. Exp. Med.* **116**, 565.

Priest, R. E., Koplitz, R. M., and Benditt, E. P. (1960). *J. Exp. Med.* **112**, 225.

Puche, R. C., and Romano, M. C. (1971). *Calcif. Tissue Res.* **7**, 103.

Quintarelli, G., and Dellovo, M. C. (1966). *Histochemie* **7**, 141.

Rabinovitch, A. L., and Gibson, M. A. (1972). *Teratology* **6**, 51.

Rasio, E. A., Soeldner, J. S., and Cahill, G. F., Jr. (1965). *Diabetologica* 1, 125.

Ray, R. D., Asling, C. W., Simpson, M. E., and Evans, H. M. (1950). *Anat. Rec.* 107, 253.

Ray, R. D., Asling, C. W., Walker, D. G., Simpson, M. E., Li, C. H., and Evans, H. M. (1954). *J. Bone Joint. Surg., Amer. Vol.* 36, 94.

Reichlin, S., and Haddad, H. M. (1963). *J. Lab. Clin. Med.* 61, 44.

Reiss, M., Fernandes, J. E., and Golla, Y. M. L. (1946). *Endocrinology* 38, 65.

Rendall, J. L., Delcher, H. K., and Lebovitz, H. E. (1972). *Biochem. Biophys. Res. Commun.* 46, 1425.

Renner, R., Hepp, K. D., Humbel, R. E., and Froesch, E. R. (1973). *Horm. Metab. Res.* 5, 56.

Reynolds, J. J. (1966). *Exp. Cell Res.* 41, 174.

Richards, R. K., and Kueter, K. (1941). *Endocrinology* 29, 990.

Riekstnience, E., and Asling, C. W. (1966). *Proc. Soc. Exp. Biol. Med.* 234, 258.

Rigal, W. M. (1964). *Proc. Soc. Exp. Biol. Med.* 117, 794.

Robbins, P. W., and Lipman, F. (1956). *J. Amer. Chem. Soc.* 78, 6409.

Robbins, P. W., and Lipman, F. (1957). *J. Biol. Chem.* 229, 837.

Rodén, L. (1970). *In* "Chemistry and Molecular Biology of the Intercellular Matrix" (E. A. Balazs, ed.), Vol. 2, pp. 797–821. Academic Press, New York.

Root, A. W., Bongiovanni, A. M., and Eberlein, W. R. (1969). *J. Pediat.* 75, 826.

Rosenberg, L. (1973). *Fed. Proc., Fed. Amer. Soc. Exp. Biol.* 32, 1467.

Rosenberg, L., Johnson, B., and Schubert, M. (1965). *J. Clin. Invest.* 44, 1647.

Rubinstein, H. S., and Solomon, M. L. (1941a). *Endocrinology* 28, 112.

Rubinstein, H. S., and Solomon, M. L. (1941b). *Endocrinology* 28, 229.

Salmon, W. D. (1960a). *J. Lab. Clin. Med.* 56, 673.

Salmon, W. D. (1960b). *J. Lab. Clin. Med.* 56, 682.

Salmon, W. D. (1972). *In* "Growth and Growth Hormones" (A. Pecile and E. E. Müller, eds.), Int. Congr. Ser. No. 244, pp. 180–191. Excerpta Med. Found., Amsterdam.

Salmon, W. D. (1973). *In* "Advances in Human Growth Hormone Research," DHEW Publ. No. (NIH) 74-612, pp. 76–94. US Govt. Printing Office, Washington, D.C.

Salmon, W. D., and Daughaday, W. H. (1957). *J. Lab. Clin. Med.* 49, 825.

Salmon, W. D., and Daughaday, W. H. (1958). *J. Lab. Clin. Med.* 51, 167.

Salmon, W. D., and DuVall, M. R. (1970a). *Endocrinology* 86, 721.

Salmon, W. D., and DuVall, M. R. (1970b). *Endocrinology* 87, 1168.

Salmon, W. D., and Hosse, B. R. (1971). *Proc. Soc. Exp. Biol. Med.* 136, 805.

Salmon, W. D., Bower, P. H., and Thompson, E. Y. (1963). *J. Lab. Clin. Med.* 61, 120.

Salmon, W. D., von Hagen, M. H., and Thompson, E. Y. (1967). *Endocrinology* 80, 999.

Salmon, W. D., DuVall, M. R., and Thompson, E. Y. (1968). *Endocrinology* 82, 493.

Salter, J. M., and Best, C. H. (1953). *Brit. Med. J.* 2, 353.

Samaan, N., Fraser, R., and Dempster, W. J. (1963). *Diabetes* 12, 339.

Samaan, N., Brown, J., Fraser, R., and Trayner, I. (1965). *Brit. Med. J.* 1, 1153.

Schatton, J., and Schubert, M. (1954). *J. Biol. Chem.* 211, 565.

Schlesinger, B., and Fisher, O. D. (1951). *Lancet* 2, 289.

Schoeffling, K., Ditschuneit, H., Petzoldt, R., Beyer, J., Pfeiffer, E. F., Sirek, A., Geerling, H., and Sirek, O. V. (1965). *Diabetes* 14, 658.

Schooley, R. A., Friedkin, A. S., and Evans, E. S. (1966). *Endocrinology* 79, 1053.

Schubert, M. (1964). *Biophys. J.* **4,** 119.

Schubert, M. (1966). *Fed. Proc., Fed. Amer. Soc. Exp. Biol.* **25,** 1047.

Schubert, M., and Hammerman, D. (1965). *In* "The Amino Sugars" (R. W. Jeanloz and E. A. Balazs, eds.), Vol. 2A, p. 257. Academic Press, New York.

Schwartz, P. L., Wettenhall, R. E. H., Troedel, M. A., and Bornstein, J. (1970). *Diabetes* **19,** 465.

Scott, J. E., and Stockwell, R. A. (1967). *J. Histochem. Cytochem.* **15,** 111.

Scow, R. O., Simpson, M. E., Asling, C. W., Li, C. H., and Evans, H. M. (1949). *Anat. Rec.* **104,** 445.

Seno, N., and Anno, K. (1961). *Biochim. Biophys. Acta* **49,** 407.

Serafini-Fracassini, A., and Smith, J. W. (1974). *In* "The Structure and Biochemistry of Cartilage," pp. 1–236. Churchill, London.

Sheikholislam, B. M., Lebovitz, H. E., and Stempfel, R. S. (1966). *Proc. 48th Meet. Endocrine Soc.* Abstract.

Shephard, T. H. (1971). *J. Embryol. Exp. Morphol.* **25,** 347.

Silberberg, M., and Silberberg, R. (1965). *Growth* **29,** 311.

Silberberg, M., and Silberberg, R. (1972). *In* "The Biochemistry and Physiology of Bone" (G. H. Bourne, ed.), 2nd ed., Vol. 3, pp. 410–484. Academic Press, New York.

Silberberg, R., and Hasler, M. (1972). *Growth* **36,** 17.

Silberberg, R., Hasler, M., and Silberberg, M. (1965). *Amer. J. Pathol.* **46,** 289.

Silberberg, R., Hasler, M., and Silberberg, M. (1966). *Anat. Rec.* **155,** 577.

Silbert, J. E., DeLuca, S., and Spencer, A. F. (1970). *In* "Chemistry and Molecular Biology of the Intercellular Matrix" (E. A. Balazs, ed.), Vol. 2, pp. 929–934. Academic Press, New York.

Silbert, J. H. (1964). *J. Biol. Chem.* **239,** 1310.

Simpson, M. E., Asling, C. W., and Evans, H. M. (1950). *Yale J. Biol. Med.* **23,** 2.

Sissons, H. A. (1972). *In* "The Biochemistry and Physiology of Bone" (G. H. Bourne, ed.), 2nd ed., Vol. 3, pp. 145–180. Academic Press, New York.

Slater, J. D. H., Samaan, N., Fraser, R., and Stillman, D. (1961). *Brit. Med. J.* **1,** 1712.

Sledge, C. B. (1973). *Fed. Proc., Fed. Amer. Soc. Exp. Biol.* **32,** 1503.

Solomon, J., and Greep, R. O. (1959). *Endocrinology* **65,** 158.

Solomon, S. S., Fenster, L. F., Ensinck, J. W., and Williams, R. H. (1967). *Proc. Soc. Exp. Biol. Med.* **126,** 166.

Soyka, L. F., and Crawford, J. D. (1965). *J. Clin. Endocrinol. Metab.* **25,** 469.

Spiro, R. G. (1967a). *J. Biol. Chem.* **242,** 1915.

Spiro, R. G. (1967b). *J. Biol. Chem.* **242,** 1923.

Spiro, R. G. (1967c). *J. Biol. Chem.* **242,** 4813.

Spiro, R. G., and Spiro, M. J. (1971). *J. Biol. Chem.* **246,** 4919.

Steelman, S. L., Morgan, E. R., Cuccaro, A. J., and Glitzer, M. S. (1970). *Proc. Soc. Exp. Biol. Med.* **133,** 269.

Steelman, S. L., Glitzer, M. S., Ostlind, D. A., and Mueller, J. F. (1971). *Recent Progr. Horm. Res.* **27,** 97.

Steinke, J., Sirek, A., Lauris, V., Lukens, F. D. W., and Renold, A. E. (1962). *J. Clin. Invest.* **41,** 1699.

Stempfel, R. S., Sheikholislam, B. M., Lebovitz, H. E., Allen, E., and Franks, R. C. (1968). *J. Pediat.* **73,** 767.

Stidworthy, G., Masters, Y. F., and Shetlar, M. R. (1958). *J. Gerontol.* **13,** 10.

Stockwell, R. A., and Scott, J. E. (1965). *Ann. Rheum. Dis.* **24,** 341.
Stoolmiller, A. C., Horwitz, A. L., and Dorfman, A. (1972). *J. Biol. Chem.* **247,** 3525.
Strawich, E., and Nimni, M. E. (1971). *Biochemistry* **10,** 3905.
Strickland, A. L., and Sprinz, H. (1973). *Amer. J. Obstet. Gynecol.* **115,** 471.
Suzuki, S., and Strominger, J. L. (1960a). *J. Biol. Chem.* **235,** 257.
Suzuki, S., and Strominger, J. L. (1960b). *J. Biol. Chem.* **235,** 267.
Suzuki, S., and Strominger, J. L. (1960c). *J. Biol. Chem.* **235,** 274.
Szirmai, J. A. (1963). *J. Histochem. Cytochem.* **11,** 24.
Szirmai, J. A. (1966). *Ann. Rheum. Dis.* **25,** 374.
Szirmai, J. A., VanBoven-de Tyssonsk, E., and Gardell, S. (1967). *Biochim. Biophys. Acta* **136,** 331.
Tatum, A. H., and Lebovitz, H. E. (1975). *Fed. Proc., Fed. Amer. Soc. Exp. Biol.* **34,** Abstr. 3077.
Tell, G. P. E., Cautrecasas, P., VanWyk, J. J., and Hintz, R. L. (1973). *Science* **180,** 312.
Temin, H. M. (1966). *J. Nat. Cancer. Inst.* **37,** 167.
Temin, H. M. (1967). *J. Cell. Physiol.* **69,** 377.
Temin, H. M., Smith, G. L., and Dulak, N. C. (1974). *In* "Control of Proliferation in Animal Cells" (B. Clarkson and R. Baserga, eds.), Vol. 1, pp. 19–26. Cold Spring Harbor Lab., Cold Spring Harbor, New York.
Tesler, A., Robinson, H. C., and Dorfman, A. (1966). *Arch. Biochem. Biophys.* **116,** 458.
Thompson, J. S., and Urist, M. R. (1973). *Clin. Orthop. Relat. Res.* **90,** 201.
Thorngren, K. G., and Hansson, L. I. (1973). *Acta Endocrinol. (Copenhagen)* **74,** 24.
Toole, B. P. (1973). *Science* **180,** 302.
Underwood, L. E., Hintz, R. L., Voina, S. J., and VanWyk, J. J. (1972). *J. Clin. Endocrinol. Metab.* **35,** 194.
Uthne, K. (1973). *Acta Endocrinol. (Copenhagen)* **73,** Suppl. 175, 1.
Uthne, K., and Uthne, T. (1972). *Acta Endocrinol. (Copenhagen)* **71,** 255.
Uthne, K., Reagan, C. R., Gimpel, L. P., and Kostyo, J. L. (1974). *J. Clin. Endocrinol. Metab.* **39,** 548.
Van den Brande, J. L., VanWyk, J. J., Weaver, R. P., and Mayberry, H. E. (1971) *Acta Endocrinol. (Copenhagen)* **66,** 65.
VanWyk, J. J., Hall, K., Van den Brande, J. L., and Weaver, R. P. (1969). *Biochim. Biophys. Acta* **192,** 560.
VanWyk, J. J., Hall, K., Van den Brande, J. L., and Weaver, R. P. (1971). *J. Clin. Endocrinol. Metab.* **32,** 389.
VanWyk, J. J., Hall, K., Van den Brande, J. L., Weaver, R. P., Uthne, K., Hintz, R. L., Harrison, J. H., and Mathewson, P. (1972). *In* "Growth and Growth "Hormones" (A. Pecile and E. E. Müller, eds.), Int. Congr. Ser. No. 244, pp. 155–167. Excerpta Med. Found., Amsterdam.
VanWyk, J. J., Underwood, L. E., Hintz, R. L., Voina, S. J., and Weaver, R. P. (1973). *In* "Advances in Human Growth Hormone Research" (S. Raiti, ed.), DHEW Publication No. (NIH) 74-612, pp. 25–49. US Govt. Printing Office, Washington, D.C.
VanWyk, J. J., Underwood, L. E., Hintz, R. L., Clemmons, D. R., Voina, S. J., and Weaver, R. P. (1974). *Recent Progr. Horm. Res.* **30,** 259.

Varon, S., Nomura, J., Perez-Polo, J. R., and Shooter, E. M. (1972). *In* "Methods and Techniques of Neurosciences" (R. Fried, ed.), pp. 203–229. Decker, New York.

Vaughan, J. M. (1970). *In* "Physiology of Bone," pp. 212–215. Oxford Univ. Press (Clarendon), London and New York.

Wagner, E. M., and Scow, R. O. (1957). *Endocrinology* **60,** 419.

Wettenhall, R. E. H., Schwartz, P., and Bornstein, J. (1969). *Diabetes* **18,** 280.

Whitehead, R. G., and Weidmann, S. M. (1959). *Biochem. J.* **72,** 667.

Whitehouse, M. W., and Boström, H. (1961). *Biochem. Pharmacol.* **7,** 135.

Whitehouse, M. W., and Boström, H. (1962). *Biochem. Pharmacol.* **11,** 1175.

Whitehouse, M. W., and Lash, J. W. (1961). *Nature (London)* **189,** 37.

Wiedemann, E., and Schwartz, E. (1972). *J. Clin. Endocrinol. Metab.* **34,** 51.

Wilkins, L. (1957). "The Diagnosis and Treatment of Endocrine Disorders in Childhood and Adolescence," 2nd ed. Thomas, Springfield, Illinois.

Winterburn, P. J., and Phelps, C. F. (1971). *Biochem. J.* **121,** 711.

Wong, P. Y.-K., Majeska, R. J., and Wuthier, R. E. (1975). *Fed. Proc., Fed. Amer. Soc. Exp. Biol.* **34,** Abstract 2477.

Wu, A., Grant, D. B., Hembley, J., and Levi, A. J. (1974). *Clin. Sci. Mol. Med.* **47,** 359.

Yablon, I. G., Franzblau, C., and Leach, R. E. (1974). *J. Bone Joint Surg., Amer. Vol.* **56,** 322.

Yalow, R. S., Hall, K., and Luft, R. (1975). *J. Clin. Invest.* **55,** 127.

Yde, H. (1968). *Acta Endocrinol. (Copenhagen)* **57,** 557.

Yde, H. (1969a). *Acta Med. Scand.* **186,** 293.

Yde, H. (1969b). *Acta Endocrinol. (Copenhagen)* **62,** 49.

Zingg, A. E., and Froesch, E. R. (1973). *Diabetologia* **9,** 472.

Zondek, E. (1936). *Lancet* **2,** 842.

Steroid Hormone *Receptors*

ETIENNE-EMILE BAULIEU, MICHEL ATGER,*
MARTIN BEST-BELPOMME,† PIERRE CORVOL,**
JEAN-CLAUDE COURVALIN, JAN MESTER,
EDWIN MILGROM,* PAUL ROBEL,‡ HENRI ROCHEFORT,§
AND DENISE DE CATALOGNE

*Unité de Recherches sur le Métabolisme Moléculaire et la Physio-Pathologie
des Stéroides de l'Institut National de la Santé et de la Recherche Médicale
(Inserm U 33), Département de Chimie Biologique, Faculté de Médecine de
Bicêtre, Université Paris-Sud, Bicêtre, France*

* And Inserm U 135.
† Present address: Biologie Animale, Paris VI, 12 rue Cuvier, 75005-Paris, France.
** Inserm U 47, 17 rue du Fer à Moulin, 75005-Paris, France.
‡ And ER 125 Cnrs.
§ Inserm U 58, 34000-Montpellier, France.

I. Introduction

Hormones are messengers. Their information content is determined strictly by their chemical structure. A given steroid establishes in the "milieu intérieur" a low concentration, which is capable of provoking effect(s) in a set of designated "target" cells. Specificity is a common feature of most components of the endocrine system, and here it is clear that only cells possessing a discriminating system capable of recognizing the steroid may be responsive. This system is a "receptor," provided that the "information" implicated by the interaction of the hormone with the specific cellular structure provokes in turn a change in the functioning of a part of the cellular machinery which will lead to the overall hormonal response, the hormone no longer playing a role after the triggering. The obligatory complex structure of the nature of the receptor is indicated in Fig. 1.

Steroid hormones show different kinds of activities when examined at

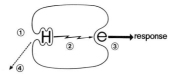

Fig. 1. Phenomenological "minimum" portrait of a receptor. A receptor has a "receptive" or "discriminating" binding site (r) ① of high affinity and specificity for the hormone (H). Transduction or coupling ② follows, influencing the functioning of the "executive" or "effector" site (e) ③, which may be a catalytic site [transforming substrate (S) into product (P) (see Fig. 2; top] or a binding site (for instance, with nucleic acid or protein). Then, ipso facto, the binding in the r site is the last interaction of the hormone obligatorily implicated in the hormonal response, and the hormone will have to leave afterward ④, being eventually replaced by incoming molecules.

Notes: There is no alternative model with two separate units, binding and catalytic, since this case is accounted for in this "portrait": the binding unit for steriod would have an e site interaction with the catalytic unit. It should also be realized that no information is available concerning the executive counterpart of the e site, which could help to define the model better. The problem of acceptor site vs e site is treated in Fig. 2. Elsewhere (Baulieu, 1975a) an "inactivation" site has been proposed to account for the effect of progesterone on its *receptor*. It is believed that the concept is applicable to other hormones. Therefore, step ④ does not necessarily mean dissociation of the ligand following the reverse reaction of the binding (XI). It may be related to any sort of "inactivation" of the *receptor*, reversible or not [see a discussion of mechanisms for inactivation in Baulieu (1975a), and on *receptor* "cycle" in Sections VI, C and IX, C, 5].

the physiological level. Differences may be also classified in terms of gross biological responses. For instance, the tropic effects of testosterone upon prostate and seminal vesicles, or of estradiol on the uterus have, while physiologically different, something in common since both involve cell growth and eventually cell division. In other target organs, such as muscle or kidney, androgens also promote cellular growth, but no DNA synthesis or cell division occurs in most cases. In cells in culture, such as hepatoma tumor cells (HTC), glucocorticosteroids induce no growth change but induce the synthesis of only a few proteins. Elsewhere, as in certain fibroblasts in culture, glucocorticosteroids participate in mitogenic effects, but they are cellulolytic in the case of thymocytes or lymphoma cells. Studies of the development of male secondary sex organs and hypothalamus in mammals and of the oviduct in avians and batracians suggest that hormones such as estradiol or testosterone can promote the formation of morphologically and functionally stabilized new type of cells, enough to justify thinking in terms of "differentiation" processes.

A basic question is whether or not there are different mechanisms behind these various modes of responses of target cells to steroid hormones, and more particularly whether the receptors are different, or, on the contrary, the steroid receptors are essentially the same in all cases with expected "small" differences at the molecular level. In the latter case, there is indeed a possibility that the differences between systems will be found in the other characteristics of the responsive machinery, as determined by the genes, the state of differentiation, and various environmental factors including nutrients, hormones, and nerves. Then the steroid hormones would essentially be standardized, providing a set of specific "master keys" for a series of locks, and always playing the same role regardless of the controlled functions. In other words, the steroid itself and the "receptive" part of the receptor would be specific for connecting the control system and the target cells, while the "executive" part of the receptor would be engaged in a predetermined response mechanism. According to the particular case, it could consist, for example, of specific protein synthesis, overall protein synthesis for growth, changes of DNA synthesis, or gene expression leading to differentiation.

Currently, with a few exceptions and reservations to which we shall come back later, all steroid hormone *"receptors"* appear to be physicochemically similar and also "specific" in that they show high affinity and narrow specificity for binding the corresponding hormones. They are intracellular proteins reached by the steroids in the extranuclear compartment of the target cells, and the hormone–*receptor* complexes ultimately interact with some nuclear structure ("acceptor"). This translocation is compatible with most biochemical data pointing to an early effect of many steroid hormones involving the transcriptional level of the genetic apparatus. If it is definitely established that steroid hormones enter target cells and form complexes with intracellular high-affinity proteins (*receptors*) situated secondarily in the nucleus, it is fair to say that in spite of *many supporting arguments*, there is no definitive proof that these specific intracellular binding proteins *are* truly receptors fulfilling all the criteria summarized above and shown in Fig. 1. In particular, it is not known whether the executive site interacts with one or more macromolecules (nucleic acid or protein) to switch the target machinery, or whether it is a catalytic site, the *receptor* therefore being an enzyme involved with the production of a sort of "second messenger." It is also not known whether the nuclear acceptor is interacting with the executive site or corresponds to another part of the *receptor* (see Fig. 2).

The word "receptor" is used here in italics (*receptor*) in order to indicate that, until conclusive progress is made, the only definitive evidence at present is that pointing to highly selective hormone binding systems in target cells.

II. Historical Background

Steroid hormones are concentrated and retained by target organs. This important finding was made possible through the use of highly labeled hormones, hexestrol (a synthetic estrogen) in goats and estradiol (a natural estrogen) in the rat (Glasscock and Hoekstra, 1959; Jensen and Jacobson, 1960). The untransformed hormone is itself present in the target tissues (Jensen and Jacobson, 1962), a result arguing against the hypothesis that steroid transformation is directly engaged in the hormonal activity in the target cell. It follows that *in vitro* binding experiments are relevant, and, early, the macromolecular and proteic nature of the binding was indicated (Talwar *et al.*, 1964) and defined quantitatively and qualitatively (Toft *et al.*, 1967; Baulieu *et al.*, 1967). At the same time, as shown after *in vivo* injection of hormones, the remarkable usefulness of gradient ultracentrifugation was established for *receptor* estradiol complexes of the rat uterus (Toft and Gorski, 1966), and the "8 S" value, easy to distinguish from many protein sedimentation coefficients, had already become a valuable marker for *receptor* characterization.

Important too was the discovery that hormones accumulate in nuclei of target cells. Evidence came from radioautography of toad bladder preparations exposed to radioactive aldosterone (Edelman *et al.*, 1963; Porter *et al.*, 1964), and from the extraction of the rat uterus a radioactive estradiol protein complex with a sedimentation coefficient of 5 S was extracted from nuclei with ≥ 0.3 M KCl-containing solutions (Jungblut *et al.*, 1967). It was then ascertained that the 8 S hormone *receptor* found in the soluble fraction of tissue extracts (cytosol) could be dissociated into 4 S complexes by high salt (Erdos, 1968; Rochefort and Baulieu, 1968; Korenman and Rao, 1968; Truong and Baulieu, 1971). This led to a discussion of the relationship of the cytosol and nuclear binding systems. At the same time, it was shown that when target cells (uterus) are reached by the hormone (estradiol), there is a decrease of the cytosol *receptor* while the hormone *receptor* complexes appear ("neonuclear") and increase in the nucleus. "Reconstitutive" experiments with hormone-labeled cytosol and "empty" nuclei led to the description of a "two-step mechanism" involving the hormone-induced transfer of the *receptor* from cytoplasm to the nucleus (Jensen *et al.*, 1968; Gorski *et al.*, 1968). This concept was formulated quite soon after other related experiments (Brecher *et al.*, 1967). Moreover, it was observed that the cytosol *receptor* could be "transformed" into the 5 S form characteristic of the nuclear *receptor* (without the presence of the nucleus) in a hormone-dependent temperature-accelerated process (Jensen *et al.*, 1971b). Detailed studies with corticosteroids (Higgins *et al.*, 1973a; Milgrom *et al.*, 1973a) demonstrated a transconformation of the *receptor*, hormone dependent and temperature and salt accelerated, resulting in an increase of affinity for polyanions including DNA, and this was termed "activation." However, the detailed mechanism of *receptor* transformation or activation is still not understood. The precise involvement of DNA (Harris, 1971; Musliner and Chader, 1971; Toft, 1972), chromatin protein (O'Malley *et al.*, 1972; Bresciani *et al.*, 1973), and ribonucleoprotein (Liang and Liao, 1974) in the "acceptor" characteristics of nuclei for the cytosol *receptor* is still a matter of controversy. At the time of this review, there is no definitive answer as to exactly what or even "where" the acceptor is.

In fact, doubts have been, and indeed still are, so largely shared by workers in this field that, in addition to biochemical efforts, parallel lines of research have evolved largely in order to determine whether the intracellular specific binding protein *receptors* are really the best candidates for the function of receptor. Systematic investigations have confirmed the high affinity, which is well suited for the normal low concentrations of physiological hormones, and have shown nice correlations between biological activity and affinities of different steroids, and even of nonsteroidal hormonally active compounds. Also, *receptors* are present in all target tissues whereas nonresponsive tissues or cells do not contain significant amounts of these binding proteins, regardless of whether their absence or the very low value is normal (nontarget organ) (Jensen and Jacobson, 1962) or pathological (Hollander and Chui, 1966; Jensen *et al.*, 1967a) and eventually genetically determined (Gehring *et al.*, 1971; Sibley and Tomkins, 1974). Other correlations between *receptor* presence and hormone response have been obtained in pathological or experimental cases (mostly breast cancer) (Jensen *et al.*, 1971a). Therefore, it is almost certain that the presence of the binding proteins that we call *receptors* is one of the necessary steps in conditioning the hormone response of the cells, although obviously the *receptors* cannot be the only parts genetically or pathologically affected in all circumstances. Besides, *receptors* are not "inert," since ontogenic developmental processes (Clark and Gorski, 1970) and hormonal controls (Baulieu and Jung, 1970; Milgrom *et al.*, 1970, 1973c; O'Malley *et al.*, 1970) have been described and are currently being very carefully studied. In fact, correlations of *receptor* content with physiology really open the path to long awaited studies of hormonal "receptivity" in molecular terms. The notion of cellular *receptor* plurality has also come up recently (Jung-Testas and Baulieu, 1974). Finally, experiments at the subcellular level, where the RNA-synthesizing nuclear machinery has been exposed to hormone *receptor* complexes, have *directly* suggested the obligatory involvement of the *receptor*, even if the molecular details are far from being understood (Raynaud-Jammet and Baulieu, 1969; Mohla *et al.*, 1972).

Among other aspects of *receptor* history, but still of undetermined importance, one can mention (a) the finding of an entry step of steroid into uterine cells (Milgrom *et al.*, 1973b), which may or may not be related to the attachment of the estradiol *receptor* to the membrane; (b) the evaluation of the relative importance of free and bound hormones in target cells (Rennie and Bruchovsky, 1972); (c) the description of an "intermediary step" for *receptor* placed "between" the cytosol *receptor* and the KCl-extractable nuclear *receptor* (Swaneck *et al.*, 1970); and (d) the finding (initially in chick liver, using estradiol) of an "insoluble" nuclear *receptor* (Lebeau *et al.*, 1973), which, indeed, can be solubilized by mild trypsin proteolytic treatment (Lebeau *et al.*, 1974). Since the "soluble" and "insoluble" *receptors* c and d have the same affinity and specificity as the more conventional cytosol- and KCl-extractable nuclear *receptors*, they may be the same entity but placed in different environments during a sequence of events.

It is of great importance to establish the significance of the cellular *receptor* distribution and the processes of inactivation and/or return to cytoplasm (a metabolism-dependent step according to Ishii *et al.*, 1972; Bell and Munck, 1973). Finally, among nonhistone chromatin (NHC) proteins, a very high affinity and rare binding protein has been observed (Alberga *et al.*, 1971b), which remains of undetermined significance.

To conclude, it has been definitely established that there are intracellular specific protein *receptors* for binding steroid hormones, all properties of which are compatible with the assumption that they are receptors, though a formal demonstration is still lacking. Steroid hormones regulate protein and nucleic acid synthesis and are involved in the functioning, growth replication, and differentiation of cells; the difficulty in assessing whether or not *receptors* are the "true" receptors lies at the frontier of modern biology, and its successful resolution will probably necessitate the combined talents of steroidologists and cell biologists. Much is awaited from large-scale purification of steroid *receptors*, and these in turn will provide invaluable tools for further progress. Recent observations are encouraging (Truong *et al.*, 1973; Sica *et al.*, 1973a,b; Sherman *et al.*, 1974; Smith *et al.*, 1975).

Several reviews and books have been published; these can be consulted by the reader, since this presentation is by choice and necessity incomplete and partial (André and Rochefort, 1974; Baxter and Forsham, 1972; Diczfalusy, 1970, 1971, 1972; Edelman and Fanestil, 1970; Edelman and Ismail-Beigi, 1974; Gorski *et al.*, 1968; Hechter and Halkerston,

1964; Jensen and DeSombre, 1972a,b; King and Mainwaring, 1974; Liao and Fang, 1969; Meuller *et al.*, 1972; O'Malley *et al.*, 1969; O'Malley and Means, 1973, 1974; O'Malley and Hardman, 1975; Pasqualini, 1975; Raspé, 1971; Segal and Scher, 1967; Thomas, 1973; Westphal, 1971). Recent surveys from this laboratory include Baulieu *et al.*, (1971), Baulieu, (1974a,b, 1975b), and Milgrom and Baulieu (1974).

III. ESTROGEN *Receptors*

The story of the estrogen *receptors* is almost the history of steroid receptors. The discovery of the intracellular *receptors* followed *in vivo* experiments where animals were given highly radioactive (tritium-labeled) estradiol (Jensen and Jacobson, 1960, 1962; Gupta, 1960) or hexestrol (Glascock and Hoekstra, 1959). Selective retention of radioactivity was found in estrogen target organs (uterus, vagina, anterior pituitary). As was the case in the discovery of estradiol itself 50 years ago, the female hormone was the first studied when the time came to elucidate mechanisms of action.

A. CYTOSOL *Receptor* OF THE MAMMALIAN UTERUS

Most of the studies have been performed using rat or calf uterus. In addition, the mouse, pig, rabbit, and human have been studied, yielding similar results.

The stage was set in the search for a binding macromolecule when it was demonstrated that, after estradiol injection, it is estradiol itself which is retained in the target cells (studies with immature or castrated adult rats, using ^{3}H-labeled estradiol, including the 17α-labeled species: Jensen and Jacobson, 1962).

1. *Physicochemical Properties of Cytosol Receptor*

The macromolecular estradiol-binding substance present in the uterine cytosol fraction was initially detected by gel filtration (Talwar *et al.*, 1964). The use of gradient sedimentation analysis (Toft and Gorski, 1966) indicated an approximate 8–10 S range of sedimentation coefficient for the *receptor* in a medium of low ionic strength. This is of great practical interest because, after high-affinity labeling by radioactive estrogen, one can easily distinguish the "8 S peak" from other proteins (sedimenting in the 3–5 S region) after several hours of ultracentrifugation at low temperature in 5 to 20% sucrose or 5 to 25% glycerol gradients. Early studies in a soluble system gave quantitative information concerning binding (Baulieu *et al.*, 1967), as well as did a similar study using the gradient technique (Toft *et al.*, 1967), and showed that binding specificity was probably an *intrinsic* property of the *receptor* molecule. Identical binding is obtained regardless of how the cytosol is labeled, and the same results are reported after injection of radioactive hormone, after exposure of uterus or pieces of uterus *in vitro* or in incubation of the soluble extract (Toft and Gorski, 1966; Toft *et al.*, 1967; Erdos, 1968; Rochefort and Baulieu, 1968; Korenman and Rao, 1968; Jensen *et al.*, 1968, 1969a; Shyamala and Gorski, 1969; Steggles and King, 1970; Alberga *et al.*, 1971a).

It was found that high ionic strength (e.g., 0.3 M KCl) causes reversible dissociation of the cytosol *receptor* to a 4–5 S unit (Erdos, 1968; Korenman and Rao, 1968; Rochefort and Baulieu, 1968; Jensen *et al.*, 1969a) showing the same binding parameters (Truong and Baulieu, 1971). In a medium of ionic strength close to that existing under physiological conditions, e.g., 0.15 M KCl, a large fraction of the *receptor* sediments at approximately 6 S (Rochefort and Baulieu, 1971). It is not known to what extent the measured sedimentation constants represent the intracellular reality or whether they can possibly reflect artificial association with macromolecules in the medium. This question remains unresolved in light of experiments demonstrating heterogeneity of the sedimentation peaks (Vonderhaar *et al.*, 1970) and the influence of agents, such as mercaptoethanol (Rochefort and Baulieu, 1971) and heparin (Chamness and McGuire, 1972), or the effect of dilution of the cytosol (Stancel *et al.*, 1973) etc. Other "4 S" forms of the uterine cytosol *receptor* have been obtained after treatments involving Ca^{2+} ions (which may act through the activation of an enzyme: Puca *et al.*, 1971a), or with trypsin under mild conditions (Erdos, 1971). These two "4 S" forms of approximately 60,000 MW are not identical (Puca *et al.*, 1972) and differ from the KCl 4–5 S "subunit" (Rat *et al.*, 1974; Soulignac, 1974). It has been observed that under a series of (poorly controlled) conditions, such as ammonium sulfate precipitation, freezing, gel filtration through various sorts of chromatographic columns, "aggregates" are found. Some of them may be related to interaction with ribonucleoprotein particles of possible physiological interest (Liang and Liao, 1974), but surely others are artifactual. They are nevertheless extremely difficult to avoid or eventually to reverse. Partially proteolyzed *receptors* (calcium 4 S or trypsin 4 S forms) do aggregate much less, in contrast to the KCl subunit of the cytosol *receptor* [or to the 5 S form obtained after extraction of nuclei (see later)].

2. *Affinity and Specificity of Cytosol Receptor*

Almost all methods that can be used to obtain equilibrium dissociation constants (K_D) at 0°–4°C have been exploited, and most results give approximately 0.1 nM for the *receptor*–estradiol complex. Attempts to measure *receptor* affinity at higher temperatures do not exclude the undesirable possibility that proteolysis or other alteration may occur with nonpurified preparations. Some "abnormal" results have been obtained. For instance, complexes of higher affinity have been found after warming the human (Hähnel, 1971) or the rabbit (Cowan *et al.*, 1975) cytosol at 37°C. However, all 4–5 S fractions described above have the same affinity as the "native" 8 S *receptor*.

Affinity of the *receptor* for steroidal and nonsteroidal estrogens run parallel to their biological activities (Jensen, 1965; Baulieu *et al.*, 1967; Korenman, 1970; Ellis and Ringold, 1971; Jensen and DeSombre, 1972), justifying the names of estrophile or estrophilin (Gorell *et al.*, 1974). Derivatives of estradiol, such as estrone, estriol, 17-deoxyestradiol, 16α-estradiol (3,16α-dihydroxy-1,3,5-estratriene) have an affinity between one-half (for estrone) and one-tenth estradiol. Incidentally, it is quite remarkable that, when estradiol, estrone, and estriol are compared, the rate of dissociation of uterine *receptor* steroid complexes is similar for the three steroids, but the rate of association is slower for the two lower affinity ones (estrone and estriol) than for estradiol (Geynet *et al.*, 1972a) (see Section III, A, 3). Even though the results have never been well documented, it is probable that, when a short chain is linked to the 17β-oxygen of estradiol, it still allows high affinity (e.g., 17β-acetate, 17β-methoxy). 17α-Ethynylestradiol (more than estradiol itself) and some other 17α-alkylated derivatives bind well to *receptor*.

In contrast, any modification of ring A seems to be deleterious to affinity. 3-Methoxyestradiol exemplifies the deteriorating effect of blocking the phenol group, and 3-deoxyestradiol also binds very little. Among other compounds of special interest is the high affinity of 7α-methylestradiol, which allows one to predict the use of various 7α-derivatives in affinity chromatography. It is also remarkable that if 11β- and 11α-hydroxyestradiol and the 17-ethynyl analogs do not bind to the *receptor*, the 11β- and 11α-methoxy 17-ethynyl derivatives bind with high affinity, one being a strong estrogen and its α-epimer a powerful antiestrogen (Raynaud *et al.*, 1973; J. P. Raynaud, unpublished observations, 1975).

In the androgen series, there is binding of testosterone and 19-nor derivatives to the uterine estrogen *receptor* binding site, as far as competition experiments against ^{3}H-labeled estradiol can determine. However, the affinity is rather low (10^{-3} of the estradiol affinity) for nortestosterone derivatives, androstanolone and 5α-androstanediol, and even lower (10^{-4} affinity) for testosterone (Rochefort and Lignon, 1974; Van Kordelaar et al., 1975a; Ruth et al., 1975). These last results may explain the androgen-induced nuclear accumulation of estrogen receptor (Rochefort et al., 1972). Δ^5-Androstene-$3\beta,17\beta$-diol is quite active (Poortman et al., 1975). Some androgen derivatives are progestagens used in contraceptive pills and bind somewhat to the estrogen receptor (Van Kordelaar et al., 1975a,b). On the other hand, neither progesterone C_{21} derivatives, including those used as progestagens for contraception, nor corticosteroids bind to the receptor, although chlormadinone acetate has been seen as a competitor (Ellis and Ringold, 1971).

Among nonsteroidal compounds, diethylstilbestrol and hexestrol (transmeso +) have higher affinity than estradiol, and from a discussion concerning its "flexible" conformation with reference to the structure of estradiol itself, some asymmetrical methyl derivatives of diethylstilbestrol have been synthesized, and they retain high affinity (Hospital et al., 1972). The problem of correlating the affinity of nonsteroidal estrogens to their structure is still not well understood (Geynet et al., 1972b), although it should be of great importance for a better prediction of the estrogenic and antiestrogenic properties of drugs.

3. Association and Dissociation

The kinetic parameters of the binding reaction of the uterine receptor-estradiol were studied at temperatures between 0°C and 30°C, when the receptor molecule is sufficiently stable (Geynet et al., 1972a; Best-Belpomme et al., 1970; Truong and Baulieu, 1971; Sanborn et al., 1971; Mester and Robertson, 1971). High association rate constant and low dissociation rate were observed as expected from values obtained at equilibrium. However, the results led to the conclusions that although the association reaction appears to follow the simple scheme

$$R \ (receptor) + H \ (hormonal \ ligand) \rightleftarrows RH \ (complex)$$

the dissociation proceeds eventually according to a two-step pattern. This may be interpreted owing to the existence of two forms of the RH complex, one dissociating relatively fast (rate constant at 20°C = 1.8×10^{-4} sec^{-1} for estradiol), the other dissociating considerably more slowly (rate constant at 20°C = 3.1×10^{-5} sec^{-1} for estradiol) (values taken from Geynet et al., 1972a). This discrepancy remains as yet unresolved. An example of a "simple" (kinetically) receptor was recently described (Korach and Muldoon, 1974): the rat pituitary cytosol receptor-hormone complex dissociates according to a one-step mechanism following the scheme

$$R + H \underset{k_{-1}}{\overset{k_{+1}}{\rightleftharpoons}} RH$$

and the calculated equilibrium constant $k + 1/k - 1$ is in agreement with the value experimentally measured at equilibrium. In most cases (and specifically with uterine *receptor*) the ratio, even taking the first (faster) slope of dissociation, gives an association constant (at least) one order of magnitude higher than the direct determination (Baulieu, 1973).

4. Chemical Structure of the Receptor and Characteristics of the Binding Reaction

The destructive effect of proteinases (Noteboom and Gorski, 1965; Toft and Gorski, 1966) and the inhibition of estradiol binding by SH group blocking agents (Shyamala and Gorski, 1969; Jensen *et al.*, 1967b; Puca and Bresciani, 1970) as well as the protective effect of the reducing agent mercaptoethanol (Mester *et al.*, 1970) suggest that the *receptor* molecule contains an essential protein portion and that SH groups are important for its binding activity, although they may not be directly involved with the binding (Truong, 1970). Moreover, one can find conditions where the estradiol binding is intact, but the *receptor* ability to interact with the "acceptor" is altered by SH blocking agents (Milgrom *et al.*, 1973b).

The effect of mild trypsin treatment (Erdos, 1968), which leaves the binding of estrogen by the *receptor* intact, has been mentioned before. In addition to the change of structure shown by the decrease of sedimentation coefficient and of molecular weight (Soulignac *et al.*, 1974), the "trypsin 4 S form" shows less ability to aggregate and cannot be "activated" for interacting with an acceptor (Sala-Trepat and Reti, 1974; André and Rochefort, 1973b; A. Alberga, unpublished observations, 1973). These results are compatible with the loss of a protein part engaged in binding other macromolecules. The effect(s) of calcium ion have been related to the activity of a *receptor* transforming factor, likely a proteolytic enzyme (Puca *et al.*, 1971b). It has been reported that the subunits of the "trypsin" and "calcium" 4 S forms are different (Erdos and Fries, 1974). Other studies on possibly specific uterine protease have been presented (Notides *et al.*, 1973).

No other hydrolytic enzyme has been definitively proved to interfere with the hormone binding by the *receptors*, even though several reports have indicated partial effects of nucleases, phospholipases, and glycosidases (Little *et al.*, 1973; Cidlowski and Muldoon, 1974; Hähnel *et al.*, 1974).

There is no evidence as to whether or not the *receptor* molecule possesses an enzymic activity itself, and binding of estrogens does not result in their chemical transformation. The binding is of noncovalent character: the hormone is easily extracted by organic solvents (Jensen *et al.*, 1966; Maurer and Chalkley, 1967). Although some authors reported augmentation of binding by agents containing the imidazole ring (purine nucleotide) and free bases (Vonderhaar *et al.*, 1970), studies involving work with rabbit uterine cytosol treated previously by charcoal led to the conclusion that small molecules are not necessary as cofactors for the binding reaction (Mester and Robertson, 1971). The cytoplasmic *receptor* molecule is progressively inactivated at 37°C (Mester *et al.*, 1970). This process may be due to an endogenous enzyme, since at 45°C the entire loss occurs within the first 10 minutes and represents approximately only 30% of the initial binding. The remaining binding sites are stable at this temperature (Truong, 1970; Puca *et al.*, 1971b). Partial protection of the *receptor* against thermal inactivation is achieved by occupying the binding sites with the hormone (Rochefort and Baulieu, 1971). The nuclear *receptor* appears stable at 45°C (Puca and Bresciani, 1969). The pH optimum for binding lies between 7 and 9, and progressive inactivation is observed outside this range (Mester *et al.*, 1970; Notides, 1970). Partial renaturation occurs if the pH is readjusted to the optimal range (Soulignac *et al.*, 1974).

"Basic" microsomal *receptors* (Little *et al.*, 1972) have been detected and may be biosynthetic precursors of "native" *receptors* (Little *et al.*, 1975).

5. *Purification of Estrogen Receptor*

Two basic approaches have been utilized in the attempts to purify the estrogen *receptor*.

Classical methods of purification, such as ammonium sulfate precipitation, gel filtration and polyacrylamide gel electrophoresis, have been applied to nuclear KCl-soluble extracts obtained after incubation of ^{3}H-labeled estradiol–cytosol mixture with KCl-containing, buffer-extracted nuclei of calf uterus. In other words, the authors (Gorell *et al.*, 1974) have, for the purification of a cytosol material, used specific activation by estradiol to obtain selective binding by the nuclei. Preliminary results have been published, including electrophoretic mobility.

Other groups have chosen to purify a stabilized form of the cytosol *receptor*, either the 4 S calcium (Sica *et al.*, 1973a,b) or the 4 S trypsin (Truong *et al.*, 1973; Truong and Baulieu, 1974), using mainly affinity chromatography. Different adsorbents have been produced, and in one step a 10,000-fold purification has been obtained currently (Truong *et al.*, 1975b). The main problems are found at the level of stability of the *receptor*, and the problems of the yields of the fixation on affinity material and of the elution from it, as well as the large-scale preparation, remain technically difficult. However, it is very likely that, at the time of the printing of this review, other publications will be available indicating progress in this field.

B. (NEO)NUCLEAR *Receptor* OF THE MAMMALIAN UTERUS

1. *Relationship between the Cytosol and the Nuclear Forms of the Estrogen Receptor in Uterus*

The incorporation of estradiol into the nucleus of target cells is very rapid. *In vivo* injections and *in vitro* incubations of tissues or cells have shown that it takes a few minutes (up to 30–45 maximum) to obtain a plateau at 37°C (Gorski *et al.*, 1968; Anderson *et al.*, 1973). In fact, it is remarkable that radioautographic data (Stumpf, 1968; Jensen *et al.*, 1969a) have not clearly demonstrated specific "grains" in the cytoplasm [recent data obtained with a clone of mammary cells (Weiller *et al.*, 1974) give evidence for specific binding sites in the cytoplasm (S. Weiller, unpublished observation, 1975)].

It is certain that, in target cells of the uterus, most radioactivity in the nucleus after exposure to ^{3}H-labeled estradiol is protein bound, and indeed it is unchanged radioactive estradiol itself. The movement of estradiol–*receptor* complexes is demonstrated by the shift from the cytosol fraction to the nuclear extract when the temperature is increased from 0° to 25° or 37°C. This is confirmed by radioautographic data and by *in vitro* cell-free experiments exposing the nucleus to labeled cytosol. They indicate a two-step mechanism, which can be summarized as follows: the hormone combines first in the cytoplasm with the protein *receptor* of high affinity. Transfer to the nucleus is shown by a decrease of cytosol binding sites (Jensen *et al.*, 1968; Gorski *et al.*, 1968; Rochefort and Baulieu, 1968, 1969; Brecher *et al.*, 1967) and by an increase of estradiol–*receptor* complexes in the nucleus, which are extractable by KCl (0.25 *M* and above) containing buffer. There were no estradiol binding sites that could be extracted by the same buffer from nuclei in the absence of hormone, and it follows that "neonuclear" *receptor*–hormone complexes have been generated (Alberga *et al.*, 1971a; Rochefort and Baulieu, 1972). The *receptor* does not have affinity for the nucleus in cells deprived of hormone, since it is found strictly in the cytosol. The presence of hormone gives the *receptor* the capacity to bind to some nuclear "acceptor" structures implicating a passage through the nuclear membrane. The step is temperature dependent, but it may take place very slowly at 0°C. In acellular experiments, exposure of the *receptor* even at low temperature to a relatively high-salt medium (e.g., 0.15 *M* KCl) favors "activation" (Rochefort and Baulieu, 1972), suggesting that under physiological conditions, temperature and salt concentration may be optimal. It is then very probable that the "transformation" (Jensen *et al.*, 1971b) of the *receptor* is an essential step in hormone action. Isotope dilution experiments have suggested that it is really the (cytosol) *receptor* that is required for the transfer, since the radioactive hormone–*receptor* complexes have been found in the nuclear fraction even after their incubation with nuclei in the presence of nonradioactive hormone in large amounts (Rochefort and Baulieu, 1972). The effects *in vitro* of cytosol *receptor* on the nuclear RNA polymerase activity (see Section IX, A) plea also for the role of the transfer of hormone–*receptor* complexes to the nuclei and therefore of the activation (transformation) of the *receptor* (Jensen *et al.*, 1972).

Even after acceptance of these conclusive data, several controversies remain. It is not known whether the intact 8 S protein or a part (subunit) of it is transferred intact (Jensen *et al.*, 1971b; Rochefort and Baulieu, 1972) or whether there is addition of a nuclear (Jungblut *et al.*, 1971b) or cytoplasmic (Notides and Nielsen, 1974; Yamamoto, 1974) protein moiety. Another difficulty that needs to be resolved is whether or not the uptake by the nucleus is cell (organ) specific. The uterus cytosol *receptor* can be bound not only to uterine nuclei, but to other nuclei from nontarget organs and even to glass beads (Clark and Gorski, 1970). A series of experiments have indicated a limited capacity (which is presumably specific) for uterine nuclei to bind the *receptor*–hormone complexes (King *et al.*, 1971), but incubations of tissues have shown no limitation for binding to the nucleus provided there is availability of cytosol *receptor* (Williams and Gorski, 1971). Recently, it has been reported that there is neither specificity nor limitation of acceptor sites in uterine nuclei (Chamness *et al.*, 1973, 1974). This has been determined by utilizing nuclei of different sources and a *receptor* preparation of a fixed amount in which the concentration of complexes is modified by changing the hormone concentration (but not the protein concentration). DNA is probably implicated in the binding of the *receptor* in uterine nuclei (Harris, 1971; Musliner and Chader, 1971). In binding experiments, a limited number of sites have been found for a uterine *receptor* on DNA corresponding to 500–1000 per cell and therefore to ~2 for 10^7 nucleotide pairs (King and Gordon, 1972). However, the role of interfering proteins in those saturation curves may have led to artifacts (André and Rochefort,

1974). Indeed, binding of the *receptor* to various DNAs and polynucleotides (A. Alberga, unpublished observations, 1973) does not favor the specificity of the acceptor sites that have been studied. However, nonspecific binding to DNA (which may hide specific interaction) could be of great functional importance, as suggested in other systems for regulatory proteins interacting with nonoperator DNA.

Quantitatively, neonuclear *receptor* complexes found after estradiol administration may not account for all cytosol *receptor* binding sites. In other words, the nuclear bound hormone (representing transferred *receptor*) never attained the level expected from the number of cytosol sites (Mester and Baulieu, 1975). It seems as though only a part of the *receptor* could be transferred to the nucleus. When the dose of estrogen administered is high, there is more transfer, and even more decrease in the cytosol, but an apparent return to the cytoplasm and subsequent increase to the cytosol sites takes place very rapidly (Jensen and De-Sombre, 1972b; Mester and Baulieu, 1975). Indeed, whatever the amount of injected estradiol, one finds the same quantity of nuclear estrogen–*receptor* complexes after 3–6 hours. This is a result that apparently correlates well with the dose-response curves of certain estradiol effects (J. N. Anderson *et al.*, 1973, 1974). The possible role for the excess of *receptor* in cytoplasm is not known, and interactions with extranuclear components have not been excluded.

2. *Other Nuclear Receptors*

In addition to the cytosol–neonuclear *receptor* system, a nonhistone chromatin (NHC) protein has been found in calf uterine extracts. It is present in nuclei even in the absence of hormone, and it is of exceptionally high affinity ($K_D \leq 10\ fM$) (Alberga *et al.*, 1971b). The number of sites calculated per cell on the basis of DNA is very small (≤ 10 per cell), and its possible insertion in the mechanism of the action of estradiol is still not understood. It has also been found in dimethylbenzanthracene (DMBA)-induced tumors of mammary gland in the rat (A. Alberga, unpublished observations, 1973), but not in tissues that are not targets for estradiol (spleen, liver, lung, etc.). A set of very high affinity nuclear binding sites have been also detected by de Hertogh *et al.* (1973).

Binding of estradiol to the nuclear membrane of bovine endometrium has been described (Jackson and Chalkley, 1974a). A "lysosol" *receptor* present in lysosomal protein (Hirsch and Szego, 1974) has been reported recently; this *receptor* which would transfer to the nucleus.

The "insoluble" *receptor* described in chick estrogen target tissues (Lebeau *et al.*, 1973) also exists in the rat uterus and is operationally defined by its nonextractability with KCl-containing buffer. Its increase after the injection of estradiol to the rat has been reported (Mester and Baulieu, 1975). However, it requires more characterization. It may correspond to the fraction of uterine estradiol early defined by Alberga and Baulieu (1968) as non-ether-extractable.

C. Entry of Estradiol into Uterine Cells

The entry of estradiol into uterine cells (and likewise of any steroid into its target cells) is classically supposed to be a diffusion process (non-limited, not specific) through the lipoprotein plasma membrane. However, recent work with rat uterus has indicated the possibility of a step of limited capacity, showing different relative affinities for estradiol and diethylstilbestrol in comparison with the cytosol *receptor*. This is compatible with a protein-mediated process that is not energy dependent and differs from active transport (Milgrom *et al.*, 1973b). A specific "gate" for steroid hormone entering cells could be considered as a target for pharmacological manipulation of great interest. It is not known whether the (cytosol) *receptor* (e.g., attached to the external membrane and functionally different from its soluble state) is implicated in such a transfer phenomenon, and the possibility that component(s) present between uterine cells may play a role has not been excluded. One may recall that an interaction of the cytoplasmic estradiol *receptor* with the cell membrane has also been postulated for other reasons (Jackson and Chalkley, 1974b).

D. Amount of Uterine *Receptors* and Regulation

The number of *receptors* present in actual target cells is difficult to assess. In most organs, no radioautographic data are available that would indicate the kind of cells labeled by estrogens. Data relating the number of binding sites to (cytosol) protein or to DNA are then difficult to evaluate. Moreover, precautions should be taken for avoiding destruction by enzymic proteolysis or heat inactivation (even the technique used for fractionation of tissue is of importance).

In the uterus, most cells appear to be targets for estrogen. When expressed in terms of number of binding sites per cell (assuming 6.7 pg of DNA per cell), the *receptor* concentration in rat uterine cytosol under various physiological states can be calculated using the data of Feherty *et al.*, (1970), Gorski *et al.* (1971), Sarff and Gorski (1971), Mester *et al.* (1974), and Michel *et al.* (1974). In the immature animal the *receptor* concentration first rises to a maximum of 20,000–60,000 sites/cell at the age of about 10 days, declining subsequently to a level of ~15,000–20,000 sites/cell at 20–22 days (40–50 gm body weight). After puberty, the values vary between a minimum just after estrus (2000 sites/cell) and a maximum at proestrus (20,000 sites/cell). The existence of this maximum (Feherty et al., 1970; Shain and Barnea, 1971) has been controversial (Lee and Jacobson, 1971). In pregnancy (Mester et al., 1974) the maximum cytosol *receptor* level coincides with the implantation of embryos (day 5) and reaches 40,000 sites/cell in the endometrium (approximately 0.8 pmole of cytosol per milligram of protein*), while the myometrium levels (on a DNA basis) are approximately one-third of endometrial levels. Experiments with castrated rats have indicated that estradiol increases the cytosol *receptor* in both myometrium and endometrium (on a DNA basis) and that progesterone alone can also elevate the endometrial *receptor* whereas it abolishes almost completely the estradiol-induced increase of the *receptor* in myometrium (Mester et al., 1974). These experiments, aimed at reproducing physiological changes, may lead to a better understanding of the hormonal conditions for implantation.

The nuclear levels of estrogen *receptor* have been determined (Clark et al., 1972), and they vary during the estrous cycle, following the variations of ovarian estrogen secretion. The maximum (proestrus) level was 1.29 pmoles per milligram of DNA, corresponding to ~5000 sites/cell; the maximum value at metestrus was 0.22 pmoles per milligram of DNA, 900 sites/cell. Then variations in both the cytosol and the nuclear *receptor* concentrations closely follow the pattern of estrogen secretion during the cycle (this would indicate either induction of synthesis or activation by the ligand). Finally, that estradiol influences and regulates its own *receptor* under physiological conditions is, in addition to results reported above, suggested also by the effect of castration, which decreases the *receptor* level (Feherty et al., 1970; Steggles and King, 1970). However, it is not known whether or not the development of the receptor from birth to puberty results from estrogen secretion.

It should be pointed out that the biochemical evaluation of uterine estrogen *receptor* may mask further complexity of their regulation. The effects of progesterone on estradiol distrubution in the different uterine cells have been revealed by radioautographic studies of Tachi et al. (1972): estradiol accumulation is decreased in the luminal epithelial cells, but not in glandular cells.

Besides *receptor* measurements performed under various physiological conditions, acute experiments have been undertaken. When immature

---

* Expression of *receptor* sites per milligram of protein naturally depends quite extensively on the physiological state and the type of tissue (e.g., myometrium vs endometrium) considered.

(20–23 days old) rats were injected with physiological doses of estradiol (Sarff and Gorski, 1971), the initial decrease in the *receptor* cytosol concentration was accompanied by a parallel increase in the amount of nuclear estradiol (Anderson *et al.*, 1973) and was followed by a period of replenishment between 4 and 24 hours after the hormone treatment. The final receptor concentration exceeds the initial level by approximately 50%. The replenishment is blocked by cycloheximide, and therefore it is probably dependent on protein synthesis (Sarff and Gorski, 1971; Mester and Baulieu, 1975; Cidlowki and Muldoon, 1974). However, certain observations (Jensen *et al.*, 1968; Mester and Baulieu, 1975) have indicated that after the injection of a supraphysiological dose of estradiol (1 μg) into the rat, there is a 90% decrease in the amount of the cytosol *receptor*, which then returns to the cytoplasm, and this last step is not suppressible by cycloheximide. On the other hand, during replenishment an increase of the *receptor* level that is not dependent on protein systhesis has been observed and may be due to activation (Sarff and Gorski, 1971). It should also be indicated that Paton (1969) has observed that DNP and other metabolic inhibitors decrease the amount of cytosol *receptor*. Finally, after estradiol administration, the decrease of cytosol *receptor* cannot be accounted for by the complexes found in nuclei (Mester and Baulieu, 1975). If protein synthesis is blocked by cycloheximide and a newly synthetized cytosol *receptor* does not appear, one sees the decrease in nuclear complexes as though there were some kind of inactivation (M. Luu Thi and E. Milgrom, unpublished observations, 1973).

It has also been indicated that during lactation (Leung, 1974; Chatkoff and Julian, 1973) there is an increase of *receptor* in the uterus. The suggestion that it may be due to prolactin is not supported by the observations (Cidlowski and Muldoon, 1974; Vignon and Rochefort, 1974) that hypophysectomy does not indicate a pituitary dependence for initiation and maintenance of cytoplasmic estrogen *receptor* levels and that prolactin is inactive.

E. The Human Uterus

In the human uterus, estrogen cytosol *receptor* has been detected early (Wyss *et al.*, 1968). It has been studied in some detail (Mester *et al.*, 1970; Hähnel, 1971; Evans and Hähnel, 1971; Notides *et al.*, 1973). Nuclear *receptors* have also been described (Evans and Hähnel, 1973). Investigation of the variations of cytosol *receptor* concentration in the endometrium over the menstrual cycle has indicated the presence of higher *receptor* levels during the proliferative phases than in secretory phases. However, owing to considerable variability between individuals as well as to the difficulty in collecting material from healthy normal subjects, there is a controversy concerning the exact pattern of *receptor* concentrations during the cycle (Robertson *et al.*, 1971; Evans *et al.*, 1974; Trams *et al.*, 1973; Evans and Hähnel, 1973). Highest levels found in the cytosol endometrium correspond to approximately 15,000 binding sites per cell (Robertson *et al.*, 1971).

F. Estrogen *Receptors* in Other Organs and Species

1. *In Mammals*

a. Fallopian Tubes. In the monkey (Brenner *et al.*, 1974), the monitoring of artificial cycles has indicated that progesterone may be involved in the decrease of the amount of the cytosol *receptor* in a way similar to that in the rat uterus (Mester *et al.*, 1974; Hsueh *et al.*, 1975). The cytoplasmic *receptors* in the human (Robertson and Landgren, 1975) and the rabbit (Muechler *et al.*, 1974) fallopian tubes have also been described.

b. Vagina. (Feherty, 1972). In the rat, a high-affinity estrogen *receptor* has been found in the cytoplasm of vaginal tissue.

c. Mammary Gland. Estrogen *receptors* in the mammary gland were described in the rat (Sander, 1968) and mouse (Puca and Bresciani, 1968, 1969). The concentration of cytosol estrogen *receptors* increases during lactation in the rat (Shyamala and Nandi, 1972; Wittlif *et al.*, 1972; Hsueh *et al.*, 1973); this rise appears to be prolactin-induced. The correlation between estrogen sensitivity and nonsensitivity of tumors induced by DMBA and the presence of *receptor* is satisfactory (Nomura *et al.*, 1974).

d. Certain Tumor Cells. These cells in culture retain high-affinity estrogen *receptors* (Jung-Testas and Baulieu, 1974; Mester *et al.*, 1973; Jung-Testas and Bayard, 1975).

e. Anterior Pituitary and Hypothalamus. In both male and female rats, cytosol estrogen *receptors* have been described (Eisenfeld and Axelrod, 1967; Kato, 1970a,b, Kato *et al.*, 1970; Ginsburg *et al.*, 1972; Friend and Leavitt, 1972; Cidlowski and Muldoon, 1974; Maurer, 1974). Localization and variation of the estrogen-concentrating cells have been shown to coincide with the estrogen-dependent neuroendocrine control systems (Pfaff and Keiner, 1973; Ginsburg *et al.*, 1975).

f. Corpus Luteum. In the rabbit, the corpus luteum (estrogen dependent) contains estrogen *receptors* that show variations with the cycle (level highest at mid-luteal phase, decline prior to regression of corpora lutea), while in the human (nonestrogen dependent luteal tissue) no estrogen *receptors* could be demonstrated (Chung Lee *et al.*, 1971; Scott and Rennie, 1971).

g. *Male.* High-affinity estrogen *receptor* sites are also present in the testis, epididymis, and prostate (Mulder *et al.*, 1974; Jungblut *et al.*, 1971a).

h. *Other Tissues.* Estrogen *receptors* are present also in certain tissues not apparently concerned with reproduction: rat liver (Eisenfeld, 1974), hamster kidney (Li *et al.*, 1974), pineal gland (Pedroza-Garcia *et al.*, 1974), pancreas (Sandberg *et al.*, 1973), and eosinophiles (Tchernitchin *et al.*, 1975).

2. *In Nonmammalian Species*

High-affinity estrogen *receptors* were described in the immature *chick oviduct* cytosol and nuclei (Cox *et al.*, 1971; Palmiter *et al.*, 1973; Harrison and Toft, 1975; Best-Belpomme *et al.*, 1975). Their characteristics again resemble those of the uterine *receptors*. Interestingly enough, in the mature chick oviduct (i.e., laying hen), there are extremely few ($\sim 10^2$) estrogen cytosol *receptor* binding sites per cell. Practically all the *receptors* ($\sim$7000 sites/cell) are associated with the nuclear fraction in contrast to, for example, the adult rat uterus, where comparable levels of estrogen *receptors* exist both in the cytosol and nuclear fraction.

The *chick and amphibian liver*, also a target organ for estrogens, does contain high-affinity nuclear *receptors* (Mester and Baulieu, 1972; Lebeau *et al.*, 1973; Ozon and Bellé, 1973a; Gschwendt and Kittstein, 1974), but no such *receptors* were found in the cytosol fraction. Here only a more weakly binding macromolecule (K_D 10^{-9} M) was found (Arias and Warren, 1971; Zelson and Wittliff, 1974). Moreover, in the cell-free experiments, the nuclear uptake of estradiol was not enhanced in the presence of the chick liver cytosol fraction.

Another interesting aspect of the chick liver and oviduct *receptors* is the extractability of the nuclear form. Only a part ($\sim$50%) of their total amount is extractable by a medium of high-ionic strength; the "residual" "insoluble" binding material exhibits typical *receptor* characteristics, i.e., high affinity ($K_D \lesssim 1$ nM at 37°C), estrogen specificity, and protein character (Lebeau *et al.*, 1973). Solubilization of this form of the *receptor* can be achieved by mild trypsin treatment (Lebeau *et al.*, 1974). A 4 S molecule retaining its binding properties is then released from the nuclear residue. The physiological importance of this "insoluble" estrogen receptor remains to be explored.

IV. Progesterone *Receptors*

Progesterone *receptors* have been studied principally in the mammalian (mostly rodents) uterus and in the chick oviduct. In both cases (Milgrom *et al.*, 1970; O'Malley *et al.*, 1970), as probably in vagina from uptake experiments (Podratz and Katzman, 1968), estrogens can induce their synthesis. This provides an interesting opportunity to study, in progesterone-deprived animals, a large amount of *receptor* in the absence of the bound hormone, a convenient feature for physicochemical studies and investigations of the hormonal control of *receptor* concentration.

Progesterone–*receptor* complexes have generally a faster dissociation rate than the estradiol and androgen analogs. The hormonal specificity of the *receptor* is much narrower than that of progesterone-binding plasma protein, such as corticosteroid-binding globulin (CBG) (Westphal, 1971), from which they must be eventually distinguished in biological extracts (Milgrom and Baulieu, 1970a; Sherman *et al.*, 1970).

A. The Chick Oviduct System

In vitro administration of ^{3}H-labeled progesterone to chicks has indicated retention of radioactivity in oviduct (O'Malley *et al.*, 1968, 1969). It is found to be mainly distributed between the cytosol and the nuclear fractions of homogenates, with a progressive increase with time in the latter. *In vitro* studies have clearly distinguished the *receptor* protein from CBG (O'Malley *et al.*, 1970; Sherman *et al.*, 1970). These were generally done using gradients at different ionic strengths and gel filtration.

Fractionation of 120,000 g cytosol by $(NH_4)_2SO_4$, agar filtration, and DEAE-cellulose chromatography (elution by KCl), and sucrose gradient give 2500-fold purification. After DEAE chromatography, the *receptor* appears to be dissociated in an equimolecular amount of two forms, A and B, eluting at 0.10 and 0.25 M KCl, respectively, and of the same affinity as the steroids and not interconvertible. Only B binds to chromatin; A has high affinity for DNA, but B has not (Schrader and O'Malley, 1972). As yet, the structure of the two "subunits" has been reported only for the chick oviduct progesterone *receptor*. From the response to progesterone of different cell types (goblet, tubular, and probably ciliary), the plurality of progesterone *receptors* in this system cannot be excluded. Moreover, uncontrolled partial proteolysis in estrogen-treated tissue could also be operative.

The cytosol *receptor* is tissue specific (not found in heart, spleen, liver, and diaphragm) and hormone specific. It is increased by estrogen, as in the avidin response to progesterone. These characteristics indicate that it probably plays a role in progesterone action.

The cytosol *receptor* transfer to the nucleus is progesterone dependent (O'Malley and Toft, 1971), and organ nuclear specificity for this interaction has been described (Steggles *et al.*, 1971). *In vitro* studies with progesterone-³H labeled oviduct cytosol and chromatin preparations of chick oviduct and spleen (nontarget organ) have indicated selectivity of the target chromatin for binding the radioactive hormone–*receptor* complexes. This has been observed only with component B of the cytosol *receptor* (not with A), and reconstitution experiments, in which "artificial" chromatins have been obtained by exchanging histones and nonhistone chromatin proteins of target and nontarget tissues, point to some acidic proteins [more particularly fraction AP 3 (Feil *et al.*, 1972)] as a possible acceptor (Steggles *et al.*, 1971).

Affinity of the *receptor* for progesterone corresponds to a K_D of approximately 1 nM. Many steroids have been tested (Smith *et al.*, 1974), and only a few have higher affinity than progesterone itself.

Recent research (Strott, 1974) indicates that 5α-pregnanedione is bound to the nuclear *receptor* after incubation at 37°C of oviduct tissue previously labeled with progesterone-³H at 0°C. Since both the affinity of 5α-pregnanedione for the *receptor* and its activity for inducing avidin synthesis are significant, its occurrence is of unclear significance. As with androstanolone in the case of androgens, its role would be better understood if one could know more about 5α-reductase activity and distribution. Presently one cannot distinguish between the possibility that it plays a role in expressing progesterone action, or the possibility that it is only a metabolite binding an active site by pure stereochemical chance and possibly an intermediary compound along the route of the detoxifying metabolism of the hormone after its action (interaction with receptor). In the uterus of different mammals, detailed investigations do not support an important role for 5α-pregnanedione in progesterone action. 5β-Reduced, 20 hydroxy, and 3 hydroxy derivatives of progesterone bind very little.

19-Norprogesterone has higher affinity than progesterone. Among progestagens, 19-nor-4-androstene derivatives (such as ethisterone or norethindrone) and 19-nor-13β-ethyl-4-gonen derivatives (such as norgestrel) have high affinity, attributable in part to the 17α-ethynyl group, since 19-nor-testosterone, for instance, shows very low binding.

Interesting negative results include the findings that A-norprogesterone, 17-hydroxyprogesterone, 17-acetoxyprogesterone and derivatives, such as chlormadinone and medroxyprogesterone, and cortisol have low affinity, whereas deoxycorticosterone binds well. Testosterone (and most androgens) and estradiol (and estrogens) do not have much affinity for the *receptor*. Recently, the binding of ATP to the *receptor* has been described (Moudgil and Toft, 1975).

B. Progesterone *Receptors* in the Mammalian Uterus

Specific progesterone binding components have been found in the uterus of mammals; these components show all the common features of *receptors* and are distinct from plasma proteins. They were first observed in the estrogen-primed guinea pig (Milgrom *et al.*, 1970; Corvol *et al.*, 1972; Faber *et al.*, 1972b) and rabbit (Faber *et al.*, 1972a, 1973; Rao and Wiest, 1971; Rao *et al.*, 1973; McGuire and Dedella, 1971), and in calf uterus cytosol (Best-Belpomme, 1974; Wagner *et al.*, 1972). High affinity ($K_D \sim 1$ nM at $0°$–$4°C$) and specificity for progesterone and progestational compounds have been observed (glucocorticosteroids are not bound, but deoxycorticosterone has some affinity). The protein nature (binding disintegrated by protease but not by nucleases), the sedimentation coefficient of the cytosol *receptor* in low-salt medium (more in the 6–7 S range for guinea pig, and around 8 S in rabbit), and sensitivity of the binding to SH-blockers and to temperature increase have been observed. More recently the same conventional *receptor* has been obtained in the hamster (Leavitt *et al.*, 1974), rat (Feil *et al.*, 1972) and human (Rao *et al.*, 1974; Young and Cleary, 1974) uterus. With the use of the progestagen derivative R 5020 of a higher affinity than progesterone, which does not bind much to plasma and other nonspecific proteins, a comparison between rat, rabbit, guinea pig, and human *receptor* has indicated their similarities (Philibert and Raynaud, 1974). The sheep *receptor* has also been compared to that in other species (Kontula, 1975).

The question of binding of metabolites may be different in mammalian uterus and chick oviduct. Even if incubation studies have indicated that metabolism may take place in uterus (Armstrong and King, 1971; Milgrom and Baulieu, 1970a), evidence favors a unique role for progesterone itself.

The binding specificity of human (Smith *et al.*, 1974) and other mammalian (Kontula *et al.*, 1975) *receptors* is very similar to that of the chick oviduct *receptor* (see above). However, there are differences that are probably related mainly to the region of the site interacting with ring D of steroids. Deoxycorticosterone is relatively less bound than in the chick, but conversely the 17-acetoxy derivatives of progesterone, including the active medroxyprogesterone and chlormadinone, bind to the *receptor* almost as well as progesterone itself. Finally 19-nor steroids display a dramatic enhancement of affinity for the mammalian *receptor* when compared to the corresponding 19-methyl compounds.

Nuclear *receptor* has been relatively difficult to study, possibly because the transfer of progesterone–*receptor* complex to nuclei has been generally studied in an estrogen-primed uterus, which shows a great deal of proteolytic activity. However, from radioautographic studies (Warembourg and Milgrom, 1971; Stumpf and Madhabananda, 1973) and other recent findings (Hsueh *et al.*, 1974), it appears that the same *receptor* transfer as with other steroids occurs in the case of progesterone, in uterus as well as in chick oviduct.

C. PHYSICOCHEMICAL ASPECTS OF PROGESTERONE *Receptors*

Progesterone *receptors* are relatively favorable for purification since they may be induced by estrogens and found in relatively great abundance, unoccupied by endogenous ligand. Moreover, the rate of dissociation of progesterone is faster than that of other hormones from their own *receptors*, and this gives an operational facility in the case of affinity chromatography and more generally for exchange techniques.

When the cytosol *receptor* of the chick oviduct has been studied, the two major 4 S "subunits" (see Section V, A) show differences, B being more stable (e.g., in solutions without thioglycerol). This B fraction has been purified 3000-fold (Schrader and O'Malley, 1972) and was recently obtained in homogeneous form (Kuhn *et al.*, 1975) by ion exchange, adsorption and gel chromatography, or alternatively by affinity chromatography. A single polypeptide chain of 117,000 MW has been described (N-terminal, lysine), binding 1 progesterone molecule; the pI was 4.8. It binds to nuclei and chromatin, but not to DNA. A steroid-binding "subunit" formed with divalent cations, especially Ca^{2+}, has been reported (Sherman *et al.*, 1974). Its sedimentation coefficient is 2.6 S, the Stocke radius 21 Å, and the MW about 20,000. Recently, the *receptor* has been studied by electrophoresis in highly cross-linked polyacrylamide gel, and a molecular weight of 113,000 was observed (Sherman *et al.*, 1975).

In mammalian uteri, after estradiol induction, *receptors* always have a 6–8 S sedimentation coefficient in low-salt medium, whereas in castrated animals or during diestrus or pregnancy, many receptors appear to have a 4 S sedimentation coefficient. In the rat, rabbit, sheep, and guinea pig, 0.3 M KCl transforms the 6–8 S into 4–5 S (Faber *et al.*, 1973; Kontula, 1975), and the reported MW in rabbit is 60,000 (Rao *et al.*, 1973). In the human, the purified *receptor* from myometrium and endometrium migrates with a sedimentation coefficient between 3.8 and 4.5 S (Verma and Laumas, 1973; Young and Cleary, 1974; Kontula *et al.*, 1973), and

7 S is occasionally seen. The molecular weight is approximately 56,000–67,000, and the Stokes radius is 33–31 Å with a frictional ratio of 1.26–1.22 (Verma and Laumas, 1973). Recent results (O'Malley, 1975, personal communication) obtained using affinity chromatography with 11-deoxycorticosterone derivatives, give MW ~ 110,000 and a sedimentation coefficient of 3.7 S.

D. VARIATIONS OF PROGESTERONE *Receptor(s)* AND REGULATION

1. *Variations during the Estrous Cycle and the Beginning of Pregnancy in the Guinea Pig Uterus*

Changes of cytosol *receptor* have been measured by an exchange technique (Milgrom *et al.*, 1972a) evaluating their total concentration (occupied or not by the hormone). The highest amount of *receptor* is found in proestrus (~ 40,000 binding sites per cell). There is then a fast decrease during estrus and proestrus to attain 16-fold lower level at diestrus (Milgrom *et al.*, 1972b).

In proestrus, the *receptor* is 6.7 S, with a shoulder in the 4–5 S region as in castrated animals primed with estradiol (Milgrom *et al.*, 1970, 1971). There appears to be a progressive decay of the 6.7 S binder from proestrus to diestrus. It is composed only of *receptor* protein sensitive to PHMB, and binds specifically progestagens. In the 4.5 S region of the cytosol, there is a mixture of *receptor* and of other uncharacterized binding macromolecules. These variations of the sedimentation coefficient do not reflect an aggregation–dissociation equilibrium due to concentration variations or an artifact due to partial proteolysis. Their functional meaning is not understood.

The *receptor* at the beginning of pregnancy is very similar to that of nonpregnant animals, and at day 7 (implantation time) the concentration is very low. This points to the possible physiological importance of progesterone secreted several days before implantation at the pre- and periovulatory period, when the *receptor* concentration is highest.

2. *Hormonal Control*

The variations during the estrous cycle imply the probable existence of hormonal mechanisms (Milgrom *et al.*, 1973c). The rise of *receptor* after estrogen injection, observed in preliminary experiments, points to the existence of a positive control. The fact that estrogen-deprived animals (castrated at various periods of the cycle or prepubertal guinea pigs) had higher levels of *receptor* than diestrus animals indicated the possible existence of another, probably negative, control.

After estradiol, the concentration of progesterone *receptor* (per cell) at 6 hours is already double the basal level (3000–4000 binding sites per cell, and peaks at about 1 day with an 8-fold increase ($\sim$ 30,000 sites/cell). The 6.7 S form is greater (relatively to the 4 S) with a high amount of induced *receptor*. When cycloheximide or actinomycin D is injected 15 minutes before estrogen, there is a marked inhibition of progesterone-*receptor* induction. Conversely, if these compounds are injected at the time of peak concentration, there is no effect on the slow decrease observed without metabolic inhibitors.

These experiments suggest that after injection of estradiol there is a rise in the concentration of the progesterone *receptor*, dependent on RNA and protein synthesis, while there is subsequently a slow decrease, apparently not dependent on RNA and protein synthesis. It is probable that this decrease mainly reflects the inactivation of the *receptor* since the rate of synthesis as judged by inhibitor experiments is then very slow. If this assumption is correct, the half-life of the *receptor* molecule is about 5 days.

If progesterone is injected in physiological amounts after estrogen induction of the *receptor*, the latter concentration falls to very low values 24 hours afterward, contrary to what is observed in the absence of this progesterone administration. This effect of progesterone is due neither to masking of sites as indicated by the amount of unlabeled progesterone found in the uterus (furthermore this "endogenous" progesterone was taken into account when measuring *receptor*), nor to an accumulation in the nuclei of steroid–*receptor* complexes. The variation in *receptor* concentration is probably due to a modification of the rate of inactivation (and is not changed by administration of cycloheximide 15 minutes before progesterone). It is possible that the decrease of *receptor* is related to the transfer of the *receptor* from the cytosol to the nucleus under the influence of progesterone itself, but in spite of experiments suggesting a relatively fast "disappearance" of the nuclear *receptor* in *in vitro* tests, no definitive conclusion can be drawn at the present time.

Finally, the effects of estradiol and progesterone are compatible with the changes observed during the estrous cycle. Uncertainties remain regarding the mechanism of activation and inactivation and may be solved only when the actual measurement of the *receptor* protein is possible, rather than with the present techniques using binding properties. The available results do not indicate whether all *receptor* molecules bound in the nuclei are inactivated or only a fraction of them. They do not even determine whether the observed variations take place in individual cells or are due to variations of cell populations in the uterus. Preliminary radioautographic studies of progesterone-³H localization in the guinea pig uterus have shown that although some heterogeneity exists cells of all types bind the hormone (Warembourg and Milgrom, 1971). The cellular complexity of the uterus and the differential reactivity of the various cells to progesterone have been reasons for a study in the guinea pig showing that the *receptor* properties are essentially the same in endometrium and myometrium (Atger *et al.*, 1974).

However, the situation when *receptor* concentration is low can reflect either a static situation with low synthesis and inactivation or a dynamic state with a fast turnover. In this respect a low *receptor* concentration could eventually be related to a situation where the hormone is very active and produces a rapid turnover of the *receptor*.

E. The Story of the Rat Uterus and the Problem of Corticosteroid-Binding Globulin

A cytosol protein binding progesterone with high affinity and limited capacity was initially found in the rat uterus (Milgrom and Baulieu, 1970a). It was rapidly observed that its binding property (same high affinity for both progesterone and corticosterone), physicochemical properties, and immunological reactivity indicated that it was indeed either plasma corticosteroid-binding globulin (CBG), transcortin, or a CBG-like protein. Gross contamination of extracts by blood was excluded by hemoglobin measurement and washing experiments. The variations in concentration of the CBG-like protein are remarkable: it is more abundant in the adult than in the prepubertal uterus, is increased vastly in the uterus by estradiol priming, and is absent in nontarget organs (kidney, diaphragm). These characteristics are indeed compatible with a role in the mechanisms of progesterone action, and studies indicate that (at least part of) the CBG-like protein found in the uterine extract could indeed be of intracellular origin, not a simple contaminant by extracellular fluid, as is easier to postulate (Milgrom and Baulieu, 1970b). Indeed, if the CBG-like protein of uterine cytosol binds cortisol and progesterone equally well, it can be observed that when intact uterus cells are exposed *in vivo* or *in vitro* (slice incubations), either to progesterone or to cortisol, results are very different: only progesterone (or a metabolite) is found to have easy access to the binding protein, and not much cortisol (or metabolite) can reach it. This strong but indirect evidence for the intracellular location of CBG in rat uterine cells has recently received some further immunological support (Rosenthal *et al.*, 1974) in the guinea pig. Moreover, the presence of CBG-like protein has also been found in soluble extracts of deciduoma, 5-day pregnant rat uterus, pseudopregnant rat uterus (Reel *et al.*, 1971), rabbit uterus (Faber *et al.*, 1973) (from which it cannot be washed out by perfusion) and in human endometrium extract (Rao *et al.*, 1974; Kontula *et al.*, 1973; Haukkamaa and Luuk-kainen, 1974). Techniques for measuring *receptors* should therefore always take into account such CBG-like protein (F. Bayard, S. Damilano, and P. Robel, unpublished observations, 1975).

Studies during pregnancy in the rat show that a progesterone binding component of the uterus cytosol, possibly identical to the CBG-like protein, decreases just before parturition (Davies and Ryan, 1973; Davies *et al.*, 1974) and may be related to its triggering.

The presence of a large amount of CBG-like protein in the uterus, in addition to the *receptor*, may not be trivial in terms of mechanisms of action of hormones, and its presumable localization must receive more attention, as must also the relationship between estrogen-CBG increases in the plasma and uterus.

F. PROGESTERONE *Receptors* IN OTHER ORGANS AND SPECIES

Progesterone *receptors* have been detected in vagina (Attramadal, 1973) and mammary glands (Atger *et al.*, 1974) of guinea pig and in the mammary gland of lactating rats and women (normal and tumoral). They have still not been found in hypothalamus (Atger *et al.*, 1974).

Progesterone *receptors* in the guinea pig vagina and cervix are subject to regulation by estrogen (Atger *et al.*, 1974). In the hamster uterus, the cyclic variation and hormonal control of progesterone *receptor* are very similar to what are found in the guinea pig (Leavitt *et al.*, 1974).

In rat, mouse, and rabbit, it has been confirmed (Feil *et al.*, 1972; Rao and Wiest, 1971; Faber *et al.*, 1972a) that the concentration of *receptor* in the uterus is increased by the administration of estrogen. The same observation has been made in chick oviduct (O'Malley *et al.*, 1970). It has also been shown (Faber *et al.*, 1972a) that in rat and mouse during proestrus the *receptor* is in a 7 S form whereas 4 S is found in diestrus. In the rat, whatever the hormonal state, radioautography has indicated a nuclear progesterone binding in muscle and stroma cells, but not in luminal and glandular epithelium (Tchernitchin *et al.*, 1973). However, if competition studies with progesterone and corticosteroids and binding studies with radioactive corticosteroids are not conducted, one cannot definitively determine what sort of binding protein is responsible for the retention of hormones (in fact, there is no indication that CBG may proceed to the nucleus of target cells). In the castrated rabbit, the *receptor* is 4 S and shifts to 8 S after estrogen injection.

Finally, from all results, it seems that in many species there exists a situation similar to that described in the guinea pig, and it has been suggested that *receptor* regulation be used as a target for new contraceptive methods (Baulieu, 1975a).

In any case, progesterone *receptors* should always be characterized with special care, not only because of possible CBG contamination, but also because of the "secondary" binding of progesterone by other steroid *receptors* (see next paragraph). High affinity for progesterone should be obtained, corresponding to $K_D \sim 1$ nM and definitively higher than that for nonprogestational compounds.

The gluco- and mineralocorticosteroid *receptors* as well as androgen *receptors* bind progesterone with an affinity far from negligible, 10^{-1} to 10^{-2} times the "physiological" steroid. Progesterone analogs or derivatives are similarly bound. The biological significance of this "secondary" binding of progesterone to other *receptors* is unknown, and in fact it is not even formally demonstrated that progesterone binds to the same sites as corticosteroids or androgens. Progesterone, and even more certain derivatives such as cyproterone acetate, is antiandrogenic in some target cells. Progesterone is also an antimineralocorticosteroid in kidney, and it is an antiinducer (antiglucocorticosteroid) of tyrosine aminotransferase in the HTC cells, in which it does not locate in the nucleus in the form of hormone–*receptor* complexes (Section VI, C).

Amphibian oocytes respond to progesterone and also to a series of C_{21} or C_{19} steroids by maturation, in preparation for meiosis. While indirect evidence points to a membrane localization of a *receptor* (Smith and Ecker, 1971), recent work (Ozon and Bellé, 1973b; Iacobelli et al., 1974) has indicated that *Pleurodeles* and *Xenopus laevis* oocytes display a larger number of high-affinity binding sites (*receptor*) for progesterone in the fractions of homogenates containing melanosomes. The hormonal specificity of the binding is reasonably parallel to the biological activities of the steroids, and therefore is remarkably wide (testosterone and cortisol are bound and active).

V. ANDROGEN *Receptors*

Uptake and retention of androgens by male accessory organs was observed when low doses of highly radioactive testosterone were administrated to castrated rats (Bruchovsky and Wilson, 1968; Tveter and Attramadal, 1968). In ventral prostate and seminal vesicles a metabolite of testosterone, androstanolone or 5α-dihydrotestosterone (DHT), was found attached to *receptor* in nuclei (Anderson and Liao, 1968; Bruchovsky and Wilson, 1968). At the same time, it was demonstrated in organ culture that testosterone is transformed into androstanolone and other

5α-reduced metabolites at the target tissue level and that some of these metabolites (androstanolone first of all) are active per se (Baulieu *et al.*, 1968). Since the formation of the neonuclear *receptor* is possibly central to steroid action at the cellular level, it is logical to conclude that the formation of metabolite from testosterone in target cells may be a very important step in at least certain cases. No corresponding metabolic step has been established for other steroids. Some related problems, insofar as binding by the *receptor* is concerned, will be discussed later.

A. Cytosol *Receptor* in the Rat Ventral Prostate

The rat ventral prostate has been the most popular target organ for studying androgen *receptors*. Early radioautographic data (Sar *et al.*, 1969; Tveter and Attramadal, 1969) indicated the localization of the hormone in nuclei of epithelial cells. Rare "grains" have been found in other ventral prostate cells, and also in cell nuclei from other lobes of the prostate.

1. *Physicochemical Properties*

A soluble androgen *receptor* has been identified in the 105,000 g supernatant fraction of the rat prostate homogenate after labeling of the tissue *in vivo*, or after incubation of slices or of the cytosol with the radioactive steroid. Recent results indicate why it was difficult to obtain clear-cut results with intact adult rats. Most sites are occupied by androstanolone (Robel *et al.*, 1975), and, contrary to what apparently occurs in the rat uterus for the estrogen *receptor*, there are no available free sites that can be bound at 0°C. In any case, the *receptor* is present mainly in the nucleus *in vivo* (Tveter and Attramadal, 1968; Anderson and Liao, 1968), possibly because testosterone is continuously secreted (whereas estrogen and progesterone secretions are cyclic with periods of unoccupied *receptors*). The *receptor* is clearly observed when the cytosol of adult rats is obtained from an animal castrated 24–48 hours before sacrifice (Mainwaring, 1969; Baulieu and Jung, 1970). This is because almost all endogenous androgens have disappeared from the binding sites and the regression of prostate is still minimal, and subsequently the number of *receptor* sites per milligram of protein has not appreciably decreased (Baulieu and Jung, 1970). The *receptor* is very unstable and thermolabile, so that all operations must be conducted strictly at low temperature (0°C). The use of EDTA, mercaptoethanol, and glycerol has a protective effect (Mainwaring, 1969; Baulieu and Jung, 1970). Incubation of cytosol with ^{3}H-labeled androstanolone in the nanomolar range and subsequent analysis on linear sucrose or glycerol low salt-containing gradients have demonstrated the presence of an 8–10 S specific binding protein (Mainwaring, 1969: Baulieu and Jung, 1970; Unhjem et al., 1969) corresponding to an estimated molecular weight of 220,000–280,000. A significant amount of bound androgen is also present in the 4 S region, after the labeling of cytosol, but competition studies show that only the 8–10 S binding has a limited capacity. The absence of a plasma protein-binding androgen with high affinity in the rat (Mercier-Bodard et al., 1970) facilitates the interpretation of gradient analysis. Similar specific complexes with a sedimentation constant of 3.5 S have been described (Fang et al., 1969).

One can deduce from proteolytic enzyme digestion that the specific 8–10 S macromolecule is a protein (but resistant to other hydrolytic enzymes: Mainwaring, 1969; Baulieu and Jung, 1970). The involvement of cysteine and tyrosine in the binding sites is evoked by the inhibitory effect of SH-blocking agents and N-bromosuccinimide (Mainwaring, 1969; Baulieu and Jung, 1970). Protamine sulfate precipitation (Mainwaring, 1969) and isoelectric focusing, pI 5.8 (Mainwaring and Mangan, 1973), show that it is an acidic protein. Treatment of the 8–10 S receptor by high salt (0.4 M KCl) results in its reversible conversion into a 4–5 S macromolecule (Baulieu and Jung, 1970; Mainwaring, 1970). An irreversible conversion to a 4 S component can be obtained by heating it for 10 minutes at 30°C (Liao et al., 1973b).

The plurality of androgen receptors has been suggested by ammonium sulfate fractionation of rat ventral prostate cytosol (Fang and Liao, 1971). One fraction, "β," precipitated at 35–40% ammonium sulfate concentration, is strictly specific for androstanolone and for a nuclear transfer of the hormone receptor complex (Liao et al., 1973b). Another fraction, α, precipitated at high ammonium sulfate concentration, is less substrate specific and also binds testosterone, estradiol and progesterone. Although there is general agreement that the protein sedimenting at low concentration of ammonium sulfate is the actual receptor protein (Fang and Liao, 1971; Mainwaring and Peterken, 1971; Verhoeven, 1974), the strict androstanolone specificity of the β protein has been questioned (Verhoeven, 1974; Blondeau et al., this volume). Recently, the use of microisoelectric focusing techniques has suggested a large heterogeneity of the androgen receptor (Goldman and Katsumata, 1974), and partial purification has been obtained by DNA-cellulose chromatography (Irving and Mainwaring, 1974).

2. Amount, Affinity, and Specificity of Receptor

It is interesting that the hormone specificity of the 8 S receptor of ventral prostate cytosol is shared by many other androgen receptors found in different species and/or different organs.

Recently the binding constants of rat ventral prostate cytosol *receptors* for androstanolone have been reported by several groups (Töpert *et al.*, 1974; Verhoeven, 1974; Blondeau and Corpéchot, 1974; Boesel and Shain, 1974; Bruchovsky and Craven, 1975; C. Bonne, unpublished observations, 1975). Studies have been conducted on cytosol prepared from young adult rats of several strains castrated 24 hours before sacrifice. The reported K_D are between 0.4 and 3 nM, and the number of specific binding sites are in the range 20–300 fmoles per milligram of protein. The affinity for testosterone is ≤ 3 times lower than for androstanolone.

However, during binding studies, even if most of them are performed at 0° or 4°C for a relatively short period of time (e.g., 2 hours), some steroid metabolism may proceed (including high speed supernatant) and modify the relative amounts of 17β-hydroxyl and 17-ketonic compounds or of 3α-hydroxyl and 3-ketonic derivatives. If the "cytosol" contains membranes (endoplasmic reticulum), Δ^4-3-ketone can be reduced to 5α-derivatives. Some studies reporting the relative affinity of various compounds must be critically interpreted in this respect (Michel and Baulieu, 1975). In any case, the *receptor* binding site is distinct from 5α-reductase, not only because the affinity of the latter is much lower, but also because the two proteins can be easily separated by physical means (Mainwaring, 1970). Even with some reservations (due to enzymic activities *in vitro*), it now seems well established that the main structural features of active androgens are the planar A ring (Δ^4 or 5α-structure) and the presence of a 3-ketone and of a 17β-hydroxyl group (Baulieu and Jung, 1970; Liao *et al.*, 1973a). 19-Nortestosterone is bound but its 7α-methyl derivative is even better. 7α-Methyltestosterone is also active. The 5β-reduced compounds are not bound at all (and do not display any androgenic activity). 3β- and 3α-Hydroxy compounds are not bound or only weakly per se (but they may be metabolized to 3-ketone), and 3-deoxy compounds are very weakly bound. There is no binding of 17α-hydroxy derivatives (e.g., epitestosterone), but the 17α-methyl derivatives of 17β-hydroxy steroids maintain approximately the same affinity as the parent compounds. Another interesting aspect is that even 5α-androstanolone has more affinity than testosterone, the polyunsaturated steroids of the 19-nortesterone series as the trienic $\Delta^{4,9,11}$ derivatives from Roussel-UCLAF (Bucourt *et al.*, 1971). These are not reduced by the 5α-reductase and are bound with a higher affinity than androstanolone. Therefore, as indicated also by detailed studies with β-protein (Liao *et al.*, 1973a) one has rather a stereochemical view of the binding than a theory concerning electronic requirements.

The 8–10 S *receptor* also binds steroids of series other than androgens (Baulieu and Jung, 1970). For instance, from competition experiments progesterone has an apparent affinity approximately 0.1–0.3 that of androstanolone. Another interesting aspect is that androgens can be competed by estradiol, probably at the binding site level even through no formal demonstration is available, with an apparent affinity approximately 20 times weaker than that of androstanolone itself. The latter result may explain why the direct binding of ^{3}H-labeled estradiol to the *receptor* has not been observed by a gradient ultracentrifugation technique. Diethystilbestrol is much less active than estradiol for competing androgen binding in rat ventral prostate cytosol.

Several antiandrogens, testosterone derivatives such as 17α-methyl B-nortestosterone or SKF 7690 (Hansson and Tveter, 1971b), R 2956 (Baulieu and Jung, 1970), or BOMT (Mangan and Mainwaring, 1972), as well as other steroidal (pregnane derivatives) antiandrogens, such as cyproterone acetate (Fang and Liao, 1969; Baulieu and Jung, 1970) or spironolactones (C. Bonne, unpublished observations, 1975), and even nonsteroidal antiandrogens, such as flutamide (Liao *et al.*, 1974), have been shown to displace androstanolone from its *receptor* binding sites.

3. *Microsomal Binding*

Recently, the binding of androgens to a microsomal fraction of rat ventral prostate has been studied (Robel *et al.*, 1974). High affinity and (very) low capacity have been demonstrated, with a steroid-binding specificity different from that of the cytosol *receptor*. This result may indicate that it is not the same binding protein, even though it could be that differences are due to a different environment (e.g., polypeptide chain on ribosomes before release). However, metabolic transformations may also have influenced the apparent specificity of this binding. "Basic" microsomal *receptors* have also been reported by Little *et al.* (1973).

B. Neo(nuclear) *Receptor* in the Rat Ventral Prostate

The androstanolone binding protein, extractable by buffered 0.4–0.6 *M* KCl from labeled nuclei after exposure of tissues *in vivo* or *in vitro* to radioactive testosterone or androstanolone, migrates in salt-containing sucrose gradient centrifugation with a sedimentation coefficient of 3.0 S (Fang *et al.*, 1969; Jung and Baulieu, 1971). If nuclei are isolated 72 hours after castration of the rats and then incubated with ^{3}H-labeled androstanolone, there is no retention of the hormone in a protein-bound form. However, when nuclei are exposed to ^{3}H-labeled androstanolone cytosol complexes, there is then a formation of a soluble nuclear radioactive fraction sedimenting at 3 S (Baulieu and Robel, 1970; Jung and Baulieu, 1971). As in the case of estrogens, even though fewer experiments deal with this, evidence suggests that prostate nuclei have sites that can retain the specific androstanolone–protein complexes, but not the protein moiety alone. It has been observed that the cytosol protein which transfers to the nucleus is the 8–10 S *receptor* (Jung and Baulieu, 1971) or the 3.5 S β-protein (Fang and Liao, 1971) and that testosterone is a poor substitute for androstanolone (Jung and Baulieu, 1971). Whereas the formation of the androstanolone–cytosol *receptor* complexes can occur at 0°C, the interaction of these complexes with the nuclear acceptors is a temperature-dependent step (Liao *et al.*, 1973b). No direct experiment has yet demonstrated the relationship of this temperature dependency to the "activation" of the steroid *receptor* complexes, as shown in other systems.

The transfer of ^{3}H-labeled androstanolone–*receptor* complexes into prostatic chromatin has been studied *in vitro* in the cell-free reconstituted system (Mainwaring and Peterken, 1971). The transfer of complexes is tissue specific, maximal in chromatin isolated from androgen-dependent tissues. Androgenic steroids *in vivo* may maintain the tissue-specific nature of chromatin in androgen-dependent tissues by the selective induction of nuclear protein synthesis. Alternatively, it has been proposed that the nuclear retention of androgen in target tissues may be due, at least in part, to the binding of the cytoplasmic ^{3}H-labeled androstanolone–*receptor* complex by nuclear ribonucleoprotein particles (Liao *et al.*, 1973b). Experiments on *receptor* binding to DNA have been reported (Mainwaring and Peterken, 1971), as well as effects of hormone and *receptor* on DNA-polymerase activity (Mainwaring, 1973). The stimulation *in vitro* of both nuclear prostatic RNA polymerase A and B activities by prostatic 5α-dihydrotestosterone *receptor* complexes has recently been documented (Davies and Griffiths, 1974).

C. Androgen *Receptors* in Other Organs and Species

1. *In the Rat*

Seminal vesicles have an androgen *receptor* (Tveter and Unhjem, 1969; Stern and Eisenfeld, 1969). Intracellular *receptors* for androstanolone have also been studied in some detail in *epididymis* cytosol and nuclei and were shown to be very similar to the corresponding *receptors* of ventral prostate (Hansson and Tveter, 1971a; Blaquier, 1971; Ritzen *et al.*, 1971; Tindall *et al.*, 1972). Its ontogeny has also been studied (Calandra *et al.*, 1974). Some peculiarities of epididymis nuclei have been reported insofar as the binding of hormone cytosol *receptor* complexes is concerned (Blaquier and Calandra, 1973). The epididymal *receptor* has to be distinguished from another "androgen-binding protein" (ABP) present in rat

testis (French and Ritzen, 1973), secreted from Sertoli cells into efferent
duct fluid, and found in epididymis (French and Ritzen, 1973; Hansson
et al., 1973). This separation can be achieved by polyacrylamide gel
electrophoresis sucrose gradient, ultracentrifugation, and Sephadex G-200
filtration. In addition, the *receptor* is more sensitive to heat, charcoal, and
sulfhydryl reagent inactivation than ABP. Both proteins have a greater
affinity for androstanolone than for testosterone (approximately 10 times
greater for the *receptor* than for ABP). Globally, ABP resembles very
much the human plasma protein SBP (Mercier-Bodard *et al.*, 1970). In
seminiferous tubules of adult rats, there is also a *receptor* for testosterone
(Mulder *et al.*, 1975). Evidence has also been presented for the presence of
androgen *receptors* in rat *preputial gland* cytosol (Bullock and Bardin,
1972), *pituitary* (Jouan *et al.*, 1971, 1973; Sar and Stumpf, 1973; Naess
et al., 1975), and *hypothalamus* (Jouan *et al.*, 1971; Naess *et al.*, 1975).

A cytosol *receptor* has been described in rat *levator ani muscle* (Jung
and Baulieu, 1972). In this muscle there is not much androstanolone *in
vivo* (intact adults) (Robel *et al.*, 1974), and cytosol labeling experiments
showed more affinity for testosterone than for androstanolone. In *skeletal
muscles* of the thigh (Michel and Baulieu, 1974, 1975), there is also a
cytosol *receptor* of high affinity for testosterone and androstanolone,
which can be competed for by estradiol and cyproterone acetate, and
this finding reopens the study of the "direct" action of androgens on muscles (Michel and Baulieu, 1975). In *bone marrow* (Valladares and
Minguell, 1975) there is a *receptor* extractable from nuclei and binding
testosterone. In the *skin* (Eppenberger and Hsia, 1972) there is also an
androgen *receptor*. In the *uterus* of immature (Giannopoulos, 1971;
Rochefort and Lignon, 1974) and mature (Heyns, 1974) rats, there is
a *receptor* that again apparently binds more testosterone than androstanolone. Finally, in the rat *liver*, indications of an androstanolone *receptor* have been reported (Roy *et al.*, 1974), while specific binding for
Δ^4-androstanedione has been found in liver nuclei (J. A. Gustafsson and
A. Stenberg, unpublished observations, 1974).

2. *In Other Species*

Androgen *receptors* have been demonstrated in *mouse, rabbit* (Mainwaring and Mangan, 1973), and *human* (normal and pathological) *prostate* (Hansson *et al.*, 1971; Mainwaring and Milroy, 1973), *guinea pig*
(Mainwaring and Mangan, 1973) and *rabbit* (Danzo *et al.*, 1973), *epididymis*, in *mouse kidney* (Bullock and Bardin, 1972; Attardi and Ohno,
1974) and *submaxillary gland* (Wilson and Goldstein, 1972), in *guinea
pig levator ani muscle* (where androstanolone is present) (Mainwaring
and Mangan, 1973), in *calf uterus* (Jungblut *et al.*, 1971a) and *pig semi-*

nal vesicles (Hansson *et al.*, 1973), and also in the cytosol and nuclei
of androgen-dependent *mouse mammary tumors,* the S 115 carcinoma
(Mainwaring and Mangan, 1973; Gordon *et al.*, 1974; Jung-Testas and
Baulieu, 1974). In the latter case, testosterone itself can promote the
transfer of the *receptor* to the nucleus. It is also the case with *mouse
fibroblasts* L-929 cells (Jung-Testas and Bayard, 1975) and *human fibroblasts* (Meyer *et al.*, 1975; A. Groyer and P. Robel, unpublished observations, 1975). There is also a *receptor* in the hamster *sebaceous gland*
(C. Bonne, unpublished observations 1975). In the *erythropoietic spleen*
of the *mouse,* which responds to phenylhydrazine hemolysis (Hadjian
et al., 1974), the *receptor* is not present before the anemia and also seems
to disappear late in the evolution. There is also a *receptor* in a tumor
of the Syrian hamster *vas deferens* (Norris *et al.*, 1974) and in the *cock
comb* and *wattle* (Dube and Tremblay, 1974), where it may be difficult
to find owing to the viscosity problem. Indeed, in the cock a receptor
is found in many tissues, including the *spleen, pancreas,* and *muscles*
(Dube and Tremblay, 1974). Androgen *receptor* has been described in
the chick oviduct (Harrison and Toft, 1973).

D. Regulation, Genetic Control and Plurality of Androgen *Receptors*

Castration of rats leads to a decrease of the prostatic cytosol androgen-
binding sites at least up to 4 days after bilateral orchiectomy, regardless
of what is expressed per milligram of cytosol proteins or on a per cell
basis (Baulieu and Jung, 1970; Mainwaring and Mangan, 1973; Verhoeven, 1974), even though it had not been demonstrated that removal of
testosterone supply is responsible until recent experiments by Blondeau *et
al.* (this volume). Indeed, a late reappearance of cytosol *receptors* 8-10
days after castration is observed (Sullivan and Strott, 1973; Blondeau
et al., this volume). This reappearance of *receptor* is not mediated by
adrenal or pituitary factors (Sullivan and Strott, 1973) and might be
related to changes of prostatic proteolytic activity (Mainwaring and
Mangan, 1973; Blondeau *et al.*, this volume).

Androgen binding varies in rat skin during the hair cycle (Eppenberger
and Hsia, 1972). There is no difference in the number of binding *receptor*
sites in the male and in the female mouse kidney, but apparently there
is an increase (expressed per milligram of cytosol protein) at sexual
maturity (in females) (Attardi and Ohno, 1974). There are also androgen · *receptors* before puberty in thigh muscles of rats of both sexes
(Michel and Baulieu, 1975).

The testicular feminization (TFM) syndrome provides an interesting opportunity for studies of the possible absence or abnormality of *receptor* in animals nonresponsive to androgens. In these feminized XY organisms androgen activity is defective, but androgen production and 5α-reductase are normal or subnormal. *Receptor* studies are not available in *man*, but a series of reports have been published dealing with the *rat* and the *mouse* TFM syndromes (Bullock and Bardin, 1972; Attardi and Ohno, 1974; Gehring *et al.*, 1971). In the rat *preputial gland* and the mouse *kidney* of TFM animals, there is a decrease in the number of *receptor* sites. The androgen *receptor* has not been found in TFM rat liver (Roy *et al.*, 1974). However, it has been indicated that in the cytoplasmic extract of *submaxillary* glands of TFM-Y mice there is high-affinity, large-capacity androstanolone binding which is even greater than in normal animals (Wilson and Goldstein, 1972). Even though detailed experiments have not been done, it may be envisaged that the (low) binding found in androgen target organs of TFM animals belongs to "abnormal" *receptors* (Attardi and Ohno, 1974). Since it has been suggested (Ohno *et al.*, 1973) that the TFM mutation does not represent a *receptor* gene deletion, one could even expect to find an altered *receptor* in TFM cells rather than complete absence, and the hormonal control of an abnormal binding system has been studied (Attardi and Ohno, 1974). It is not known whether the TFM locus specifies the androgen *receptor* itself or regulates its activity.

Finally, there is also a genetic implication in the suggestion that testosterone action may be mediated in different tissues through different metabolites and eventually different *receptors* (Baulieu, 1974b). For instance, *if* estrogens express part of the testosterone message at the hypothalamic level, presumably it is through a *receptor* different from the androstanolone-binding protein, and such an estrogen *receptor* is not under the control of the TFM locus. At other levels, for example, in muscles, kidney, or bone marrow, *if receptors* are different from ventral prostate binding sites, it follows that they could be partly independent from the gene of the TFM locus. Recent observations (Imperato-McGinley *et al.*, 1974) indicate not all androgen-dependent tissues depend on the transformation of testosterone to androstanolone for their development. However, the significance of such findings has not yet been established. This may be a matter of the respective affinities of the two androgens for the same *receptor* as well as a question of different *receptors*. Finally, as previously stated (see Section V, A, 2), much work is necessary before one can assess differential binding specificity at the *receptor* level and then propose differentially specific pharmacological androgens for different targets.

VI. GLUCOCORTICOSTEROID *Receptors*

Glucocorticosteroid *receptors* have been found in numerous tissues of adult animals as well as in the embryo and the fetus (Ballard *et al.*, 1974; Giannopoulos *et al.*, 1974; Feldman, 1974). A great deal of work was initially done with the thymus (Munck and Brinck-Johnsen, 1968). The first indication for a *receptor* protein came from studies of the kinetics of release of radioactive hormone from isolated thymocytes labeled by radioactive glucocorticoids and transferred into a large amount of a buffer containing no hormone. Thereafter, detailed studies were done also with cells grown in culture, particularly hepatoma tumor cells (HTC), of which a stable line has been carefully analyzed (Samuels and Tomkins, 1970), fibroblasts, and lymphoma cells. Owing to its relatively large size and easy purification of nuclei, the rat liver has also been extensively studied.

A. CYTOSOL *Receptor*

In the cases just mentioned, as well as in many other systems, the cytosol *receptor* appears to be a macromolecule, at least in part protein since the binding of a hormone is destroyed by the proteolytic enzyme pronase. In all instances, in a 5–20% sucrose gradient, the *receptor* sedimentation coefficient is between 6 and 8 S in low salt medium ($\leq 0.1\ M$), and between 3.5 and 4.5 S in high KCl concentration solutions (0.25–1 M). Changes of the sedimentation coefficient in the presence of KCl have been interpreted as suggestive of the dissociation of an oligomeric protein into subunits. The binding of the steroids to the receptor may require SH groups since SH-blocking agents are inhibitors. The affinity of the hormone for the *receptor* is high, the K_D being close to 1 nM at 0°C (Ballard *et al.*, 1974; Baxter and Tomkins, 1971; Fu *et al.*, 1973; Funder *et al.*, 1973a,b; Giannopoulos, 1973; Lippman *et al.*, 1973b; Schaumburg and Crone, 1971; Schaumburg, 1972a,b). The association rate constant is high, 10^6 to $10^7\ M^{-1}\ sec^{-1}$ at 0°C, and the dissociation rate constant is low, 10^{-2} to $10^{-3}\ M$ at 0°C (Baxter and Tomkins, 1971; Koblinsky *et al.*, 1972; Lippman *et al.*, 1973b; Pratt and Ishii, 1972; Shyamala, 1973a) number of reported *receptor* binding sites per cells falls in the range of two orders of magnitude 10^3 to 10^5. This large range may be attributed to (1) the techniques that have been used, considering that most determinations have been obtained in crude preparation; (2) the physiopathological states of animals, since occupation of sites by endogenous hormone may or may not have been considered (however, there are also possible differences according to age and other physiological parameters) ; (3) eventual intrinsic differences between *receptors* of various tissues (Baxter and Tomkins, 1971; Schaumburg and Bojesen,1968).

1. *Partial Purification of Cytosol Receptor*

The more detailed purification efforts reported to date deal with the rat liver *receptor*. Two groups (Beato *et al.*, 1970b, 1972; Beato and Feigelson, 1972; Koblinsky *et al.*, 1972; Filler and Litwack, 1973; Litwack *et al.*, 1973; Morey and Litwack, 1969; Singer *et al.*, 1973) have been involved in this work. In the first group, the glucocorticosteroid *receptor*, designated fraction G, is obtained by column chromatography. It binds dexamethasone more than the natural hormones cortisol and corticosterone, which correlates with the known respective biological activities of these compounds (Beato and Feigelson, 1972). Other binding fractions, D and B, do not appear to be *receptors*, B probably being transcortin. The molecular weight of fraction G in high salt is around 66,000, and the "8 S form" (in low salt) has been estimated at 200,000. The isoelectric point is between 4.3 and 5.1. In the other group (Litwack *et al.*, 1973), several glucocorticosteroid-binding fractions have also been obtained from rat liver cytosol. Fraction II represents the *receptor*. Binders I and III bind glucocorticosteroid metabolites, and binder IV has been identified as transcortin. Binder II appears to be very similar to compound G, with a molecular weight of 66,000 and two identical subunits and a sedimentation coefficient of 4.5 S. However, the reported isoelectric point is 6.7. The K_D for dexamethasone is 0.1–0.6 nM and for cortisol about 10 nM. Only binder II goes to the nucleus, in contrast to binder III (MW 7000) and ligandin (MW 40,000). Nuclear extracts have been obtained after transfer of the cytosol *receptor* either *in vivo* or *in vitro*, and the protein has been shown to be identical to the cytosol compound II. Antibodies against binder II do not cross-react with other binding fractions. Recently, a binder I B has been eluted from DEAE-Sephadex A-50 column chromatography, just after ligandin, of MW 30,000 (Litwack and Rosenfield, 1974). Its relationship with the other binding proteins is unknown.

2. *Binding Specificity of Receptor*

Affinities of glucocorticosteroids *receptors* for natural and synthetic derivatives have been measured in numerous tissues and have also been compared to biological activities in glucocorticosteroid-sensitive cells cultured *in vitro*. Corroborating biological observations *in vivo*, triamcinolone acetonide and dexamethasone have generally higher affinity for the *receptor* than either of the naturally occurring steroids corticosterone and cortisol. These latter steroids may or may not have (a question not yet resolved) differential affinity for the *receptor* correlated with the pattern of adrenal corticosteroid production in the given species. In most cases mineralocorticosteroids, aldosterone and deoxycorticosterone, have a certain affinity for the glucocorticosteroid receptor (1/10–1/50). Moreover, compounds such as progesterone and cortexolone (deoxycortisol) also have some affinity for the *receptor*, but do induce a very low amount of response, and can be antiinducer when used in competition against active glucocorticosteroid (Kaiser *et al.*, 1972). It has been reported that progesterone bound to the cytoplasmic glucocorticosteroid *receptor* of HTC cells or mammary tumors does not translocate to nuclei. Testosterone and estradiol have affinities 10^{-3} times less than glucocorticosteroids.

The classification of steroids, as tested for tyrosine aminotransferase (TAT) induction in the HTC system in culture, is interesting because it leads to hypotheses concerning *receptor* functioning. Optimum inducers can maximally induce the rate of synthesis, and there might be greatest-affinity compounds, such as dexamethasone, or relatively low-affinity compounds, such as aldosterone (Samuels and Tomkins, 1970). The correlation between binding affinity and steroid concentration for TAT induction is very good. Suboptimal inducers, such as cortexolone, can only increase enzyme to a submaximal but characteristic level, whatever the concentration of steroid in this system, and therefore they may compete against an optimal inducer for full induction. (If one takes an allosteric model implicating "active" and "inactive" forms of the *receptor*, there will be relatively less affinity for the active form and more for the inactive with suboptimal inducers than those with optimal inducers). Antiinducers, such as testosterone and 17α-methyltestosterone, cannot induce the enzymes at all, but "competitively" inhibit induction by optimal and suboptimal inducers and bind to the *receptor* (essentially to the inactive form in case of an allosteric model). Finally, there are compounds that neither promote induction of TAT nor act as antiinducer, and presumably do not interfere with the *receptor*. Similar results have been obtained in other systems (Chader and Reif-Lehrer, 1972; Lippman *et al.*, 1973a,b).

B. Distribution and Ontogeny

Physiological and physiopathological data indicate that glucocorticosteroids act upon many cells in the organism (adult as well as embryonic or fetal). Therefore, it is not surprising that glucocorticosteroid *receptors* have been found in most tissues where they have been looked for. Systematic studies have been performed mainly in the rat and in the rabbit. Many references can be found on Table I.

In the adult rat, on the basis of DNA and protein contents—which do not always go together (Table II)—liver, thymus, and kidney come first. Lungs do not have a *receptor* early in the fetus, but the increase at the end of gestation seems to be of great functional importance (Giannopoulos *et al.*, 1972). On occasion, it has been difficult to detect a *receptor* in sex organs, such as prostate and uterus. When the *receptor* has been analyzed by ultracentrifugation, a 7–8 S hormone complex has been found in all tissues, with occasional varying amounts of 4 S complexes. Also, specificity for glucocorticosteroids was essentially the same in all cases. Affinity for a given steroid, when it has been compared in different tissues, may have varied by a factor of 10, but the results are probably not significant, considering the techniques which have been used.

Besides changes from fetus to adult, aging has been studied (Roth, 1974, 1975). For instance, the number of sites decreases in muscle, brain, epididymal fat pad, and spleen leukocytes between the second and third months and the twenty-fifth month in the rat. Conversely, there is an increase in liver binding. The mechanism of these variations in glucocorticosteroid *receptors* is unknown, and it is not clear whether there may be some relationship with an adaptation of the organs or of the organism to nutritional changes, stresses, etc.

"New" target organs are presumably of great interest in research. There are fetal lung (mentioned already), and muscles and bones that react dramatically to corticosteroid therapy. Quite remarkable too, is the distribution of radioactivity observed autoradiographically and biochemically in the brain after injection of radioactive corticosterone to the rats (McEwen *et al.*, 1970, 1972). Hypothalamus is labeled, but not as much as hippocampus, septum, and amygdala. This finding has been extended to other species (Rotsztejn *et al.*, 1975). Here it seems that the discovery of *receptors* may have led to the discovery of new regulatory pathways. There may be heterogeneity of *receptors* (CBG excluded) in the brain as indicated by preferential binding of dexamethasone or corticosterone, according to the zone.

Indeed, comparison between the concentration and the affinity of *receptors* in different crude extracts is difficult. For instance, studies with cytosol of normal liver cells, Zajdela hepatoma, and HTC cells have led to the suggestion of positive and negative modulators of *receptor* binding (Defer *et al.*, 1974).

Another case where glucocorticosteroid *receptors* are difficult to analyze is the kidney, which also contains mineralocorticosteroid *receptors* binding aldosterone and deoxycorticosterone, and also dexamethasone and

TABLE I

DATA FROM STUDIES ON GLUCOCORTICOID RECEPTORS

| | Rat: juvenile buffalo rat (Ballard et al., 1974) | | Rabbit: New Zealand white rabbit | | | | |
| | | | Juvenile (pmoles/mg protein) | | Fetal (pmoles/mg protein) | | Fetal (pmoles/mg DNA) |
	Pmoles/mg DNA	Pmoles/mg protein	Ballard et al. (1974)	Giannopoulos et al. (1974)	Ballard et al. (1974)	Giannopoulos et al. (1974)	Giannopoulos et al. (1974)
Liver	10.62	0.64	0.12	0.12	0.12	0.17	0.49
Skeletal muscle	3.14	0.06	0.03	0.01	0.14	0.21	0.95
Heart	2.91	0.26	0.13	0.01	0.17	0.19	0.69
Kidney	1.38	0.23	0.16	0.05	0.24	0.46	1.83
Testis	1.23	0.10	0.22	—	—	—	—
Thymus	0.95	0.45	0.65	0.08	0.08	0.22	0.35
Small intestine	0.00	0.00	0.20	0.03	0.12	0.7	0.80
Stomach	0.56	0.08	0.19	—	—	—	—
Spleen	0.26	0.07	0.27	0.16	—	—	—
Lung	0.09	0.02	0.53	0.25	0.43	0.51	1.62
Brain	2.53	0.19	0.12	—	0.08	0.08	0.41
Uterus	0.00	0.00	—	—	—	—	—
Prostate	0.00	0.00	—	—	—	—	—
Placenta	—	—	—	—	—	0.25	1.78

TABLE II

ORGANS OR CELLS IN WHICH THE GLUCOCORTICOSTEROID RECEPTORS
HAVE BEEN DESCRIBED

Organ and cell	References
Skin	Ballard *et al.*, 1974; Giannopoulos *et al.*, 1974
Placenta	Ballard *et al.*, 1974; Giannopoulos *et al.*, 1974
Heart	Ballard *et al.*, 1974; Baxter and Forsham, 1972; Funder *et al.*, 1973c; Giannopoulos *et al.*, 1974
Intestine	Ballard *et al.*, 1974; Baxter and Forsham, 1972; Giannopoulos *et al.*, 1974; Henning *et al.*, 1975
Pancreas	Simonsson, 1972
Liver	Ballard *et al.*, 1974; Beato and Feigelson, 1972; Beato *et al.*, 1969, 1970a,b; Giannopoulos *et al.*, 1974; Litwack and Rosenfield, 1974; Milgrom *et al.*, 1973a; Morey and Litwack, 1969; Rosen and Milholland, 1972; Schaumburg, 1972b; Singer *et al.*, 1973; Van der Meulen and Sekeris, 1973
Kidney	Ballard *et al.*, 1974; Funder *et al.*, 1973c; Giannopoulos *et al.*, 1974; Rousseau *et al.*, 1972a
Lung	Ballard *et al.*, 1974; Giannopoulos *et al.*, 1972, 1974
Retina (chick)	Chader, 1973; Moscona and Piddington, 1966, 1967; Reif-Lehrer, 1968; Reif-Lehrer and Chader, 1969
Skeletal muscle	Ballard *et al.*, 1974; Baxter and Forsham, 1972; Giannopoulos *et al.*, 1974; Mayer *et al.*, 1975; Simpson and White, 1973
Smooth muscle	Baxter and Forsham, 1972
Bone	Feldman *et al.*, 1975
Stomach	Baxter and Forsham, 1972
Mammary gland (and tumor)	Tucker *et al.*, 1971; Shyamala, 1973b, 1974, 1975
Testes	Baxter and Forsham, 1972
Brain	Ballard *et al.*, 1974; Geilach and McEwen, 1972; McEwen *et al.*, 1970
Hippocampus	Rotsztejn *et al.*, 1975
Pituitary	Harrison *et al.*, 1975:[a] Rotsztejn *et al.*. 1975
Leukocytes	Simonsson, 1972
Lymphoid tissue	Baxter *et al.*, 1971; Kirkpatrick *et al.*, 1972; Lippman *et al.*, 1973a; Rosenau *et al.*, 1972; Schaumburg and Crone, 1971
Thymus	Augustyn and Brunkhorst, 1972b; Ballard *et al.*, 1974; Giannopoulos *et al.*, 1974; Kaiser *et al.*, 1972, 1973; Koch *et al.*, 1972; Munck and Brinck-Johnsen, 1968; Schaumburg, 1972a,b; Schaumburg and Bojesen, 1968; Wira and Munck, 1970
Fibroblasts and L cells	Hackney *et al.*, 1970; Ishii *et al.*, 1972; Lippman and Thompson, 1973, 1974; Pratt and Ishii, 1972
HeLa cells	Melnykovych and Bishop, 1969, 1971
Lymphoma S 49	Baxter *et al.*, 1971; Rosenau *et al.*, 1972
Hepatoma tumor cells	Baxter and Tomkins, 1970, 1971; Lippman and Thompson, 1973, 1974; Singer *et al.*, 1973

[a] In the cell line studied, a limited entry of glucocorticosteroids, distinct from cytosol *receptor*, has been described.

cortisol. Moreover, there is the presence of CBG. As already seen, liver tissue also displays some binding complexity.

C. Relationships between Cytosol and Nuclear *Receptors*

Even if many aspects of *receptor* transfer have initially been observed with estrogens, the glucocorticosteroid *receptors* have also been studied in detail insofar as the problems of distribution, activation, and transfer to nucleus are concerned. They are found in the cytosol fraction only in the absence of hormone (in HTC cells, Baxter *et al.*, 1971) or in rat liver after adrenalectomy (Milgrom *et al.*, 1973a) while present in both the cytosol and in the nucleus after exposure to steroid (Baxter *et al.*, 1971; Beato *et al.*, 1969; Levinson *et al.*, 1972; Milgrom *et al.*, 1973a). *In vitro* experiments with cells first incubated at 0°C and then at 37°C (Higgins *et al.*, 1973a) and with subcellular systems where nuclei and cytosol preparations are mixed together (Milgrom *et al.*, 1973a) have clearly indicated the necessity of the binding of hormone to allow transfer and then "activation" of the *receptor*. The change is accelerated by brief heating at 20°–30°C and high ionic strength, or both, even at a cold temperature.

When activated, the *receptor* can bind to the nucleus even at 0°C, provided the salt concentration is lower than 0.2 *M*. The appearance of the nuclear *receptor* is parallel to the decrease of the cytosol *receptor* in cellular or subcellular systems, or in *in vivo* experiments, and then leads to the concept of a transfer of the *receptor* from an extranuclear compartment to the nucleus. The nuclear acceptor which binds the activated hormone *receptor* complexes may include DNA, since after treatment by DNase, no binding is observed. Conversely, the binding of the hormone *receptor* preparation to various DNAs shows no convincing specificity on the part of the DNA. *In vitro* binding studies with corticosteroid *receptors* from HTC and liver cells have, however, shown conclusive evidence for the specificity of the interaction of the *receptor* with DNA (Beato *et al.*, 1973; Higgins *et al.*, 1973a,b,c; Kalimi *et al.*, 1973). On the other hand, nuclear binding sites for glucocorticosteroid *receptors* have been reported in nontarget tissues (Higgins *et al.*, 1973b; Lippman and Thompson, 1973). After "saturation" of nuclear binding sites in intact HTC cells, for instance, it was still possible to bind an important additional amount of *receptor* in a secondary *in vitro* incubation of the "charged" nuclei with a *receptor* containing cytosol (Higgins *et al.*, 1973b). Therefore, owing to contradictory results, the significance as well as the mutual relationship of *in vitro*- and *in vivo*-detected nuclear binding sites for the *receptor* still remains to be established. For instance, experiments where crude preparations of HTC (cytosol and nuclei of HTC cells) and rat uterus were mixed (Higgins *et al.*, 1973b,c) are difficult to evaluate and do not conclusively demonstrate acceptor specificity.

Other experiments have taken advantage of different glucocorticosteroid *receptors* from different cells (Lippman and Thompson, 1973), as, for instance, HTC cells responding by enzyme induction to glucocorticosteroids and L cells (mouse fibroblasts), which show a general decrease of macromolecular synthesis. Differences in nuclear acceptor activity have been reported (Lippman and Thompson, 1973). Hybrids from HTC and L cells (Lippman and Thompson, 1974) respond to glucocorticosteroid as well as L cells, but do not show an HTC-type response. However, it has been stated that both parental cytoplasmic *receptors* are present, as well as the two classes of nuclear acceptor sites (supposedly able to discriminate among the *receptors*). Moreover, hybrids between HTC cells and steroid-resistant L cells (not containing L-cell *receptor*) contain the HTC *receptor*, but again show no HTC response (and no L response), indicating that it is not the "negative response" of L cells which dominates the hybrid.

It is also with glucocorticosteroids that some aspects of the *receptor* cycle in target cells have been studied. In HTC cells, the *receptor* has a long half-life and this slow turnover necessarily distinguishes it from the posttranscriptional repressor postulated in this HTC system (Tomkins *et al.*, 1969). If the *receptor* is located in the extranuclear part of the cells in the absence of hormone and transfers largely to the nucleus in the presence of hormone, the corticosteroid is released in changing the cells to a nonhormone-containing medium, and there is an exit of hormone with a return to the *receptor* binding sites in the cytoplasm (Rousseau *et al.*, 1973). This return does not require protein synthesis. Working with mouse L-929 cells in culture (Ishii *et al.*, 1972), it has been observed that in the presence of radioactive triamcinolone acetonide at 37°C, the amount of bound cytoplasmic steroids which appear constant for several hours depends on *receptor* sites being continually inactivated and then probably recycled. It seems that there might be an active component for the reentry of binding sites in the cytoplasm. Energy deprivation reduces the binding of steroid in the supernatant fraction but increases the *receptor* in the nuclear fraction as though the release of the *receptor* from the particular fraction is inhibited by lack of oxygen, cyanide, or DNP.

Recent work (Jung-Testas and Bayard, 1975) points to an "insoluble" fraction, similar to the one described by Lebeau *et al.* (1973) for estrogens and it may be precisely engaged in the nuclear block in absence of energy sources (Middlebrook *et al.*, 1975). Therefore, one may propose that the cell is continuously regenerating (and inactivating) *receptors*, instead of suggesting a simple application of the law of mass action for dissociation of the nuclear hormone–*receptor* complexes. These results may be compared to results that, in rat thymus cells (Munck *et al.*, 1972; Bell and Munck, 1973), indicate that the cytoplasmic fraction prepared from cells incubated at 37°C in the absence of oxygen binds cortisol less readily than when obtained from aerobic cells, while the binding capacity can be restored by exposure of anaerobic cells to oxygen. Again, the use of an inhibitor of protein synthesis does not change the result, and an energy-dependent step directly or indirectly implicating ATP is described. One should observe that these results essentially apply to short periods of time. In this respect they must be considered in connection with the protein synthesis-dependent replenishment of the estradiol cytosol *receptor* (Sarff and Gorski, 1971; Mester and Baulieu, 1975) and the "inactivation" of the progesterone *receptor* (Milgrom *et al.*, 1973a), which concern a longer period of time.

D. RECEPTOR DEFECTS AND STEROID RESISTANCE

Interesting correlations between the presence or the absence of *receptor* and the lack of effects of glucocorticosteroids have been observed. This is the case in human acute lymphoblastic leukemia (Lippman *et al.*, 1973a,b) and in mouse lymphoma cell lines (Hollander and Chui, 1966; Baxter *et al.*, 1971; Kirkpatrick *et al.*, 1971, 1972; Rosenau *et al.*, 1972), with a recent genetic analysis of glucocorticosteroid resistance *in vitro* (Sibley and Tomkins, 1974). A series of steroid-resistant clones have been isolated, using the line of lymphoma S-49, which is sensitive to dexamethasone; ~80% are deficient in cytosol *receptor* (r—); some (~10%) have the receptor, but no transfer of steroid complexes to nucleus (nt—) occurs; and the rest (~10%) show *receptor* and normal transfer (d—). These results strongly support a hypothesis that would attribute an important role to *receptors* in hormone action. Not only do merely 10% of those nonresponsive with *receptor* normally reach the nucleus, but among those, a detailed analysis may have indicated in some cases a small but nevertheless detectable abnormality of dexamethasone binding (increased affinity). Therefore, the percentage of detected abnormalities of the *receptor* that could explain steroid resistance is (surprisingly) very high.

VII. MINERALOCORTICOSTEROID *Receptors*

Aldosterone, the principal mineralocorticosteroid, is secreted in very low amounts and is present in extremely low concentration in the plasma of mammals. In addition to its very important activity of sodium retention at the kidney level, it may affect other cells in the body. Physiological *in vivo* experiments have encountered great difficulties in a clear evaluation of certain frontiers between the so-called glucocorticosteroid and mineralocorticosteroid activities. A study of the *receptors* may throw some light on this important problem. As already cited, it is with aldosterone that it was shown for the first time by radioautography that an active steroid hormone eventually locates in the nuclei of target cells (toad bladder, *in vitro*, Edelman *et al.*, 1963; Bogoroch, 1969).

A. Isolation and Characterization of Aldosterone *Receptor* in Rat Kidney

The rat kidney has been carefully studied on the basis of selective uptake and binding of aldosterone to cytosol and nuclear protein after injection of low doses of radioactive hormone to adrenalectomized animals (Fanestil and Edelman, 1966). The plasma concentration of radioactive steroid to obtain saturation of nuclear sites when increasing doses of injected radioactive hormone was in good agreement with the concentration required for maximal antinatriuresis.

As in many other steroid target organs, no binding was observed in microsomal and mitochondrial fractions (Fanestil, 1968). However, specific binding has recently been described at the plasma membrane level (Forte, 1972).

Kidney cytosol contains at least two classes of specific aldosterone-binding proteins as indicated by Scatchard analysis. The higher-affinity component probably represents the mineralocorticosteroid *receptor* sites, properly specific, called type I. Its K_D at $0°C$ is approximately 5 nM, and at $37°C$, 0.5 nM (Rousseau *et al.*, 1972a; Funder *et al.*, 1973a). Another high affinity set of sites has K_D at $0°C$ approximately 65 nM, and at $37°C$, 25 nM: it is called type II. The number of sites of type II *receptor* is similar to the value determined by dexamethasone binding, and competition studies indicate high affinity for dexamethasone and corticosterone; this site may in fact be the glucocorticosteroid *receptor* sites to which aldosterone also binds (Table III). In fact, there is even a type III binding system in the kidney cytosol to which aldosterone binds very feebly, dexamethasone hardly at all, and corticosterone very well, as expected for a plasma CBG contaminant (Funder *et al.*, 1973b). Study of the aldosterone *receptor* has indicated better stability in glycerol-containing media (Marver *et al.*, 1972); two peaks are obtained by ultracentrifugation in the 8–9 S region and in the 4–5 S region in hypotonic low-salt medium. The addition of 0.3 M KCl in the buffer apparently gives

TABLE III

RELATIVE AFFINITIES OF RAT KIDNEY CYTOSOL STEROID-BINDING PROTEINS

	Mineralo-receptor	Gluco-receptor	CBG	Hormone concentration in plasma (nM)
Aldosterone	100[a]	50	∼0	0.2
Deoxycorticosterone	80	40	30	0.4
Corticosterone	2	100[a]	100[b]	100
Dexamethasone	∼0	4300	∼0	—

[a] K_D of *receptors* approximately 1 nM at 0°C.

[b] K_D of corticosteroid-binding globulin (CBG) approximately 10 nM at 0°C.

a single 4 S peak. These studies have been confirmed by a gel filtration technique (Ludens and Fanestil, 1971; Morris and Davis, 1973). The protein nature of the receptor and its susceptibility to SH-blocking agents have been demonstrated (Herman *et al.*, 1968). Attempts to purify it by affinity chromatography have not been successful to date, even though interesting technical observations have been recorded in the course of this work (Ludens *et al.*, 1973). Recent work uses ion-exchange chromatography (Agarwal, 1975).

Nuclear binding of ³H-labeled aldosterone has been studied after *in vivo* injection of the hormone (Fanestil and Edelman, 1966; Herman *et al.*, 1968; Swaneck *et al.*, 1970), and also after incubation of isolated nuclei with ³H-aldosterone–*receptor* complexes (Marver *et al.*, 1972). Untransformed aldosterone is present in the nucleus, bound to macromolecular complexes (Swaneck *et al.*, 1970). An easily solubilizable nuclear fraction is extractable by 0.1 M Tris 3 mM $CaCl_2$ buffer, and its sedimentation rate is 3 S. It has been called "soluble nuclear." After this low-salt extraction, the same buffer, but containing 0.3 or 0.4 M KCl, applied to residual nuclear pellet removes another protein sedimenting somewhat faster (4 S), certainly not a histone (Swaneck *et al.*, 1970; Edelman, 1971), and called "chromatin-bound *receptor*." It is interesting that time-course experiments with rat kidney slices have indicated a sort of serial relationship between the cytosol, the soluble nuclear, and the chromatin-binding systems (Marver *et al.*, 1972). Entering the tissue, aldosterone-³H successively binds to the cytosol and then the soluble nuclear complex appears, and finally chromatin binding. This sequence suggests a three-step mechanism (Marver *et al.*, 1972; Edelman, 1971). The nuclear transfer is temperature-dependent and does not occur in the absence of cytosol.

B. Specificity of Aldosterone-Binding Proteins in Kidney

The specificity of binding sites for a wide range of steroids is indistinguishable on cytosol and nuclear proteins. Mineralocorticosteroids, such as (d)-aldosterone, 9α-fluorocortisol, 6α-methylprenisolone and deoxycorticosterone, have the highest affinity. There is also some binding, of lower affinity, of 18-hydroxydeoxycorticosterone, 18-hydroxycorticosterone (Feldman and Funder, 1973), and glycyrrhetic acid (Corvol et al., 1974). Sites I bind glucocorticosteroids to a certain degree, but not estradiol and isoaldosterone (aldosterone with a 17α chain instead of the 17β chain of pregnane steroids) (Funder et al., 1973b; Herman et al., 1968; Swaneck et al., 1970). Antimineralocorticosteroid spironolactone (SC-1, 426) (Fanestil, 1968; Herman et al., 1968; Swaneck et al., 1970) inhibits the binding of aldosterone to chromatin sites, when it is in a molar ratio with aldosterone, antagonizing the sodium transport effect. Recent studies with SC-26,304 (Marver et al., 1974), a spironolactone of higher affinity for the receptor and available in the radioactive form, indicate that its binding occurs presumably at the same cytosol *receptor* sites as aldosterone, but the ^{3}H-labeled SC-26,304 *receptor* complexes exhibit 3 S and 4 S sedimentation coefficients in low-salt and high-salt media, respectively (when the aldosterone-^{3}H complexes treated in parallel fashion have 8.5 S and 4 S in low salt and 4.5 S in high salt). Moreover, in *in vivo* as well as in *in vitro* slice experiments, and in reconstitution studies with prelabeled cytosol and purified nuclei or chromatin, ^{3}H-labeled SC-26,304 does not give specific nuclear complexes. These results may indicate that the change of sedimentation coefficients of antialdosterone complexes with reference to those of aldosterone are possibly related to a lack of the "activation" necessary for nuclear uptake.

The respective concentrations of corticosterone, deoxycorticosterone, and aldosterone in rat plasma and the affinities of *receptor* I for these steroids indicate that the mineralocorticosteroid *receptors* could be preferentially occupied by deoxycorticosterone if another competing binding mechanism is not in operation (Funder et al., 1973b). It seems that plasma transcortin may play that role.

Incidentally, mineralocorticosteroid *receptors* are the same in salt-sensitive and salt-resistant rats (which have hypertension) (Funder et al., 1974).

C. Mineralocorticosteroid *Receptors* in Other Organs and Species

In the rat, aldosterone-binding proteins have been detected from the cytosol of kidney, *duodenal mucosa, spleen, liver* (Swaneck et al., 1969), and *parotid gland* (Funder *et al.*, 1972). However, the possibility that aldosterone-³H binds principally to glucocorticosteroid binding sites in the spleen and liver has not yet been systematically explored. The presence of aldosterone binding proteins in the kidney of *guinea pig fetus* at midgestation has been reported (Pasqualini and Sumida, 1971).

The binding of aldosterone-³H has been studied in whole *toad bladder* (Sharp *et al.*, 1966) and in nuclei from the *mucosal cells* of this tissue (Ansiello and Sharp, 1968; Alberti and Sharp, 1969; Sharp and Alberti, 1971). These early studies have indicated two sets of binding proteins with high affinity for aldosterone. Aldosterone-³H was readily displaced from both sets by known steroid agonists and by spironolactone. The physiological role of the highest affinity *receptor* (K_D on the order of the 10 pM) is obscure, since it should be saturated at concentrations of hormone too low to provoke sodium transport (Sharp and Alberti, 1971). Studies with this system have permitted a classification of steroids according to their interaction with mineralocorticosteroid *receptors* and their activity on sodium transport (Alberti and Sharp, 1970). There is also indication that a characteristic latent period before stimulation of sodium transport is not attributable to a delay in the binding of the hormone within the tissue since the chromatin is reached a few minutes before physiological action is seen (Sharp *et al.*, 1966).

Studies of aldosterone binding have been hampered by the fact that the kidney may present the problem of heterogeneity of steroid *receptor* sites. However, studies with different zones of the kidney have not yet shown significant differences. Toad bladder, for its part, requires a large quantity of material. However, the two most often used target tissues respond quickly and quantitatively to administration of mineralocorticosteroids, and therefore remain among the best in which one can correlate binding phenomena and hormone action.

Recent studies (Lassman and Mulrow, 1974) have indicated the lack of deoxycorticosterone-binding protein in the *brain* of rats resistant to deoxycorticosterone-induced hypertension when this protein is present in hypothalamus of sensitive rats and also in the cortex of resistant rats. Available data raised the question that it may be related to the brain glucocorticosteroid *receptor* (McEwen *et al.*, 1972; Stevens *et al.*, 1971).

VII. Ecdysone, Vitamin D, and Thyroid Hormones

A. Ecdysone *Receptors*

The many effects of ecdysone in insect development have led to a search for corresponding *receptors*. However, early attempts have been hampered by the lack of α-hormone of high specific activity. Radioauto-graphic studies (Emmerich, 1969; Claycomb et al., 1971) have suggested nuclear uptake in cells of salivary glands. Since β-ecdysone (a metabolite formed from α) has been implied in hormone action, the lack of highly labeled β-derivatives is still a difficulty. However, with α-ecdysone-³H injected in vivo, a "transport" protein has been identified (Butterworth and Berendes, 1974). Recently, the nuclear localization and the cyto-plasm to nuclear transfer of "specifically bound" (limited number of sites) radioactive material have been observed in glands of Drosophila by radioautography after injection of highly labeled α-ecdysone-³H (C. Le Goascogne and H. Berendes, unpublished observations), which has also been reported in imaginal discs (Yund and Fristrom, 1975) and in β-ecdy-sone-sensitive cell clones whereas no β-ecdysone receptor was detectable in β-ecdysone-resistant clones (Best-Belpomme and Courgeon, 1975).

B. VITAMIN D Receptors

Recent findings concerning the formation and role of vitamin D metab-olites have attracted much attention. It is rather interesting that in intes-tine, where 1α-25-dihydroxycalciferol appears to be the active compound, there is a receptor system very similar to that found in conventional ste-roid hormone target tissues. As shown recently, (Fraser and Kodicek, 1970; Norman and Henry, 1974; De Luca, 1974; Brumbaugh and Haus-sler, 1974a), cholecalciferol and metabolites can be considered as steroid hormones. Receptor work is found in the following references (Brum-baugh and Haussler, 1974a,b; Lawson and Wilson, 1974; Tsai and Nor-man, 1973; Chen and De Luca, 1973; Lawson et al., 1971).

C. THYROID HORMONE Receptors

Although they belong to another chemical series, thyroid hormones are the only hormones, besides steroids, to have well established intracellular receptors. There were few publications since the early studies of Tata (1962) until the findings of Oppenheimer et al. (1972), who indicated specific nuclear binding in rat liver. However, the matter is currently being carefully probed (Oppenheimer, 1975). "Activated" steroid receptor complexes and triiodothyronine receptor complexes bind to DNA (McLeod and Baxter, 1975). Unlike steroids, thyroid hormones do not seem to influence receptor distribution between cytoplasm and nucleus of target cells, and the cytosol-binding system(s) is still of undetermined significant (Dillman et al., 1974; DeGroot and Torresani, 1975).

IX. *Receptors* and Hormone Action: Steroid *Receptors* in
Target Cell Nuclei

In most cases steroid hormone *receptors* are found in the cytosol of
homogenates of hormone-deprived target cells (see exceptions in Section
III, B, 2). The current data suggesting that *receptors* are indeed located
in the cytoplasm of target cells come only from radioautographic studies
(S. Weiller, unpublished observations, 1975). Even so, one cannot exclude
the possibility that *receptors* are not really cytosoluble and detached from
cytoplasmic particles during homogenization. In any case, after injection
of hormone into the whole animal or after incubation of the tissues or
cells at 20°–37°C with the corresponding steroids, a large fraction of the
steroid *receptor* complexes is found in the nuclei (Jensen, 1965; Noteboom
and Gorski, 1965).

The increased affinity for the nucleus of "activated" steroid *receptor*
complexes designates an acceptor as being responsible for the binding.
"Acceptor" does not necessarily designate the cellular structure responsible for switching the cell machinery after the interaction with steroid
receptor complexes. In other words, the *receptor* site interacting with the
acceptor may theoretically be different from the executive site (Fig. 2),
even if the simplest and most likely possibility is that they are one and
the same. Therefore, one uses the word acceptor as an operational definition to physically designate the attachment of hormone–*receptor* complexes in nuclei. Other questions deal with the fate of the *receptor* in
the nucleus, its eventual recycling to cytoplasm and/or inactivation, and
the correlated problem of departure of the hormone from its site of action.

A. *Receptor* "Transformation" or "Activation"

Three parameters have been studied in relation with the modifications
of hormone *receptors* interacting with nuclei: these are changes of the
sedimentation coefficient, novel affinity for nuclear "acceptor" acquired
under specific conditions, and stimulation of RNA polymerase activity
in isolated nuclei. The overall change of *receptor* is designated as "transformation" or "activation."

It has been observed that the sedimentation coefficient of the estradiol
nuclear *receptor* is about 5 S in 0.3–0.4 M KCl, while the cytosol *receptor*
is 4 S in the same medium (Jensen *et al.*, 1969b). It has not been decided
whether this change of sedimentation coefficient is related to a purely
conformational change or if it is related to the addition of a subunit of
40,000–50,000 MW (Yamamoto and Alberts, 1974; Notides and Nielsen,

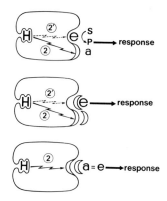

Fig. 2. Acceptor (a) and executive (e) sites of the *receptor*: some theoretical possibilities. (I, *top*). e is catalytic, and is distinct from a. The *receptor* is an enzyme (by its e site), and the localization of the hormone–*receptor* complexes in the nucleus corresponds to the presence of an acceptor that interacts with the site a. Then the e and the a sites are distinct. Activation follows the binding of H and modifies the a site, ② leading to interaction with acceptor. Whether or not activation influences the e site is optional ②' .

(II, *middle*). e is binding, and is distinct from a. The hormone–*receptor* complex binds, for instance, to a protein or a nucleic acid in a specific manner, and the response is switched on. However, the nuclear acceptor is distinct, eventually nonspecific; as in I, activation follows the binding of H and modifies the a site, ②, leading to interaction with acceptor. Whether or not there is influence of the e site by activation is optional, ②'.

(III, *bottom*). e is binding, and is the same as a. The *receptor* binds, for instance, to either a protein or a nucleic acid and, since e and a are the same, activation leads to binding to acceptor and to switching the response. The (nuclear) structure, which is at the same time acceptor and executive, may not be specific [specific would mean here a unique or limited class of protein or nucleic structure(s)].

Notes: Whatever is the case (I, II, or III), there is a possibility that the acceptor structure is not narrowly specific, corroborating the characteristics of "acidophilic activation" of the *receptor* (Milgrom *et al.*, 1973a). The function of the interaction of the acceptor with the *receptor* could be, for instance, to designate to the *receptor* some preferential positioning. Results in nonestrogenic sensitive mammary tumors (Shyamala, 1973b) and mutants of lymphoma cells (Gehring and Tomkins, 1974) show binding of hormone, but not of *receptor,* to nucleus. They indicate that the a site of the *receptor* and/or the nuclear acceptor may be decisive for hormone action, but they do not designate any of the possibilities between I, II, and III.

1974). In subcellular systems (cytosol plus nuclei), as well as in intact cells where there is a rapid transfer of the hormone *receptor* into the nucleus at 20°–37°C, the 4 S → 5 S transformation of the hormone–cytosol *receptor* complex has been parallelly observed. These observations have been correlated by the possibility of obtaining a 4 S → 5 S change *in vitro* by heating the hormone containing cytosol (high ionic strength) (Jensen and De Sombre, 1972b). Since the estradiol–*receptor* complexes have acquired a capacity to bind the nuclei, the concept which relates the change of the sedimentation coefficient to the increased affinity for nuclear acceptor has gained acceptance. Finally, with estrogens, a third indication of transformation of the *receptor* has been observed, since there is increased incorporation of radioactivity from labeled triphosphate nucleosides into RNA by isolated target (uterus or prostate) nuclei exposed to *receptor*-containing cytosol-hormone (estradiol or androstanolone) mixture (Raynaud-Jammet and Baulieu, 1969; Davies and Griffith, 1974; Arnaud *et al.*, 1971; Mohla *et al.*, 1972). Recent results with purified uterine *receptor* (Mohla *et al.*, 1975) and with the chick oviduct estrogen systems (B. W. O'Malley, unpublished observation, 1975) confirm these observations. Here, like the changes in sedimentation coefficient and affinity for acceptor, the effect is hormone dependent.

Similarly, facts observed with other systems confirm the overall concept of transformation or activation of the *receptor,* but also raise some doubts about the obligatory linkage between the three parameters already cited. For instance, the nuclear transfer of the prostatic *receptor* of androstanolone is accelerated by preheating, but the yield does not change (Mainwaring and Irving, 1973). Similarly, the transfer or the binding of the glucocorticosteroid *receptor* of HTC (Rousseau *et al.*, 1972b) or of rat liver (Milgrom *et al.*, 1973a) to nuclei or chromatin of the corresponding cells is accelerated by preheating, including that in a low-salt medium. No changes of sedimentation coefficients have been reported in the latter case. Increased affinity for nuclei and for DNA has been reported after transitory exposure to high ionic strength of the corticosteroid *receptor* of liver and HTC, even at 0°C (Rousseau *et al.*, 1972b; Milgrom *et al.*, 1973a). This latter observation brings into question the significance of the change in sedimentation coefficient reported above for the estrogen *receptor*, since, even at low temperature, 16–18 hours of centrifugation in 0.4 M KCl medium may be sufficient for activation. Therefore, the proposed relationship between the change of sedimentation coefficient and activation is not completely satisfactory. Under reported experimental conditions, the affinity of the *receptor* is increased not only for a physiological acceptor such as the nucleus or homologous chromatin, but also for homologous and heterologous DNAs and even for a series of polyanions [RNAs and substituted dextrans (Milgrom *et al.*, 1973a; A. Alberga, unpublished observations, 1973)]. One might hypothesize that "acidophilic" activation (Milgrom *et al.*, 1973a) may be due to an increase of positive charge at the surface of the *receptor* molecule, the hormone stabilizing the appropriate conformation.

B. Nuclear "Acceptor"

The nature of the acceptor is still unknown. *In vitro* steroid–*receptor* complexes in many experiments involving temperature and/or salt exposure, are capable of interacting with DNA (Mainwaring and Peterken, 1971; Rousseau *et al.*, 1972b; Milgrom *et al.*, 1973a; André and Rochefort, 1973a; King and Gordon, 1972; Toft, 1972; Yamamoto and Alberts, 1972; Musliner and Chader, 1971, 1972; Clemens and Kleinsmith, 1972), certain acidic protein(s) of chromatin (Spelsberg *et al.*, 1971, 1972), and ribonucleoproteins (Liao *et al.*, 1973b). However, it has not been demonstrated that these interactions are of physiological significance. For instance, the fact that it is possible to bind any steroid *receptor* to *any* eukaryotic DNA (and even to many other polyanions) leaves some doubt about the specificity of the observed phenomenon.

In some experimental conditions, "saturation" of nuclear or chromatin binding sites has been observed when increasing the amount of *receptors* (or, more precisely, *receptor*-containing cytosol preparations). Then a high affinity (K_D of the order of 10^{-10} M) and a relatively small number of acceptor sites (corresponding to a few hundred or thousand per target cell) have been reported (Mainwaring and Peterken, 1971; Rousseau *et al.*, 1972b; King and Gordon, 1972; O'Malley *et al.*, 1973; Higgins *et al.*, 1973b; Halimi *et al.*, 1973). However, no clear demonstration has been given, for instance, for the noncompetition by noncharged *receptors* (which cannot be activated) and even of competition by (nonlabeled) hormone *receptor* complexes. One can add *in vitro* as much steroid *receptor* to nuclei already charged *in vivo* as to "empty" nuclei (Higgins *et al.*, 1973c). Other authors (Chamnes *et al.*, 1974; Milgrom and Atger, 1975) found that the acceptor sites of nuclei cannot be saturated with *receptors* of estrogens and glucocorticosteroids. This would suggest the interference of nonspecific macromolecules in experiments where "saturation" has been observed. The limitation of nuclear binding observed *in vivo* after injection of hormone may be due to a deficit of cytosol *receptor* in the corresponding cells. The experiments of Williams and Gorski (1971) have indicated that in intact uterine cells there is a sort of partition between extranuclear and nuclear hormone–*receptor* complex implicating no high-affinity, low (limiting)-capacity nuclear acceptor sites; this conclusion has been reached independently in *in vivo* uptake experiments by de Hertogh *et al.* (1973).

Indeed, there is even a controversy concerning the specificity of target cell nuclei for being or containing the acceptor in *in vitro* experiments, since certain authors (Mainwaring and Peterken, 1971; Spelsberg *et al.*, 1971, 1972; Jensen and DeSombre, 1972b) believe that this is so, while others (Chamness *et al.*, 1973) do not. It is possible that, until now, experimental conditions have not been appropriate for letting one see the specificity, but it may also be recalled that all mechanisms, for explaining hormone action, as shown in Fig. 2, do not implicate such selectivity.

C. Fate of the *Receptor* and of the Hormone

No general picture has yet emerged.

1. Unconventional views have stated that lysosomes play a role in hormone transport in target nuclei (Szego, 1974) or that a cytosol 5 S *receptor* delivers hormone to a nuclear membrane *receptor* (Jackson and Chackley, 1974a).

2. In the uterine estradiol system, in physiological hormone concentration, an excess of cytosol binding sites seem to be unoccupied by hormones. But this is not the case of the prostate, where all the sites are occupied by androgen. Whether this different situation is related to the different plasma concentrations of hormones (cycling estrogens lower than constant androgen) to a limited number of nuclear sites, or to another reason is an open question. When the hormone is increased in the uterine system, more cytosol *receptor* moves to the nucleus, but it rapidly returns to the cytoplasm (Mester and Baulieu, 1975; Jensen and DeSombre, 1972b), and, after 3–6 hours (Anderson *et al.*, 1973), there is a maximum number of KCl-extractable hormone–*receptor* complexes, regardless of the amount of hormone administered.

3. There may be some destruction of the *receptor* since the transfer of the cytosol *receptor* to the nucleus cannot account for the decrease of the cytosol *receptor* in the case of a high dose of estradiol (Mester and Baulieu, 1975). Moreover, in the nucleus, there might be some masking or degradation of *receptor*, which may eventually explain the results obtained in the case of progesterone (Milgrom *et al.*, 1973c).

4. Three sorts of nuclear *receptors* have been detected in target nuclei: "soluble" nuclear, KCl-extractable, and "insoluble." The soluble is operationally defined by extractability from purified nuclei using solutions of low ionic strength: it has been found in the case of aldosterone in kidney (Edelman, 1971) and of estradiol in chick liver (Mester and Baulieu, 1972). It has not been definitively determined whether it is only the experimental conditions and species differences that make this low-salt extraction more successful in certain cases than in others. Therefore, whether or not the soluble differs from the more classical KCl-extractable *receptors* is a matter for future work. The KCl-extractable *receptor*, also called chromatin-bound by Swaneck *et al.* (1970), has been discussed in each steroid *receptor* section. It has been operational in developing

the concept of transformation or activation of *receptor* (see above). Finally, in considering the "insoluble" *receptor,* seen with estrogens (Lebeau *et al.,* 1973; Mester and Baulieu, 1975) and confirmed with corticosteroids (Middlebrook *et al.,* 1975; Jung-Testas and Baulieu, 1975), it must again be described as an operationally defined fraction, extensive buffer extraction being unable to remove specific binding sites from target nuclei. It is not yet known whether the various percentages of "insoluble" binding sites in different cases should be related to experimental conditions or to some physiologically important differences. Solubilization of a portion of this *receptor* by mild trypsin treatment has indicated a similarity with trypsin-treated cytosol *receptor* (Lebeau *et al.,* 1974), and recent kinetic studies with cultured cells (Middlebrook *et al.,* 1975) have suggested also a possible relationship with the cytosol *receptor.* Therefore, one cannot exclude the possibility that the insoluble *receptor* is the same as the cytosol *receptor* becoming nuclear (neonuclear), which would then be inserted successively into a KCl-extractable and then an "insoluble" environment, possibly in relation to its functioning (RNA polymerases were called "soluble" or "aggregated," and it turned out that they are related to nontranscribing and transcribing states).

5. The suppression of sources of energy by nitrogen exposure or metabolic inhibitors (Ishii *et al.,* 1972; Munck *et al.,* 1972) gives a decrease of binding sites in the cytoplasm. This effect has been attributed to some kind of intervention occurring on the return of the *receptor* from the nucleus, as if there were a reactivation of a "used" nuclear *receptor.* If this hypothesis is valid, the *receptor* could release the hormone in the nucleus, return to the cytoplasm and then again be reactivated, and thus enable a new binding of hormone. Actually, very little is understood concerning a possible *receptor* cycle in target cells.

X. Steroid Hormones and Prevision of Hormone Dependence of Human Cancer

The role of hormone *receptors* in physiopathological processes remains to be established, even if the first results concerning their variations and controls have been reported. More will come soon. In this chapter, progress in the human cancer field are summarized.

Since the observation of Beatson in 1896 showing the remission of advanced breast cancer after ovariectomy, the observations of Huggins *et al.* (1941) on prostatic carcinoma treated by castration and estrogen have established that a number of human malignancies are hormone dependent. Mammary, endometrial, prostatic, and renal cancers and lymphoblastic leukemias have already been classified as such. The development of the disease may depend on hormonal secretion and regress after its suppression, obtainable physically (e.g., by surgery) or by hormonal treatment (e.g., leading to pituitary inhibition). In other cases, administered steroids would antagonize another hormone effect at the target level (e.g., androgen-antagonizing estrogen) or elsewhere, the steroid would have a cellulolytic effect (e.g., glucocorticosteroids on lymphocytes). However, from the overall experience with breast cancer, a gross evaluation estimates that only 30% of the tumors are sensitive to hormones, and even those often become secondarily hormone resistant. For these reasons, it is important to be able to predict with a certain degree of accuracy which patients can benefit from hormonal therapeutics. Most of these treatments are quite serious, such as adrenalectomy or hypophysectomy for breast cancer; or massive corticosteroid therapy in leukemias. So, obviously, the goal is to try to avoid them in patients who cannot benefit. No histological criterion yet exists that can be used to determine those who can and those who cannot be helped by hormonal therapeutics. However, the presence of *receptors* indicates that a tissue may be hormone responsive, and their absence excludes such a possibility. Several authors have undertaken investigations, particularly with studies concerning breast cancer and acute lymphoid leukemias.

A. BREAST CANCER

As early as 1961 (Folca *et al.*, 1961), hexestrol-^{3}H was injected into breast cancer patients for whom adrenalectomy was indicated. More radioactivity was found in the breasts of the 4 patients responding favorably to the hormonal surgery than in the 6 other patients who did not improve. A systematic effort was then undertaken, which initially measured estradiol-^{3}H incorporation *in vitro* in tumor slices (the specificity being assessed by subtracting a value obtained in presence of an excess of nonradioactive hormone or antihormone (Jensen *et al.*, 1967a). Secondarily, the cytosol *receptor* was directly measured, using charcoal technique, electrophoresis, or ultracentrifugation (Feherty *et al.*, 1971; Jungblut *et al.*, 1972; McGuire, 1973). Characteristics of human breast cancer *receptors* were found to be very similar to those of other target tissues in the human and other mammals (Engelsman *et al.*, 1973; Korsten and Persijn, 1972).

Essentially, it was found that approximately half of the patients showed the presence of an estradiol *receptor*, with probably a somewhat higher percentage in postmenopausal women, even though it is difficult to assess the validity of the difference because in most cases the endogenous hormone was taken not into account. In all reports, there is a positive correlation between the presence of *receptor* and responses to hormonal treatment regardless of the therapeutics (McGuire, 1973; Engelsman *et al.*, 1973; Hähnel and Twaddle, 1973; Jensen *et al.*, 1971a; Jensen and DeSombre, 1972b). No relationship between the presence of *receptor* and any histological pattern was found [however, Terenius *et al.* (1974) reported correlation between amount and "cellularity], and there was no parallelism with effects of chemotherapy or local surgery. Basically, it should be emphasized that the presence of *receptors*, even in a high amount, indicates only that there are cells that are possibly susceptible to estrogen stimulation. A positive result does not eliminate nonresponsiveness to hormone therapy. On the other hand, an absence of the *receptor* excludes the possibility of hormonal response, but the limit of sensitivity under which one decides that *receptor* is "not present" is still a matter of controversy (J. P. Raynaud, unpublished observations, 1975). The probable heterogeneity of many tumors permitted the prediction that if hormone-sensitive cells are either killed or repressed by hormonal treatment, other cells will not be influenced. In some rare cases, *receptors* were not detected, but hormonal therapeutics were successful. Different explanations can be offered for such observations, which are "false negative" for *receptors*. It is therefore very important to establish that the methodology is quite discriminating. Difficulties may come from the inevitable contamination by noncancerous tissue and from neglect of a small clone of estrogen-sensitive cells.

Glucocorticosteroid *receptors* have been described in mammary tissue including in experimental tumors (Tucker *et al.*, 1971; Shyamala 1973b; Gardner and Wittliff, 1973a,b). While progesterone binds to glucocorticosteroid *receptors*, independent progesterone *receptors* have also recently been described, in particular using the synthetic progestagen R 50 20 (Horwitz and McGuire, 1975; J. P. Raynaud, unpublished observations, 1975). It is present only when there is estrogen *receptor*, as in approximately 50% of these cases, as though it was an index of the well established estrogen induction (Milgrom *et al.*, 1973c), and it may become an important index of hormone sensitivity (Horwitz and McGuire, 1975). Androgen *receptor* has recently been detected in some mammary cancers (Maass, 1975).

B. ENDOMETRIAL CARCINOMA

As in normal endometrium, estrogen and progesterone *receptors* are now found in endometrial carcinoma (Pollow *et al.*, 1975).

C. Acute Lymphoid (Lymphoblastic) Leukemia

Glucocorticosteroid *receptors* have been detected in lymphoblast cells of untreated patients. The concentration of these *receptors* is very low in normal lymphocytes (Lippman *et al.*, 1973a,b). It is known that after treatment with cortisone derivatives there are leukemias that respond favoraby to hormonal treatment and others that become irreversible. There is a good correlation with the presence of glucocorticosteroid *receptor* in the first case and with their absence in the second. A test of response to glucocorticosteroids *in vitro* (inhibition of thymidine incorporation into DNA) runs parallel to the binding data. Considering the complexity of the steps involved in the mechanisms of action of glucocorticosteroids, it is astonishing that such a close parallelism has been observed (see also genetic results with lymphoma cells (Sibley and Tomkins, 1974)).

If more work is still needed, one can predict that the evaluation of the hormone *receptors* in malignancies will come to be used systematically in clinical medicine. Studies of the presence of *receptors,* and also of the amount, nuclear transfer, binding of different hormone derivatives and of plurality of *receptors* are the immediate areas for future work in this field.

X. Detection and Characterization of
Steroid *Receptor* Interactions

In this section, only a brief list of pertinent references is given, since theoretical and practical arguments are practically impossible to summarize (see also O'Malley and Hardman, 1975).

A. Theory

Reviews are available that discuss the steroid–*receptor* interaction as noncovalent, reversible, and following the law of mass action (Baulieu *et al.*, 1970; Baulieu, 1974a; Best-Belpomme and Dessen, 1973; Rodbard, 1973; Baulieu and Raynaud, 1970). In general, binding affinity at 4°C corresponds to approximately 12 kcal/mole. The contribution of entropy is probably not important, but studies at elevated temperatures have been difficult. Recent papers (Kahn, 1975; Birnbaumer *et al.*, 1974) give references related to other hormone *receptors*. An "allosteric" model of the *receptor*, based on dose/effect relationships of glucocorticosteroids, is found in Samuels and Tomkins (1970) and Baxter and Tomkins (1970). The relation between steroid concentration and TAT induction evokes a cooperative mechanism. Since no cooperativity is found in the steroid–*receptor* interaction, and apparently not in nuclear binding of hormone–*receptor* complexes, cooperativity could eventually be due either to the activation process or to (one of) the reaction(s) linking the nuclear binding to enzyme induction. Syn- and antiandrogenic effects of progestins may also be explained by such a concept (Mowszowicz *et al.*, 1975).

The model of *receptor* shown in Fig. 1 is indeed suited for allosteric functioning. Recently, it has been observed that the binding of estradiol and of estrone to the calf uterus estrogen *receptor* does not generate the same interaction with DNA (A. Alberga, unpublished observations, 1973). Applications of this result to more or less potent hormones, and to agonist and antagonist compounds, are educed in Baulieu (1975a,b).

B. SPECIFICITY

The "quadruple" specificity (Baulieu *et al.*, 1971) of *receptors* includes (1) high affinity (necessary for discriminating and binding the corresponding ligand in low concentration); (2) limited number of sites (different from practically unlimited interactions with most macromolecules which have no biological relevance to hormones); (3) hormone specificity (binding of the natural corresponding hormone and of derivatives with affinities parallel to activities); and (4) organ specificity (*receptor* "only" in target cells).

It should be realized that "saturability," as determined in most experimental *in vitro* conditions, depends more on high affinity than on low capacity. It has been found that certain *receptors* with normal affinity for "their" hormones ($K_D = 0.1$–1 nM) also show tight binding ($K_D \sim 10$ nM) for other natural (and artificial) steroids that are physiologically unrelated (apparently). This is so in the case of androgen *receptors* that show affinity for estradiol and progesterone and of glucocorticosteroid *receptors* that bind progesterone. Indeed, high affinity does not always go along with "agonistic" biological activity, since (see also Section XII, B and Fig. 3, I α) identical equilibrium constants may correspond to a totally different activation of the executive site. For instance, 11β- and 11α-methoxyestradiol have approximately the same affinity for the rat uterus *receptor*, but the former is a strong estrogen and the latter is an antiestrogen with very weak estrogenic effect (J. P. Raynaud, unpublished observations, 1975). Correlations between binding studies and biological activities are nevertheless very important for the study of the *receptor,* as seen in the early difficult research for the catecholamine *receptor* (Cuatrecasas *et al.,* 1974).

Finally, lack of detection of the *receptor* in a given tissue should be interpreted cautiously. Not only technical aspects (for instance, undue heating or deteriorating media) may be involved, but the *receptor* may also be masked by nonspecific binding (Cuatrecasas *et al.,* 1974; Baulieu *et al.,* 1970). The *receptor* may be present only in a few disseminated cells or in discrete areas (for instance in the brain). It is still unknown if, while most ordinary target cells contain 5×10^3 to 5×10^4 sites per cell, there are populations with only a few 10 to 10^2 sites per cell, which could then be difficult to measure.

C. Techniques for Measurement

Several reviews have been published (Baulieu *et al.,* 1970; Baulieu, 1974a,b; O'Malley and Hardman, 1975).

To measure binding at equilibrium, equilibrium dialysis is used. In fact, most experiments deal with pseudoequilibrium techniques and therefore involve the separation of bound from unbound steroid. The most important methods use salt (Mayes and Nugent, 1968) or protamine sulfate precipitation (Steggles and King, 1970), adsorption of complexes on hydroxyapatite (Erdos *et al.,* 1970), DEAE-cellulose (Santi *et al.,* 1973), gel chromatography (Pearlman and Crépy, 1967), and separation by ultrafiltration, ultracentrifugation (Toft and Gorski, 1966), and electrophoresis (French *et al.,* 1974; Wagner *et al.,* 1972), and adsorption of unbound hormone by charcoal (Nugent and Mayes, 1966; Binoux and Odell, 1973) or steroid antibody (Castañeda and Liao, 1975; Fishman and Fishman, 1974).

The principle of "differential dissociation" (Milgrom and Baulieu, 1969) is applicable to pseudoequilibrium methods on the ground of simple physical principles.

Kinetics of binding are more difficult to evaluate, and some theoretical and experimental observations have already been made (Best-Belpomme *et al.,* 1970; Truong and Baulieu, 1971; Geynet *et al.,* 1972a).

For physiological experiments (Milgrom *et al.,* 1972b; Anderson *et al.,* 1972; Katzellenbogen *et al.,* 1974) and purification of *receptors* (Truong *et al.,* 1975a), exchange methods have been worked out in order to evaluate all binding sites present whether they are free or organized. They consist in setting experimental conditions for replacing a ligand (usually nonradioactive) with another ligand (usually radioactive) without altering the *receptor* sites. Each case, unfortunately, is unique, and the method should be adapted to specific experimental conditions.

D. GRAPHICAL REPRESENTATIONS AND CALCULATIONS

The hyperbolic curve of bound hormone vs unbound hormone of a standard reaction, $H + R \leftrightarrows HR$, can be linearized according to Scatchard (1949), applying Eadie's concept to nonenzymic binding protein. Purified *receptors* and *receptor*-containing mixtures with negligible amounts of other binding systems are conveniently treated by the Scatchard plot. Techniques based on "differential dissociation" eliminate eventually much "nonspecific" rapidly dissociating binding and may reduce the complexity and finally allow the use of linearization methods.

Nonspecific binding can be subtracted by the use of isotope dilution with certain precautions (Rosenthal, 1967; Blondeau and Robel, 1975). Complex binding systems must be analyzed with other techniques (Baulieu and Raynaud, 1970; Thompson and Kotz, 1971; Hunston, 1975; Raynaud, 1973; Rodbard, 1973). Evaluation of binding parameters of a competing ligand may also be difficult (Best-Belpomme and Dessen, 1973).

XII. CONCLUSIONS: ARE *Receptors* THE "REAL" RECEPTORS?
COMPLEXITY AND PHYSIOPHARMACOLOGICAL INTEREST

A. *Receptors* MAY BE RECEPTORS

Are the specific intracellular binding proteins designated *receptors* the likely candidates to be "real" receptors (Fig. 1). The affirmative arguments are very strong, although we have already mentioned that no decisive proof yet exists.

The "quadruple" specificity of steroid *receptors* has already been discussed and is very suggestive per se. Two parameters, the number of sites per cell and organ specificity, have already been studied quantitatively, and it appears to be certain that the *receptor* content of target cells is not inert.

There are various concentrations of *receptors* as studied ontogenetically (Clark and Gorski, 1970; Giannopoulos et al., 1972) or under physiological or experimental hormonal conditions (Baulieu and Jung, 1970; O'Malley and Toft, 1971; Milgrom et al., 1970, 1973d). Also the naturally occurring (Gehring et al., 1971) or experimentally obtained (Sibley and Tomkins, 1974) genetic abnormalities, as well as the pathological findings (Jensen et al., 1971a; Lippman et al., 1973a), indicate that there is never a hormonal response without a *receptor*, and that, in most cases, nonresponsive cells lack *receptors*. However, presently, there is no evaluation of the "newest" nuclear *receptors,* as the "insoluble" (Lebeau *et al.,* 1973) or the higher-affinity (Alberga *et al.,* 1971b) forms in correlation with biological responses (see also Karlson, 1971).

That *receptor* transfer, even partial, into nuclei of target cells is compatible with most indirect evidence concerning the mechanism of steroid action suggests (but does not demonstrate) that transcription is implicated. At the molecular level, the strict hormone dependency of "acidophilic activation" (Milgrom *et al.,* 1973a) or "transformation" (Jensen and DeSombre, 1972b) as indicated by increased affinity for polyanions make the *receptor* a reactive protein well suited for a specific regulatory mechanism. Correlations between the amount of nuclear KCl extractable hormone–*receptor* complexes and the degree of response have been obtained in the uterus system (Katzenellengoben and Gorski, 1972; Anderson *et al.,* 1973) and cultured cells (Baxter *et al.,* 1971). However, at this time, not only is the executive site not known, but its nature, binding or catalytic, remains undetermined (Fig. 2) like the nuclear acceptor. To date, not even the turnover of the hormone in target cells can be described.

The apparent half-life of cytosol *receptor,* long in hormone-deprived tissue ($\sim$5 days, Sarff and Gorski, 1971; Milgrom *et al.,* 1973c), is shorter in the presence of hormone (Milgrom *et al.,* 1973c),* and the first elements suggesting some complex *receptor* cycle in target cells have been presented (Ishii *et al.,* 1972; Bell and Munck, 1973) and will have to be considered in order to understand the regulatory function of *receptors.*

Finally, there is no evidence against the possibility that the cytosol $\rightarrow$KCl-extractable neonuclear *receptor* system is an obligatory piece of the responding target cells, and perhaps even is "the" *receptor,* but conversely the existence of another "final" binding entity which is the last to interact with the hormone (Fig. 1) is not excluded, as should be true for the *receptor.* Moreover, some other additional interaction (Baulieu *et al.,* 1971), for instance at the level of a translational event in the cytoplasm (Shao *et al.,* 1975), may coexist with the transcriptional changes.

B. THE COMPLEXITY OF STEROID HORMONE *Receptors* IS OF
  PHARMACOLOGICAL AND PHYSIOLOGICAL INTEREST

There is already complexity if one considers the different forms of one given steroid *receptor.* Besides, there might be two *receptors* per cell for one hormone. This is the case when there is an estrogen (E) and an

---

* A regulatory effect of hormone on its *receptor* has also been observed with insulin *receptors* (Roth, 1973).

androgen (A) *receptor,* the latter also binding estradiol. This has been demonstrated recently with cultured cell lines such as MI_1 (derived from Shionogi SC-115), an androgen-dependent mammary tumor in mice in which estrogen antagonizes the androgen-promoted growth (Jung-Testas and Baulieu, 1974) and L-929 mouse fibroblast cells (Jung-Testas and Bayard, 1975). Since two *receptors* have also been demonstrated in homogenates of prostate, uterus, and breast tissue, the same situation may exist in many normal and abnormal cells, even though the cellular complexity has precluded a formal demonstration in the organs. Since the affinity of estradiol for the E *receptor* is higher than for the A *receptor,* it may be envisaged that the E *receptor* may be operative at low concentration of hormone, whereas the A *receptor* becomes active when the hormone is more abundant. In case the two *receptors* for the same hormone mediate opposite activities (for instance, via two different genes), this is a mechanism for different effects of the same hormonal ligand at varying concentrations. Another possibility may be that the complexes of the two different *receptors* with estradiol compete for the same genetic sites, with which their interactions would be radically different (Fig. 3, II).

Moreover, the E sites bind diethylstilbestrol similarly to estradiol, but the A sites have much higher affinity for the natural estradiol than for the synthetic diethylstilbestrol. It follows that a double *receptor* system may be capable of "dissociating" the effects of the two estrogens, which have similar activities when considered only via the estrogen receptor.

For the two different classes of hormones, such as androgens and estrogens, the above-mentioned observations also indicate that their own *receptors,* of approximatively identical affinity for the two respective steroids, can be present in the same cells. This may, for example, be of physiological interest in the case of the couple estradiol–progesterone. Data show that estradiol modulates the synthesis of the progesterone *receptor* (O'Malley *et al.,* 1970; Milgrom *et al.,* 1970, 1973c) and conversely that progesterone changes the concentration of the estrogen *receptor* (Mester *et al.,* 1974; Hsueh *et al.,* 1975). Therefore *a* possibility is that these regulations occur in the same cells, which "must" therefore, respectively, contain two *receptors* for progesterone and estradiol (these do not bind the reciprocal hormone). The same reasoning holds true for the synthesis of ovalbumin in tubular cells of chick oviduct by estradiol and progesterone (P. Pennequin and R. Schmike, unpublished observations, 1974). Consequently, the mechanism for hormonal agonism (priming effects or synergistic effects) or hormonal antagonism, may be discussed as in the case of the biphasic effect of one hormone as argued above. The two hormone–*receptor* complexes may have their own and different responsive correspondents in the genetic apparatus (Fig. 3, III) or may

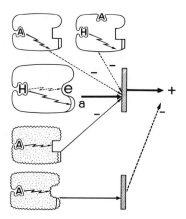

FIG. 3. Antihormone and *receptor(s)*. Three drawings are presented, for picturing antihormone (A) activity. Hormone H *receptor* (Larger drawing) is similar to type II in Fig. 2.

(I, two top drawings). A binds to the *receptor*. Two possibilities (α and β) are seen. (α) A binds *to the r site*, but the coupling mechanism for switching on sites a or e, or both, is disturbed. For instance, the A-*receptor* complex can be weak and the rate of dissociation of A is faster than the rate of dissociation of H; then, the *receptor* either does not reach the nucleus or may, in the nucleus, be left without ligand, very sensitive to destructive processes. Another possibility is that the A-*receptor* complex does not bind very strongly to the chromatin and is released faster than the H-*receptor* complex. It is seen that these mechanisms could be operative in the case of antagonists which are also weak agonists. A different eventuality is an alkylating ligand "blocking" the *receptor*.

(β) A binds to the *receptor* elsewhere than to the r site (noncompetitive inhibitor), and consequently the coupling between the r site and the e or a site, or both sites, is disturbed. α and β can be discussed in terms of two *receptor* conformations, one favoring the binding of H and the other the binding of A.

II and III (stippled drawings) show two eventualities introducing a second *receptor* for A. (II, above). A *receptor* for A competes with the H *receptor* for interaction with the executive and/or the acceptor part of the gene machinery. The assumption is that this competition between hormone–*receptor* complexes abolishes the effect of H because the A-*receptor* complex is not effective at the chromatin level.

(III, bottom). The *receptor* of A has its own executive and/or acceptor counterparts in the gene machinery and produces an effect of its own, antagonistic to the effect of H. Many other possible antagonistic mechanisms implicating the *receptor* could be represented. For instance, one may envisage modifying the *receptor*–chromatin interaction (e.g., by altering directly and a or e sites, or both, of the *receptor*, by alkylating or intercalating agents in DNA) or changing the stability, transfer, "recycling," and/or resynthesis of the *receptor*, etc.

interfere with a single system (Fig. 3, II). Incidentally, two antagonistic hormones may alternatively bind only to a single *receptor*, either competing for the same site (Fig. 3, I α) or binding two distinct sites (Fig.

716   ETIENNE-EMILE BAULIEU ET AL.

3, I β). It is also clear that agonist and antagonist effects may be produced at the *receptor* level, but via other mechanisms, such as changes in its cellular distribution, modification of its half-life, etc. The same effects may also be due to other defects of the cellular machinery, "elsewhere" than at the receptor level, "before" (for instance, at the entry of hormone) or "after" it. Finally, it is not excluded that synergy and antagonism involve the simultaneous participation of different cell types. An analysis of these possibilities may be of pharmacological interest (Baulieu, 1975b), as shown in other systems (Axelrod, 1974).

ACKNOWLEDGMENTS*

We thank, A. Alberga, F. Bayard, J. P. Blondeau, C. Corpéchot, S. Damilano, A. Groyer, I. Jung-Testas, M. C. Lebeau, C. Le Goascogne, M. Luu Thi, G. Michel, H. Truong, and S. Weiller, from this laboratory, who allowed us to cite work in progress. We have also reported an unpublished experiment done in collaboration with H. Berendes (Nimègue) who died on May 29, 1975, and have mentioned personal communications from B. W. O'Malley (Baylor University), J. P. Raynaud (Roussel-Uclaf), P. Pennequin and R. Schimke (Stanford University), and J. A. Gustafsson and S. Sternberg (Karolinska Institutet).

We are indebted to A. Atger, M. Leblondel, G. Marcadier, and D. Prod'homme for secretarial assistance.

Work from these laboratories is supported partially by the CNRS, the DGRST, the Ford Foundation, and Roussel-Uclaf.

REFERENCES

Agarwal, M. K. (1975). *Nature (London)* **254**, 623.
Alberga, A., and Baulieu, E. E. (1968). *Mol. Pharmacol.* **4**, 311.
Alberga, A., Jung, I., Massol, N., Raynaud, J. P., Raynaud-Jammet, C., Rochefort, H., Truong, H. and Baulieu, E. E. (1971a). *Advan. Biosci.* **7**, 45.
Alberga, A., Massol, N., Raynaud, J. P., and Baulieu, E. E. (1971b). *Biochemistry* **10**, 3835.
Alberti, K. G. M. M., and Sharp, G. W. G. (1969). *Biochim. Biophys. Acta* **192**, 335.
Alberti, K. G. M. M., and Sharp, G. W. G. (1970). *J. Endocrinol.* **48**, 563.
Anderson, J. N., Clark, J. H., and Peck, E. J. (1972). *Biochem. J.* **126**, 561.
Anderson, J. N., Peck, E. J., and Clark, J. H. (1973). *Endocrinology* **92**, 1488.
Anderson, J. N., Peck, E. J., and Clark, J. H. (1974). *Endocrinology* **95**, 174.
Anderson, K. M., and Liao, S. (1968). *Nature (London)* **219**, 277.
Anderson, N. S., III, Fanestil, D. D., and Ludens, J. H. (1974). *J. Steroid Biochem.* **5**, Abstr. 166.
André, J., and Rochefort, H. (1973a). *FEBS (Fed. Eur. Biochem. Soc.) Lett.* **29**, 135.
André, J., and Rochefort, H. (1973b). *FEBS (Fed. Eur. Biochem. Soc.) Lett.* **32**, 330.
André, J., and Rochefort, H. (1974). *Eur. J. Obstet. Gynecol. Reprod. Biol.* **4**, 67.

*July, 1975: This review is dedicated to the memory of Gordon Tomkins, who died, depriving us of his marvelous intelligence and friendship.

Ansiello, D. A., and Sharp, G. W. G. (1968). *Endocrinology* **82**, 1163.

Arias, F., and Warren, J. C. (1971). *Biochim. Biophys. Acta* **230**, 550.

Armstrong, D. T., and King, E. R. (1971). *Endocrinology* **89**, 191.

Arnaud, M., Beziat, Y., Guilleux, A., Hough, A., Hough, D., and Mousseron-Canet, M. (1971). *Biochim. Biophys. Acta* **232**, 117.

Atger, M., Baulieu, E. E., and Milgrom, E. (1974). *Endocrinology* **94**, 161.

Attardi, B., and Ohno, S. (1974). *Cell* **2**, 205.

Attramadal, A. (1973). *Acta Endocrinol. (Copenhagen), Suppl.* **177**, 248.

Augustyn, J. M., and Brunkhorst, W. K. (1972a). *Biochim. Biophys. Acta* **264**, 557.

Augustyn, J. M., and Brunkhorst, W. K. (1972b). *Biochim. Biophys. Acta* **264**, 566.

Axelrod, J. (1974). *Science* **184**, 1340.

Ballard, P. L., Baxter, J., Higgins, S. J., Rousseau, G. G., and Tomkins, G. M. (1974). *Endocrinology* **94**, 998.

Baulieu, E. E. (1973). *In* "Receptors for Reproductive Hormones" (B. W. O'Malley and A. R. Means, eds.), p. 80. Plenum, New York.

Baulieu, E. E. (1974a). *Proc. Int. Congr. Endocrinol., 4th, 1972* Int. Congr. Ser. No. 256, p. 30.

Baulieu, E. E. (1974b). *In* "Physiology and Genetics of Reproduction" (E. M. Coutinho and F. Fuchs, eds.), Vol 4, p. 113. Plenum, New York.

Baulieu, E. E. (1975a). *Eur. J. Obstet. Gynecol. Reprod. Biol.* **4**, 161.

Baulieu, E. E. (1975b). *J. Amer. Med. Ass.* **234**, 404.

Baulieu, E. E., and Jung, I. (1970). *Biochem. Biophys. Res. Commun.* **38**, 599.

Baulieu, E. E., and Raynaud, J. P. (1970). *Eur. J. Biochem.* **13**, 293.

Baulieu, E. E., and Robel, P. (1970). *In* "Some Aspects of the Aetiology and Biochemistry of Prostatic Cancer" (K. Griffiths and C. G. Pierrepoint, eds.), p. 74. Alpha Omega Alpha, Cardiff, Wales.

Baulieu, E. E., Alberga, A., and Jung, I. (1967). *C. R. Acad. Sci.* **265**, 354.

Baulieu, E. E., Lasnitzky, I., and Robel, P. (1968). *Nature (London)* **219**, 1155.

Baulieu, E. E., Raynaud, J. P., and Milgrom, E. (1970). *Acta Endocrinol. (Copenhagen), Suppl.* **147**, 104.

Baulieu, E. E., Alberga, A., Jung, I., Lebeau, M. C., Mercier-Bodard, C., Milgrom, E., Raynaud, J. P., Raynaud-Jammet, C., Rochefort, H., Truong, H., and Robel, P. (1971). *Recent Progr. Horm. Res.* **27**, 351.

Baxter, J. D., and Forsham, P. H. (1972). *Amer. J. Med.* **53**, 573.

Baxter, J. D., and Tomkins, G. M. (1970). *Proc. Nat. Acad. Sci. U.S.* **65**, 709.

Baxter, J. D., and Tomkins, G. M. (1971). *Proc. Nat. Acad. Sci. U.S.* **68**, 932.

Baxter, J. D., Harris, A. W., Tomkins, G. M., and Cohn, M. (1971). *Science* **171**, 189.

Beato, M., and Feigelson, P. (1972). *J. Biol. Chem.* **247**, 7890.

Beato, M., Homoki, J., and Sekeris, C. E. (1969). *Exp. Cell Res.* **55**, 107.

Beato, M., Braendel, W., Biesewig, D., and Sekeris, C. E. (1970a). *Biochim. Biophys. Acta* **208**, 125.

Beato, M., Schmid, W., Braendel, W., and Sekeris, C. E. (1970b). *Steroids* **16**, 207.

Beato, M., Schmid, W., and Sekeris, C. E. (1972). *Biochim. Biophys. Acta* **263**, 764.

Beato, M., Kalimi, M., Konstam, M., and Feigelson, P. (1973). *Biochemistry* **12**, 3372.

Beatson, G. T. (1896). *Lancet* **2**, 104.

Bell, P. A., and Munck, A. (1973). *Biochem. J.* **136**, 97.

Best-Belpomme, M. (1974). *J. Steroid Biochem.* **5**, Abstr. 148.

Best-Belpomme, M., and Courgeon, A. M. (1975). *C. R. Acad. Sci.* **280**, 1397.

Best-Belpomme, M., and Dessen, P. (1973). *Biochimie* **55**, 11.

Best-Belpomme, M., Fries, J., and Erdos, T. (1970). *Eur. J. Biochem.* **17**, 425.

Best-Belpomme, M., Mester, J., Weintraub, H., and Baulieu, E. E. (1975). *Eur. J. Biochem.* **57**, 537.

Binoux, M. A., and Odell, W. D. (1973). *J. Clin. Endocrinol. Metab.* **36**, 303.

Birnbaumer, L., Pohl, S. L., and Kaumann, A. J. (1974). *Advan. Cyclic Nucleotide Res.* **4**, 239.

Blaquier, J. A. (1971). *Biochem. Biophys. Res. Commun.* **45**, 1076.

Blaquier, J. A., and Calandra, R. S. (1973). *Endocrinology* **93**, 51.

Blondeau, J. P., and Corpéchot, C. (1974). *J. Steroid Biochem.* **5**, Abstr. 154.

Blondeau, J. P., and Robel, P. (1975). *Eur. J. Biochem.* **55**, 375.

Blondeau, J. P., Robel, P., Corpéchot, C., Le Goascogne, C., and Baulieu, E. E. (1975). This volume, p. 319.

Boesel, R. W., and Shain, S. A. (1974). *Biochem. Biophys. Res. Commun.* **61**, 1004.

Bogoroch, R. (1969). *In* "Autoradiography of Diffusible Substances" (L. J. Roth and W. E. Stumpf, eds.), p. 99. Academic Press, New York.

Brecher, P. I., Vigersky, R., Wotiz, H. S., and Wotiz, H. H. (1967). *Steroids* **10**, 635.

Brenner, R. M., Resko, J. A., and West, N. B. (1974). *Endocrinology* **95**, 1094.

Bresciani, F., Nola, E., Sica, V., and Puca, G. M. (1973). *Fed. Proc., Fed. Amer. Soc. Exp. Biol.* **32**, 2126.

Bruchovsky, N., and Craven, S. (1975). *Biochem. Biophys. Res. Commun.* **62**, 837.

Bruchovsky, N., and Wilson, J. D. (1968). *J. Biol. Chem.* **243**, 2012.

Brumbaugh, P. F., and Haussler, M. R. (1974a). *J. Biol. Chem.* **249**, 1251.

Braumbaugh, P. F., and Haussler, M. R. (1974b). *J. Biol. Chem.* **249**, 1258.

Bucourt, R., Nedelec, L., Torelli, V., Gasc, J. C., and Vignau, M. (1971). *Proc. Int. Congr. Horm. Steroids, 3rd, 1970* Int. Congr. Ser. No. 219, Abstr. 125.

Bullock, L. P., and Bardin, C. W. (1972). *J. Clin. Endocrinol. Metab.* **35**, 935.

Butterworth, F. M., and Berendes, H. D. (1974). *J. Insect. Physiol.* **20**, 2195.

Calandra, R. S., Podesta, E. J., Rivarola, M. A., and Blaquier, J. A. (1974). *Steroids* **24**, 507.

Castañeda, E., and Liao, S. (1975). *J. Biol. Chem.* **250**, 883.

Chader, G. J. (1973). *J. Neurochem.* **21**, 1525.

Chader, G. S., and Reif-Lehrer, L. (1972). *Biochim. Biophys. Acta* **264**, 186.

Chamness, G. C., and McGuire, W. L. (1972). *Biochemistry* **11**, 2466.

Chamness, G. C., Jennings, A. W., and McGuire, W. L. (1973). *Nature (London)* **241**, 458.

Chamness, G. C., Jennings, A. W., and McGuire, W. L. (1974). *Biochemistry* **13**, 327.

Chatkoff, M. L., and Julian, J. A. (1973). *Biochem. Biophys. Res. Commun.* **51**, 1015.

Chen, T. C., and DeLuca, H. F. (1973). *J. Biol. Chem.* **248**, 4890.

Chung Lee, Keyes, P. L., and Jacobson, H. I. (1971). *Science* **173**, 1032.

Cidlowski, J. A., and Muldoon, T. G. (1974). *Endocrinology* **95**, 1621.

Clark, J. H., and Gorski, J. (1970). *Science* **169**, 76.

Clark, J. H., Anderson, J., and Peck, E. J. (1972). *Science* **176**, 528.

Claycomb, W. C., Lafond, R. E., and Villee, C. A. (1971). *Nature (London), New Biol.* **234**, 302.

Clemens, L. E., and Kleinsmith, L. (1972). *Nature (London), New Biol.* **237**, 204.

Corvol, P., Falk, R., Freifeld, M., and Bardin, C. W. (1972). *Endocrinology* **90**, 1464.

Corvol, P., Ulmann, A., Michaud, A., and Ménard, J. (1975). *Res. Steroids* **6**, 65–75.

Cowan, R. A., Kim, U. H., and Mueller, G. C. (1975). *Steroids* **25**, 135.

Cox, R. F., Catlin, G. H., and Carey, N. H. (1971). *Eur. J. Biochem.* **22**, 46.

Cuatrecasas, P., Tell, G. P. E., Sica, V., Parikh, I., and Chang, K. I., (1974). *Nature (London)* **247**, 92.

Danzo, B. J., Orgebin-Crist, M. C., and Toft, D. O. (1973). *Endocrinology* **92**, 310.

Davies, I. J., and Ryan, K. J. (1973). *Endocrinology* **92**, 394.

Davies, I. J., Challis, S. R. G., and Ryan, K. J. (1974). *Endocrinology* **95**, 165.

Davies, P., and Griffiths, K. (1974). *J. Endocrinol.* **62**, 385.

Defer, N., Dastugue, B., and Kruh, J. (1974). *Biochimie* **56**, 1549.

DeGroot, L. J., and Torresani, J. (1975). *Endocrinology* **96**, 357.

DeHertogh, R., Ekka, E., Vanderheyden, I., and Hoet, J. J. (1973). *J. Steroid Biochem.* **4**, 289, 301, 313.

DeLuca, H. F. (1974). *Fed. Proc., Fed. Amer. Soc. Exp. Biol.* **33**, 2211.

Diczfalusy, E., ed. (1970). *Acta Endocrinol. (Copenhagen), Suppl.* **147**.

Diczfalusy, E., ed. (1971). *Acta Endocrinol. (Copenhagen), Suppl.* **158**.

Diczfalusy, E., ed. (1972). *Acta Endocrinol. (Copenhagen), Suppl.* **168**.

Dillman, W., Surks, M. I., and Oppenheimer, J. H. (1974). *Endocrinology* **95**, 492.

Dube, J. Y., and Tremblay, R. R. (1974). *Endocrinology* **95**, 1105.

Edelman, I. S. (1971). *Advan. Biosci.* **7**, 267.

Edelman, I. S., and Fanestil, D. D. (1970). *In* "Biochemical Actions of Hormones" (G. Litwack, ed.), Vol. 1, p. 324. Academic Press, New York.

Edelman, I. S., and Ismail-Beigi, F. (1974). *Recent Progr. Horm. Res.* **30**, 235.

Edelman, I. S., Bororoch, R., and Porter, G. A. (1973). *Proc. Nat. Acad. Sci. U.S.* **50**, 1169.

Eisenfeld, A. J. (1974). *J. Steroid Biochem.* **5**, 328.

Eisenfeld, A. J., and Axelrod, J. (1967). *Biochem. Pharmacol.* **16**, 1781.

Ellis, D. S., and Ringold, H. J. (1971). *In* "The Sex Steroids" (K. W. McKerns, ed.), p. 73. Appleton, New York.

Emmerich, H. (1969). *Nature (London)* **221**, 954.

Engelsman, E., Persijn, J. P., Korsten, C. B., and Cleton, F. J. (1973). *Brit. Med. J.* **2**, 750.

Eppenberger, U., and Hsia, S. L. (1972). *J. Biol. Chem.* **247**, 5463.

Erdos, T. (1968). *Biochem. Biophys. Res. Commun.* **32**, 338.

Erdos, T. (1971). *Proc. Int. Congr. Steroids, 3rd, 1970* Int. Congr. Ser. No. 219, p. 364.

Erdos, T., and Fries, J. (1974). *Biochem. Biophys. Res. Commun.* **58**, 932.

Erdos, T., Best-Belpomme, M., and Bessada, R. (1970). *Anal. Biochem.* **37**, 244.

Evans, L. H., and Hähnel, R. (1971). *J. Endocrinol.* **50**, 209.

Evans, L. H., and Hähnel, R. (1973). *J. Endocrinol.* **56**, 503.

Evans, L. H., Martin, J. D., and Hähnel, R. (1974). *J. Clin. Endocrinol.* **38**, 23.

Faber, L. E., Sandmann, M. L., and Stavely, H. E. (1972a). *J. Biol. Chem.* **247**, 5648.

Faber, L. E., Sandmann, M. L., and Stavely, H. E. (1972b). *J. Biol. Chem.* **247**, 8000.

Faber, L. E., Sandmann. M. L., and Stavely, H. E. (1973). *Endocrinology* **93**, 74.

Fanestil, D. D. (1968). *Biochem. Pharmacol.* **17**, 2240.

Fanestil, D. D., and Edelman, I. S. (1966). *Proc. Nat. Acad. Sci. U.S.* **56**, 872.

Fang, S., and Liao, S. (1969). *Mol. Pharmacol.* **5**, 428.

Fang, S., and Liao, S. (1971). *J. Biol. Chem.* **246**, 16.

Fang, S., Anderson, K. M., and Liao, S. (1969). *J. Biol. Chem.* **244**, 6584.

Feherty, P. (1972). Ph.D. Thesis, University of London.

Feherty, P., Robertson, D. M., Waynforth, B. H., and Kellie, A. E. (1970). *Biochem. J.* **120,** 836.

Feherty, P., Farrer-Brown, G., and Kellie, A. E. (1971). *Brit. J. Cancer* **25,** 697.

Feil, P. D., Glasser, S. R., Toft, D. O., and O'Malley, B. W. (1972). *Endocrinology* **91,** 738.

Feldman, D. (1974). *Endocrinology* **95,** 1219.

Feldman, D., and Funder, J. W. (1973). *Endocrinology* **92,** 1389.

Feldman, D., Dzials, R., Kochler, R., and Stern, P. (1975). *Endocrinology* **96,** 29.

Filler, R., and Litwack, G. (1973). *Fed. Proc., Fed. Amer. Soc. Exp. Biol.* **32,** Abstr. 1691.

Fishman, J., and Fishman, J. H. (1974). *J. Clin. Endocrinol. Metab.* **39,** 603.

Folca, P. J., Glasscock, R. F., and Irvine, W. T. (1961). *Lancet* **2,** 796.

Forte, L. R. (1972). *Life Sci.* **11,** 461.

Fraser, D. R., and Kodicek, E. (1970). *Nature (London)* **228,** 764.

French, F. S., and Ritzen, E. M. (1973). *Endocrinology* **93,** 88.

French, F. S., Weddington, S. C., and Nayfeh, S. N. (1974). *J. Biol. Chem.* **249,** 6597.

Friend, J. P., and Leavitt, W. W. (1972). *Acta Endocrinol. (Copenhagen)* **69,** 230.

Fu, C. S., Kaiser, N., Milholland, R. J., and Rosen, F. (1973). *Fed. Proc., Fed. Amer. Soc. Exp. Biol.* **32,** Abstr. 1691.

Funder, J. W., Feldman, D., and Edelman, I. S. (1972). *J. Steroid Biochem.* **3,** 209.

Funder, J. W., Feldman, D., and Edelman, I. S. (1973a). *Endocrinology* **92,** 994.

Funder, J. W., Feldman, D., and Edelman, I. S. (1973b). *Endocrinology* **92,** 1005.

Funder, J. W., Duval, D., and Meyer, P. (1973c). *Endocrinology* **93,** 1300.

Funder, J. W., Duval, D., Meyer, P., and Dhal, L. K. (1974). *Endocrinology* **94,** 1739.

Gardner, D. G., and Wittliff, J. L. (1973a). *Biochim. Biophys. Acta* **320,** 617.

Gardner, D. G., and Wittliff, J. L. (1973b). *Brit. J. Cancer* **27,** 441.

Gehring, U., and Tomkins, G. M. (1974). *Cell* **3,** 59.

Gehring, U., Tomkins, G. M., and Ohno, S. (1971). *Nature (London), New Biol.* **232,** 106.

Geilach, J. L., and McEwen, B. D. (1972). *Science* **175,** 1133.

Geynet, C., Millet, C., Truong, H., and Baulieu, E. E. (1972a). *C. R. Acad. Sci.* **275,** 1551.

Geynet, C., Millet, C., Truong, H., and Baulieu, E. E. (1972b). *Gynecol. Invest.* **3,** 2.

Giannopoulos, G. (1971). *Biochem. Biophys. Res. Commun.* **44,** 943.

Giannopoulos, G. (1973). *J. Biol. Chem.* **248,** 3876.

Giannopoulos, G., Mulay, S., and Solomon, S. (1972). *Biochem. Biophys. Res. Commun.* **47,** 411.

Giannopoulos, G., Hassan, Z., and Solomon, S. (1974). *J. Biol. Chem.* **249,** 2424.

Ginsburg, M., Morris, I. D.. Maclusky, N. J., and Thomas, P. J. (1972). *J. Endocrinol.* **55,** XX.

Ginsburg, M., Maclusky, N. J., Morris, I. D., and Thomas, P. J. (1975). *J. Endocrinol.* **64,** 443.

Glasscock, R. F., and Hoekstra, W. G. (1959). *Biochem. J.* **72,** 673.

Goldman, A. S., and Katsumata, M. (1974). *J. Steroid Biochem.* **5,** abst. 153.

Gordon, J., Smith, J. A., and King, R. J. B. (1974). *Mol. Cell. Endocrinol.* **1,** 259.

Gorell, T. A., DeSombre, E. R., and Jensen, E. V. (1974). *Fed. Proc., Fed. Amer. Soc. Exp. Biol.* **33,** 1511 (Abstr. 1624).

Gorski, J., Toft, D. O., Shyamala, G., Smith, D., and Notides, A. (1968). *Recent Progr. Horm. Res.* **24,** 45.

Gorski, J., Sarff, M., and Clark, J. (1971). *Advan. Biosci.* **7,** 5.

Gschwendt, M., and Kittstein, W. (1974). *Biochim. Biophys. Acta* **361,** 84.

Gupta, G. N. (1960). Ph.D. Thesis, University of Chicago, Illinois.

Hackney, J. F., Gross, S. R., Aronow, L., and Pratt, W. B. (1970). *Mol. Pharmacol.* **6,** 500.

Hadjian, A. J., Kowarski, A., Dickerman, H. W., and Migeon, C. J. (1974). *J. Steroid Biochem.* **5,** Abstr. 213.

Hähnel, R. (1971). *Steroids* **17,** 105.

Hähnel, R., and Twaddle, E. (1973). *Cancer Res.* **33,** 559.

Hähnel, R., Twaddle, E., and Brindle, L. (1974). *Steroids* **24,** 489.

Halimi, M., Beato, M., and Feigelson, P. (1973). *Biochemistry* **12,** 3365.

Hansson, V., and Tveter, K. J. (1971a). *Acta Endocrinol. (Copenhagen)* **66,** 745.

Hansson, V., and Tveter, K. J. (1971b). *Acta Endocrinol. (Copenhagen), Suppl.* **155,** 148.

Hansson, V., Tveter, K. J., Attramadal, A., and Torgersen, O. (1971). *Acta Endocrinol. (Copenhagen)* **68,** 79.

Hansson, V., Djöseland, O., Reusch, E., Attramadal, A., and Törgersen, O. (1973). *Steroids* **22,** 19.

Harris, G. S. (1971). *Nature (London), New Biol.* **231,** 246.

Harrisson, R. W., and Toft, D. O. (1973). *Biochem. Biophys. Res. Commun.* **55,** 857.

Harrison, R. W., and Toft, D. O. (1975). *Endocrinology* **96,** 199.

Harrison, R. W., Skrivseth, S., and Orth, D. N. (1975). *Biochemistry* **14,** 1304.

Hankkamaa, M., and Luukkainen, T. (1974). *J. Steroid Biochem.* **5,** 447.

Hechter, O., and Halkerston, I. D. K. (1964). *In* "The Hormones" (G. Pincus, K. V. Thimann, and E. B. Astwood, eds.), Vol. 5, p. 697. Academic Press, New York.

Henning, S. J., Ballard, P. L., and Kretchmer, N. (1975). *J. Biol. Chem.* **250,** 2073.

Herman, T. S., Fimognari, G. M., and Edelman, I. S. (1968). *J. Biol. Chem.* **243,** 3849.

Heyns, W. (1974). *J. Steroid Biochem.* **5,** Abstr. 215.

Higgins, S. J., Rousseau, G. G., Baxter, J. D., and Tomkins, G. M. (1973a). *J. Biol. Chem.* **248,** 5866.

Higgins, S. J., Rousseau, G. G., Baxter, J. D., and Tomkins, G. M. (1973b). *J. Biol. Chem.* **248,** 5873.

Higgins, S. J., Rousseau, G. G., Baxter, J. D., and Tomkins, G. M. (1973c). *Proc. Nat. Acad. Sci. U.S.* **70,** 3415.

Hirsch, P. C., and Szego, C. M. (1974). *J. Steroid Biochem.* **5,** 533.

Hollander, N., and Chui, Y. W. (1966). *Biochem. Biophys. Res. Commun.* **25,** 291.

Horwitz, K. B., and McGuire, W. L. (1975). *Steroids* **25,** 497.

Hospital, M., Busetta, B., Bucourt, R., Weintraub, H., and Baulieu, E. E. (1972). *Mol. Pharmacol.* **8,** 438.

Hsueh, A. J., Peck, E. J., and Clark, J. H. (1973). *J. Endocrinol.* **58,** 503.

Hsueh, A. J., Peck, E. J., and Clark, J. H. (1974). *Steroids* **24,** 599.

Hsueh, A. J., Peck, E. J., and Clark, J. H. (1975). *Nature (London)* **254,** 337.

Huggins, C., Stevens, R. E., and Hodges, C. V. (1941). *Arch. Surg. (Chicago)* **43**, 209.

Hunston, D. L. (1975). *Anal. Biochem.* **63**, 99.

Iacobelli, S., Hanocq, J., Baltus, E., and Brachet, J. (1974). *Differentiation* **2**, 129.

Imperato-McGinley, J., Guerreo, L., Gautier, T., and Peterson, R. E. (1974). *Science* **186**, 1213.

Irving, R., and Mainwaring, W. I. P. (1974). *J. Steroid Biochem.* **5**, 711.

Ishii, D. N., Pratt, W. B., and Aronow, L. (1972). *Biochemistry* **11**, 3896.

Jackson, V., and Chalkley, R. (1974a). *J. Biol. Chem.* **249**, 1615.

Jackson, V., and Chalkley, R. (1974b). *J. Biol. Chem.* **249**, 1627.

Jensen, E. V. (1965). *Proc. Int. Congr. Endocrinol., 2nd, 1964* Int. Congr. Ser No. 83, p. 420.

Jensen, E. V., and DeSombre, E. R. (1972a). *In* "Biochemical Actions of Hormones" (G. Litwack, ed.), Vol. 2, p. 215. Academic Press, New York.

Jensen, E. V., and DeSombre, E. R. (1972b). *Annu. Rev. Biochem.* **41**, 103.

Jensen, E. V., and Jacobson, H. I. (1960). *In* "Biological Activities of Steroids in Relation to Cancer" (G. Pincus and E. P. Vollmer, eds.), p. 161. Academic Press, New York.

Jensen, E. V., and Jacobson, H. I. (1962). *Recent Progr. Horm. Res.* **18**, 387.

Jensen, E. V., Jacobson, H. I., Flesher, J. W., Saha, N. N., Gupta, G. N., Smith, S., Colucci, V., Shiplacoff, D., Neumann, H. G., DeSombre, E. R., and Jungblut, P. W. (1966). *In* "Steroid Dynamics" (G. Pincus, J. F. Tait, and T. Nakao, eds.), p. 133. Academic Press, New York.

Jensen, E. V., DeSombre, E. R., and Jungblut, P. W. (1967a). *In* "Endogenous Factors Influencing Host-tumor Balance" (L. R. W. Wissler, T. L. Dao, and S. Wood, eds.), Vol. 68, p. 15. Univ. of Chicago Press, Chicago, Illinois.

Jensen, E. V., Hurst, D. J., DeSombre, E. R., and Jungblut, P. W. (1967b). *Science* **158**, 385.

Jensen, E. V., Suzuki, T., Kawashima, T., Stumpf, W. E., Jungblut, P. W., and DeSombre, E. R. (1968). *Proc. Nat. Acad. Sci. U.S.* **59**, 632.

Jensen, E. V., DeSombre, E. R., Jungblut, P. W., Stumpf, W. E., and Roth, L. J. (1969a). *In* "Autoradiography of Diffusible Substances" (L. J. Roth and W. E. Stumpf, eds.), p. 81. Academic Press, New York.

Jensen, E. V., Suzuki, T., Numata, M., Smith, S., and DeSombre, E. R. (1969b). *Steroids* **13**, 417.

Jensen, E. V., Block, G. E., Smith, S., Kyser, K., and DeSombre, E. R. (1971a). *Nat. Cancer Inst., Monogr.* **34**, 55.

Jensen, E. V., Numata, M., Brecher, P. I., and DeSombre, E. R. (1971b). *Biochem. Soc. Symp.* **32**, 133.

Jensen, E. V., Mohla, S., Gorell, T., Tanaka, S., and DeSombre, E. R. (1972). *J. Steroid Biochem.* **3**, 445.

Jouan, P., Samperer, S., Thieulant, M. L., and Mercier, L. (1971). *J. Steroid Biochem.* **2**, 223.

Jouan, P., Samperer, S., and Thieulant, M. L. (1973). *J. Steroid Biochem.* **4**, 65.

Jung, I., and Baulieu, E. E. (1971). *Biochimie* **53**, 807.

Jung, I., and Baulieu, E. E. (1972). *Nature (London), New Biol.* **237**, 24.

Jung-Testas, I., and Baulieu, E. E. (1974). *C. R. Acad. Sci.* **279**, 671.

Jung-Testas, I., Bayard, F., and Baulieu, E. E. (1975). *Nature (London)* (in press).

Jungblut, P. W., Hätzel, I., DeSombre, E. R., and Jensen, E. V. (1967). *Colloq.*

Ges. Physiol. Chem. **18,** 58.

Jungblut, P. W., Hughes, L., Görlich, U., Gowers, U., and Wagner, R. K. (1971a). *Hoppe Seyler's Z. Physiol. Chem.* **352,** 1603.

Jungblut, P. W., Hughes, A., Little, M., McCann-Hughes, S., Rosenfeld, G. C., and Wagner, R. K. (1971b). *Advan. Biosci.* **7,** 137.

Jungblut, P. W., Hughes, S., Hughes, A., and Wagner, R. K. (1972). *Acta Endocrinol. (Copenhagen)* **70,** 185.

Kahn, C. A. (1975). *Methods Membrane Biol.* **3** (in press).

Kaiser, N., Milholland, R. J., Turnell, R. W., and Rosen, F. (1972). *Biochem. Biophys. Res. Commun.* **49,** 516.

Kaiser, N., Milholland, R. J., and Rosen, F. (1973). *J. Biol. Chem.* **248,** 478.

Kalimi, M., Beato, M., and Feigelson, P. (1973). *Biochemistry* **12,** 3365.

Karlson, P. (1971). *Advan. Biosci.* **7,** 389.

Kato, J. (1970a). *Acta Enlocrinol. (Copenhagen)* **63,** 577.

Kato, J. (1970b). *Acta Endocrinol. (Copenhagen)* **64,** 687.

Kato, J., Atsumi, Y., and Muramatsu, M. (1970). *J. Biochem. (Tokyo)* **67,** 871.

Katzenellenbogen, B. S., and Gorski, J. (1972). *J. Biol. Chem.* **247,** 1299.

Katzenellenbogen, J. A., Johnson, H. J., Carlson, K. E., and Myers, H. N. (1974). *Biochemistry* **13,** 2986.

King, R. J. B., and Gordon, J. (1972). *Nature (London), New Biol.* **240,** 185.

King, R. J. B., and Mainwaring, W. I. P. (1974). "Steroid-Cell Interactions." Butterworth, London.

King, R. J. B., Beard, V., Gordon, J., Pooley, A. S., Smith, J. A., Steggles, A. W., and Vertes, M. (1971). *Advan. Biosci.* **7,** 21.

Kirkpatrick, A. F., Milholland, R. J., and Rosen, F. (1971). *Nature (London), New Biol.* **232,** 216.

Kirkpatrick, A. F., Kaiser, N., Milholland, R. J., and Rosen, F. (1972). *J. Biol. Chem.* **247,** 70.

Koblinsky, M., Beato, M., Kalimi, M., and Feigelson, P. (1972). *J. Biol. Chem.* **247,** 7897.

Koch, P. A., Neuklis, J. C., Holland, C. A., Kennedy, C. A., Weaver, R. C., and Litwack, G. (1972). *Endocrinology* **90,** 1600.

Kontula, K. (1975). *Acta Endocrinol. (Copenhagen)* **78,** 593.

Kontula, K., Jänne, O., Luukkainen, T., and Vihko, R. (1973). *Biochim. Biophys. Acta* **328,** 145.

Kontula, K., Jänne, O., Vihko, R., de Jager, E., de Visser, J., and Zeelen, F. (1975). *Acta Endocrinol. (Copenhagen)* **78,** 574.

Korach, K. S., and Muldoon, T. G. (1974). *Biochemistry* **13,** 1932.

Korenman, S. G. (1970). *Endocrinology* **87,** 1119.

Korenman, S. G., and Rao, B. R. (1968). *Proc. Nat. Acad. Sci. U.S.* **61,** 1028.

Korsten, C. B., and Persijn, J. P. (1972). *Z. Klin. Chem. Klin. Biochem.* **10,** 1.

Kuhn, R. W., Schrader, W. T., and O'Malley, B. W. (1975). *Fed. Proc., Fed. Amer. Soc. Exp. Biol.* **34,** Abst. 2311.

Lassman, M. N., and Mulrow, P. J. (1974). *Endocrinology* **94,** 1541.

Lawson, D. E. M., and Wilson, P. W. (1974). *Biochem. J.* **144,** 573.

Lawson, D. E. M., Bell, P. A., Pelc, B., Wilson, P. W., and Kodicek, E. (1971). *Biochem. J.* **121,** 673.

Leavitt, W. W., Toft, D. O., Strott, C. A., and O'Malley, B. W. (1974). *Endocrinology* **94,** 1041.

Lebeau, M. C., Massol, N., and Baulieu, E. E. (1973). *Eur. J. Biochem.* **36**, 294.

Lebeau, M. C., Massol, N., and Baulieu, E. E. (1974). *FEBS (Fed. Eur. Biochem. Soc.) Lett.* **43**, 107.

Lee, C., and Jacobson, H. I. (1971). *Endocrinology* **88**, 596.

Leung, B. S. (1974). *J. Steroid Biochem.* **5**, Abstr. 1164.

Levinson, B. B., Baxter, J. D., Rousseau, G. G., and Tomkins, G. M. (1972). *Science* **175**, 189.

Li, J. S., Talley, D. J., Li, S. A., and Villee, C. A. (1974). *Endocrinology* **95**, 1134.

Liang, T., and Liao, S. (1974). *J. Biol. Chem.* **249**, 4671.

Liao, S., and Fang, S. (1969). *Vitam. Horm. (New York)* **27**, 17.

Liao, S., Liang, T., Fang, S., Castañeda, E., and Shao, T. (1973a). *J. Biol. Chem.* **248**, 6154.

Liano, S., Liang, T., and Tymoezko, J. L. (1973b). *Nature (London), New Biol.* **241**, 211.

Liao, S., Howell, D. K., and Chang, T. M. (1974). *Endocrinology* **94**, 1205.

Lippman, M. E., and Thompson, E. B. (1973). *Nature (London)* **246**, 352.

Lippman, M. E., and Thompson, E. B. (1974). *J. Biol. Chem.* **249**, 2483.

Lippman, M. E., Halterman, R. H., Leventhal, B. G., Perry, S., and Thompson, E. B. (1973a). *J. Clin. Invest.* **52**, 1715.

Lippman, M. E., Halterman, R., Perry, S., Leventhal, B., and Thompson, E. B. (1973b). *Nature (London), New Biol.* **242**, 157.

Little, M., Rosenfeld, G. C., and Jungblut, P. W. (1972). *Hoppe-Seyler's Z. Physiol. Chem.* **353**, 231.

Little, M., Szendo, P. I., and Jungblut, P. W. (1973). *Hoppe Seyler's Z. Physiol. Chem.* **354**, 1599.

Little, M., Szendo, P. I., Teran, C., Hughes, A., and Jungblut, P. W. (1975). *J. Steroid Biochem.* **6**, 493.

Litwack, G., and Rosenfield, S. A. (1974). *J. Steroid Biochem.* **5**, Abstr. 164.

Litwack, G., Filler, R., Rosenfield, S. A., Lichtash, N., Wishman, C. A., and Singer, S. (1973). *J. Biol. Chem.* **248**, 7481.

Ludens, J. H., and Fanestil, D. D. (1971). *Biochim. Biophys. Acta* **244**, 360.

Ludens, J. H., DeVries, J. R., and Fanestil, D. D. (1973). *J. Biol. Chem.* **247**, 7533.

Maass, H. (1975). *Acta Endocrinol. (Copenhagen), Suppl.* **193**, 160.

McEwen, B. S., Weiss, J. M., and Schwartz, L. S. (1970). *Brain Res.* **17**, 471.

McEwen, B. S., Magnus, C., and Wallach, G. (1972). *Endocrinology* **90**, 217.

McGuire, W. L. (1973). *J. Clin. Invest.* **52**, 73.

McGuire, W. L., and Dedella, C. (1971). *Endocrinology* **88**, 1099.

McLeod, M., and Baxter, J. D. (1975). *Biochem. Biophys. Res. Commun.* **62**, 177.

Mainwaring, W. I. P. (1969). *J. Endocrinol.* **45**, 531.

Mainwaring, W. I. P. (1970). *Biochem. Biophys. Res. Commun.* **40**, 192.

Mainwaring, W. I. P. (1973). *Symp. Norm. Abnorm. Growth Prostate. 1973* pp. 577–599.

Mainwaring, W. I. P., and Irving, R. (1973). *Biochem. J.* **134**, 113.

Mainwaring, W. I. P., and Mangan, F. R. (1973). *J. Endocrinol.* **59**, 121.

Mainwaring, W. I. P., and Milroy, E. J. G. (1973). *J. Endocrinol.* **57**, 371.

Mainwaring, W. I. P., and Peterken, B. M. (1971). *Biochem. J.* **125**, 285.

Mangan, F. R., and Mainwaring, W. I. P. (1972). *Steroids* **20**, 331.

Marver, D., Goodman, D., and Edelman, I. S. (1972). *Kidney Int.* **1**, 210.

Marver, D., Stewart, J., Funder, J. W., Feldman, D., and Edelman, I. S. (1974). *Proc. Nat. Acad. Sci. U.S.* **71**, 1431.

Maurer, R. A. (1974). *Brain Res.* **67,** 175.

Maurer, H. R., and Chalkley, G. R. (1967). *J. Mol. Biol.* **27,** 431.

Mayer, M., Kaiser, N., Milholland, R. J., and Rosen, F. (1975). *J. Biol. Chem.* **250,** 1207.

Mayes, D., and Nugent, C. A. (1968). *J. Clin. Endocrinol. Metab.* **28,** 1169.

Melnykovych, G., and Bishop, C. F. (1969). *Biochim. Biophys. Acta* **177,** 579.

Melnykovych, G., and Bishop, C. F. (1971). *Endocrinology* **88,** 450.

Mercier-Bodard, C., Alfsen, A., and Baulieu, E. E. (1970). *Acta Endocrinol. (Copenhagen)* **64,** Suppl. 147, 204.

Mester, J., and Baulieu, E. E. (1972). *Biochim. Biophys. Acta* **261,** 236.

Mester, J., and Baulieu, E. E. (1975). *Biochem. J.* **146,** 617.

Mester, J., and Robertson, D. M. (1971). *Biochim. Biophys. Acta* **230,** 543.

Mester, J., Robertson, D. M., Feherty, P., and Kellie, A. E. (1970). *Biochem. J.* **120,** 831.

Mester, J., Brunelle, R., Jung, I., and Sonnenschein, C. (1973). *Exp. Cell Res.* **81,** 447.

Mester, J., Martel, D., Psychoyos, A., and Baulie, E. E. (1974). *Nature (London)* **250,** 776.

Meyer, W. J., Migeon, B. R., and Migeon, C. J. (1975). *Proc. Nat. Acad. Sci. U.S.* **72,** 1469.

Michel, G., and Baulieu, E. E. (1974). *C. R. Acad. Sci.* **279,** 671.

Michel, G., and Baulieu, E. E. (1975). *J. Endocrinol.* **65,** 31.

Michel, G., Jung, I., Baulieu, E. E., Aussel, C., and Uriel, J. (1974). *Steroids* **24,** 437.

Middlebrook, J. L., Wong, M. D., Ishii, D. N., and Aronow, C. (1975). *Biochemistry* **14,** 180.

Milgrom, E., and Atger, M. (1975). *J. Steroid Biochem.* **6,** 487.

Milgrom, E., and Baulieu, E. E. (1969). *Biochim. Biophys. Acta* **194,** 602.

Milgrom, E., and Baulieu, E. E. (1970a). *Endocrinology* **87,** 276.

Milgrom, E., and Baulieu, E. E. (1970b). *Biochem. Biophys. Res. Commun.* **50,** 723.

Milgrom, E., and Baulieu, E. E. (1974). *MTP Int. Rev. Sci., Physiol. Ser. 1* **8,** 203.

Milgrom, E., Atger, M., and Baulieu, E. E. (1970). *Steroids* **16,** 741.

Milgrom, E., Atger, M., and Baulieu, E. E. (1971). *Advan. Biosci.* **7,** 235.

Milgrom, E., Atger, M., Perrot, M., and Baulieu, E. E. (1972a). *Endocrinology* **90,** 1071.

Milgrom, E., Perrot, M., Atger, M., and Baulieu, E. E. (1972b). *Endocrinology* **90,** 1064.

Milgrom, E., Atger, M., and Baulieu, E. E. (1973a). *Biochemistry* **12,** 5198.

Milgrom, E., Atger, M., and Baulieu, E. E. (1973b). *Biochim. Biophys. Acta* **320,** 267.

Milgrom, E., Luu Thi, M., Atger, M., and Baulieu, E. E. (1973c). *J. Biol. Chem.* **248,** 6366.

Milgrom, E., Luu Thi, M., and Baulieu, E. E. (1973d). *Acta Endocrinol. (Copenhagen), Suppl.* **180,** 380.

Mohla, S., DeSombre, E. R., and Jensen, E. V. (1972). *Biochem. Biophys. Res. Commun.* **46,** 661.

Mohla, S., DeSombre, E. R., and Jensen, E. V. (1975). *Fed. Proc., Fed. Amer. Soc. Exp. Biol.* **34,** Abstr. 577.

Morey, K. S., and Litwack, G. (1969). *Biochemistry* **8,** 4813.

Morris, D. J., and Davis, R. P. (1973). *Steroids* **21**, 383.

Moscona, A. A., and Piddington, R. (1966). *Biochim. Biophys. Acta* **121**, 409.

Moscona, A. A., and Piddington, R. (1967). *Science* **158**, 496.

Moudgil, V. K., and Toft, D. O. (1975). *Proc. Nat. Acad. Sci. U.S.* **72**, 901.

Mowszowicz, I., Bieber, D. E., Chung, K. W., Bullock, L. P., and Bardin, C. W. (1975). *Endocrinology* **95**, 1589.

Muechler, E. K., Flickinger, G. L., and Mikhail, G. (1974). *Fert. Steril.* **25**, 893.

Mueller, G. C., Vonderhaar, B., Kim, U. H., and Le Mahieu, M. (1972). *Recent Progr. Horm. Res.* **28**, 1.

Mulder, E., Van Beurden-Lamers, W. M. O., DeBoer, W., and Mechielsen, M. J. (1974). *J. Steroid Biochem.* **5**, Abstr. 158.

Mulder, E., Peters, M. S., DeVries, J., and Van der Molen, H. J. (1975). *Cell* **2**, 171.

Munck, A., and Brinck-Johnsen, T. (1968). *J. Biol. Chem.* **243**, 5556.

Munck, A., Wira, C., Young, D. A., Mosher, K. M., Hallaham, C., and Bell, P. A. (1972). *J. Steroid Biochem.* **3**, 567

Musliner, T. A., and Chader, G. J. (1971). *Biochem. Biophys. Res. Commun.* **45**, 998.

Musliner, T. A., and Chader, G. J. (1972). *Biochim. Biophys. Acta* **262**, 256.

Naess, O., Attramadal, A., and Aakvaag, A. (1975). *Endocrinology* **96**, 1.

Nomura, Y., Abe, Y., and Inokuchi, K. (1974). *Gann* **65**, 523.

Norman, A. W., and Henry, H. (1974). *Recent Progr. Horm. Res.* **30**, 431.

Norris, J. S., Gorski, J., and Kohler, P. O. (1974). *Nature (London)* **248**, 422.

Noteboom, W. D., and Gorski, J. (1965). *Arch. Biophys. Biochem.* **111**, 559.

Notides, A. C. (1970). *Endocrinology* **87**, 987.

Notides, A. C., and Nielsen, S. (1974). *J. Biol. Chem.* **249**, 1886.

Notides, A. D., Hamilton, D. E., and Rudolph, J. H. (1973). *Endocrinology* **93**, 210.

Nugent, C. A., and Mayes, D. M. (1966). *J. Clin. Endocrinol. Metab.* **26**, 1116.

Ohno, S., Christian, L., Attardi, B. J., and Kan, J. (1973). *Nature (London), New Biol.* **245**, 92.

O'Malley, B. W., and Hardman, J. G., eds. (1975). "Methods in Enzymology," Vol. 36. Academic Press, New York.

O'Malley, B. W., and Means, A. R., eds. (1973). *Advan. Exp. Med. Biol.* **36**.

O'Malley, B. W., and Means, A. R. (1974). *Science* **183**, 610.

O'Malley, B. W., and Toft, D. O. (1971). *J. Biol. Chem.* **246**, 117.

O'Malley, B. W., Kirschner, M. A., and Bardin, C. W. (1968). *Proc. Soc. Exp. Biol. Med.* **127**, 521.

O'Malley, B. W., McGuire, W L., Kohler, P. O., and Korenman, S. G. (1969). *Recent Progr. Horm. Res.* **25**, 105.

O'Malley, B. W., Sherman, M. R., and Toft, D. O. (1970). *Proc. Nat. Acad. Sci. U.S.* **67**, 501.

O'Malley, B. W., Spelsberg, T. C., Schrader, W. T., Chytil, F., and Steggles, A. W. (1972). *Nature (London)* **235**, 141.

O'Malley, B. W., Schrader, W. T., and Spelsberg, T. C. (1973). *Advan. Exp. Med. Biol.* **36**, 174.

Oppenheimer, J. H. (1975). *N. Engl. J. Med.* **292**, 1063.

Oppenheimer, J. H., Koerner, D., Schwartz, H. L., and Surks, M. I. (1972). *J. Clin. Endocrinol. Metab.* **35**, 330.

Ozon, R., and Bellé, R. (1973a). *Biochim. Biophys. Acta* **297**, 155.

Ozon, R., and Bellé, R. (1973b). *Biochim. Biophys. Acta* **320**, 588.

Palmiter, R. D., Catlin, G. H., and Cox, R. F. (1973). *Cell Differentiation* **2**, 163.

Pasqualini, J., ed. (1975). *J. Steroid Biochem.* **6** (in press).

Pasqualini, J. R., and Sumida, C. (1971). *C. R. Acad. Sci.* **273**, 1061.

Paton, D. M. (1969). *Arch. Int. Pharmacodyn. Ther.* **181**, 118.

Pearlman, W. H., and Crépy, O. (1967). *J. Biol. Chem.* **242**, 182.

Pedroza-Garcia, E., Cardinali, D. P., Laborde, N. P., Garcia-Bienere, W., Nagle, C. A., and Rosner, J. M. (1974). *Neuroendocrinology* **14**, 174.

Pfaff, D., and Keiner, M. (1973). *J. Comp. Neurol.* **151**, 121.

Philibert, D., and Paynaud, J. P. (1974). *Endocrinology* **94**, 627.

Podartz, K. C., and Katzman, P. A. (1968). *Fed. Proc., Fed. Amer. Soc. Exp. Biol.* **27**, 497.

Pollow, K., Lübbert, H., Boquoi, E., Kreuzer, G., and Pollow, B. (1975). *Endocrinology* **96**, 319.

Poortman, J., Prenen, J. A. C., Schwarz, F., and Thijssen, J. H. H. (1975). *J. Clin. Endocrinol. Metab.* **40**, 373.

Porter, G. A., Bogoroch, R., and Edelman, I. S. (1964). *Proc. Nat. Acad. Sci. U.S.* **52**, 1326.

Pratt, W. B., and Ishii, D. N. (1972). *Biochemistry* **11**, 1401.

Puca, G. A., and Bresciani, F. (1968). *Eur. J. Cancer* **3**, 475.

Puca, G. A., and Bresciani, F. (1969). *Nature (London)* **223**, 745.

Puca, G. A., and Bresciani, F. (1970). *Res. Steroids* **4**, 247.

Puca, G. A., Nola, E., Sica, V., and Bresciani, F. (1971a). *Biochemistry* **10**, 3760.

Puca, G. A., Nola, E., Sica, V., and Bresciani, F. (1971b). *Biochemistry* **10**, 3769.

Puca, G. A., Nola, E., Sica, V., and Bresciani, F. (1972). *Biochemistry* **11**, 4157.

Rao, R. B., and Wiest, W. G. (1971). *Proc. Int. Congr. Horm. Steroids, 3rd, 1970* Int. Congr. Ser. No. 210, Abst. 153.

Rao, R. B., Wiest, W. G., and Allen, W. M. (1973) *Endocrinology* **92**, 1229.

Rao, R. B., Wiest, W. G., and Allen, W. M. (1974). *Endocrinology* **95**, 1275.

Raspe, G., ed. (1971). "Advances in the Biosciences," Vol. 7. Pergamon, Oxford.

Rat, R. L., Vallet-Strouve, C., and Erdos, T. (1974). *Biochimie* **56**, 1387.

Raynaud, J. P. (1973). *Comput. Programs Biomed.* **3**, 63.

Raynaud, J. P., Bouton, M. M., Gallet-Bourquin, D., Philibert, D., Tournemine, C., and Azadian-Boulanger, A. (1973). *Mol. Pharmacol.* **9**, 520.

Raynaud-Jammet, C., and Baulieu, E. E. (1969). *C. R. Acad. Sci.* **268**, 3211.

Reel, J. R., Vandewark, S. D., Shih, Y., and Callantine, M. R. (1971). *Steroids* **18**, 441.

Reif-Lehrer, L. (1968). *Biochim. Biophys. Acta* **170**, 263.

Reif-Lehrer, L., and Chader, G. J. (1969). *Biochim. Biophys. Acta* **192**, 310.

Rennie, P., and Bruchovsky, N. (1972). *J. Biol. Chem.* **247**, 1546.

Ritzen, E. M., Nayfeh, S. N., French, F. S., and Dobbins, M. C. (1971). *Endocrinology* **89**, 143.

Robel, P., Blondeau, J. P., and Baulieu, E. E. (1974). *Biochim. Biophys. Acta* **373**, 1.

Robertson, D. M., and Landgren, B. M. (1975). *J. Steroid Biochem.* **6**, 511.

Robertson, D. M., Mester, J., Reilly, J., and Steele, S. J. (1971). *Acta Endocrinol. (Copenhagen)* **68**, 534.

Rochefort, H., and Baulieu, E. E. (1968). *C. R. Acad. Sci.* **267**, 662.

Rochefort, H., and Baulieu, E. E. (1969). *Endocrinology* **84**, 108.

Rochefort, H., and Baulieu, E. E. (1971). *Biochimie* **53**, 893.

Rochefort, H., and Baulieu, E. E. (1972). *Biochimie* **54**, 1303.

Rochefort, H., and Lignon, F. (1974). *Eur. J. Biochem.* **48**, 503.

Rochefort, H., Lignon, F., and Capony, F. (1972). *Biochem. Biophys. Res. Commun.* **47**, 662.

Rodbard, D. (1973). In "Receptor for Reproductive Hormones" (B. W. O'Malley and A. K. Means, eds.), p. 289. Plenum, New York.

Rosen, F., and Milholland, R. J. (1972). *Fed. Proc., Fed. Amer. Soc. Exp. Biol.* **31**, 6229.

Rosenau, W., Baxter, J. D., Rosseau, G. G., and Tomkins, G. M. (1972). *Nature (London), New Biol.* **237**, 20.

Rosenthal, H. E. (1967). *Anal. Biochem.* **20**, 525.

Rosenthal, H. E., Paul, M. A., and Sandberg, A. A. (1974). *J. Steroid Biochem.* **5**, 219.

Roth, G. S. (1974). *Endocrinology* **94**, 82.

Roth, G. S. (1975). *Fed. Proc., Fed. Amer. Soc. Exp. Biol.* **34**, 183.

Roth, J. (1973). *Metab., Clin. Exp.* **22**, 1059.

Rotsztejn, W. H., Normand, M., Lalonde, J., and Fortier, C. (1975). *Endocrinology* **97**, 223.

Rousseau, G. G., Baxter, J. D., Funder, J. W., Edelman, I. S., and Tomkins, G. M. (1972a). *J. Steroid Biochem.* **3**, 219

Rousseau, G. G., Benson, M. C., Garcea, R. L., Ito, J., and Tomkins, G. M. (1972b). *Proc. Nat. Acad. Sci. U.S.* **69**, 1892.

Rousseau, G. G., Baxter, J. D., Higgins, S. J., and Tomkins, G. M. (1973). *J. Mol. Biol.* **79**, 539.

Roy, A. K., Milin, B. S., and McMinn, D. M. (1974). *Biochim. Biophys. Acta* **354**, 213.

Ruh, T. S., Wassilak, S. G., and Ruh, M. F. (1975). *Steroids* **25**, 257.

Sala-Trepat, J. M., and Reti, E. (1974). *Biochim. Biophys. Acta* **338**, 92.

Samuels, H. H., and Tomkins, G. M. (1970). *J. Mol. Biol.* **52**, 57.

Sanborn, B. M., Rao, B. R., and Korenman, S. G. (1971). *Biochemistry* **10**, 4955.

Sandberg, A. A., Kindani, R. Y., Varkarakis, M. J., and Murphy, G. P. (1973). *Steroids* **22**, 259.

Sander, S. (1968). *Acta Endocrinol. (Copenhagen)* **58**, 49.

Santi, D. V., Sibley, C. H., Perriand, E. R., Tomkins, G. M., and Baxter, J. D. (1973). *Biochemistry* **12**, 2412.

Sar, M., and Stumpf, W. E. (1973). *Science* **179**, 389.

Sar, M., Liao, S., and Stumpf, W. (1969). *Fed. Proc., Fed. Amer. Soc. Exp.* **28**, 707.

Sarff, M., and Gorski, J. (1971). *Biochemistry* **10**, 2557.

Scatchard, G. (1949). *Ann. N.Y. Acad. Sci.* **51**, 660.

Schaumburg, B. P. (1972a). *Biochim. Biophys. Acta* **261**, 219.

Schaumburg, B. P. (1972b). *Biochim. Biophys. Acta* **263**, 414.

Schaumburg, B. P., and Bojesen, E. (1968). *Biochim. Biophys. Acta* **170**, 172.

Schaumburg, B. P., and Crone, M. (1971). *Biochim. Biophys. Acta* **237**, 494.

Schrader, W. T., and O'Malley, B. W. (1972). *J. Biol. Chem.* **247**, 51.

Scott, R. S., and Rennie, P. I. C. (1971). *Endocrinology* **89**, 297.

Segal, S. J., and Scher, W. (1967). *In* "Cellular Biology of the Uterus" (R. M. Wynn, ed.), p. 114. Appleton, New York.

Shain, S. A., and Barnea, A. (1971). *Endocrinology* **89**, 1270.

Shao, T. C., Castañeda, E., Rosenfield, R. L., and Liao, S. (1975). *J. Biol. Chem.* **250**, 3095.

Sharp, G. W. G., and Alberti, K. G. M. (1971). *Advan. Biosci.* **7**, 281.

Sharp, G. W. G., Kowack, C. L., and Leaf, A. (1966). *J. Clin. Invest.* **45**, 450.

Sherman, M. R., Corvol, P. L., and O'Malley, B. W. (1970). *J. Biol. Chem.* **245**, 6085.

Sherman, M. R., Atienza, S. B. P., Shansky, J. R., and Hoffman, L. M. (1974). *J. Biol. Chem.* **249**, 5351.

Sherman, M. R., Miller, M. K., and Diaz, S. C. (1975). *Fed. Proc., Fed. Amer. Soc. Exp. Biol.* **34**, Abstr. 1930.

Shyamala, G. (1973a). *Fed. Proc., Fed. Amer. Soc. Exp. Biol.* **32**, Abstr. 1291.

Shyamala, G (1973b). *Biochemistry* **12**, 3085.

Shyamala, G (1974) *J. Biol. Chem.* **249**, 2160.

Shyamala, G. (1975). *Biochemistry* **14**, 437.

Shyamala, G., and Gorski, J. (1969). *J. Biol. Chem.* **244**, 1097.

Shyamala, G., and Nandi, S. (1972). *Endocrinology* **91**, 861.

Sibley, C. H., and Tomkins, G. M. (1974). *Cell* **2**, 221.

Sica, V., Nola, E., Parikh, I., Puca, G. A., and Cutrecasas, P. (1973a). *Nature (London), New Biol.* **244**, 36.

Sica, V., Parikh, I., Nola, E., Puca, G. A., and Cuatrecasas, P. (1973b). *J. Biol. Chem.* **248**, 6543.

Simonsson, B. (1972). *Acta Physiol. Scand.* **86**, 398.

Simpson, P., and White, A. M. (1973). *Biochem. Pharmacol.* **22**, 1195.

Singer, S., Becker, J. E., and Litwack, G. (1973). *Biochem. Biophys. Res. Commun.* **52**, 943.

Smith, H. E., Smith, R. G., Toft, D. O., Neergaard, J. R., Bunows, E. P., and O'Malley, B. W. (1974). *J. Biol. Chem.* **249**, 5924.

Smith, L. D., and Ecker, R. E. (1971). *Develop. Biol.* **25**, 233.

Smith, R. G., Iramain, C. A., Buttram, V. C., Jr., and O'Malley, B. W. (1975). *Nature (London)* **253**, 271.

Soulignac, O. (1974). Thèse pour le Doctorat en Médecine, Université Paris Sud, Faculté de Médecine de Bicêtre.

Soulignac, O., Truong, H., and Baulieu, E. E. (1974). *C. R. Acad. Sci.* **278**, 2955.

Spelsberg, T. C., Steggles, A. W., and O'Malley, B. W. (1971). *J. Biol. Chem.* **246**, 4188.

Spelsberg, T. C., Steggles, A. W., Chytil, F., and O'Malley, B. W. (1972). *J. Biol. Chem.* **247**, 1368.

Stancel, G. M., May Tek Leung, K., and Gorski, J. (1973a). *Biochemistry* **12**, 2130.

Steggles, A. W., and King, R. J. B. (1970). *Biochem. J.* **118**, 695.

Steggles, A. W., Spelsberg, T. C., and O'Malley, B. W. (1971). *Biochem. Biophys. Res. Commun.* **43**, 20.

Stern, J., and Eisenfeld, A. J. (1969). *Science* **166**, 233.

Stevens, W., Grossner, B. I., and Reed, D. J. (1971). *Brain Res.* **35**, 602.

Strott, C. A. (1974). *Endocrinology* **95**, 826.

Stumpf, W. E. (1968). *Endocrinology* **83**, 777.

Stumpf, W. E., and Madhabananda, S. (1973). *J. Steroid Biochem.* **4**, 477.

Sullivan, J. M., and Strott, C. A. (1973) *J. Bol. Chem.* **248**, 3202.

Swaneck, G. E., Highland, E., and Edelman, I. S. (1969). *Nephron* **6**, 297.

Swaneck, G. E., Chu, L. H., and Edelman, I. S. (1970). *J. Biol. Chem.* **245**, 5382.

Szego, C. M. (1974). *Recent Progr. Horm. Res.* **30**, 171.

Tachi, C., Tachi, S., and Lindner, H. R. (1972). *J. Reprod. Fert.* **31**, 59.

Talwar, G. P., Segal, S. J., Evans, A., and Davidson, O. W. (1964). *Proc. Nat. Acad. Sci. U.S.* **52**, 1059.

Tata, J. R. (1962). *Recent Progr. Horm. Res.* **18**, 221.

Tchernitchin, A., Tseng, L., Stumpf, W. E., and Gurpide, E. (1973). *J. Steroid Biochem.* **4**, 451.

Tchernitchin, A., Tchernitchin, X., Robel, P., and Baulieu, E. E. (1975). *C. R. Acad. Sci.* **280**, 1477.

Terenius, L , Johansson, H., Rimsten, A., and Thoren, L. (1974). *Cancer* **33**, 1364.

Thomas, M. (1973). *J. Endocrinol.* **57**, 333.

Thompson, C. J., and Klotz, I. M. (1971). *Arch. Biochem. Biophys.* **147**, 178.

Tindall, D. J., French, F. S., and Nayfeh, S. N. (1972). *Biochem. Biophys. Res. Commun.* **49**, 1391.

Toft, D. (1972). *J. Steroid Biochem.* **3**, 515.

Toft, D., and Gorski, J. (1966). *Proc. Nat. Acad. Sci. U.S.* **55**, 1574.

Toft, D., Shyamala, G., and Gorski, J. (1967). *Proc. Nat. Acad. Sci. U.S.* **57**, 1740.

Tomkins, G. M., Gelehrter, T. D., Granner, D., Martin, D., Jr., Samuels, H., and Thompson, C. B. (1969). *Science* **166**, 1474.

Töpert, M., Zabel, I., and Ziegler, M. (1974). *Anal. Biochem.* **62**, 514.

Trams, G., Engle, B., Lehmann, F., and Maass, H. (1973). *Acta Endocrinol. (Copenhagen), Suppl.* **72**, 351.

Truong, H. (1970). Ph.D. Thesis es Science, Paris.

Truong, H., and Baulieu, E. E. (1971). *Biochim. Biophys. Acta* **237**, 167.

Truong, H., and Baulieu E. E. (1974). *FEBS (Fed. Eur. Biochem. Soc.) Lett.* **46**, 321.

Truong, H., Geynet, C., Millet, C., Soulignac, O., Bucourt, R., Vignau, M., Torelli, V., and Baulieu, E. E. (1973). *FEBS (Fed. Eur. Biochem. Soc.) Lett.* **35**, 289.

Truong, H., Soulignac, O., and Baulieu, E. E. (1975a). *C. R. Acad. Sci.* **280**, 2245.

Truong, H., Millet, C., and Redeuilh, G. (1975b). *10th FEBS Meet 1975* Abstr. 395.

Tsai, H. C., and Norman, A. W. (1973). *J. Biol. Chem.* **248**, 5967.

Tucker, H. A., Larson, B. L., and Gorski, J. (1971). *Endocrinology* **89**, 152.

Tveter, K. J., and Attramadal, A. (1968). *Acta Endocrinol. (Copenhagen)* **59**, 218.

Tveter, K. J., and Attramadal, A. (1969). *Endocrinology* **85**, 350.

Tveter, K. J., and Unhjem, O. (1969). *Endocrinology* **84**, 963.

Unhjem, O., Tveter, K. J., and Aakvaag, A. (1969). *Acta Endocrinol. (Copenhagen)* **62**, 153.

Valladares, L., and Minguell, J. (1975). *Steroids* **25**, 13.

Van der Meulen, N., and Sekeris, C. E. (1973). *FEBS (Fed. Eur. Biochem. Soc.) Lett.* **33**, 184.

Van Kordelaar, J. M. G., Brockman, M. M. M., and Van Rossum, J. M. (1975a). *Acta Endocrinol. (Copenhagen)* **78**, 145.

Van Kordelaar, J. M. G., Vermoken, A. J. M., de Weerd, C. J. M., and Van Rossum, J. M. (1975b). *Acta Endocrinol. (Copenhagen)* **78**, 165.

Verhoeven, G. (1974). Ph.D. Dissertation, Leuven.

Verma, U., and Laumas, K. R. (1973). *Biochim. Biophys. Acta* **317**, 403.

Vignon, F., and Rochefort, H. (1974). *C. R. Acad. Sci.* **278**, 103.

Vonderhaar, B. K., Kim, U. H., and Mueller, G. C. (1970). *Biochim. Biophys. Acta* **215**, 125.

Wagner, R. K., Görlich, L., and Jungblut, P. W. (1972). *Hoppe-Seyler's Z. Physiol. Chem.* **353**, 1603.

Warembourg, M., and Milgrom, E. (1971). *C. R. Acad. Sci.* **273**, 891.

Weiller, S., Le Goascogne, C., and Baulieu, E. E. (1974). *C. R. Acad. Sci.* **278**, 769.

Westphal, U. (1971). *Endocrinol.* **4**.

Williams, D., and Gorski, J. (1971). *Biochem. Biophys. Res. Commun.* **46**, 268.

Wilson, J. D., and Goldstein, J. L. (1972). *J. Biol. Chem.* **247**, 7342.

Wira, C., and Munck, A. (1970). *J. Biol. Chem.* **245**, 3436.

Wittliff, J. L., Gardner, D. G., Batterna, W. L., and Gilbert, P. J. (1972). *Biochem. Biophys. Res. Commun.* **48**, 119.

Wyss, R. M., Le Roy Heinrichs, W. M., and Herrman, W. L. (1968). *J. Clin. Endocrinol. Metab.* **28**, 1227.

Yamamoto, K. R. (1974). *J. Biol. Chem.* **249**, 7068.

Yamamoto, K. R., and Alberts, B. M. (1972). *Proc. Nat. Acad. Sci. U.S.* **69**, 2105.

Yamamoto, K. R., and Alberts, B. M. (1974). *J. Biol. Chem.* **249**, 7076.

Young, P. C. M., and Cleary, R. E. (1974). *J. Clin. Endocrinol. Metab.* **39**, 425.

Yund, M. A., and Fristrom, J. W. (1975). *Develop. Biol.* **43**, 287.

Zelson, P. R., and Wittliff, J. L. (1974). *J. Steroid Biochem.* **5**, Abstr. 1162.

ADDENDUM

Since the submission of the manuscript (July 29, 1975), many additional publications have appeared. Here follows a comprehensive list of some of them which may be useful to the reader. The list has been compiled from documents available to the authors up to October 1, 1975.

A. GENERAL REVIEW

An interesting general review on "Cellular receptors and mechanisms of action of steroid hormones" has appeared (Liao, 1975).

B. ESTROGEN *Receptors*

Several papers concerning the interaction of estradiol *receptor* with DNA have been published. Three deal with the problem of the apparent nonsaturability of *receptor* binding to DNA (André and Rochefort, 1975; Yamamoto and Alberts, 1975; Alberga *et al.*, 1975). The latter reference points also to the possible heterogeneity of estradiol binding units in terms of binding to DNA activity. Another report (Puca *et al.*, 1975) studies nuclear "acceptor" by immobilizing various nuclear protein fractions to an agarose matrix, and a fraction of basic protein(s) is shown to have specific, high affinity sites for the *receptor*.

The importance of such studies on *receptor*–DNA interactions is clear when one takes into account the already discussed stimulation of RNA synthesis in isolated uterine nuclei by estradiol *receptor* complexes (Mohla *et al.*, 1975). The significance of nuclear estradiol, bound to "chromatin" presumably through the *receptor*, is discussed in several instances. Stormshak *et al.* (1975) have studied a "refractoriness" state after prolonged exposure to estrogen which appears to be independent of binding and translocation of the hormone to the nucleus; Katzenellenbogen and Ferguson (1975) have shown that antiestrogen action does let a considerable ^{3}H-labeled estradiol binding in the nucleus to occur while estradiol action is suppressed. Clemens *et al.* (1975) find nuclear 4 S estradiol *receptors* of low affinity which are transformed in the nucleus into 5 S complexes of higher affinity. New data have appeared on human endometrium *receptors*. Tseng and Gurpide (1975) show a decrease of estradiol *receptors* under progestin influence. Bayard *et al.* (1975) describe the variations of estrogen and progesterone *receptors* over the menstrual cycle in normal individuals. The results follow the characteristics already described in animal models: preferential cytoplasmic localization of the *receptor* when the hormone is low, and nuclear *receptor* in case of high hormone level; increase of estrogen *receptor* during the first point of the cycle and then profound decrease after ovulation; preovulatory increase of the progesterone *receptor* followed by decrease.

Linkie (1975) and Kato (1975) have reported on an estradiol *receptor* in hypothalamus and pituitary and Ginsburg *et al.* (1975) in the brain of the rat, while Davies *et al.* (1975) have observed an estradiol *receptor* in the human fetal pituitary and brain tissues. Korach and Muldoon (1975) find an interaction of low affinity of the estrogen *receptor* with androstanolone, confirming previous studies with the uterus *receptor*, and the recently observed activity of catechol estrogens which increase LH in male rats suggest the possibility of a *receptor* for these estrogens (Morishita *et al.*, 1975). Moreover, the work of Lasley *et al.* (1975) may reopen the problem of an eventual progesterone receptor at the hypothalamic level in showing the interaction of estradiol and progesterone on pituitary sensitivity and reserve. The estrogen cytoplasmic *receptor* concentration is increased in anterior pituitary by thyroid influence (Cidlowski and Muldoon, 1975).

Reports have suggested the presence of an estrogen *receptor* in the liver (Eisenfeld *et al.*, 1975 in the rat and the monkey and Viladiu *et al.*, 1975 in the rat).

Various tumors, especially of mammary origin, have been analyzed for *receptor* content. Chen *et al.* (1975) have studied the relation between the tumor growth and the estradiol *receptor* of the MTW9 mammary tumor. Jung-Testas *et al.* (1975) have described an estradiol *receptor* in the androgen sensitive SC-119 mice mammary tumor, which coexist with the androgen *receptor* included in the cells of the clone MI$_1$. M. Lippman *et al.* (1975) have shown the presence of estrogen *receptor* in various lines derived from human mammary cancers. Powell-Jones *et al.*

(1975a,b) have studied the effect of antiestrogens on rat DMBA mammary tumor and human breast carcinomata.

A new report on the estradiol *receptor* of rooster liver has been published (Gschwendt, 1975) with special reference to antiestrogens, while more work has been done in *Xenopus laevis* liver (Berginck and Wittliff, 1975).

C. ANDROGEN *Receptors*

Jänne *et al.* (1975) have indicated good correlations between nuclear testosterone binding in mouse kidney and the template capacity and polymerase activity.

An androgen *receptor* has been characterized in DDT_1 cells by Norris and Kohler (1975) (cells derived from a leiomyosarcoma induced in the ductus deferens of a Syrian hamster by diethylstilbestrol and testosterone). Gustafsson and Pousette (1975) have studied the cytosol of kidney, submaxillary glands, thigh and *levator ani* muscles and have found evidence for *receptor* for testosterone. Smith *et al.* (1975) have indicated that there is an androgen *receptor* in nuclei of rat testis. Krieg *et al.* (1975) reanalyzed the binding and metabolism of 3α- and 3β-androstanediols in prostate and seminal vesicles of male rats. Shain and Boesel (1975) indicate that the androgen *receptor* content decreases in the prostate of aging rats.

Recently, two documents have appeared in which will be found several indications on androgen *receptors* (Minguell and Sierralta, 1975; Goland, 1975).

D. PROGESTERONE *Receptors*

A comparative study of endometrial and myometrial progesterone *receptor* in guinea pig uterus has appeared (Luu Thi *et al.*, 1975) and in an *in vitro* system (organ culture), a comparison of endometrial progestin *receptor* and biological response of the guinea pig has been presented by Demers and Feil (1975).

Data on the purification of the progesterone binding components of chick oviduct have been published (Kuhn *et al.*, 1975), with indication of the subunit structure and function (Schrader *et al.*, 1975). An analysis of the progesterone *receptor* binding to nuclear subfraction in the oviduct nucleus has been presented (Pikler *et al.*, 1975). The interaction of the progesterone *receptor* of chick oviduct with ATP has led to systematic studies (Lohmar and Toft, 1975) and ATP affinity chromatography (Toft and Moudgil, 1975). Another study of the binding of the chick oviduct progesterone *receptor* to chromatin has been recently published (Jaffe *et al.*, 1975).

E. GLUCO- AND MINERALOCORTICOSTEROID *Receptors*

The kinetics of glucocorticosteroid binding to the cytoplasmic *receptor* of mouse L-929 fibroblast cells has been studied (Pratt *et al.*, 1975). In the same cells, together with the glucocorticosteroid *receptors*, an androgen and an estrogen *receptor* have been identified (Jung-Testas *et al.*, 1976), confirming the possible plurality of *receptors* per cell if one assumes that the L-cells in suspension culture are all the same. The glucocorticosteroid *receptor* is found also in cultured human skin fibroblasts (Brunning *et al.*, 1975; Groyer, 1975). McEwen *et al.* (1975) have studied further putative glucocorticosteroid *receptors* in the limbic brain.

Studies of the activation of cytoplasmic glucocorticosteroid *receptor* and of its binding to nuclei have been presented by Giannopoulos (1975a,b) studying the fetal rabbit lung. Working with the rat liver system, Cake and Litwack (1975) have shown an effect of theophylline on the activation and nuclear translocation of the *receptor*. Change with age in glucocorticosteroid binding to rat liver, thymus, and splenic leukocytes has been reported by Petrovic and Markovic (1975) and G. S. Roth (1975), respectively.

Specific binding sites of glucocorticosteroids to plasma membranes of rat liver have been reported by Suyemitsu and Terayama (1975).

The binding of glycyrrhetinic acid to kidney mineralocorticosteroid and glucocorticosteroid *receptors* has been shown by Ulmann *et al.* (1975).

F. OTHER ASPECTS

The question of *thyroid hormone receptors* has been discussed in an interesting review by Tata (1975). Among papers dealing with the *techniques* of binding, there is a review by Boeynaems and Dumont (1975), and theoretical considerations by Jacobs *et al.* (1975) and Blondeau and Robel (1975). A comprehensive paper by Barkley *et al.* (1975) gives a series of quantitative data for the interaction of effecting ligands with the *Lac* repressor and the repressor–operator complex, an important model system for the investigation of hormone *receptor* studies.

REFERENCES

Alberga, A., Ferrez, M., and Baulieu, E. E. (1976). *FEBS Lett.* **61** (in press).
André, J., and Rochefort, H. (1975). *FEBS (Fed. Eur. Biochem. Soc.) Lett.* **50**, 319.

Barkley, M. D., Riggs, A. D., Jobe, A., and Bourgeois, S. (1975). *Biochemistry* **14**, 1700.

Bayard, F., Damilano, S., Robel, P., and Baulieu, E.-E. (1975). *C. R. Acad. Sci.* **281**, 1341.

Bergink, E. W., and Wittliff, J. L. (1975). *Biochemistry* **14**, 3115.

Blondeau, J. P., and Robel, P. (1975). *Eur. J. Biochem.* **55**, 375.

Boeynaems, J. M., and Dumont, J. E. (1975). *J. Cycl. Nucleotide Res.* **1**, 123.

Bruning, P. F., Meyer, W. J., and Migeon, C. J. (1975). *Abstr., 57th Meet. Endocrine Soc.* p. 60.

Cake, M. H., and Litwack, G. (1975). *Biochem. Biophys. Res. Commun.* **66**, 828.

Chen, Y. T., Giladi, M., Diamond, E. J., Shen, S. K., Koprak, S., and Hollander, V. P. (1975). *Abstr., 57th Meet. Endocrine Soc.* p. 209.

Cidlowski, J. A., and Muldoon, T. G. (1975). *Endocrinology* **97**, 59.

Clemens, L. E., Lust, J., and Siiteri, P. K. (1975). *Abstr., 57th Meet. Endocrine Soc.* p. 66.

Davies, I. J., Naftolin, F., Ryan, K. J., and Siu, J. (1975). *J. Clin. Endocrinol.* **40**, 909.

Demers, L. M., and Feil, P. D. (1975). *Abstr., 57th Meet. Endocrine Soc.* p. 64.

Eisenfeld, A. J., Aten, R., Weinberger, M., and Krakoff, L. (1975). *Abstr., 57th Meet. Endocrine Soc.* p. 68.

Giannopoulos, G. (1975a). *J. Biol. Chem.* **250**, 2896.

Giannopoulos, G. (1975b). *J. Biol. Chem.* **250**, 2904.

Ginsburg, M., Greestein, B. D., Maclusky, N. J., Morris, I. D., and Thomas, P. J. (1975). *J. Steroid Biochem.* **6**, 989.

Goland, M., ed. (1975). "Normal and Abnormal Growth of the Prostate." Thomas, Springfield, Illinois.

Groyer, A. (1975). Personal communication.

Gschwendt, M. (1975). *Biochim. Biophys. Acta* **399**, 395.

Gustafsson, J. A., and Pousette, A. (1975). *Biochemistry* **14**, 3094.

Jacobs, S., Chang, K. J., and Cuatrecasas, P. (1975). *Biochem. Biophys. Res. Commun.* **66**, 687.

Jaffe, R. C., Socher, S. H., and O'Malley, B. W. (1975). *Biochim. Biophys. Acta* **399**, 403.

Jänne, O., Bullock, L. P., Jacob, S. T., and Bardin, C. W. (1975). *Abstr., 57th Meet. Endocrine Soc.* p. 174.

Jung-Testas, I., Desmond, W., and Baulieu, E. E. (1975). *Exp. Cell Res.* In press.

Jung-Testas, I., Bayard, F., and Baulieu, E. E. (1976). *Nature (London)* **259**, 136.

Kato, J. (1975). *J. Steroid Biochem.* **6**, 979.

Katzenellenbogen, B. S., and Ferguson, E. R. (1975). *Endocrinology* **97**, 1.

Korach, K. S., and Muldoon, T. G. (1975). *Endocrinology* **97**, 231.

Krieg, M., Horst, H. J., and Sterba, M. L. (1975). *J. Endocrinol.* **64**, 529.

Kuhn, R. W., Schrader, W. T., Smith, R. G., and O'Malley, B. W. (1975). *J. Biol. Chem.* **250**, 4220.

Lasley, B. L., Wang, C. F., and Yen, S. S. C. (1975). *Abstr., 57th Meet. Endocrine Soc.* p. 164.

Liao, S. (1975). *Int. Rev. Cytol.* **41**, 87.

Linkie, D. M. (1975). *Abstr., 57th Meet. Endocrine Soc.* p. 67.

Lippman, M., Bolan, G., and Huff, K. (1975). *Nature (London), New Biol.* **258**, 339.

Lohmar, P., and Toft, D. O. (1975). *Abstr., 57th Meet. Endocrine Soc.* p. 63.

Luu Thi, M., Milgrom, E., and Baulieu, E. E. (1975). *J. Endocrinol.* **66**, 349.

McEwen, B. S., Luine, V. N., Plapinger, L., and Kloet, E. R. (1975). *J. Steroid Biochem.* **6**, 971.

Minguell, J. J., and Sierralta, W. D. (1975). *J. Endocrinol.* **65**, 287.

Mohla, S., DeSombre, E. R., and Jensen, E. V. (1975). *Abstr., 57th Meet. Endocrine Soc.* p. 70.

Morishita, H., Naftolin, F., Davies, I. J., Todd, R., Ryan, K. J., and Fishman, J. (1975). *Abstr., 57th Meet. Endocrine Soc.* p. 164.

Norris, J. S., and Kohler, P. O. (1975). *Abstr., 57th Meet. Endocrine Soc.* p. 173.

Petrovic, J. S., and Markovic, R. Z. (1975). *Develop. Biol.* **45**, 176.

Pikler, G., Webster, R., and Spelsberg, T. C. (1975). *Abstr., 57th Meet. Endocrine Soc.* p. 64.

Powell-Jones, W., Davies, P., and Griffiths, K. (1975a). *J. Endocrinol.* **66**, 437.

Powell-Jones, W., Jenner, D. A., Blamey, R. W., Davies, P., and Griffiths, K. (1975b). *Biochem. J.* **150**, 71.

Pratt, W. B., Kaine, J. L., and Pratt, D. V. (1975). *J. Biol. Chem.* **250**, 4584.

Puca, G. A., Nola, E., Hibner, U., Cicala, G., and Sica, V. (1975). *J. Biol. Chem.* **250**, 6452.

Roth, G. S. (1975). *Biochim. Biophys. Acta* **399**, 145.

Schrader, W. T., Kuhn, R. W., Heuer, S. S., and O'Malley, B. W. (1975). *Abstr., 57th Meet. Endocrine Soc.* p. 332.

Shain, S. A., and Boesel, R. W. (1975). *Abstr., 57th Meet. Endocrine Soc.* p. 175.

Smith, A. A., McLean, W. S., Hansson, V., Nayfeh, S. N., and French, F. S. (1975). *Steroids* **25**, 569.

Stormshak, F., Wertz, N., and Gorki, K. (1975). *Abstr., 57th Meet. Endocrine Soc.* p. 66.

Suyemitsu, T., and Terayama, H. (1975). *Endocrinology* **96**, 1499.

Tata, J. R. (1975). *Nature (London)* **257**, 18.

Toft, D. O., and Moudgil, V. K. (1975). *Abstr., 57th Meet. Endocrine Soc.* p. 52.

Tseng, L., and Gurpide, E. (1975). *J. Clin. Endocrinol.* **41**, 402.

Ulmann, A., Menard, J., and Corvol, P. (1975). *Endocrinology* **97**, 46.

Viladiu, P., Delgado, C., Pensky, J., and Pearson, O. H. (1975). *Endocrine Res. Commun.* **2**, 273.

Yamamoto, K. R., and Alberts, B. (1975). *Cell* **4**, 301.

Subject Index

A

Acid phosphatase, from prostatic cancer, 377–378

Adenosine, 3′,5′-cyclic monophosphate, effect on prostatic cell proliferation, 90–91

Adipose tissue, phosphatidylinositol metabolism in, 565–566

Adrenalectomy, in prostatic tumor therapy, 390

Adrenals, inositide metabolism in, 553–554

Adriamycin, in prostatic cancer therapy, 161–164, 169–170

Affinity chromatography, of steroid hormone receptors, 236–237

Aldosterone, *receptor* for, 696–698

Amino acids, imbalance of, pellagra and, 505–528

Androgen(s)
  in benign prostatic hyperplasia therapy, 450–451
  binding and transport of in testis and epididymis, 283–295
  effects on prostate, 107–108
    cartilage, 616–619
    cell proliferation, 77–93
    differences between, 31–32
    in organ culture, 1–38
  gene expression and, 310–315
  metabolism of
    in benign prostate hypertrophy, 417–438
    in perfused prostate, 193–207
  prostatic binding and metabolism of, 247–264

Androgen-binding protein (ABP), in seminiferous fluid and epididymis, 289–291

Androgen-receptor proteins, in different tissues, 269–270

Androgen *receptors,* 678–686
  complexes, evaluation of, 301–304
  multiple forms of, 298–301
  occurrence of, 683–684

properties of, 679–680
  in prostate, 91–93, 682–683
  regulation of, 685–686

3β-Androstanediol, effect on prostate organ culture, 1–38

5α-Androstane-3β,17β-diol, metabolism of, in benign prostate hypertrophy, 428–429

Androstanediol, origin of, 217

Androstenediol, origin of, 217

Androstenedione
  effect on prostate organ culture, 1–38
  metabolism of, in benign prostate hypertrophy, 429

Androstanolone
  binding constants for, 327–331
  effect on prostate organ culture, 1–38
  prostatic binding constants for, 321–331
  receptor control, 331–342

Antiandrogens
  effects on prostate, 111–115
    in organ culture, 15–18
  in prostatic tumor therapy, 351–376
  in therapy of benign prostatic hyperplasia, 451–455

Antiprostatic drugs, animal models in study of, 103–135

Antisteroid antibody, characterization of, 303–304

Arginase, in test system for chemotherapeutic agents, 157–166

Autophagia, in prostatic growth, 73–77

B

Benign prostatic hyperplasia (BPH)
  androgen therapy of, 450
  androgen uptake in, 247–257
  castration effects on, 442–450
  in dogs, 456–462
  estrogen therapy of, 450
  histology and characteristics of, 440–441
  incidence of, 439–440
  nonsurgical treatment of, 439–464
  symptomatology of, 441

737

L

Leucine
  effect on enzymes of tryptophan-nico-
    tinic acid pathway, 516–517
  role in pellagra, 509
Leukemia, hormone role in, 709
Leukocytes, inositide metabolism in, 555
Liver, inositide metabolism in, 549–550
Lymphocytes, inositide metabolism in,
  551–552

M

Medrogestone, in therapy of benign
  prostatic hyperplasia, 453, 455
Mental symptoms, of pellagra, 517–521
Metabolic clearance rate (MCR), of
  steroids, determination of, 210–212
Metal ions, interaction with dihydrotes-
  tosterone-receptor complexes, 304–
  305
Microorganisms, inositide metabolism in,
  558–560
Mineralocorticosteroid *receptors*, 695–699
Mononucleotides, interaction with dihy-
  drotestosterone-receptor complexes,
  305–306
Multiplication-stimulating activity
  (MSA), effects on cartilage, 600–604
Muscle, inositide metabolism in, 554–555
Myelin, inositide metabolism in, 546
Myo-inositol lipids, 529–573
  analysis and distribution of, 539–543
  biosynthesis of, 531
  catabolism of, 531–532
  extraction and separation of, 533–536
    by chromatography, 536–538
  metabolism of, 530–532
    in erythrocytes, 552
    in liver, 549–550
    in lymphocytes, 551–552
    in muscle, 554–555
    in nervous tissue, 545–549
    in pancreas, 554
    in platelets, 552–553
    in thyroid, 550–551
  molecular species of, 538–539
  physical properties of, 543–545
  structures of, 530–531

N

Nerve growth factor, effect on cartilage,
  625
Nervous tissue, inositide metabolism in,
  545–549
Nicotinamide nucleotides, in erythro-
  cytes, in pellagra, 512–514
Nicotinic acid
  deficiency of, in pellagra, 507–508
  metabolites, excretion of, in pellagra,
    509–511
Nonsuppressible insulinlike activity
  (NSILA), effects on cartilage, 600–
  604
NSC-45388, in prostatic cancer therapy,
  161–164, 169–170
Nuclei, interaction with dihydrotestos-
  terone-receptor complexes, 308–309
Nucleolus, of prostate epithelial cells,
  RNA synthesis in, 25–27

O

Organ culture, of prostate, androgen
  effects on, 1–38

P

Pancreas, inositide metabolism in, 554
Parathyroid hormone, effects on cartilage, 625–627
Pellagra
  amino acid imbalance in, 505–528
  biochemical changes in, 509–514
  copper metabolism in, 522
  etiology of, 506–509
  leucine excess in, 515–517
  leucine-isoleucine imbalance in, 523
  leucine role in, 509
  mental changes in, 517–521
    biochemical basis, 519–521
  nicotinic acid deficiency in, 507–508
  skin in, 521–522
Perfusion, of prostate, methods for,
  195–199
Perichromatin granules, of prostate epithelial cells, RNA synthesis in, 27–29
Pigs, bracken rhizome poisoning of,
  490–492